Endoluminal Ultrasound

Vascular and Nonvascular Applications

ENDOLUMINAL ULTRASOUND
VASCULAR AND NONVASCULAR APPLICATIONS

Edited by

Ji-Bin Liu MD

Research Assistant Professor of Radiology
Jefferson Ultrasound Research and Education Institute
and Division of Diagnostic Ultrasound, Department of Radiology
Thomas Jefferson University Medical College and Hospital
Philadelphia, PA, USA

Barry B Goldberg MD

Professor of Radiology
and Director, Jefferson Ultrasound Research and Education Institute
and Division of Diagnostic Ultrasound, Department of Radiology
Thomas Jefferson University Medical College and Hospital
Philadelphia, PA, USA

Mosby

St. Louis Baltimore Boston Carlsbad Chicago Naples New York Philadelphia Portland
London Madrid Mexico City Singapore Sydney Tokyo Toronto Wiesbaden

MARTIN DUNITZ

First published in the United Kingdom in 1998 by

Martin Dunitz Ltd
The Livery House
7–9 Pratt Street
London NW1 0AE

Mosby
Dedicated to Publishing Excellence

A Times Mirror
Company

Distributed in the U.S.A. and Canada by

Mosby–Year Book
11830 Westline Industrial Drive
St. Louis, Missouri 63146

Times Mirror Professional Publishing Ltd.
130 Flaska Drive
Markham, Ontario L6G 1B8

A CIP catalogue record for this book is available from the British Library.

ISBN 1-85317-236-7

Medical illustrations by Ji-Bin Liu MD.

Composition by Scribe Design, Gillingham, Kent
Manufactured by Imago
Printed and bound in Singapore

DEDICATION

To my parents, my wife Jiwen and my daughter Joyce for their love,
encouragement, support and understanding.
To my teachers, for their inspiration and instruction.

JBL

The potential of ultrasound continues to amaze me.
This, along with the love and support of my wife Phyllis, makes whatever I do possible.

BBG

Contents

List of contributors

Archie A Alexander MD
Associate Professor of Radiology, Jefferson Ultrasound Research and Education Institute and Division of Diagnostic Ultrasound, Department of Radiology, Thomas Jefferson University Medical College and Hospital, 132 South 10th Street, Philadelphia PA 19107, USA.

Demetrius H Bagley MD
Professor of Urology and Radiology, Department of Urology, Thomas Jefferson University Medical College and Hospital, 1025 Walnut Street, Philadelphia, PA 19107, USA.

Dietrich Baumgart MD
Research Fellow, Department of Cardiology, Division of Internal Medicine, University of Essen, 45122 Essen, Germany.

Heinrich D Becker MD FCCP
Assistant Medical Director, Department of Internal Medicine, Oncology and Endoscopy, Thoraxclinic, Heidelberg, Germany.

Nicolaas Bom MSc PhD
Professor, Head of Bioengineering, Thoraxcentre, Erasmus University, NI-3000 Rotterdam, The Netherlands.

Joseph Bonn MD
Assistant Professor of Radiology, Division of Cardiovascular and Interventional Radiology, Department of Radiology, Thomas Jefferson University Medical College and Hospital, 111 South 11th Street, Philadelphia, PA 19107, USA.

Michael B Chancellor MD
Associate Professor of Urology, Division of Urology, University Surgical Association, University of Pittsburgh Medical Center, 3471 5th Avenue, Suite 700, Pittsburgh, PA, USA.

Raimund Erbel MD FESC FACC
University Professor of Medicine/Cardiology, and Director, Department of Cardiology, Division of Internal Medicine, University of Essen, Hufelandstrasse 55, 45122 Essen, Germany.

Rick I Feld MD
Assistant Professor of Radiology, Jefferson Ultrasound Research and Education Institute and Division of Diagnostic Ultrasound, Department of Radiology, Thomas Jefferson University Medical College and Hospital, 132 South 10th Street, Philadelphia PA 19107, USA.

Flemming Forsberg PhD
Head of Research, Jefferson Ultrasound Research and Education Institute, and Assistant Professor of Radiology, Division of Diagnostic Ultrasound, Department of Radiology, Thomas Jefferson University Hospital and Jefferson Medical College, 132 South 10th Street, Philadelphia PA 19107, USA.

Junbo Ge MD
Director, Intravascular Ultrasound Laboratory and Department of Cardiology, University of Essen, Hufelandstrasse 55, 45122 Essen, Germany.

Barry B Goldberg MD
Professor of Radiology and Director, Jefferson Ultrasound Research and Education Institute, and Division of Diagnostic Ultrasound, Department of Radiology, Thomas Jefferson University Medical College and Hospital, 132 South 10th Street, Philadelphia PA 19170, USA.

Günter Görge MD
Fellow, Department of Cardiology, Division of Internal Medicine, University of Essen, Hufelandstrasse 55, 45122 Essen, Germany.

Michael Haude MD
Head, Catheterization Laboratory, Department of Cardiology, Division of Internal Medicine, University of Essen, Hufelandstrasse 55, 45122 Essen, Germany.

Charles T Lancée PhD
Thoraxcentre, Erasmus University, NI-3000 Rotterdam, The Netherlands.

Anna Lev-Toaff MD
Associate Professor of Radiology, Jefferson Ultrasound Research and Education Institute and Division of Diagnostic Ultrasound, Department of Radiology, Thomas Jefferson University Medical College and Hospital, 132 South 10th Street, Philadelphia PA 19107, USA.

Fengqi Liu MD
Cardiologist, Department of Cardiology, Division of Internal Medicine, University of Essen, Hufelandstrasse 55, 45122 Essen, Germany.

Ji-Bin Liu MD
Research Assistant Professor of Radiology, Jefferson Ultrasound Research and Education Institute and Division of Diagnostic Ultrasound, Department of Radiology, Thomas Jefferson University Hospital and Jefferson Medical College, 132 South 10th Street, Philadelphia PA 19107, USA.

Judy A Lund RT RDMS
Clinical Education Specialist, Cordis–Johnson & Johnson Company, Miami Lakes, FL, USA.

Daniel A Merton BS RDMS
Technical Coordinator of Research, Jefferson Ultrasound Research and Education Institute, and Division of Diagnostic Ultrasound, Department of Radiology, Thomas Jefferson University Medical College and Hospital, 132 South 10th Street, Philadelphia PA 19107, USA.

Larry S Miller MD
Associate Professor of Medicine and Radiology, Gastroenterology Section, Temple University Hospital, 3401 North Broad Street, Philadelphia, PA 19140, USA.

Laurence Needleman MD
Associate Professor of Radiology, Jefferson Ultrasound Research and Education Institute and Division of Diagnostic Ultrasound, Department of Radiology, Thomas Jefferson University Medical College and Hospital, 132 South 10th Street, Philadelphia PA 19107, USA.

Thomas D Schiano MD
Clinical Instructor, Gastroenterology Section, Temple University Hospital, 3401 North Broad Street, Philadelphia, PA 19140, USA.

Robert M Steiner MD
Professor of Radiology, Department of Radiology, Thomas Jefferson University Medical College and Hospital, 111 South 11th Street, Philadelphia, PA 19107, USA.

Preface

Since the beginning of diagnosic ultrasound in the late 1940s and its commercialization in the mid 1960s, there have been many advances in this modality, to the point where currently one out of every three imaging studies performed worldwide is an ultrasound examination. The advances in technology have led to the development of a variety of new uses and, as with many other areas in technology, there has been a progressive miniaturization of equipment. This is particularly evident in the development of ultrasound transducers where a reduction in the size of probes has allowed for their insertion into the rectum and vagina as well as the esophagus. In the past decade we have seen the development of transducers that fit into catheters as small as 1–3 mm in diameter. Probes can now be inserted into blood vessels and naturally occurring and surgically created nonvascular lumina throughout the body. These high frequency transducers (12.5–30 MHz) have allowed the collection of information not previously available with even the most sophisticated transabdominal ultrasound, computed tomography or magnetic resonance imaging. The uniqueness of this approach has led to extensive research establishing a wide variety of uses. This should lead the way to expansion of the diagnostic capabilities of ultrasound, providing important information for decision-making relative to patient care and surgical intervention not possible before this technological advance.

The goal of this book is to cover all aspects of endoluminal ultrasound, including its historical development, physical principles, technical considerations and instrumentation as well as its clinical applications in the cardiovascular system, the genitourinary and gastrointestinal tracts, tracheobronchial tree, reproductive tract and intra-abdominal organs. In addition, endoscopic, laparoscopic and thoracoscopic ultrasound as well as transvaginal sonohysterography are included. We attempt to bring together and introduce the reader to the many established and potential uses of this technique throughout the body, using contributions from recognized experts at the forefront of this new field. At present, the clinical applications of endoluminal ultrasound are still in their early stages of development and much clinical research remains to be carried out. We hope that this book will convey new ideas and clinical applications for these new imaging modalities.

Ji-Bin Liu
Barry B Goldberg
Philadelphia, July 1997

Acknowledgements

I wish to particularly thank Barry B Goldberg, who has been my mentor and senior colleague since I began my research fellowship at Jefferson Hospital in 1987. He has never ceased to provide me with the intellectual challenge and stimulation not only to write this book with him, but also to pursue my academic and clinical interests in diagnostic ultrasound. His guidance and friendship have been invaluable to me.

When endoluminal ultrasound was used clinically for intravascular studies, Dr Goldberg was the first to encourage its use in the study of nonvascular areas. When he saw the initial high resolution endoluminal ultrasound images of the urinary tract, he immediately realized the enormous potential of the technique for a variety of nonvascular applications. I truly appreciate his contributions and encouragement during the years of research into endoluminal ultrasound as well as during the preparation of this book.

Special acknowledgments are also extended to my friends and colleagues Larry S Miller, Demetrius H Bagley and Daniel A Merton for their great support and contributions, to Mrs Phyllis Goldberg for her tireless help in correcting the manuscript, to my secretary Ms Dorethea Taplar for her assistance in preparing the manuscript, and to Fred Ross and Ken Goodman for their excellent reproductions of the photographs used in this book.

Ji-Bin Liu
Philadelphia, July 1997

We would like to thank all the authors of this book for their valuable contributions. We also thank Alan Burgess, Commissioning Editor, and Ian Mellor, Editor, of Martin Dunitz Ltd for their organizational skills and editorial support. We also acknowledge the technical support of Diasonics, Boston Scientific Corporation, Bruel & Kjaer, Endosonics, Toshiba and Hewlett-Packard. Most of all, we wish to thank our families for their understanding and support, without which this book could not have been written.

Ji-Bin Liu
Barry B Goldberg
Philadelphia, July 1997

Chapter 1 Principles and history of endoluminal ultrasound techniques

Nicolaas Bom and Charles T Lancée

INTRODUCTION

The history of intraluminal echography dates back to the very beginning of diagnostic ultrasound. Over the years many fascinating ideas and applications of catheter-tip- or gastroscopic-tube-tip-mounted transducers have been described. In the early period of diagnostic ultrasound, one of the compelling reasons for the intraluminal approach was the low sensitivity of the existing echo transducers and, therefore, the need to closely approach the organs to be studied. Image quality was poor and the techniques were considered too invasive to stimulate large-scale applications. However, with the introduction of interventional and minimally invasive surgical techniques in the last decade, a new and enthusiastic interest in endo- and intraluminal echography has arisen because of the need for better patient selection and management of the interventional procedure. For this purpose, cross-sectional information is essential.

Resolution is the parameter that requires a close approach to the organ to be studied. With higher frequency the wavelength becomes shorter. As a result the acoustic element can be small, still yielding a sufficient acoustic aperture in wavelength and thus narrow-beam characteristics. Due to the close approach to the reflecting structure, the increase of attenuation with frequency does not create a problem. The overall effect of the endoluminal approach is an improvement of image resolution.

For endoluminal echo methods the basic echo principles as known from non-invasive diagnostic ultrasound are still applicable. These principles include: sound propagation and echo reflection; attenuation; piezoelectric effect; beam formation; and the need for time/gain compensation.

Present technology includes a variety of mechanically driven as well as the electronic beam-steering catheters and ultrasonic echoendoscopes. Advantages and disadvantages, as well as the newest methods, such as the micromotor catheter technology, will be illustrated.

ECHO PRINCIPLES

Sound waves represent a pressure disturbance that is propagated with a given sound velocity through a medium such as water or human tissue. The sound velocity in blood or water is approximately 1500 m/s. Sound pulses may be reflected from distant structures. With a known sound velocity the time elapsed between transmission of the pulse and reception of the echo can be converted to a distance or depth measurement. It is this principle which is used in SONAR applications and which is also known to be used by, for instance, dolphins. An illustration of depth measurement using an echo technique under a ship is given in Fig. 1.1. If 1 s elapses between transmission of the sound pulse and reception of the echo, then—sound velocity being 1500 m/s—the depth will be 750 m.

PIEZOELECTRIC EFFECT AND SOUND BEAM

The piezoelectric effect occurs in some materials when an electric field is applied in a certain direction. When this material becomes mechanically strained, the amount of strain is proportional to the intensity of the applied field. This effect is reversible. In Fig. 1.2, rectangular piezoelectric elements are shown in compression and expansion. The element is covered at both sides with a thin silver electrode with which the electric field is applied. For proper

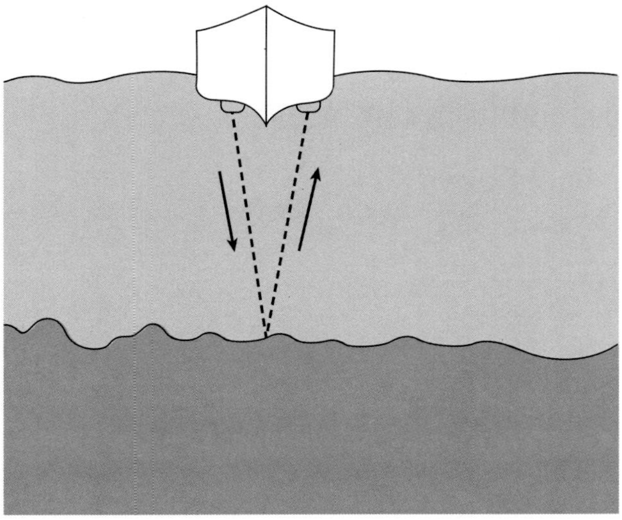

Figure 1.1 *The well-known SONAR principle for depth measurement. Reproduced with permission from Bom N, Ligtvoet CM, Principles of cardiac ultrasound, in Roelandt JRTC, Sutherland GR, Iliceto S, Linker D, eds,* Cardiac Ultrasound *(Churchill Livingstone: Edinburgh, 1993).*[31]

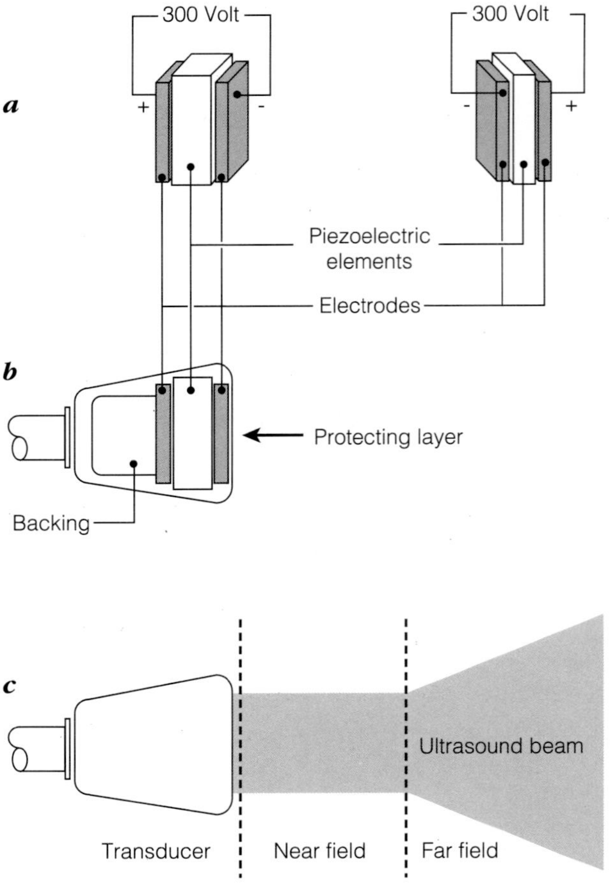

Figure 1.2 *(a) Piezoelectric elements in compression and expansion. (b) How such an element is packed in a transducer. (c) Transducer plus sound beam. Reproduced with permission from Bom N, Ligtvoet CM, Principles of cardiac ultrasound, in Roelandt JRTC, Sutherland GR, Iliceto S, Linker D, eds,* Cardiac Ultrasound *(Churchill Livingstone: Edinburgh, 1993).*[31]

resonance, the thickness of the elements has been set to an appropriate resonant size.

As illustrated in Fig. 1.2A, the piezoelectric element shrinks slightly when a voltage is applied to the electrodes. With opposite voltage the element expands slightly. Thus an alternating voltage will cause the element to vibrate. Sound pulses must be transmitted in the forward direction. Therefore, vibrations in the backward direction are attenuated or reflected forward by a backing in most transducers. The same element is used for pulse transmission and for echo reception. As with light from a torch, the sound is confined to the sound beam. The beam can be divided into a near field and a diverging far field, where the shape of the sound field depends primarily on the shape of the piezo element and the velocity in the propagation medium.

SOUND PROPAGATION AND SOUND REFLECTION

The sound waves propagate as pressure disturbances through a medium. The sound wave is a series of compressions and expansions, as illustrated in Fig. 1.3. One compression and one expansion together constitute one cycle.

An example of the pressure amplitude of an ultrasound pulse with a duration of approximately four wavelengths is shown in Fig. 1.4.

A sound pulse as used in echography may contain several wavelengths. As a result the total duration of the sound pulse and echo can be shorter for higher frequencies. This is important for the axial resolution, as will be explained later.

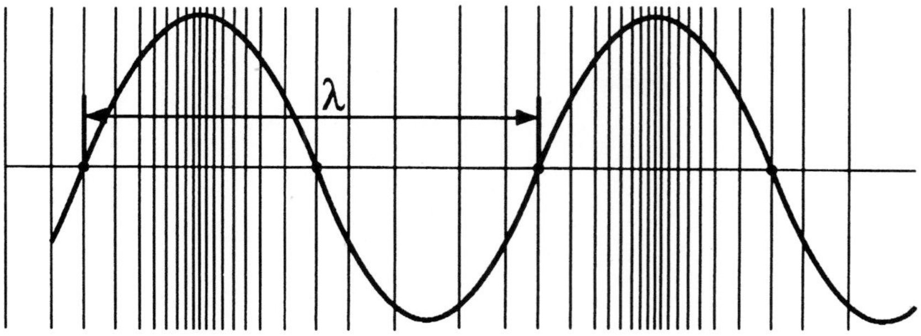

Figure 1.3 *Pressure amplitude and wavelength (λ) of a longitudinal sound wave as a function of time. Reproduced with permission from Bom N, Ligtvoet CM, Principles of cardiac ultrasound, in Roelandt JRTC, Sutherland GR, Iliceto S, Linker D, eds,* Cardiac Ultrasound *(Churchill Livingstone: Edinburgh, 1993).*[31]

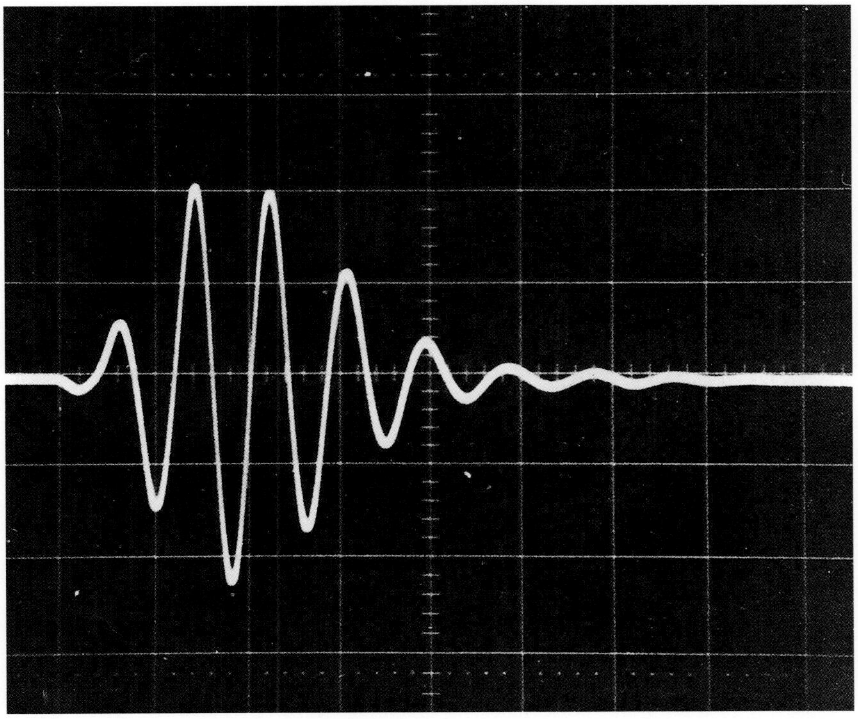

Figure 1.4 *Typical ultrasound echo at 2.24 MHz. Pressure amplitude is plotted versus time. Horizontal scale is 0.5 μs/division. Reproduced with permission from Bom N, Ligtvoet CM, Principles of cardiac ultrasound, in Roelandt JRTC, Sutherland GR, Iliceto S, Linker D, eds,* Cardiac Ultrasound *(Churchill Livingstone: Edinburgh, 1993).*[31]

Some of the important parameters of the sound pulse are (a) *the period* (this is the time it takes to complete a full cycle), (b) the peak pressure or *amplitude* of the wave (this is a measure of the strength of the sound wave), (c) *the frequency* (this is the number of cycles in 1 s) and, as indicated in Fig. 1.3, (d) *the wavelength*, λ, which is the distance the wave travels during a single cycle.

In a homogeneous medium the sound propagates along a straight line. A material may be acoustically defined by its 'acoustic impedance'. This impedance is the product of the sound velocity and the density. Reflectivity at boundaries between two media depends on their difference in acoustic impedance. Highly reflecting boundaries have big differences in acoustic impedance between the two media. Examples are interfaces between air and water or, for instance, between blood and a calcific obstruction in an artery. From each transmitted pulse only part of the acoustic energy is reflected back to the transducer as an echo. The echo can be displayed on an oscilloscope screen, where its location corresponds to the depths of the reflecting boundary.

In the example of Fig. 1.5, the reflectivity between media II and III is larger than the reflectivity between media I and II. Compare echo amplitudes E_1 and E_2.

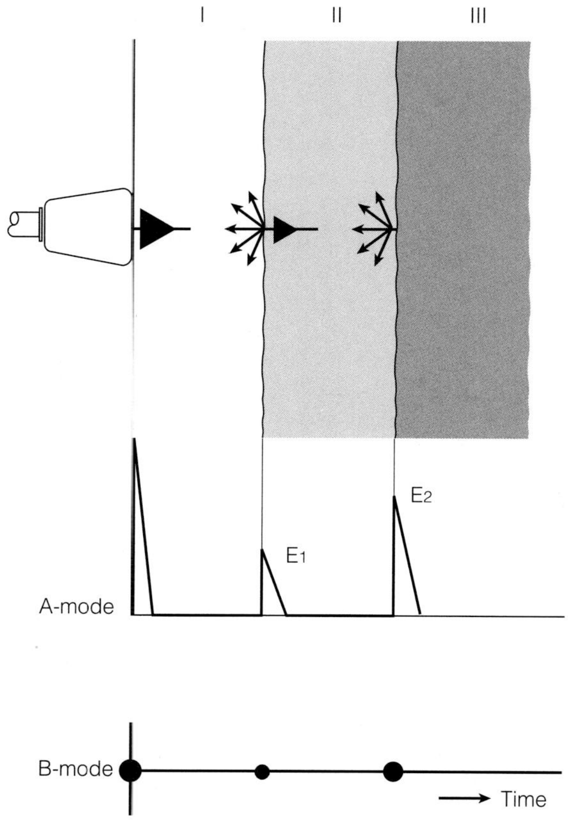

Figure 1.5 *Reflectivity at interfaces between different media. Reproduced with permission from Bom N, Ligtvoet CM, Principles of cardiac ultrasound, in Roelandt JRTC, Sutherland GR, Iliceto S, Linker D, eds,* Cardiac Ultrasound *(Churchill Livingstone: Edinburgh, 1993).*[31].

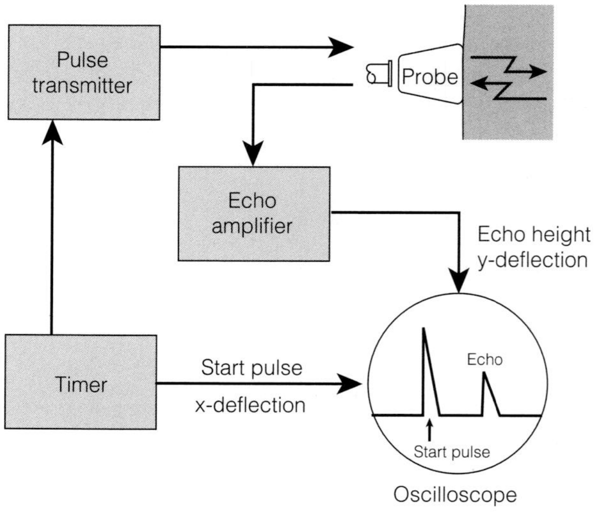

Figure 1.6 *Block diagram of an echo apparatus showing the major components for single-element echo techniques. Reproduced with permission from Bom N, Ligtvoet CM, Principles of cardiac ultrasound, in Roelandt JRTC, Sutherland GR, Iliceto S, Linker D, eds,* Cardiac Ultrasound *(Churchill Livingstone: Edinburgh, 1993).*[31]

Echoes are displayed in the amplitude mode (A-mode) and brightness mode (B-mode) as function of time (= depth). Thus, at each boundary some of the sound pulse energy is reflected and forms an echo. The remaining, diminished energy is refracted into the adjacent medium.

With ultrasound, just as in optics, the angles of incidence and reflection are the same. This means that when an ultrasound beam hits a boundary under an angle, not all acoustic energy will be returned to the probe. The echo amplitude thus depends on the angle between the sound beam and the reflecting structure. The closer the angle of incidence is to 90°, the larger the echo amplitude. This is true for specular reflections. Specular reflections are created when the interface is large compared to the wavelength. Backscatter will be caused by surface roughness, fibers and in general by structures that are small compared to the wavelength. Many tissue echoes fit into this category. In contrast to specular echoes, the amplitude of non-specular echoes is less dependent on beam angle.

These phenomena, acoustic impedance and angle of insonification, create differences in received echo intensity if the sound beam hits a variety of tissue structures. It has, for instance, been observed that, due to fiber orientation, echo intensity as received from the elastic internal lamina and the media is angle-dependent.

THE BASIC ECHO APPARATUS

As illustrated in Fig. 1.6, the core of any system is a timer. The timer sends a synchronization signal to the acoustic pulse transmitter or probe, and to the oscilloscope. The synchronization signal starts the horizontal deflection of the electron beam, and thus the spot, on the oscilloscope. At the same time the probe converts the electric pulse into a sound pulse which is transmitted into the medium. The synchronization pulse is given at a high repetition rate (500–2000/s). After the transmission of the short sound pulse the same probe is used for reception.

If an echo is received, then the amplified signal is passed on to the vertical deflection plates of the oscilloscope. The time lag between the start pulse of the oscilloscope and the received echo will be proportional to the distance between the probe and the reflecting structure. As a result the reflecting structure is 'seen' at the corresponding depth. In Fig. 1.6, the echoes are shown in A-mode.

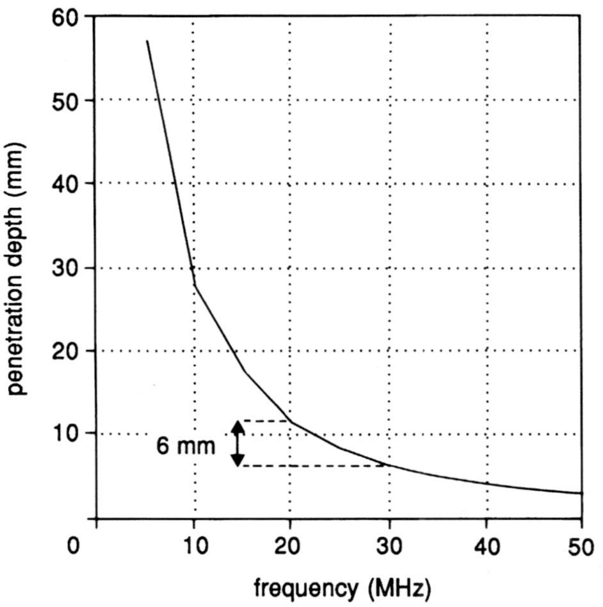

Figure 1.7 *Penetration depth as function of frequency. Reproduced with permission from Bom N, Lancée CT, Gussenhoven WJ, Li W, Ten Hoff H,, Basic principles of intravascular ultrasound imaging, in Tobis JM, York P, eds,* Intravascular Ultrasound Imaging *(Churchill Livingstone Medical Publishers: New York, 1992).*[30]

ATTENUATION AND TIME/GAIN COMPENSATION

When ultrasound waves travel through a medium, the intensity progressively weakens. This process is called attenuation. Attenuation is due to many causes; for instance, the sound energy contained in the transmitted pulse is spread over a larger area as the sound beam widens. Another important contribution to the attenuation is caused by absorption. This process is strongly dependent on the frequency, and increases with frequency. As a result, penetration depth at high frequency is limited.

As a rule of thumb, the attenuation for diagnostic ultrasound waves is 1 dB/MHz/cm. A frequency of 5 MHz can be used in diagnostic areas where penetration of 16 cm is required. In ophthalmologic applications 10 MHz can be applied, since the necessary penetration depth is only a few centimeters. As will be explained later, resolution can be improved with higher frequencies. Thus there is a tendency to use the highest possible frequency.

In Fig. 1.7, the penetration depth in blood, defined as the –20 dB level measured in reflection, illustrated as a function of frequency. As can be seen, for frequencies around 20 MHz, as used in intravascular imaging, the penetration depth becomes rather small. With the given definition, it is illustrated that a change from 20 to 30 MHz will result in a decrease of penetration depth by 6 mm.

Since the intensity of ultrasound decreases as it travels through the medium, the echo apparatus incorporates a correction mechanism by amplifying echoes from greater depth. This mechanism is a time/gain compensation circuit (TGC). In Fig. 1.8, the gain curve (a) and the echoes without TGC (b) and with TGC (c) are illustrated. The gain level between t_0 and t_1 as well as the gain ramp function between t_1 and t_2 can be selected by the operator. Some systems operate with multiple levers for 'near gain' or 'far gain'. One of the reasons for the application of TGC is to bring all significant echoes as much as possible within the limited dynamic display range of the monitor.

TWO-DIMENSIONAL IMAGE FORMATION

Today we only know real-time imaging. Real-time scanning was introduced when rapid scanning of the ultrasound beam through the cross-section became technically possible. In this way 20 or more complete cross-sectional imaging frames per second can be produced.

As will be explained later, the real-time systems are based on mechanically pivoting or rotating transducers, which rapidly sweep the sound beam through the tissue from one single entry point. This

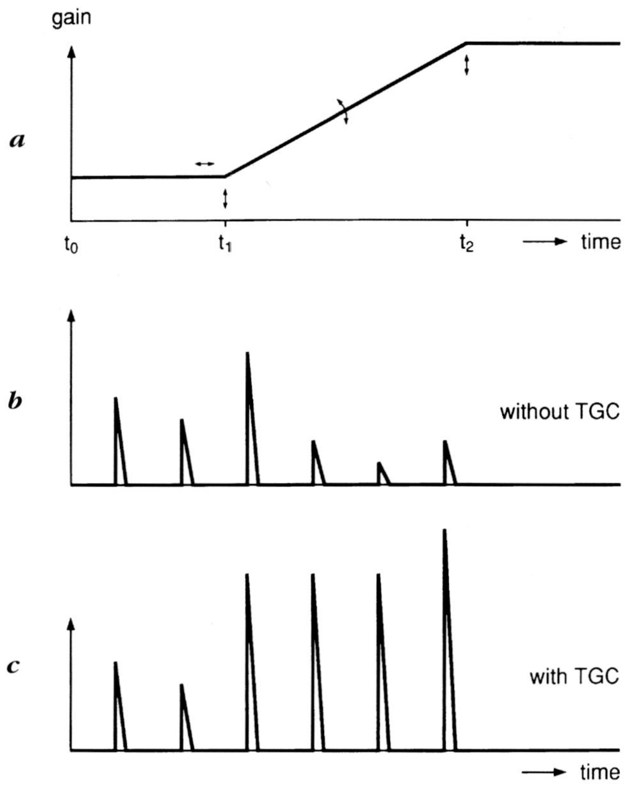

Figure 1.8 *Principle of time/gain compensation. The gain can be selected as a function of depth (a). The received echoes without gain compensation are indicated in (b). In order to compensate for attenuation, the TGC is activated; echo results are illustrated in (c). Reproduced with permission from Bom N, Ligtvoet CM, Principles of cardiac ultrasound, in Roelandt JRTC, Sutherland GR, Iliceto S, Linker D, eds,* Cardiac Ultrasound *(Churchill Livingstone: Edinburgh, 1993).*[31]

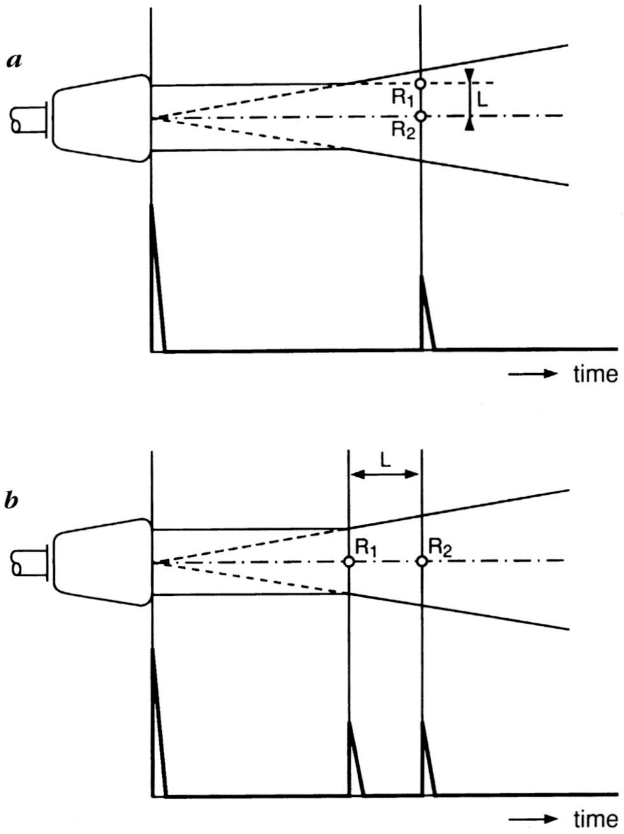

Figure 1.9 *Schematic indication of ultrasound beam and the resolution aspects in lateral (a) and axial (b) direction for reflectors positioned at distance* L. *Reproduced with permission from Bom N, Ligtvoet CM, Principles of cardiac ultrasound, in Roelandt JRTC, Sutherland GR, Iliceto S, Linker D, eds,* Cardiac Ultrasound *(Churchill Livingstone: Edinburgh, 1993).*[31]

results in a sectorial or circular real-time echo image. There also exist electronic methods to rapidly sweep the sound beam through the cross-section.

A strong advantage of the real-time scanner is the possibility of studying cardiac structures in their anatomic relationship during the interactive diagnostic study.

RESOLUTION AND SOUND BEAM

The resolution of a system is an important factor. Resolution pertains to the systems' capability of separating on the display the echoes from two closely positioned reflectors in the tissue. Depending on how the reflectors are positioned relative to each other, the sound beam and echo apparatus parameters influence the resolution. The axial resolution is the ability of the system to separate structures lying closely along the propagation direction of the sound wave: the main axis. The lateral resolution is the ability of the system to separate structures lying closely in a plane perpendicular to the main axis.

The major contribution to image quality and system resolution is made by the lateral resolution. The lateral resolution depends on the shape of the ultrasound beam produced by the transducer. This sound beam is not needle-shaped. Near the transducer the sound beam has the same width as the transducer. After a certain depth the sound beam diverges (Fig. 1.9). Both parts of the sound beam are within the region of diagnostic interest. From Fig. 1.9a it becomes clear that separation of two close reflectors R_1 and R_2 in the lateral direction requires a narrow beam. All systems are designed to produce, where possible, narrow beams by focusing methods.

Resolution in the lateral direction for intravascular imaging at 30 MHz is in the order of 0.3 mm.

Axial resolution is determined by the length of the ultrasound pulse generated by the transducer (Fig. 1.9b). Short ultrasound pulses are obtained when a high ultrasound frequency is used. However, effective penetration depth decreases with increase of frequency. Therefore, a compromise must be made between penetration depth and axial resolution. Axial resolution with intravascular echography is in the order of 0.1 mm.

Apart from pulse length and sound field, the resolution of an ultrasound system also depends on instrument parameters such as time/gain compensation. In general, an optimal resolution is achieved with a gain as low as possible.

Transducer characteristics, such as matching layer, backing, focusing or beam shape, influence resolution. In simplified explanations the sound beam is often represented as a narrow line along the beam axis.

EARLY TECHNIQUES

INTRALUMINAL MEASUREMENTS

Most of the early applications of intraluminal echography were limited to the use of ultrasound for the purpose of echo travel-time measurement. In these applications, the focus was on organ dimensions or distances. It is virtually impossible to name all the scientists who have contributed to the present technology. Therefore, the scientists briefly discussed in the following pages can only represent an incomplete selection of early workers on, in this case, endoluminal methods with some emphasis on cardiovascular applications. Early investigators applying distance measurement and their approaches are shown in Table 1.1. In the illustrations, the black area indicates the transducer element which has been mounted so that the sound beam is perpendicular to the catheter long axis.

In 1960, Cieszynski[1] built an ultrasonic catheter for intracardiac investigation, and he was able to obtain ultrasonic reflections of soft tissues during model experiments. In further experiments on dogs, he obtained good ultrasound reflections from the inner walls of the right and left ventricle as well as of the pulmonary artery. He noted that his method did not damage the animals' health. This investigator concluded that new ways of diagnosing heart failure in humans might become possible with this method. Ten years later, Kossoff[2] described a catheter tip transducer of 2 mm diameter and operating frequency of 8 MHz for measuring intracardiac septal and ventricular wall thickness with an accuracy of up to 0.1 mm. He mentioned the movement of the catheter in the cardiac chamber as one of the problems. Peronneau[3] concluded in 1968 that the cavity to be measured does not generally have the form of a 'surface of revolution', and that two opposite acoustic elements instead of one should be mounted at the tip of a catheter. Thus by adding the thickness of the catheter to the sum of the two measurements the width of the cavity is obtained. Carleton et al[4] applied a 2.5-MHz cylindrical element of 3.1 mm outer diameter and radiating through a 360° arc. He distinguished two echoes, from the shortest and longest element-to-cardiac-chamber-wall distance, from which he derived chamber diameter in experiments on dogs. He also suggested adding a forward-looking echo element.

In 1969, Stegall et al[5] introduced two transducers (0.7 × 1.5 mm) mounted at the end of a catheter-carried 'feeler gage' to determine intra-aortic and intracarotid diameter. It was a transit time system operating around 5 MHz. Another technique involved ultrasonic transit time measurement between two elements mounted at a distance apart on a catheter. This technique was described by Kardon et al.[6] The catheter had to be manipulated so that it came to rest in a certain loop inside the ventricle. In 1974, Olson and Cooke[7] described an esophageal device to monitor diameter and blood velocity at the same point along the ascending thoracic aorta. The probe was passed 1–2 cm distal to the aortic arch. Transesophageal cardiac M-mode registrations were described by Frazin et al.[8] They used a 9-mm 3.5-MHz transducer and studied cardiac structures in 38 subjects. In 1978, Hughes et al[9] increased the number of transducers from two to three to dynamically measure at 10 MHz the aortic lumen diameter.

Table 1.1 Selection of early intraluminal measurement methods.

Author	*Year*	*Method*	*Probe principle*	*Application*
Cieszynski	1960	Single-element echo	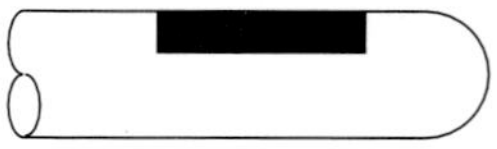	Feasibility Heart
Kossoff	1966	Single-element	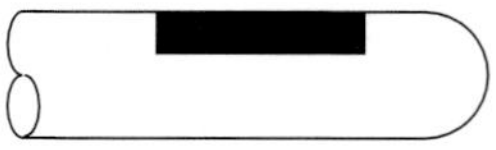	IV size Septal thickness
Peronneau	1968	Two elements		Body cavity diameter
Carleton	1968	Non-directional cylindrical element		LV diameter
Stegall	1969	Transit line	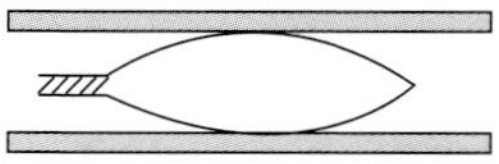	Carotid diameter
Kardon	1971	Transit time		LV diameter
Olson	1974	Doppler and echo	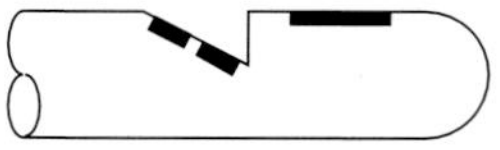	Esophageal probe
Frazin	1976	M-mode registration	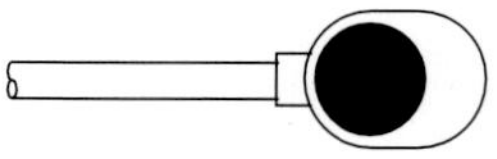	Esophageal probe
Hughes	1978	Three elements	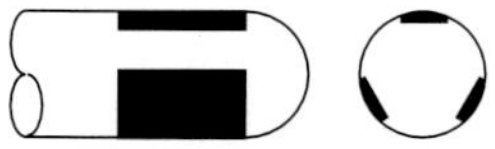	Aortic lumen

Adapted from Bom N, Ten Hoff H, Lancée CT, Gussenhoven WJ, Bosch JG, Early and recent intraluminal ultrasound devices, *Int J Cardiac Imag* 1989; **4**:79–88.[29] Reproduced by permission of Kluwer Academic Publishers.

INTRALUMINAL IMAGING

Very early in the history of diagnostic ultrasound, information was used to form a cross-sectional image. For this purpose the acoustic beam had to scan through the cross-sectional plane. In order to obtain a realistic display, the acoustic beam direction and beam deflection on the display had to be synchronized. Mechanically rotated transducers were used, such as the one described by Wild and Reid[10] in 1955 for rectal tumor location and illustrated in Table 1.2. Analyses were also made of A-mode patterns of colonic and gastric mucosa to elucidate changes characteristic of malignant transformation of these hollow organs. Watanabe et al[11] followed this up in 1968 with the description of a 'chair' for detection of prostatic cancer. Further endoscopic scanners such as the transurethral scanner were described by Holm and Northeved,[12] and the bladder scanner by Niijima.[13]

For cardiovascular applications additional early workers and their methods are further illustrated in Table 1.2. Omoto[14] used an intravenous probe with guidewire tip to study cardiac structures, and Ebina et al[15] described a miniature concave transducer for rotation inside a rubber cuff in the esophagus. Wells[16] described in 1966 a venous probe which can be considered to be the blueprint of present intravascular mechanical systems. Eggleton et al[17] approximated a cardiac cross-section by rotating a four-element

Table 1.2 Overview of early intraluminal imaging methods.

Author	*Year*	*Method*	*Probe principle*	*Application*
Wild	1955	Echoendoscope	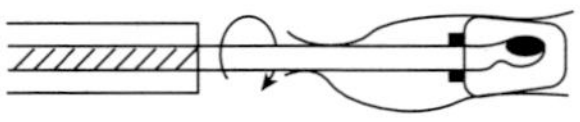	Rectal tumor location
Omoto	1962	Rotating probe C-scan	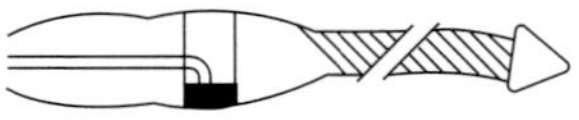	Intracardiac tomography
Ebina	1964	Transesophageal PPI scanning	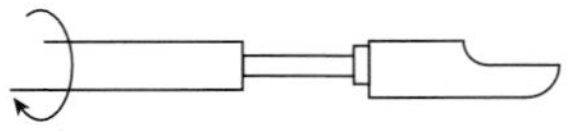	Heart and vessels
Wells	1965	Rotating mirror	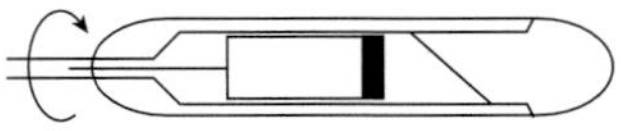	Intravenous
Eggleton	1969	Four elements EGG-triggered	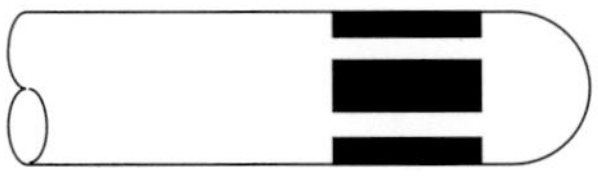	Heart
Bom	1971	32 elements Cylindrical phase array	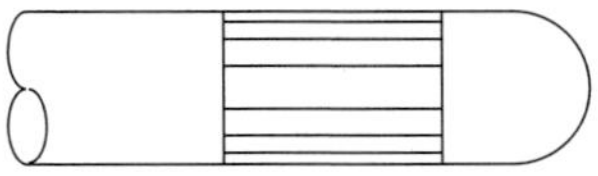	Intracardiac tomography

Adapted from Bom N, Ten Hoff H, Lancée CT, Gussenhoven WJ, Bosch JG, Early and recent intraluminal ultrasound devices, *Int J Cardiac Imag* 1989; **4**:79–88.[29] Reproduced by permission of Kluwer Academic Publishers. (PPI, plane position indicator.)

catheter. Results of his system depended on a stable state of the heart, since he accumulated data over many beats for reconstruction of a cross-section in a selected steady state. In 1971, Bom initiated a program to develop two-dimensional real-time invasive ultrasonic imaging using state-of-the-art technology. A 32-element circular phased array with an outer diameter of 3.2 mm mounted at the tip of a 9 F catheter (Fig. 1.10) was constructed.[18,19] As pointed out in the original paper, the array design was a compromise between the optimal design and the limitations imposed by technological constraints. The final design was chosen to operate at 5.6 MHz with a narrow main beam. With this catheter, real-time intraluminal images such as left ventricular and aortic cross-sections were recorded in the early 1970s.

In Table 1.3, further examples of early workers in the field of intraluminal imaging are indicated. Hisanaga[20] rotated a small transducer fixed to a

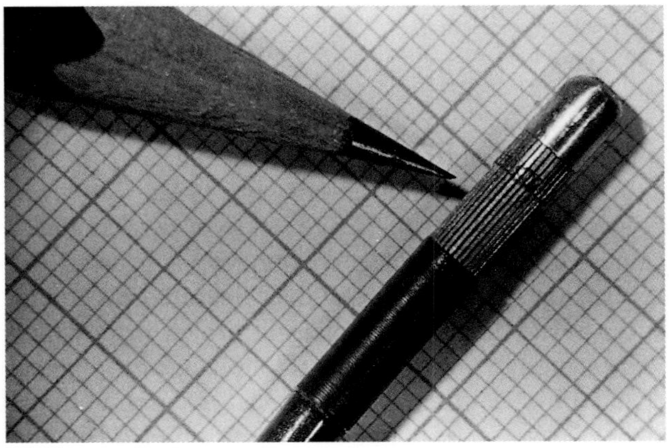

Figure 1.10 *The phased-array 32-element catheter as decribed by Bom in the early 1970s. From Bom N, Ten Hoff H, Lancée CT, Gussenhoven WJ, Bosch JG, Early and recent intraluminal devices,* Int J Cardiac Imag *1989;* **4***:79–88.*[29] *Reproduced by permission of Kluwer Academic Publishers.*

Table 1.3 Further examples of early intraluminal imaging methods.

Author	*Year*	*Method*	*Probe principle*	*Application*
Hisanaga	1977	Transesophageal rotating scanner	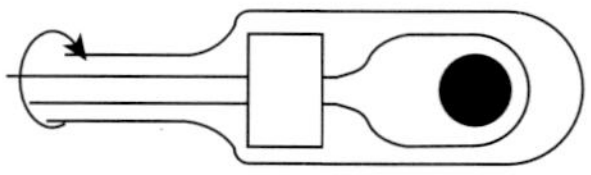	Cardiac cross-sectional images
DiMagno	1980	64 elements	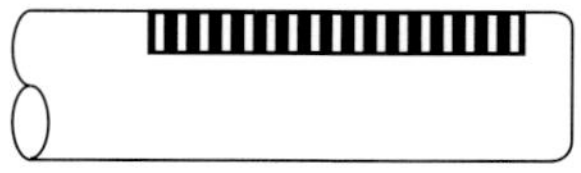	Upper abdominal organs
Bertini	1981	Distensible-tip rotating catheter	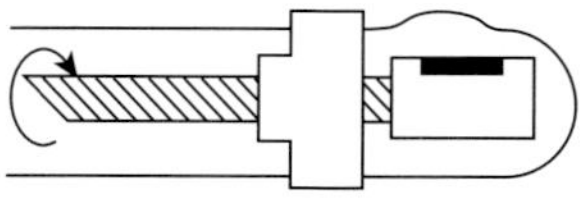	Transesophageal Cardiac
Souquet	1982	Transesophageal phase-array, two-plane	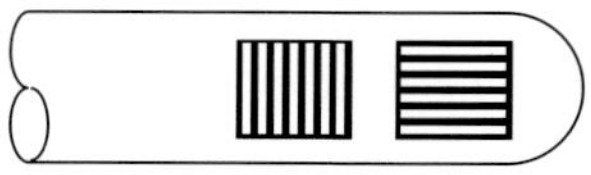	Cardiac cross-sectional images
Natori	1982	Transesophageal 5 MHz linear array	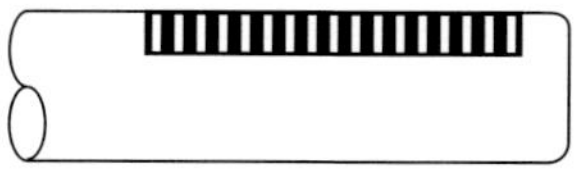	Mediastinum

Adapted from Bom N, Ten Hoff H, Lancée CT, Gussenhoven WJ, Bosch JG, Early and recent intraluminal ultrasound devices, *Int J Cardiac Imag* 1989; **4**:79–88.[29] Reproduced by permission of Kluwer Academic Publishers.

flexible shaft. It rotates at a rate of 15–50 cycles/s. Hisanaga's work can be considered very important for today's transesophageal echocardiography. DiMagno et al[21] adapted a 64-element linear array at 10 MHz. The field of view is 3 × 4 cm. Both Hisanaga and Bertini[22] and their colleagues use a distensible fluid-filled bag for contact with the esophageal wall. Souquet et al[23] introduced the phased-array principle into esophageal applications in 1982. He even suggested forming an image in two perpendicular planes. In 1985, Harui and Souquet[24] suggested the application of a fully rotatable phased-array transducer at the tip of an esophageal probe, from which stems today's vario- or multiplane esophageal techniques. Further applications of intraluminal imaging were described by Natori et al[25] and Fukuda,[26] who were interested in the diagnosis of intra-abdominal disorders. In a review article, Fukuda[27] compared the various ultrasonic endoscopes developed by American and Japanese manufacturers, as available in 1986. These include linear and radially scanning devices in the frequency range 5–10 MHz.

CURRENT INTRAVASCULAR IMAGING TECHNIQUES

The smallest presently used devices for endoluminal imaging are the intravascular catheters in the 20–30-MHz range. Intravascular echo catheters are based on two principles: electronic and mechanical rotation of the sound beam. The catheters can have an outer diameter in the order of 1 mm for coronary applications. A schematic illustration of these principles is shown in Fig. 1.11.

SINGLE-ELEMENT MECHANICAL SYSTEMS

Mechanical rotation of a single ultrasound element permits us to scan the vessel wall approximately perpendicular to the long axis of the catheter. Rotation of either the element or an acoustic reflector in front of a fixed ultrasound element causes the sound beam to rotate, thus building a cross-sectional echo image in real time. An example of an early

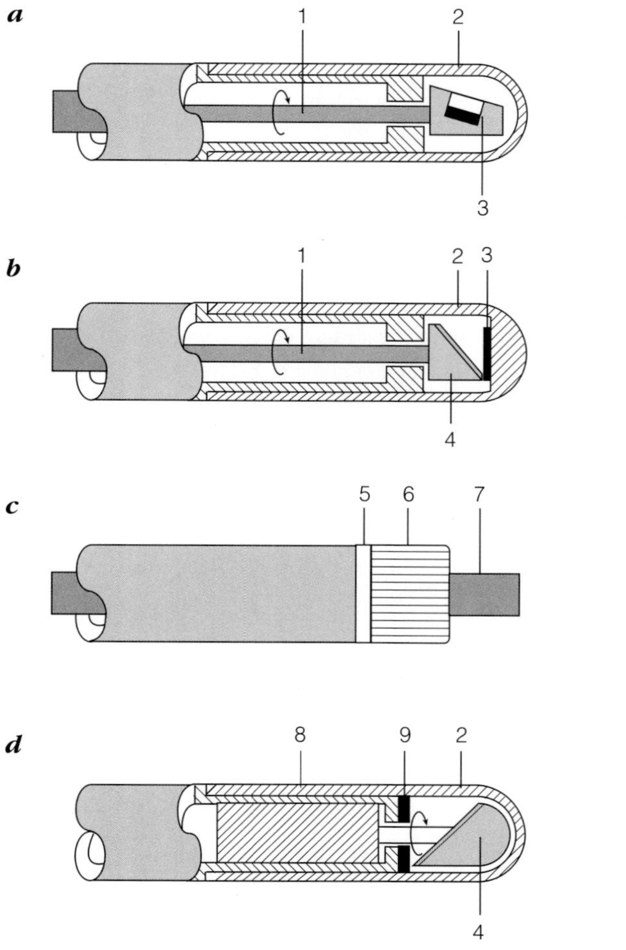

Figure 1.11 *Schematic illustration of echo catheter principles: (a) flex shaft rotation of the element; (b) flex shaft rotation of a mirror in front of the stationary transducer; (c) electronic rotation of the beam by phased-array techniques; (d) the micromotor in combination with annular transducer and rotating mirror. 1, flex shaft; 2, acoustically transparent dome; 3, transducer; 4, mirror; 5, electronic switching circuit; 6, multiple acoustic elements; 7, guidewire; 8, micromotor; 9, annular transducer. From Bom et al.*[32]

description of this type of device dates back to 1966.[16] Most mechanical systems that are presently commercially available are based on rotation of a single element or a mirror mounted in front of a fixed element in the tip of the catheter (Fig. 1.11a,b). The element or mirror is rotated by use of a long, flexible shaft driven by an external motor. With a long

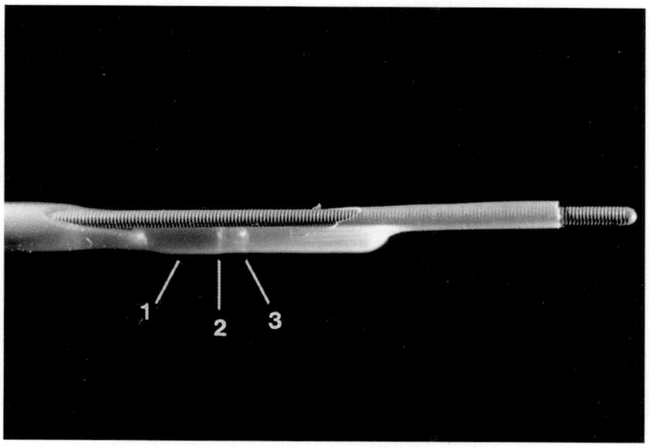

Figure 1.12 *Example of the micromotor-in-tip echocatheter with guidewire as being tested presently. Courtesy Du-MED/Endosonics. 1, micromotor; 2, element; 3, mirror. From: Bom et al*[32] *with permission.*

catheter through a tortuous path, non-uniform rotation may occur. This could cause image artifacts. The latest development to avoid these problems is substitution of the flex shaft by a micromotor in the catheter tip. The first available micromotor catheter was built for noncardiac arterial applications (Fig. 1.12). The micromotor approach will eventually allow the development of a scanning guidewire without the problems of rotating a flex shaft.

MULTI-ELEMENT ELECTRONIC SYSTEMS

The geometry of the phased-array method is illustrated in Fig. 1.11c. A large number of small transducer elements is mounted around the circumference of the catheter tip. The signal is processed and multiplexed via integrated circuits in the tip of the catheter. Signals from each individual transducer element were used for reconstruction of the cross-sectional echo image in real time by Hodgson and co-workers.[28]

Although the first commercially available catheters of this type yielded poor image quality and a large dead zone close to the surface of the catheter tip (ring-down effect), more recent catheters have shown a considerable improvement in image quality. The advantage of multi-element electronic echo catheters is the absence of any mechanical drive to rotate the

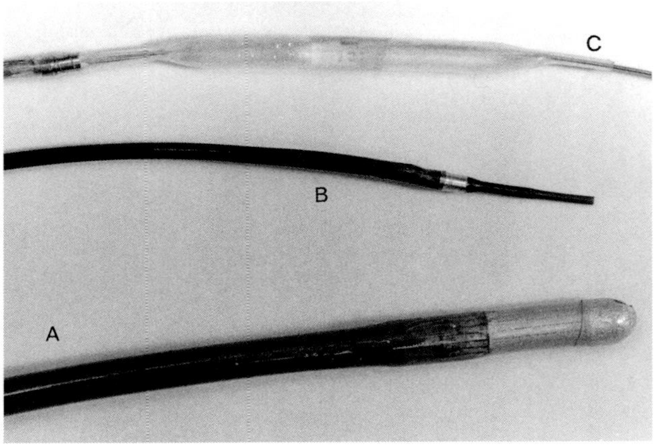

Figure 1.13 *Examples of early and recent phased-array ultrasonic catheters: (A) 32 elements, 9 Fr diameter, 5.6-MHz frequency catheter;[18] (B) the 3.5 Fr diameter, 20-MHz coronary version; (C) similar version combined with balloon capabilities. Courtesy Du-MED/Endosonics. From Bom et al[32] with permission.*

sound beam and the possibility of using a central guidewire. Significant steps forward are illustrated in Fig. 1.13.

CLINICAL RESULTS—A CASE STUDY

Whereas radiographic techniques allow optimal pathfinding for obstruction in coronary arteries by use of contrast fluid, this method does not yield volumetric or morphologic information on the plaque. Only the lumen is imaged, and a lumenogram is obtained. Intravascular ultrasound (IVUS), on the other hand, allows detection of wall pathology, detection of plaque eccentricity and study of the plaque composition. Unfortunately, study of plaque composition with IVUS remains limited to the differentiation between 'hard' plaques, which are seen as highly echogenic lesions and are likely to be composed of dense fibrous tissue (when shadowing is present, this indicates calcific deposits), and 'soft' plaques, which are lesions with low echogenicity that may consist of fibrocellular tissue, thrombus or lipid areas.

Corresponding IVUS cross-sections and angiograms obtained from a patient before and after balloon angioplasty (percutaneous transluminal angioplasty,

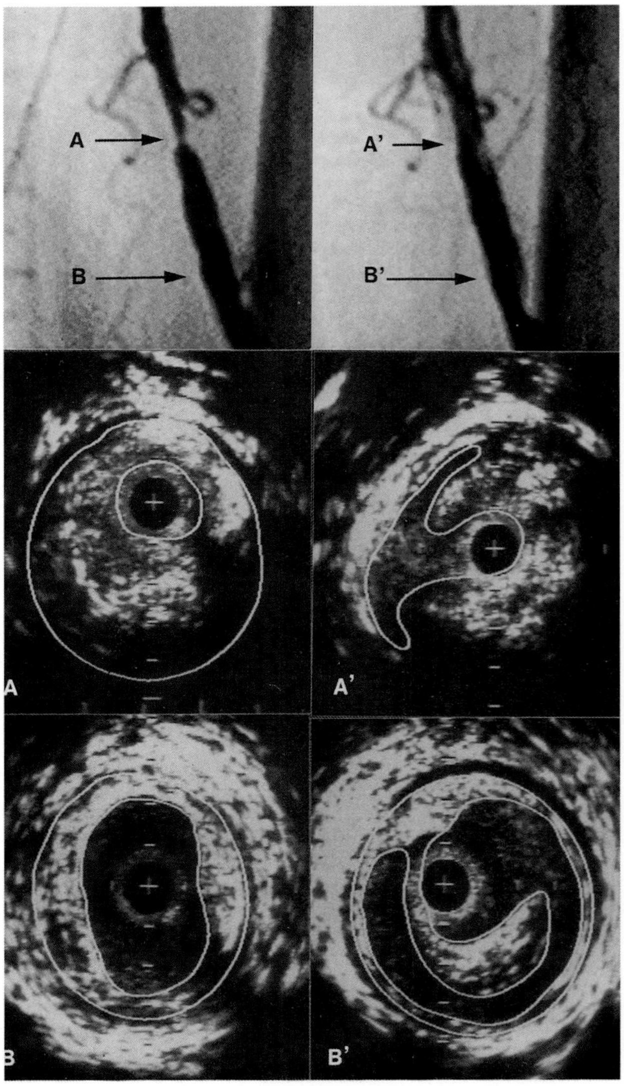

Figure 1.14 *Corresponding intravascular ultrasound cross-sections and angiograms obtained from a patient before and after balloon angioplasty of the superficial femoral artery. +, catheter. Calibration = 1 mm. Courtesy Dr EJ Gussenhoven.*

PTA) of the superficial femoral artery are illustrated in Fig. 1.14. Before PTA a tight concentric stenosis is seen on angiography. This was confirmed by IVUS (A), which revealed a more eccentric location of the lumen. Panel B shows a concentric thickening of the vessel wall, while the corresponding angiographic level appears normal. After PTA the angiogram revealed a good result, while the IVUS cross-section

(A') showed a small increase in luminal area caused by dissections. The intraluminal filling defect seen on angiography is caused by a large dissection which extends into the rather normal segments of the artery (B'). The IVUS images are contour-traced off-line, facilitating the recognition of free lumen area (inner contour) and media-bounded area (outer contour). The free lumen area at level A increased from 3.5 mm^2 to 7.8 mm^2 at level A'.

ACKNOWLEDGMENT

This chapter is in part based on previous lectures and publications by the first author on basic principles, history and technical updates. This material is documented in refrences 29, 30, 31 and 32. The permission to use this material is hereby gratefully acknowledged.

REFERENCES

1. Cieszynski T, Intracardiac method for the investigation of structure of the heart with the aid of ultrasonics, *Arch Immun Ter Dosw* 1960; **8:**551–7.
2. Kossoff G, Diagnostic applications of ultrasound in cardiology, *Australas Radiol* 1966; **X:**101–6.
3. Peronneau P, Catheter with piezoelectric transducer, US Patent No. 3,542,014 1970.
4. Carleton RA, Sessions RW, Graettinger JS, Diameter of heart measured by intracavitary ultrasound, *Med Res Engng* 1969; **May/June:**28–32.
5. Stegall HF, Pratt JR, Moser PJ, Carotid mechanics in situ, *Fed Proc* 1969; **28:**585.
6. Kardon MB, O'Rourke RA, Bishop VS, Measurement of left ventricular internal diameter by catheterization, *J Appl Physiol* 1971; **31:**613–15.
7. Olson RM, Cooke JP, A nondestructive ultrasonic technique to measure diameter and blood flow in arteries, *IEEE Trans Biomed Engng* 1974; **March:**168–71.
8. Frazin L, Talano JV, Stephanides L, Loeb HS, Kopel L, Gunnar RM, Esophageal echocardiography, *Circulation* 1976; **54:**102–8.
9. Hughes DJ, Geddes LA, Bourland JD, Babbs CF, Dynamic imaging of the aorta in-vivo with 10 MHz ultrasound. In: Metherell AF, ed., *Acoustical Imaging* 8 (Plenum Press: New York, 1980) 699–707.
10. Wild JJ, Reid JM, Ultrasonic rectal endoscope for tumor location, *Am Inst Ultrasonics Med* 1955; **4:**59.
11. Watanabe H, Kata H, Kato T et al, Diagnostic application of ultrasonography for the prostrate, *Jpn J Urol* 1968; **59:**273–9.
12. Holm HH, Northeved AA, Transurethral ultrasonic scan, *J Urol* 1974; **111:**238.
13. Niijima T, Ultrasonic diagnosis and bladder cancer staging. In: Wagai T, Omoto R, eds, *Recent advances in Ultrasound and Medicine* (Excerpta Medica: Amsterdam, 1979) 213–17.
14. Omoto R, Intracardiac scanning of the heart with the aid of ultrasonic intravenous probe, *Jap Heart J* 1967; **8:**569–81.
15. Ebina T, Oka S, Tanaka M et al, The diagnostic application of ultrasound to the disease in mediastinal organs. Ultrasono-tomography for the heart and great vessels, *Sci Rep Res Inst Tohoku Univ* 1965; **12:**199–212.
16. Wells PNT, Developments in medical electronics. In: *Proceedings of the European Symposium on Medical Electronics. World Medical Electronics* 1966; **September:**272–7.
17. Eggleton RC, Townsend C, Kossoff G et al, Computerised ultrasonic visualization of dynamic ventricular configurations. *Proceedings 8th ICMBE* Palmer House, Chicago IL (July 1969) Session 10-3.
18. Bom N, Lancée CT, Van Egmond FC, An ultrasonic intracardiac scanner, *Ultrasonics* 1972; **10:**72–6.
19. Bom N, Lancée CT, van Egmond FC, US Patent No. 1,402,192, 1973.
20. Hisanaga K, Hisanaga A, Nagata K, Yoshida S, A new transesophageal real-time two-dimensional echocardiographic system using a flexible tube and its clinical application, *Proc Jap Soc Ultrasonics Med* 1977; **32:**43–4.
21. DiMagno EP, Regan PT, Wilson DA et al, Ultrasonic endoscope, *Lancet* 1980; **i:**629–31.
22. Bertini A, Masotti L, Zuppiroli A, Cecchi F, Rotating probe for transoesophageal cross-sectional echocardiography. *J Nucl Med Allied Sci* 1984; **28:**115–21.
23. Souquet J, Hanrath P, Zitelli L, Kremer P, Langenstein BA, Schlüter M, Transesophageal phased array for imaging the heart, *IEEE Trans Biomed Engng* 1982, **BME-29:**707–12.
24. Harui N, Souquet J, Transesophageal echo cardiography scanhead, US Patent, No. 4,543,960, 1985.
25. Natori H, Tamaki S, Izumi S, Joshita Y, Kira S, Clinical application of ultrasound endoscope using linear array transducer for transesophageal ultrasonography of the disease of the mediastinum. In: Lerski A, Morley P, eds, *Ultrasound '82* (Pergamon Press: Oxford, 1983) 339–43.
26. Fukuda M, Endoscopic ultrasonography. In: Gill RW, Dadd MJ, eds, *WFUMB '85* (Pergamon Press Sydney, 1985) 13–16.
27. Fukuda M, Endoscopic sonography: use of the echoendiscope and echolaproscope in the diagnosis of intra-abdominal disorders. In: Sanders RC, Hill M, eds, *Ultrasound Annual* (Raven Press: New York, 1986) 141–70.
28. Hodgson JMcB, Graham SP, Savakus AD et al, Clinical percutaneous imaging of coronary anatomy using an over-the-wire ultrasound catheter system. *Int J Cardiac Imag* 1989; **4:**187–93.
29. Bom N, Ten Hoff H, Lancée CT, Gussenhoven WJ, Bosch JG, Early and recent intraluminal ultrasound devices, *Int J Cardiac Imag* 1989; **4:**79–88.
30. Bom N, Lancée CT, Gussenhoven WJ, Li W, Ten Hoff H, Basic principles of intravascular ultrasound imaging. In: Tobis JM, Yock P, eds, *Intravascular Ultrasound Imaging* (Churchill Livingstone Medical Publishers: New York, 1992) 7–15.

31. Bom N, Ligtvoet CM, Principles of cardiac ultrasound. In: Roelandt JRTC, Sutherland GR, Iliceto S, Linker D, eds, *Cardiac Ultrasound* (Churchill Livingstone: Edinburgh, 1993) 9–20.

32. Bom N, Li W, van der Steen AFW et al, Intravascular ultrasound: technical update 1995. In: Feyter PJ de, Mario C di, Serruys PW, eds, *Quantitative Coronary Imaging* (Barjesteh, Meeuwes & Co.: Rotterdam, 1995) 89–106.

Chapter 2 Basic physics and instrumentation of endoluminal ultrasound

Daniel A Merton and Judy A Lund

INTRODUCTION

Diagnostic ultrasound has achieved a well-deserved position as one of the most widely utilized diagnostic imaging modalities available today. Its proven safety, noninvasiveness and relative low cost contribute to its success. Recent technological improvements and advances have rapidly increased the scope and capability of ultrasound diagnoses. These improvements include the design and manufacture of the ultrasound systems and transducers. Faster and more sophisticated techniques involving ultrasound signal acquisition and processing have also been developed.

One of the most important technological developments has been the miniaturization of ultrasound transducers.[1–4] New high-frequency miniature catheter-based transducers have contributed to the development of endoluminal ultrasound imaging commonly referred to as intravascular ultrasound (IVUS) and intracoronary ultrasound (ICUS) for coronary and peripheral vascular applications or endoluminal ultrasound (ELUS) for nonvascular applications.

Endoluminal ultrasound represents an important clinical extension of the imaging capabilities of conventional percutaneous ultrasound. With the integration of miniature transducers within small plastic catheters, these probes can be placed into vascular and nonvascular lumina which could not have previously been imaged. The optimal utilization of endoluminal ultrasound requires an adequate understanding of the basic ultrasound principles and a working knowledge of the operation of the equipment being employed.

This chapter is not intended to be an all-inclusive reference source on the physics and instrumentation of diagnostic ultrasound. Should additional information be desired, the reader is encouraged to refer to one of the many excellent textbooks available that are devoted to these topics.[5–8] The purpose of this chapter is to provide the reader with a basic understanding of ultrasound physics, the techniques used for catheter-based transducers and ultrasound systems, and the skills necessary to operate an endoluminal ultrasound system. Specific applications and their unique requirements can be found in the chapters of this book devoted to individual topics.

BASIC PRINCIPLES OF ULTRASOUND

SOUND

Sound is a mechanical *wave*, or a series of compressions and expansions that move particles in a direction parallel to that of the traveling wave. The *frequency* of sound is equal to the number of cycles or oscillations that particles within a medium undergo per second. Units of frequency are the hertz (Hz), thousand hertz (kHz) and million hertz (MHz). The term *ultrasound* refers to sound at frequencies above the level of the human audible range, usually accepted as 20 Hz to 20 kHz. Typical frequencies used for conventional diagnostic ultrasound imaging range from 2 MHz to 12 MHz. The optimal frequency for a particular use depends on the specific application. Higher frequencies provide better image resolution but sacrifice tissue penetration. Lower frequencies improve penetration but lack the spatial resolution afforded by the higher frequencies. The *wavelength* is the spatial size of one wave or cycle. Wavelengths are typically measured in millimeters (mm) (Fig. 2.1). The wavelength of a typical 3.5-MHz transducer in soft tissue is about 0.43 mm. Higher frequencies have proportionately shorter wavelengths, and lower frequencies have longer

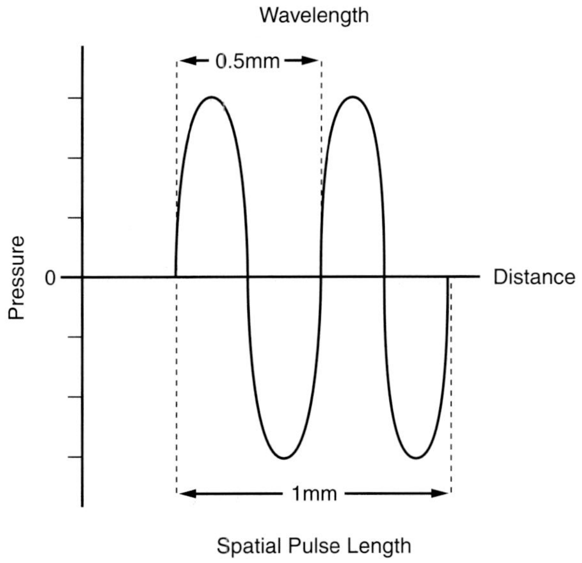

Figure 2.1 *Spatial pulse length is equal to the wavelength multiplied by the number of cycles in the pulse. In this figure, the wavelength is 0.5 mm and there are two cycles in each pulse, yielding a spatial pulse length of 1 mm.*

Table 2.1 Acoustic properties of various media

Media	*Impedance (kg/m²s)*	*Density (kg/m³)*	*Velocity (m/s)*
Air	0.0004×10^6	1.21	333
Water	1.48×10^6	1000	1480
Fat	1.38×10^6	952	1450
Soft tissue	1.63×10^6	1058	1540
Bone	7.80×10^6	2229	3500

wavelengths. Endoluminal ultrasound imaging systems use high-frequency transducers in the range of 10–30 MHz to obtain relatively high resolution over short distances.

Diagnostic ultrasound uses the *pulse-echo principle.* A *pulse* is composed of a consecutive series of waves. In diagnostic ultrasound, a pulse is transmitted into the body tissues by a sound source or *transducer.* Reflected sound waves are returned or absorbed by the body structures and produce echoes that are received by the transducer. The ultrasound system then converts the echoes into usable data in the form of a visual display on a cathode ray tube (CRT) or video screen. Doppler ultrasound is most often used to study bloodflow. Doppler ultrasound data may be in the form of an audible signal as well as a visual display.

PROPAGATION OF SOUND

Sound waves which travel through the air and ultrasound waves which travel through body tissues are both propagating mechanical pressure waves that require a medium for transmission. The density and stiffness of the medium determine the speed of propagation. *Density* is the concentration of particles within the medium and *stiffness* is the resistance of a medium to compression. Propagation speed *increases* with increasing stiffness, but *decreases* with increasing density. Usually, high levels of stiffness coincide with high density, and the stiffness of a medium has a greater effect on sound propagation. Frequency has no bearing on sound propagation speed. The temperature of the medium does have an effect, because temperature affects the medium density. The average speed of sound in air is only 333 meters per second (m/s), whereas dense body tissue, such as striated muscle, has a propagation speed of approximately 1600 m/s, and for less dense tissues, such as fat, the propagation speed is about 1450 m/s. Table 2.1 lists the acoustic properties of various media, including body tissues.

For most applications of diagnostic ultrasound, a velocity of 1540 m/s is used as an average speed of sound through body tissues. This approximation is necessary to enable the ultrasound system to determine a given reflector's distance from the transducer. In a typical scenario, a pulse is generated into the tissues and travels at a speed of 1540 m/s. As the echoes are produced from the tissues at various depths, their respective echoes return to the transducer at different times. An echo that originates from more deeply situated body tissues arrives back at the transducer later than one closer to the transducer surface. Using a simple 'time-of-flight' equation, the ultrasound system's on-board computer then calculates the depth of each returning echo. Therefore, for practical purposes, the elapsed *time* in ultrasound is equivalent to *distance* traveled. The relationship between wavelength (λ), frequency (f) and propagation speed (c) can be expressed by the equation: $\lambda = c/f$.

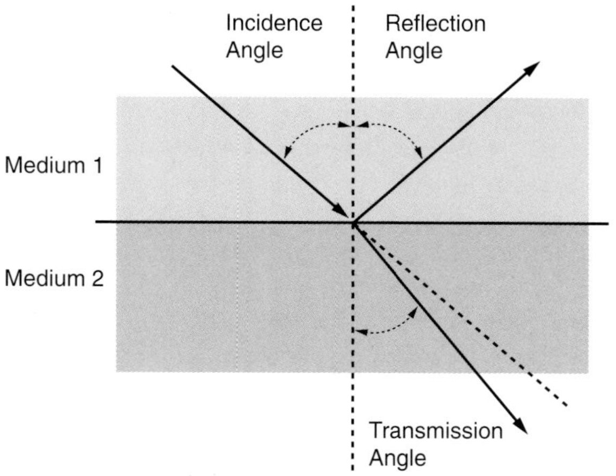

Figure 2.2 *Demonstration of sound reflection and transmission which occurs at a boundary between two different media with an oblique angle of incidence. The transmission angle is dependent on the incidence angle and the media propagation speeds. The incidence and reflection angles are equal.*

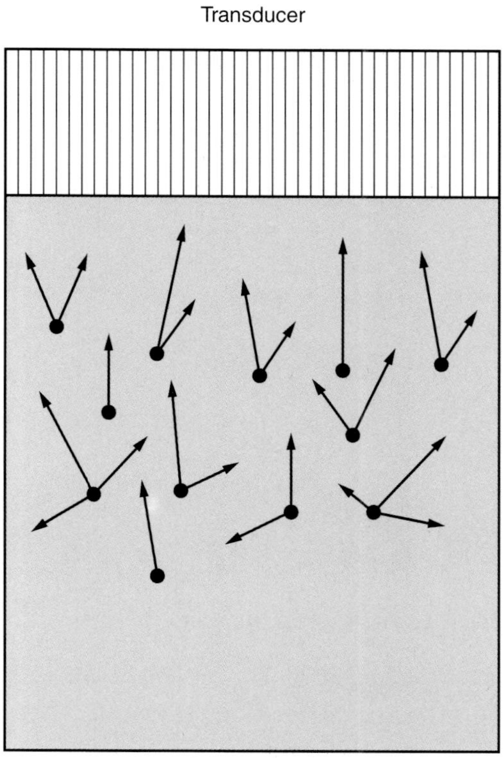

Figure 2.3 *Demonstration of echoes (arrows) produced from scatterer-type reflectors. Because they have irregular surfaces and they are relatively small compared to the wavelength, the resulting echoes travel in random directions. In practice, many of the tissues within the body are composed of scatterer reflectors, and this reduces the angle dependency for echoes to return to the transducer for the production of an image.*

SIGNAL ATTENUATION

As sound passes through a medium, it loses some of its strength or amplitude. This is referred to as signal *attenuation*. Attenuation is the reason why it is more difficult to hear a loudspeaker (a sound source) from a great distance than when you are close to the source. Attenuation results from reflection, scattering and absorption. Absorption (the conversion of sound to heat) is the primary factor contributing to sound attenuation in soft tissues. The farther the sound travels through a medium, the greater the amount of attenuation imposed on the signal's amplitude. Attenuation is measured in decibels (dB). The *attenuation coefficient* is the amount of sound attenuation per centimeter (dB/cm) of distance traveled. As the attenuation coefficient gets higher, penetration is reduced. Higher frequencies are attenuated more than lower frequencies, so the high frequencies used in most endoluminal/intravascular devices have limited penetration.

SOUND REFLECTION AND REFRACTION

The reflective properties of tissues are related to the *acoustic impedance differences* existing between two adjacent media and the *angle of incidence* between the reflector and the beam. The acoustic impedance of a given medium can be defined as a product of the propagation speed and its density. Large impedance differences or *mismatches* produce greater amplitude reflections.

The angle of reflection is equal to the angle of incidence. This statement is particularly true when dealing with *specular reflectors*, i.e. those that are relatively large (compared to the wavelength) and smooth (Fig. 2.2). *Scatterers* are reflectors that are relatively small (compared to the wavelength) or have irregular surfaces. Scatterers (as the name implies) tend to scatter the reflected sound because of their small size or irregular surfaces (Fig. 2.3). Fortunately, the majority of the body's tissues represent scatterers. Unlike with specular reflectors, the

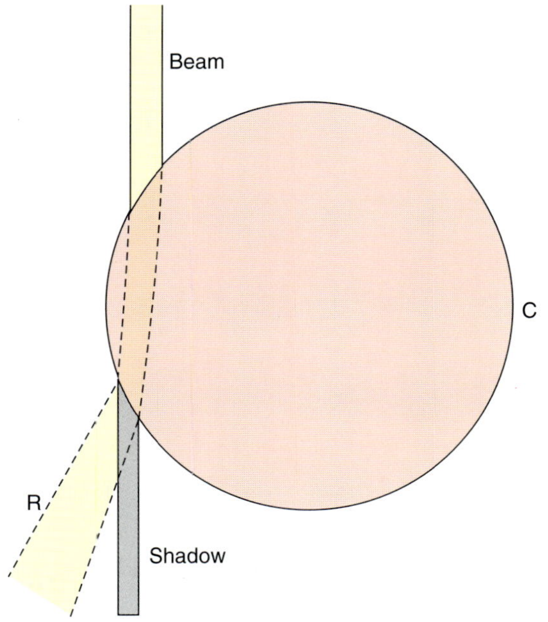

Figure 2.4 *As a sound beam enters a circular area (C) of higher propagation speed, it is refracted, and refraction (R) occurs again as it leaves. This causes deviation or 'bending' of the beam, with decreased intensity resulting in an edge shadow distal to the curved structure.*

angle of incidence is far less important for the production of echoes that return to the transducer and contribute to the formation of an image.

Refraction refers to a change in direction of travel which occurs when the sound passes from one medium into another. The difference between the media may be small (i.e. a few degrees in temperature) or large (i.e. two different tissue types). The amount of refraction that occurs when a beam passes through two media is related to the angle at which the beam strikes the interface and the difference in propagation speeds of the media (Fig. 2.2). Reflection can also occur behind the edges of spherical structures, which causes the margin shadow artifact in ultrasound imaging (Fig. 2.4).

TYPES OF DIAGNOSTIC ULTRASOUND

Various types of ultrasound are used for diagnostic imaging. The most common commercially available types of ultrasound are: A-mode; B-mode; M-mode; and Doppler ultrasound. Doppler ultrasound can be further categorized as continuous wave, pulsed wave, and color Doppler imaging (CDI).

A-mode or amplitude mode is a single point of sound that has only one dimension. Reflectors encountered along the path of the ultrasound beam cause deflections of varying heights (dependent upon signal amplitude) which are then displayed on an oscilloscope screen. This type of ultrasound has largely been replaced by B-mode ultrasound imaging but is sometimes used for ophthalmologic applications.

M-mode or motion mode is a method of evaluating the motion of structures in which the display represents a strip of data which plots the location on the vertical axis and time on the horizontal axis. M-mode is primarily used to evaluate the dynamics of cardiac wall and valve motion, such as evaluation of cardiac wall thickness and contractility as well as valvular excursion during the cardiac cycle.

B-mode or brightness mode is the most common form of diagnostic ultrasound in use today. A typical B-mode image is composed of a series of A-lines combined to form a two-dimensional image that can be depicted by a variety of display formats. B-mode is often referred to as *gray-scale ultrasound*, because the reflected echoes are displayed in shades of gray (dependent upon signal amplitude). Strong reflectors are displayed as white dots (on a black background), while progressively weaker echoes are in gradually darker shades of gray. Clear fluid that contains no reflective particles is displayed as black (echo-free). B-mode ultrasound can demonstrate motion by displaying multiple images over a very short period of time (faster than the eye can perceive). This is referred to as *real-time* ultrasound imaging.

Doppler ultrasound is used most commonly to evaluate bloodflow. It uses the Doppler principle to detect phase shifts which occur when the ultrasound signal encounters moving reflectors. The largest scatterers within moving blood are red blood cells and cell aggregates.

Continuous wave (CW) Doppler uses two separate transducers housed within a single probe case. One transducer continuously transmits the ultrasound signal, while the other transducer continuously receives the returning echoes. All reflectors moving within the sound path will be detected. CW data can be presented either audibly (via a loudspeaker), visually via a video monitor, or both audibly and visually. Although directional information may be available with a CW unit, there is no range resolution.

Therefore, if the beam encounters two overlying vessels, each signal will contribute to the data provided.

Pulsed wave (PW) Doppler, like B-mode imaging, uses the pulse-echo technique to assess bloodflow occurring at a particular distance from the transducer face. This is accomplished by *gating* the receiver time (remember; *time equals distance*). Therefore, PW Doppler, unlike CW Doppler, provides *range resolution* and can evaluate flow occurring within a specific vessel or vessel segment. As with CW Doppler, the flow information can be presented audibly, visually, or both.

Duplex Doppler ultrasound is the combination of B-mode imaging with Doppler ultrasound. Anatomic information regarding vessel location is provided by the B-mode image. In the case of a PW duplex ultrasound unit, a *sample volume* is positioned over the vessel location provided by the B-mode image. Duplex imaging provides anatomic information regarding a vessel and the surrounding tissues, while bloodflow data are acquired using the Doppler technique. This results in a powerful diagnostic tool for use in a wide variety of applications.

Color Doppler imaging provides a color display of Doppler flow information superimposed over all or part of a gray-scale image. This occurs in real time, which permits the qualitative assessment of flow over relatively large areas of the body. Most commercially available systems display the *mean Doppler frequency shift* in color detected for each pixel. A more recently available color flow mode utilizes the amplitude of the color Doppler signal to display bloodflow information. This has been termed 'color amplitude imaging' (CAI) or 'power Doppler'. For both CDI and CAI a variety of color maps are available and used, depending on the specific application and operator preference.

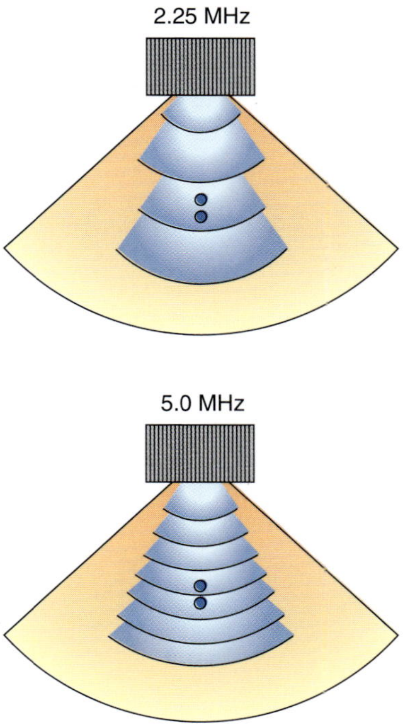

Figure 2.5 *Axial resolution along the direction of propagation with 2.25-MHz and 5.0-MHz transducers. Axial resolution is directly related to the frequency of the transducer and pulse length. In this example using the 2.25-MHz transducer, the two dots are not resolved as separate structures. Using shorter wavelengths from a 5-MHz transducer allows the two dots to be resolved as two reflectors.*

IMAGE RESOLUTION

In diagnostic ultrasound, the term resolution refers to the ability to separate echoes in space (spatial resolution), time (temporal resolution) and strength (contrast resolution). CDI has a fourth resolution component called *velocity resolution*, or the ability to discern variations in flow velocities occurring across a vessel lumen.

Spatial resolution is the ability to detect closely spaced objects, and can be further divided into axial and lateral resolution. In terms of ultrasound spatial resolution, smaller numbers imply greater resolution capabilities. *Axial resolution* refers to the resolution capabilities along the path (axis) of the ultrasound beam. Axial resolution is determined by the spatial pulse length of the ultrasound beam (Fig. 2.5). The *spatial pulse length* is equal to the wavelength multiplied by the number of cycles in a pulse. To improve axial resolution requires either a reduction in the number of cycles generated per pulse (which is done using transducer damping techniques) or increasing the transmitted frequency (wavelength decreases as frequency increases). However, remember that tradeoffs exist. Higher frequencies improve resolution but reduce penetration, whereas lower frequencies improve penetration but compromise resolution.

Lateral resolution refers to the ability to separate echoes that are positioned perpendicular to the ultrasound beam. Lateral resolution is equal to the *beam*

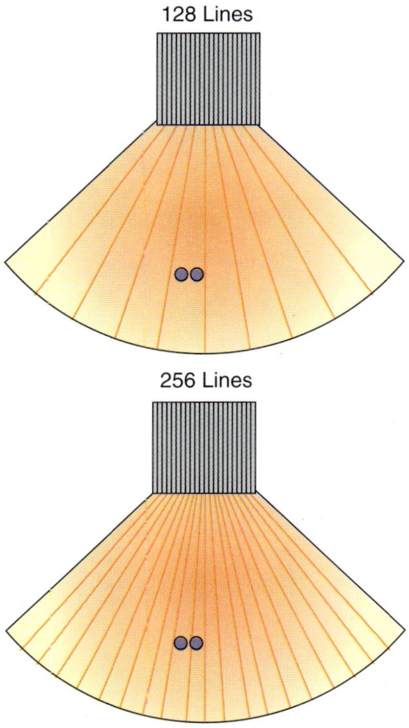

Figure 2.6 *Lateral resolution is directly related to the vector density (line density) at any given point in the image and focusing characteristics of the transducer employed. In this diagram, using a transducer with 128 lines does not resolve the two reflectors (black dots) separately. However, when a transducer with 256 lines is used, the two reflectors appear as two individual structures on an image.*

width, which is influenced by the aperture of the transducer crystal(s) and focusing properties of the unit (Fig. 2.6). A transducer with a larger effective aperture will have a greater ability to focus the beam and will, therefore, have better lateral resolution capabilities. As will be discussed later in the chapter, the beam profile changes across varying depths. Therefore, the lateral resolution capabilities of a given transducer will vary depending on the distance from the transducer surface. Some transducers have dynamic focusing abilities which allow the beam to be focused at the desired level of interest to improve lateral resolution in a selected portion of the image.

Temporal resolution is the ability to distinguish closely spaced events in time, and forms the basis of real-time ultrasound imaging. Real-time imaging allows us to evaluate moving anatomic structures and assess them over a period of time; this provides information on the dynamics of motion. Temporal resolution is determined by the imaging *frame rate*, which is the number of images displayed per second. Real-time imaging of the heart (echocardiography), for example, displays cardiac wall and valve motion in *realtime*, i.e as they actually occur in time. This is accomplished by the very rapid sequential display of single frames of data. As the transducer is moved to a different area of interest, the image is constantly refreshed to display new information about the tissues being insonated. High frame rates provide increased temporal resolution, whereas low frame rates reduce temporal resolution and may result in a mismatch of temporal data.

Factors that effect imaging frame rates are the overall depth of view, the number of scan lines being used to generate one image, and the number of focal zones used. Greater depths require a longer time between the transmission of the pulse and the receipt of the returning echo and, therefore, reduce the frame rate and temporal resolution. Generation of each scan line requires time, so that the more scan lines that are being used to create one image, the longer the time required to produce the image (and the lower the level of temporal resolution). When more focal zones are utilized, more pulses are required. Each pulse requires time to be generated, which reduces frame rates. In essence, the more a system is performing (imaging greater depths, putting more of the image in focus, improving spatial resolution, etc.), the lower the frame rate and temporal resolution.

Typical frame rates for gray-scale imaging range from about nine frames per second while imaging deep structures with multiple focal zones, to more than 30 frames/s for imaging superficial structures. For catheter-based endoluminal ultrasound devices to have sufficient frame rates, the probe or transducer elements must rotate at an adequate rate—usually about 30 rotations or frames per second. This high level of rotation is made possible by the short imaging depths typically evaluated with these devices.

Contrast resolution is directly related to the quality of the system's electronics, the transducers, and the available shades of gray that the ultrasound system uses to define tissue echogenicity. Improved contrast resolution enhances the ability to detect changes within tissue which may result from pathology or other causes.

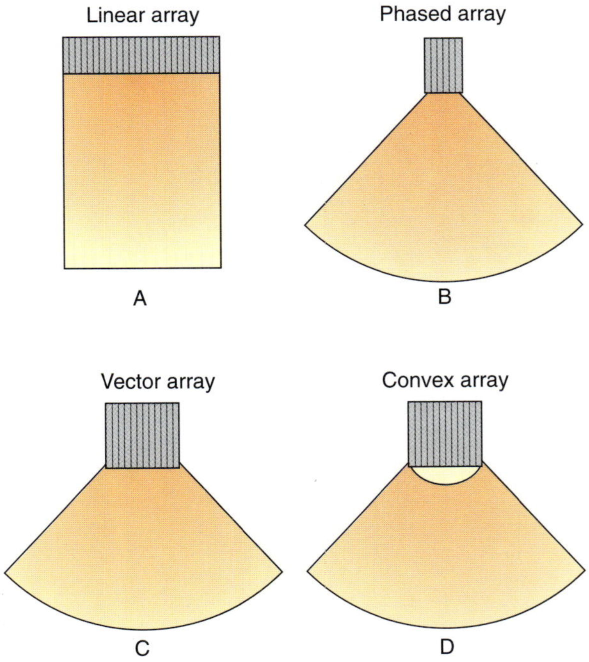

Figure 2.7 *Four common configurations of ultrasound transducers and their display formats: A, linear array; B, phased array; C, vector array; D, convex linear array.*

TRANSDUCERS

Ultrasound transducers operate on the *piezoelectric principle.* This principle states that materials such as ceramic or quartz can produce an electrical voltage when deformed by an applied pressure. This alternating pressure creates a sound wave, i.e. a *pulse.* The rate at which the voltage is applied determines the pulse repetition frequency (in hertz) of these pulses. The frequency of the ultrasound signal depends on the thickness of the piezoelectric crystal within the transducer assembly and other factors. This may be arbitrarily referred to as *transmit, fundamental,* or *output* frequency.

Many different types of transducer configurations are used to produce real-time ultrasound images (Fig. 2.7). Ultrasound probes can be divided into two types, mechanical transducers and electronic phased-array transducers. Mechanical probes generate beams projecting in different directions by moving the transducer element (or elements). This can be accomplished by moving a single element, rotating a transducer or by oscillating the element back and forth across a specified arc. A third method involves a stationary element and a moving, reflective mirror; this effectively accomplishes the same goal. The result is a pie-shaped or *sector image* which has a broad far field but a narrow near field. The major drawback with mechanically activated transducers is equipment reliability because of the many moving parts.

Electronic phased-array transducers come in several configurations. The *phased linear array* uses an electronically fired array of individual transducer elements arranged along a flat surface face to produce an image that is rectangular in shape. Another type of phased array consists of multiple elements within a single small-faced probe. Activating adjacent transducer elements with slight time delays with respect to each other effectively steers the beam across an arc; the result of this is a pie-shaped sector display of information.

A more recent development utilizes the same linear format found in a linear transducer but in this case the face of the probe is convexed slightly, which effectively diverges the beams and results in a *curved linear* display with a broad near field and even wider far field. In all cases, the transducer elements are activated (usually several at one time) in rapid sequence to provide a continuously updated (i.e. real-time) image. Phased-array transducers, while often more costly than mechanical probes, have no moving parts and are therefore less likely to have mechanical failures. Another advantage of these probes is that because the elements are electronically activated they typically provide faster frame rates and, therefore, better temporal resolution.

The benefits of the sector probe configuration (mechanical or phased) are that it has a relatively small surface which needs to be in contact with the body tissues (the *transducer face* or 'footprint'), and it provides an image with a broad field of view. The disadvantage of the sector display is a lack of image uniformity, as the diverging beams become farther and farther apart as they leave the transducer. In general, the lateral resolution capability of these probes is progressively worse the farther a structure is from the probe face. Electronic focusing of the phased array minimizes these adverse effects.

The benefits of linear transducers are improved spatial resolution, because there are no diverging beams, and a broad field of view. Their limitation is the size of the transducer face, which may limit access to certain anatomic areas. The trend in the industry and in general practice is towards the curved linear-array transducer. These probes provide good

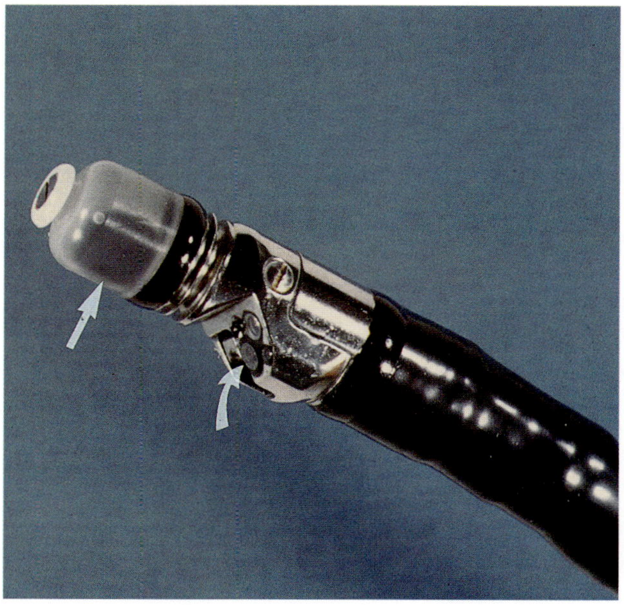

a

Figure 2.8 *(a) The working tip of an Olympus endoscope with 7.5- and 12.5-MHz mechanical ultrasound transducer (arrow) located distal to the viewing optics (curved arrow). (b) A dedicated Olympus endoscopic ultrasound imaging system. This unit is equipped with videotape recording and digital still image storage devices.*

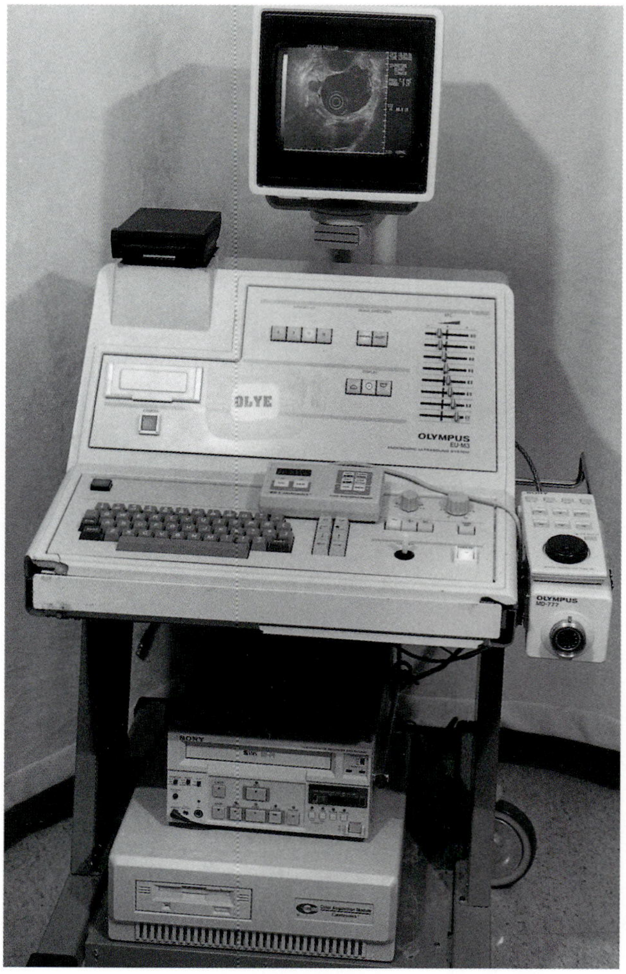

b

spatial resolution and image uniformity, have a curved surface which can be adequately applied to the body surface in most applications, and are durable enough to withstand several years of service.

DEDICATED ENDOSCOPIC ULTRASOUND INSTRUMENTATION

The most commonly used gastrointestinal (GI) endoscopic ultrasound devices are the Olympus upper GI endoscopic ultrasound probes and systems (Olympus America Inc., Melville, NY). These echoendoscopes are side-viewing instruments with a rigid tip containing the ultrasound transducer. The transducer is located in the distal part of the scope and the optics are side-viewing (Fig. 2.8). The visual optics system is conventional fiberoptics, and the tip deflection controls function as they do on conventional upper GI endoscopes. The circumferential ultrasonic section is perpendicular to the shaft axis of the instrument and allows 360° radial imaging.

The newest-generation models are lighter and easier to handle than the previous models. Side-viewing optics necessitate a blind introduction into the esophagus and, because of the rigid tip, the instrument is more difficult to pass through the pyloric channel than is a conventional duodenoscope. The instruments have a working channel which permits water to be instilled into the stomach. In addition, a balloon surrounds the ultrasound transducer which is filled with de-aerated water to provide the necessary acoustic coupling. The newer models

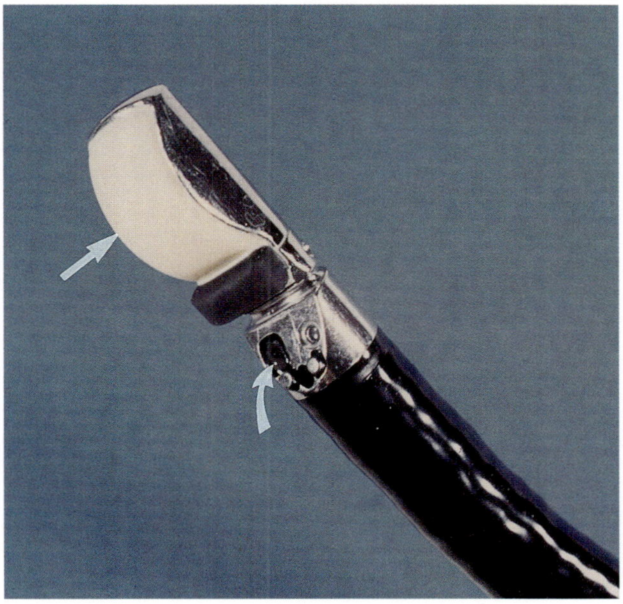

a

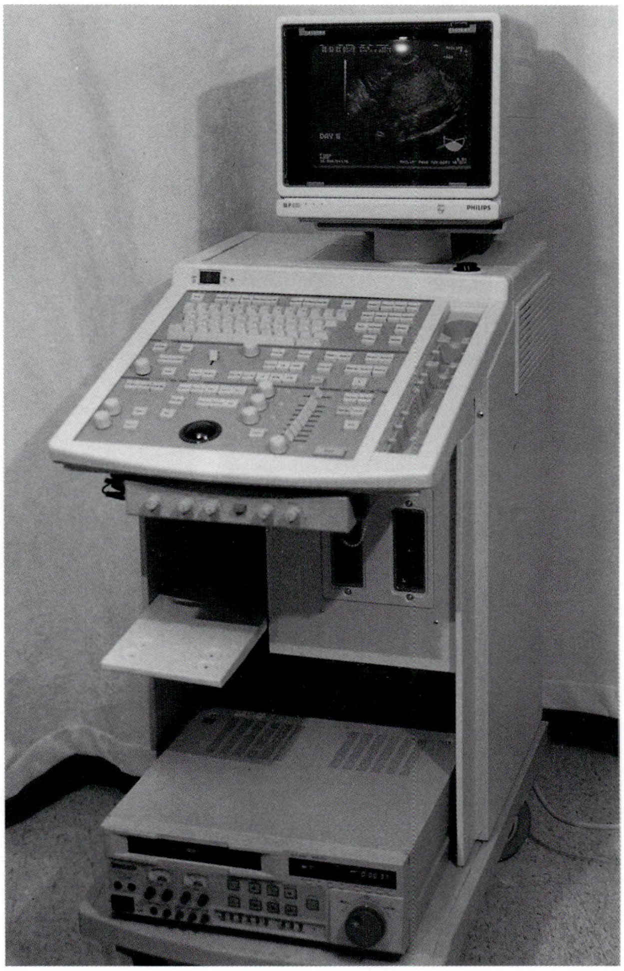

b

Figure 2.9 *(a) The working tip of a Pentax endoscope with curvilinear-array ultrasound transducer (arrow) located distal to the viewing optics (curved arrow). The convex linear-array transducer facilitates duplex and color Doppler capabilities. (b) The Pentax endoscopic ultrasound probe is utilized with the Philips P600 ultrasound unit (Philips Medical Systems, Santa Ana, CA).*

all have biopsy channels, although needle biopsy under ultrasound guidance is not possible. In addition, the frequency may be changed from 7.5 to 12 MHz. At 7.5 MHz, the focal distance is 30 mm, whereas at 12 MHz, the focal distance is 25 mm.

Other commercially available GI endoscopes permit simultaneous performance of sonography and endoscopic retrograde cholangiopancreatography (ERCP). However, because of the limited maneuverability due to the rigid tip, the performance of ERCP is hindered.

The Olympus Corporation has also designed echoendoscopes for use in the lower GI tract. These scopes function much as the upper GI endoscopes; however, the echo-colonoscope is a forward-viewing instrument with a biopsy channel. Because the optical components and accessory channels are placed next to the transducer, the sector scan is reduced from 360° to 320°. The echo-colonoscope is somewhat longer than the upper GI endoscopes and the shaft diameter is somewhat greater, as is the tip diameter.

Pentax manufactures a sector-scanning echoendoscope with a curvilinear-array transducer (Pentax Precision Instruments Corp., Orangeburg, NY). The transducer is oriented along the long axis of the scope. With this orientation, an aspiration needle can be inserted through the biopsy channel and the entire needle can be visualized with real-time ultrasound, allowing ultrasound-guided fine needle aspiration (Fig. 2.9). The scanning angle is 100°. The frequency of the Pentax transducer can be changed between 5 MHz and 7.5 MHz, with penetration capability up to 10 cm. In addition to the advantage of having the biopsy channel in the plane of the ultrasound image,

Table 2.2 Characteristics of some gastrointestinal echoendoscopes

	Pentax probe	*Olympus probe*
Type of transducer	Curved array	Mechanical
Frequency	5 and 7.5 MHz	7.5 and 12.5 MHz
Scanning plane	Long axis of endoscope	Perpendicular to endoscope
Scanning angle	100°	360°
Penetration	5–10 cm	Up to 12 cm
Ultrasound-guided biopsy	Yes	No
Duplex imaging	Yes	No
Color Doppler	Yes	No
Angle of view	105°	80°
Direction of view	60° forward	65° side–forward

this system also has CDI and duplex Doppler capabilities. The technical data and specific characteristics of the Olympus and the Pentax echoendoscopes for use in the GI are given in Table 2.2.

ENDOLUMINAL ULTRASOUND INSTRUMENTATION

The typical endoluminal ultrasound unit is a sophisticated system capable of performing ultra-high-frequency imaging. It provides a 360°, cross-sectional view of a vessel or luminal structure. These unique images are created by the combination of two very important components: (1) the catheter delivery/imaging transducer assembly, and (2) the ultra-high-frequency ultrasound imaging system.

CATHETER-BASED TRANSDUCERS

Endoluminal ultrasound images are generated using 9 MHz to 30 MHz miniature transducers incorporated into the tip of a 3 to 9-Fr interventional catheter. The relatively high-frequency ultrasound has limited tissue penetration, but it is adequate to produce high-resolution images when used in close proximity to the target tissue.

There are two basic transducer technologies used to produce endoluminal ultrasound images. One technique employs a mechanical transducer to generate the ultrasound image. Mechanical image production is accomplished by rotating either the transducer itself or an acoustic mirror (reflector). For the transducer-rotating system, a single-element transducer is fixed on the end of a drive shaft (Fig. 2.10). The transducer transmits and receives the ultrasound signal at an angle 10° from perpendicular to the axis of the catheter, which produces a cone-shaped

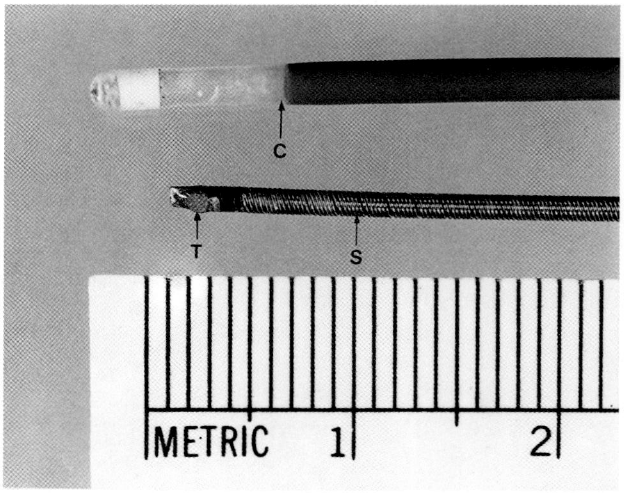

Figure 2.10 *Components of a typical catheter-based endoluminal ultrasound transducer assembly. The single-element transducer (T) is attached to the end of a drive shaft (S). The drive shaft is inserted into the flexible sterile catheter (C). The drive shaft rotates 360° within the catheter.*

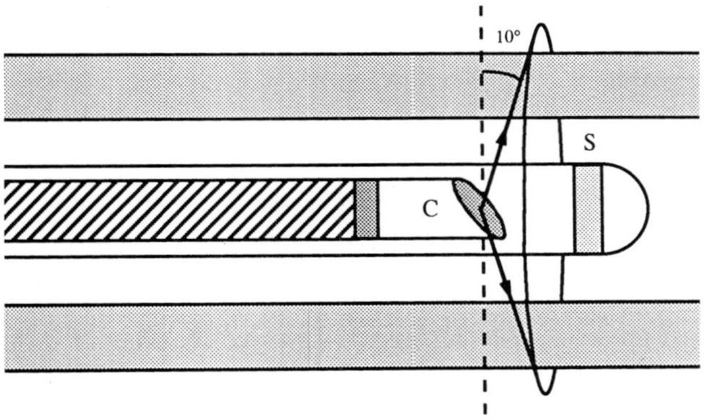

Figure 2.11 *Diagrammatic representation of a transducer-rotating ultrasound catheter transmitting and receiving the acoustic signal at an angle 10° from perpendicular to the long axis of the catheter, producing a cone-shaped imaging plane. C, transducer crystal; S, septum.*

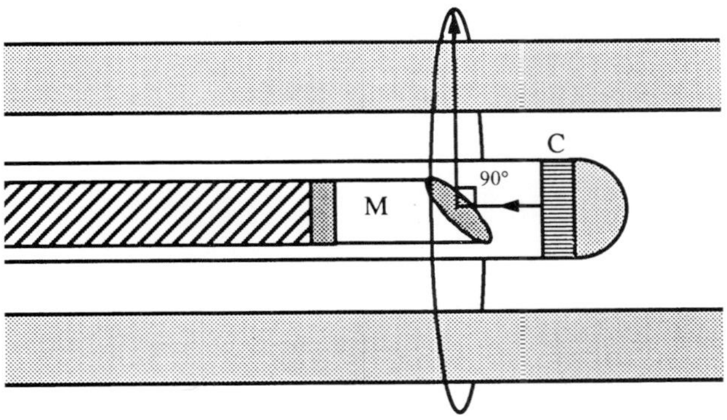

Figure 2.12 *Diagrammatic representation of a mirror-rotating ultrasound catheter probe. The stationary transducer crystal (C) transmits the sound directly towards a rotating mirror (M) which is fixed at a 45° angle. The ultrasound beam is then reflected by the mirror at a 90° angle to the long axis of the catheter, producing a true cross-sectional imaging plane.*

ultrasound beam resulting in an image of the vessel slightly forward or in front of the transducer assembly (Fig. 2.11). For the acoustic mirror reflecting system the transducer is fixed and the rotating mirror is positioned at a 45° angle to the shaft, thereby producing an image that is perpendicular to the axis of the catheter (Fig. 2.12).

The drive shaft is pre-assembled inside a sterile catheter. The catheters need be to filled with fluid (usually sterile water), which displaces the air between the rotating element and inner catheter wall, thereby acting as an acoustic coupling agent (Fig. 2.13). The preparation of the ultrasound catheter is performed as follows:

1. Fill a 1-ml syringe with sterile water (do not use saline).
2. After purging any air bubbles, carefully insert a 27 gauge needle into the catheter's chamber at the distal end of the round-tip or side-saddle catheter (Figs 2.14 and 2.15). Insert the needle so that its tip is visible on the other side of the membrane. Care should be taken not to inadvertently touch the transducer element or perforate the catheter wall with the needle. For the side-saddle catheter, this can be accomplished by gently bending the distal tip downwards, while inserting the needle (Fig. 2.15).
3. Inject water into the catheter until the tip is filled with fluid (approximately 0.5–1.0 ml) and remove needle. A continuous bubble-free column of water should be visible.
4. Using a finger, vigorously tap the distal tip of the catheter while pointing the catheter tip

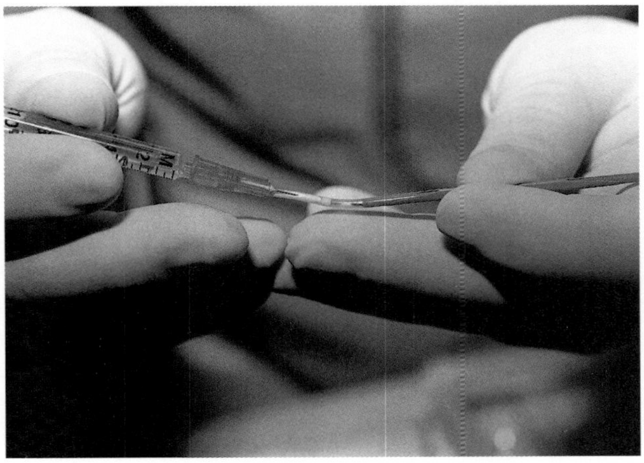

Figure 2.13 *Preparation of the miniature catheter transducer. Using a 27 gauge needle, 0.5–1.0 ml of sterile water is injected into the catheter through the membrane tip of the catheter. This effectively eliminates air trapped between the rotating transducer and inner catheter wall.*

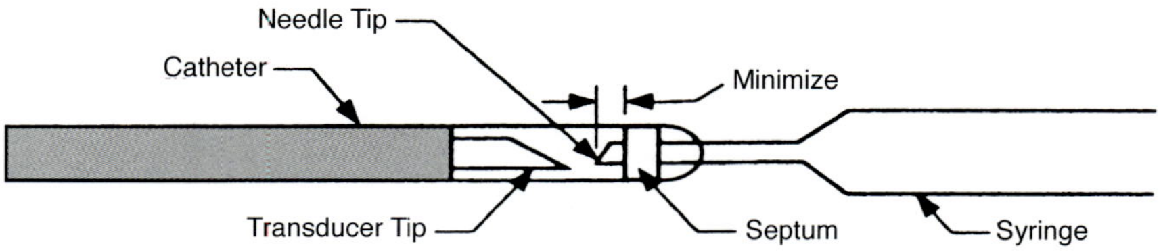

Figure 2.14 *Diagrammatic representation of the preparation technique used for a blunt-tip ultrasound catheter–transducer. Care must be exercised not to damage the transducer element with the needle tip.*

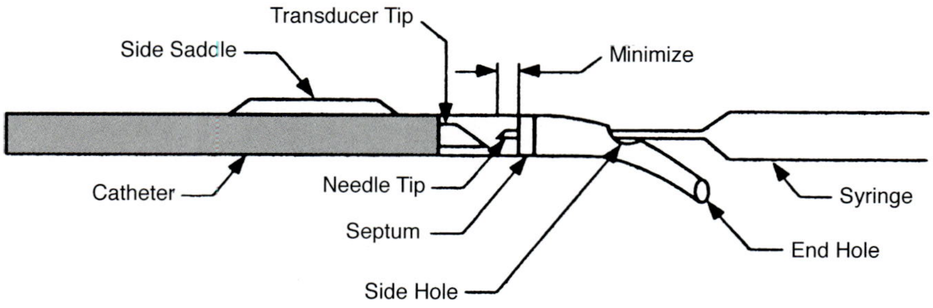

Figure 2.15 *Diagrammatic representation of the preparation technique used for a side-saddle ultrasound catheter–transducer for use with a guidewire.*

downwards. If bubbles are still present, swirl the distal 20–30 cm of the catheter in a wide circle several times quickly to create a centrifugal force that will help to remove residual air bubbles trapped near the tip of the catheter.

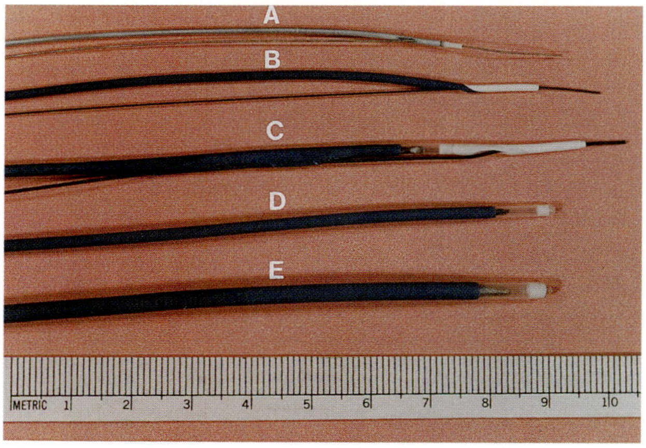

Figure 2.16 *A variety of catheter-based ultrasound transducers made by Boston Scientific Corporation: (A) 3.5 Fr over a 0.018-inch guidewire; (B) 4.8 Fr over a 0.014-inch guidewire; (C) 6.2 Fr side-saddle tip with a 0.025-inch guidewire; (D) 9 Fr blunt tip; (E) 6 Fr blunt tip. The frequencies of the transducers range from 9 to 30 MHz.*

Once connected to the ultrasound unit, the transducer is rotated inside the catheter sheath by means of a flexible shaft driven by a motor. The drive shaft doubles as an electrical cable connecting the transducer to the electronics of the ultrasound system. The catheter sheath can be configured to various specifications, depending on its intended use. For example, it may have an externally placed monorail guidewire lumen for placement into vascular structures. A typical example of this catheter–transducer system is made by Boston Scientific Corporation (Natick, MA) (Fig. 2.16). These catheter–transducers can be used with the Diasonics IVUS (Santa Clara, CA) (Fig. 2.17), the Hewlett-Packard SONOS (Andover, MA) (Fig. 2.18), the Brüel&Kjaer 3535 (Marlborough, MA) (Fig. 2.19) and the Boston Scientific ClearView (Sunnyvale, CA) (Fig. 2.20) ultrasound systems.

The second type of endoluminal ultrasound transducer is based on electronic phased-array technology. Electronic scanning is performed using an array of multiple transducer elements. The extremely small size of the electronic components prevented for a long time the incorporation of this technology into catheter-based transducers. With the recent development of a miniaturized transmit–receive electronic chip, the solid-state electronic endoluminal imaging transducer is now available. The transducer elements are placed circumferentially around the device near

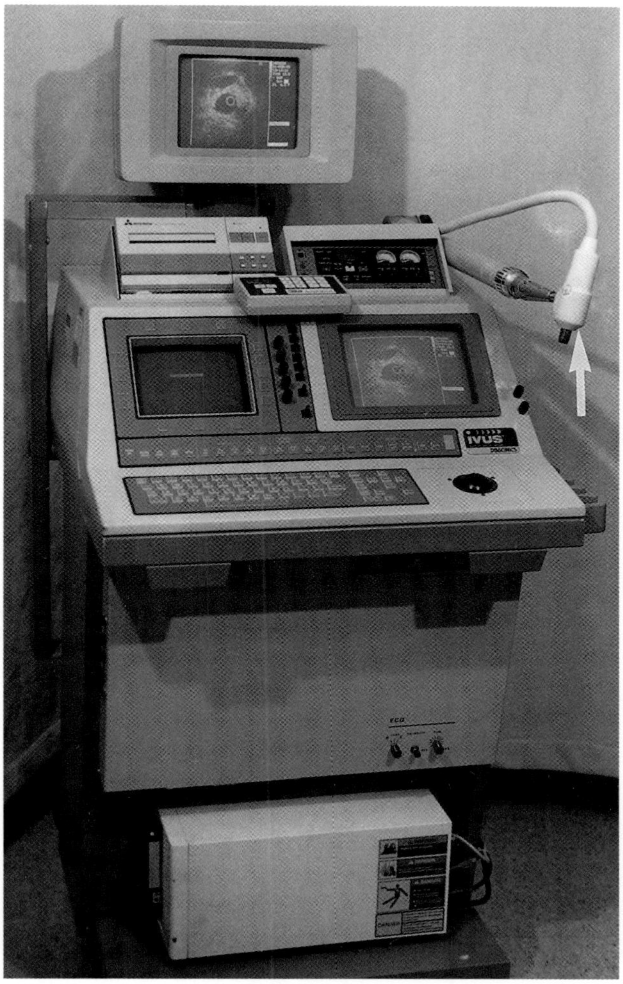

Figure 2.17 *A Diasonics IVUS ultrasound system. The extendable arm allows the motor drive (arrow) to be positioned closer to the access site and the unit to remain at a comfortable distance to permit easy operation during the examination. Two monitors (one stationary and one rotational) facilitate viewing of the image from a variety of locations by various examiners during the procedure.*

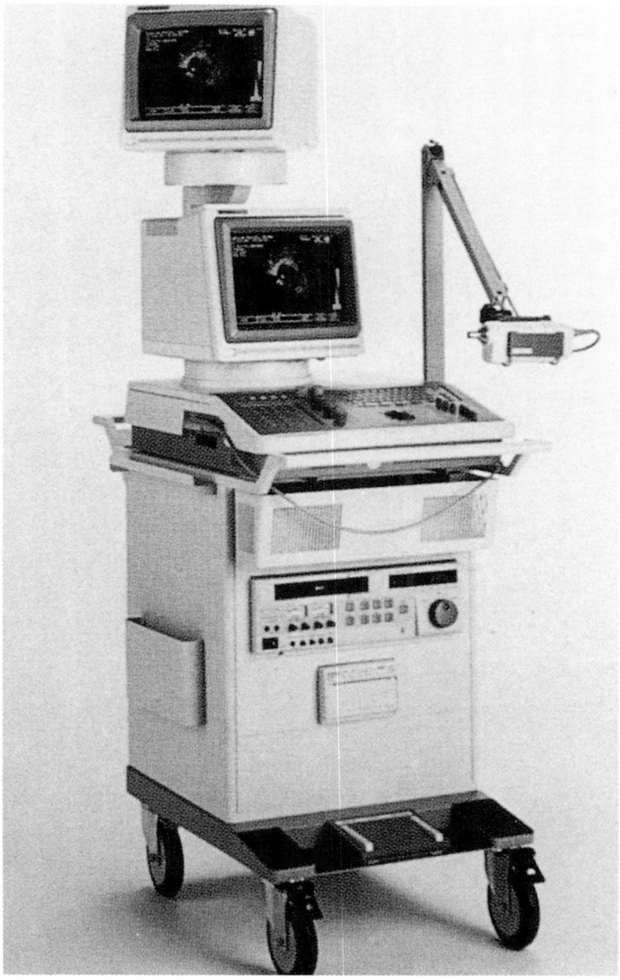

Figure 2.18 *A Hewlett-Packard SONOS 100 ultrasound machine with similar conveniences as the Diasonics system (seen in Fig. 2.17), including two monitors and a mechanical arm to which the catheter–transducer is attached. Recording devices are located under the system keyboard.*

its tip. Endosonics Corporation (Rancho Cordova, CA) produces an electronic phased-array system of this design (Figs 2.21 and 2.22).

Through a unique design and packaging technique, the components responsible for the transmission, reception and steering of the ultrasound signal are contained within the catheter tip. A four-sided 'flip-chip' carrier is used, with 64 tiny transducer elements and all associated transmit and receive circuitry within the microprobe. All interface circuitry for the 64 transducer channels is contained within the four sides, each of which handles 16 channels. The entire body of the probe assembly supports the array of transducer elements and integrated circuitry and also accommodates conventional devices such as a therapeutic balloon (Fig. 2.23). Because there are no moving parts necessary to generate 360° real-time images, a central guidewire

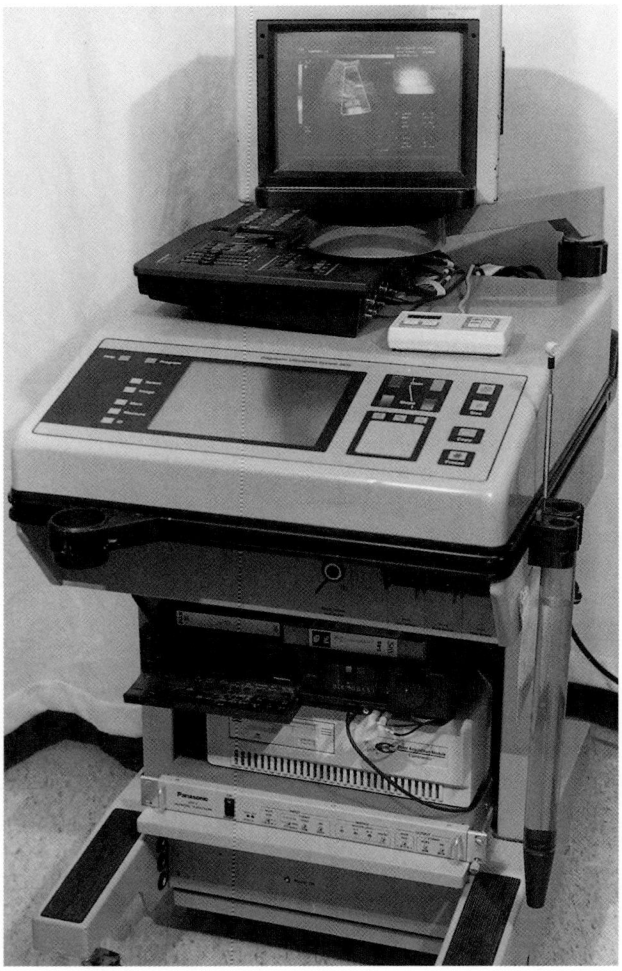

Figure 2.19 *A Brüel&Kjaer 3535 ultrasound system. This system is capable of performing endoluminal and conventional ultrasound examinations as well as laparoscopic and other intraoperative ultrasound imaging.*

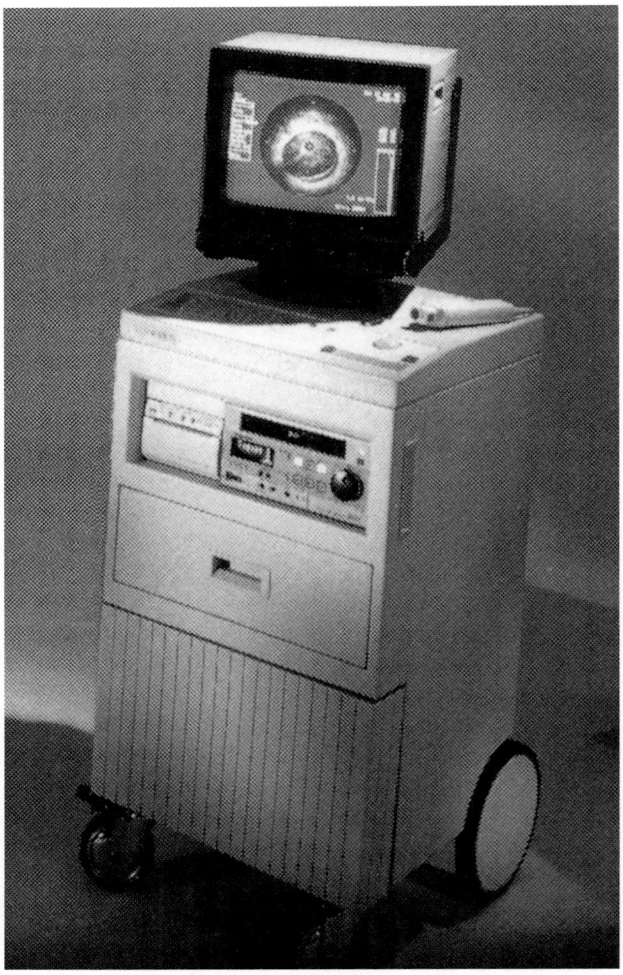

Figure 2.20 *A CVIS intravascular ultrasound system. The small size of this unit facilitates use in confined spaces such as some angiographic suites.*

is possible which can be used for special applications, such as navigation through small, tortuous vessels (Fig. 2.24).

The transducer elements are selected and controlled by an electronic signal-processing unit, which transmits voltage pulses via a transmission cable to the integrated circuitry on board the body of the probe assembly. The integrated circuitry routes the signal to the transducer elements in a predetermined sequence. The multiple-element array and digital signal-processing capabilities provide not only gray-scale imaging but also a color flow display utilizing the time-domain technique (Fig. 2.25).

All communications within the probe occur over a multiple-conductor micro-coaxial cable that is contained within a standard catheter lumen. Advanced microelectronics results in a high degree of flexibility and a relatively small-diameter catheter which facilitates intravascular ultrasonic imaging.

To accommodate a variety of applications, most of the imaging catheters are available in different sizes. The sizes can range from 2.9 Fr for intracoronary

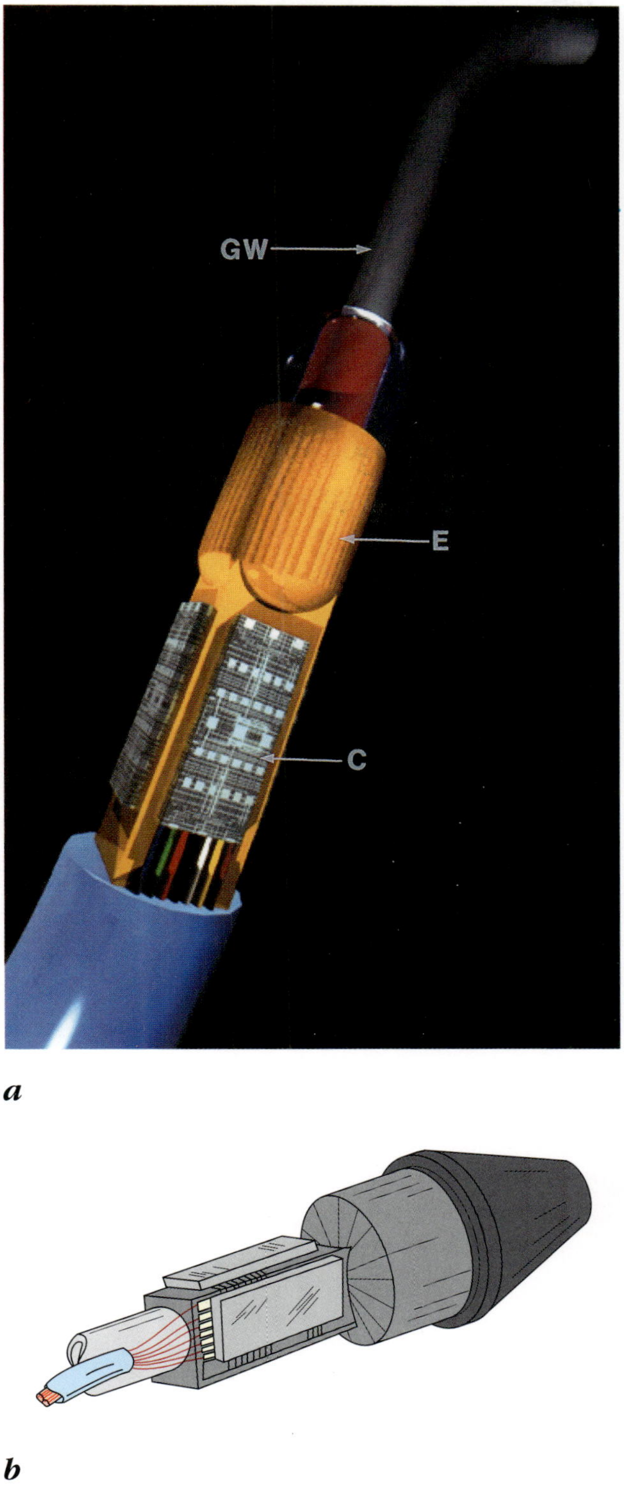

Figure 2.21 *(a) An illustration of an electronic phased-array catheter-based transducer with 64 elements (E) and four computer chips (C). A central guidewire (GW) can be used in this non-rotating transducer, assembly. (b) Diagram of the assembly of this transducer detailing its components and dimensions.*

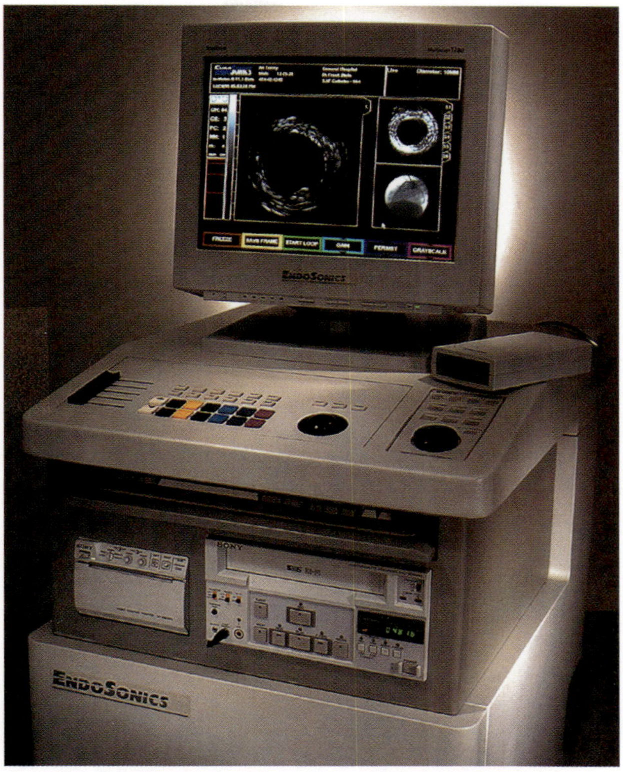

Figure 2.22 *The Endosonics intravascular ultrasound system used with the phased-array catheter-based transducer shown in Fig. 2.21.*

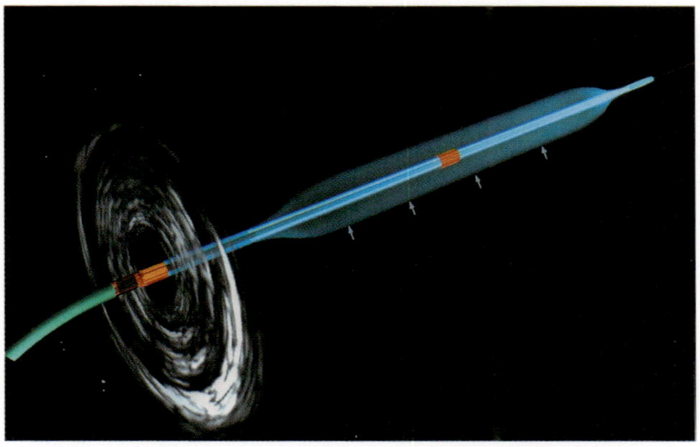

Figure 2.23 *Catheter-based transducers can be combined with a variety of therapeutic devices. In this example, a therapeutic dilation balloon (arrows) is positioned beyond the imaging transducer. This device facilitates time-efficient simultaneous diagnostic examinations and therapeutic procedures.*

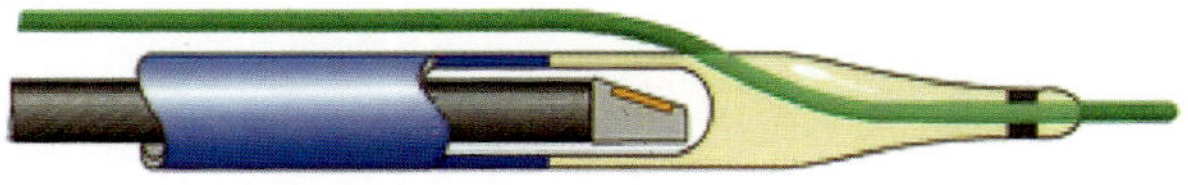

a

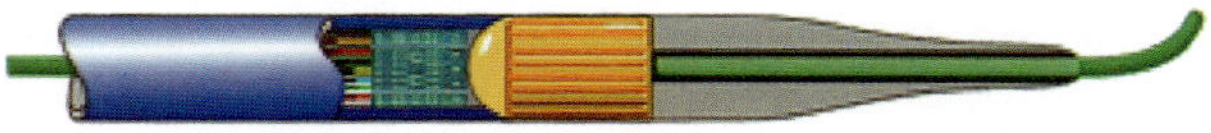

b

Figure 2.24 *Comparison of the monorail and central guidewire devices. (a) A monorail guidewire is used with a mechanical rotating catheter–transducer assembly. (b) The central guidewire is used with the electronic phased-array transducer system.*

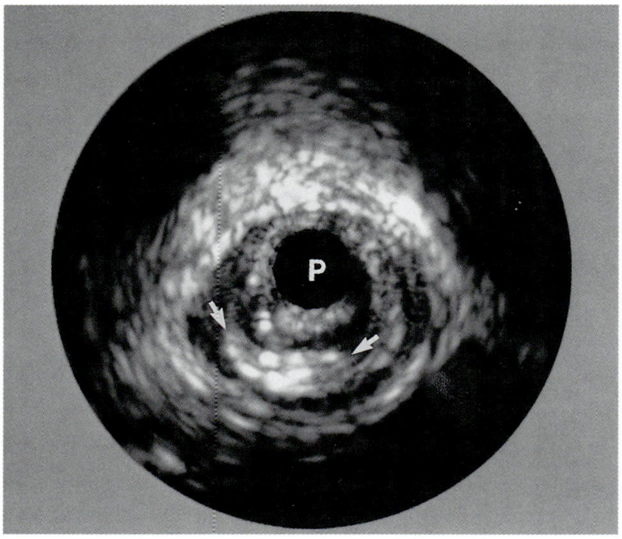

a

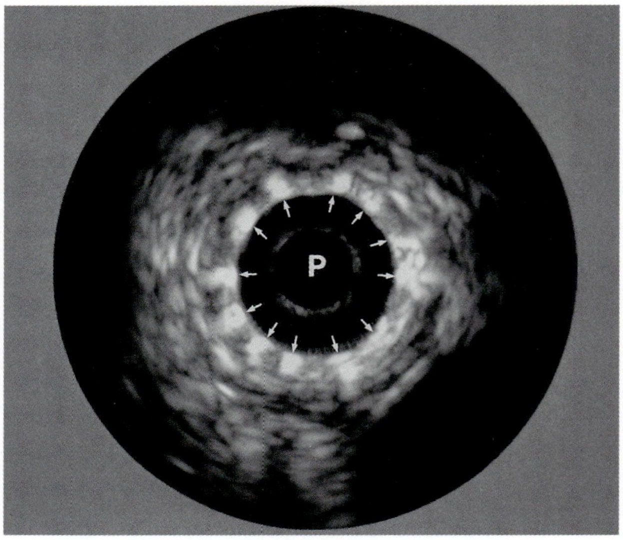

b

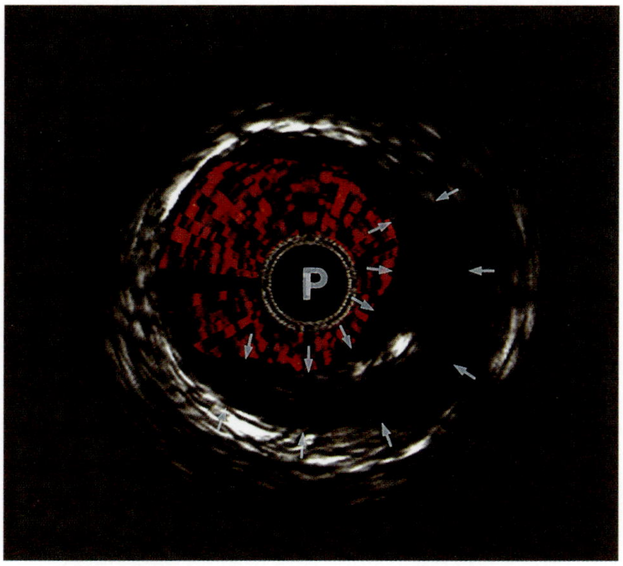

c

Figure 2.25 *Examples of intracoronary gray-scale images produced by the electronic phased-array probe assembly (P). (a) Eccentric coronary atheroma (arrows) and (b) an intracoronary stent (arrows). The stent material appears as brightly reflective echoes. (c) Color flow imaging with the phased-array catheter–probe (P) demonstrates the functional lumen (in red) and eccentric vessel wall thickening (arrows).*

applications to 9 Fr for use in nonvascular lumina, such as in the genitourinary and gastrointestinal tracts. There are a variety of catheter-tip designs which vary from manufacturer to manufacturer. For intracoronary and other vascular applications where a guidewire is required, the catheter can be configured as an over-the-wire design with a floppy tip for a monorail or rapid exchange. In some nonvascular applications or in certain applications where a guidewire is not necessary, a simple round-tip catheter is available without a guidewire port. Ultrasound catheter performance has been evaluated and rated according to three basic criteria:

1 Trackability—the ability of the imaging catheter to *follow* a guidewire to the desired location.
2 Pushability—the ability of the imaging catheter to transmit *push force* to advance the catheter through the lumen without 'buckling'.
3 Torque control—the ability to rotate one end of the imaging catheter and have the opposite end rotate equally.

ENDOLUMINAL UTRASOUND SYSTEM

A full understanding and proper use of the controls of an ultrasound system are crucial for obtaining optimal diagnostic images. Incorrect parameter adjustments will result in suboptimal image quality, which may result in inadequate or incorrect sonographic diagnoses.

It is beneficial for the user to thoroughly study the operator's manual, which is usually provided with each ultrasound system. Since every ultrasound system manufacturer has its own individual design and uses unique nomenclature for the various controls, referring to these manuals will assure a complete understanding of the functionality of each button, dial, slide-pod or similar device on the unit in question. The ideal way to become comfortable and proficient with a specific unit is to gain experience by using it.

The typical endoluminal ultrasound system utilizes an advanced high-speed mainframe computer that performs the signal processing responsible for ultra-high-frequency imaging. The ultrasound system typically consists of a mobile unit with imaging monitors and user-adjustable keyboard(s) controls. The cabinet houses the microcomputer and associated electronic components. In addition, most ultrasound platforms feature some type or types of recording devices to allow documentation of the examination results. These include videotape recorders, thermal paper printers, conventional hard-copy cameras or writeable software disks. The dynamics of a real-time examination are best documented by videotape. Still image documentation is limited to the image captured in a moment of time by the operator.

ENDOLUMINAL ULTRASOUND SYSTEM CONTROLS

Listed below are common user-adjustable parameters that are on most currently available ultrasound units. The most common name for the control is given, with other names listed in parentheses. Remember that diagnostic ultrasound uses the pulse-echo principle. Parameter adjustments can be made which affect the signal before it leaves the transducer (the pulse), after it returns to the transducer (the echo) or both. How these two sides of the pulse-echo equation are configured directly influences the display of data and, therefore, the amount of diagnostic information contained therein.

Output power (acoustic output)

This refers to the amount of acoustic power transmitted from the transducer into body tissues. The acoustic power should be increased only as a last resort to optimize image quality. The phrase 'as low as reasonably allowable' (ALARA) pertains to the prudent use of acoustic power levels during diagnostic ultrasound examinations.

Gain (master gain or overall gain)

This is a single control which increases or decreases the received echo signal strength over the entire image.

Time–gain compensation (TGC) (depth–gain compensation, DGC)

This control provides an increase in received signal strength from a given depth within the image. Typically, several 'slide-pods' or similar controls are used corresponding to a given depth on the image. The TGC should be adjusted to compensate for signal attenuation over depth, so as to make like tissues appear alike. Its purpose is to provide a balanced image in which the amplitudes of the echoes are

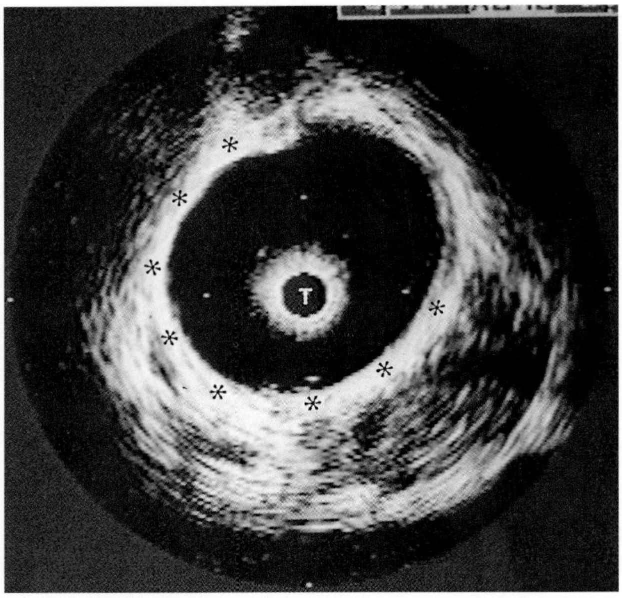

Figure 2.26 *Endoluminal ultrasound image of a bile duct with the near-field time–gain compensation set inappropriately high. The sonographic information in the near field (*) is limited by the 'white-out' as a result of the excessive gain. T, transducer.*

uniform throughout the depth of the image. Since ultrasonic energy is attenuated as it passes through tissue, more returned signal amplification (i.e. gain) must be applied to those echoes that are generated from more deeply located tissues. When the transmitted sound is not attenuated, e.g. through fluid paths, the TGC of the far field may need to be suppressed (Fig. 2.26).

Freeze-frame

The freeze-frame control can be used discretionarily. When it is activated, the real-time image display stops, or 'freezes', the image. When it is reactivated, real-time imaging is resumed. Storing an image on a hard-copy device while in freeze-frame may at times improve the quality of the document.

Field of view (FOV) (image depth)

Increased FOV is equal to increased depth visualized on the monitor and may at times result in slower frame rates. Therefore, using the shortest depth that allows complete visualization of the area of interest will maintain the highest frame rates allowable.

Dynamic range

This refers to the way in which the gray-scale information is compressed into a usable range for display. An increase in the dynamic range will yield an increase in the amount of gray shades, while decreasing the dynamic range will reduce the number of shades of gray to produce a more 'black-and-white' image.

Measurements

Specific calculation capabilities are available for use with all ultrasound imaging systems. The mode of operation for the measurement function is similar for most of the calculations. Some units allow calculations to be performed in either real-time or freeze-frame modes, while others only allow measurements to be performed on still (i.e. 'frozen') images. It is strongly recommended that measurements be done in freeze-frame mode for the most accurate caliper placement. The most frequent measurements used in endoluminal imaging are measurements of distance, area and circumference.

The ultrasound system operator should be knowledgeable on the functions available on a given system and, when necessary, be able to communicate with the physician performing the procedure. Information on image orientation, spatial relationships, dimensions, measurements and changes in parameters needs to be constantly passed between them so as to maximize the information obtained during the ultrasound examination. Although complications from the use of endoluminal vascular and nonvascular ultrasound have been very rare, care should always be taken when passing the ultrasound catheter through the various body lumina.

ARTIFACTS OF ENDOLUMINAL ULTRASOUND

Imaging artifacts can be a help or a hindrance in the interpretation of diagnostic findings. When an ultrasound signal does not pass through a structure, an

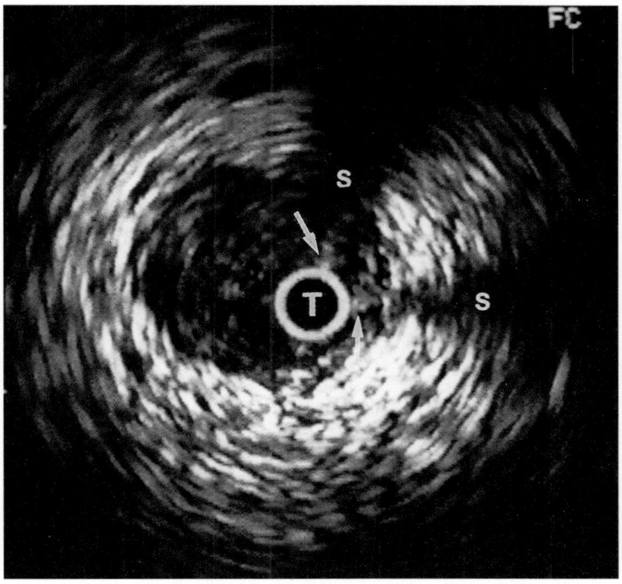

Figure 2.27 *An image obtained using the side-saddle guidewire transducer (T) during evaluation of the ureter. In this example, two guidewires are present (arrows). The location of the guidewires (obtained via fluoroscopy) can assist proper imaging orientation within the urinary tract. The guidewires also cause acoustic shadowing artifacts (S).*

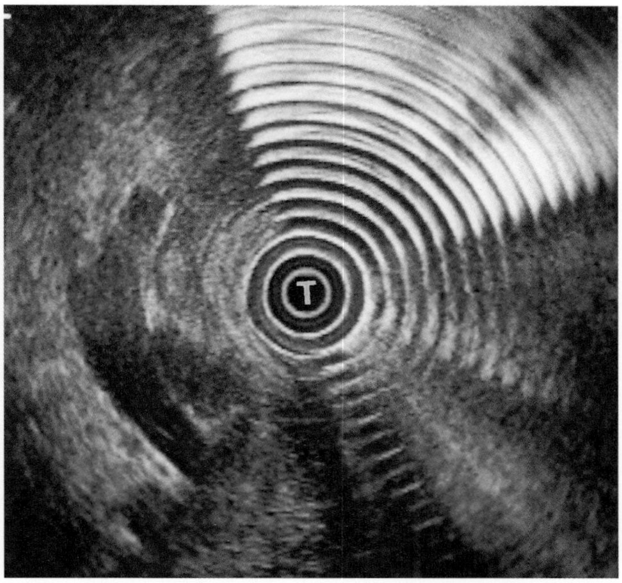

Figure 2.28 *An example of a reverberation artifact (seen between 11 o'clock and 5 o'clock) resulting from the water-filled transducer balloon and air trapped within the balloon on this endoscopic ultrasound image. T, transducer.*

acoustic shadow is produced. In some cases, these shadows may be helpful, e.g. in distinguishing between gallstones and other objects. On the other hand, shadows can also impose limitations when imaging structures (Fig. 2.27). When an ultrasound beam encounters a medium that is less attenuating, more sound energy reaches the opposite side of the medium, while at the same time the system TGC often amplifies the echo signal. This is called acoustic enhancement and is seen, for example, when imaging fluid-filled structures such as the gallbladder or simple cysts. This posterior enhancement is often beneficial in distinguishing between fluid-filled structures and anechoic solid structures.

Radial scanning ultrasound endoscopes may produce an artifact called the reverberation artifact or multiple reflection artifact. This may result in multiple concentric circles of echoes around the case housing the transducer. The case surrounding the transducer reflects the sound energy back to the transducer, and some of this energy may be reflected again. Because these sound waves have traveled twice the original distance between the transducer and the case, the case appears in the image at twice the distance from the transducer as its actual position (Fig. 2.28). Additional concentric rings are possible from third and fourth reverberations of the ultrasound beam. Reducing the overall gain setting may be helpful in minimizing these artifacts. Reverberation artifacts can also be produced by the water-filled balloon surrounding the transducer. Another type of reverberation artifact can produce a mirror image of the transducer or water-filled balloon (Fig. 2.29). This is seen when imaging within a partially distended organ such as the stomach.

When imaging structures with a non-perpendicular beam, care must be taken not to misinterpret increased wall or layer thickness, since tangential scanning may give the appearance of a thickened wall. On the other hand, overdistending the balloon surrounding the transducer may cause wall thinning due to compression of the wall with the balloon.

A dark wedged-shaped void in an ultrasound image may indicate a transducer defect such as a few elements not functioning in a multiple-element-array transducer or a tiny air bubble trapped between the element and inner sheath wall of an ultrasound catheter. Proper preparation of the catheter–transducer

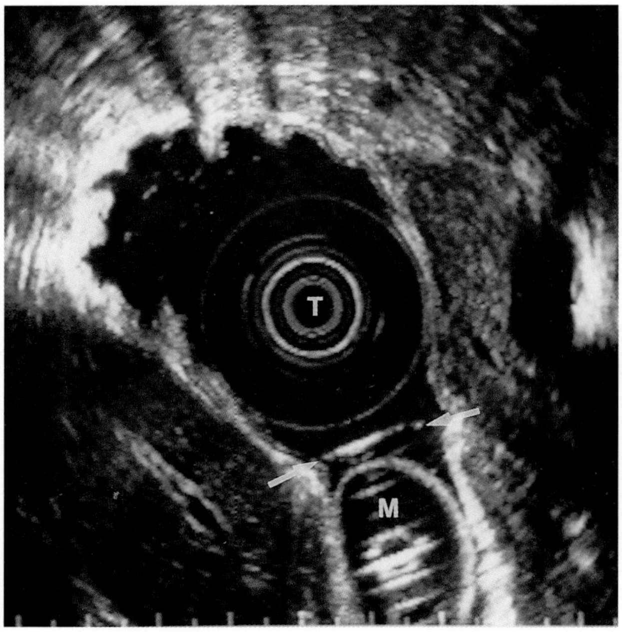

Figure 2.29 *A mirror image artifact (M) caused by a strong reflector (arrows) obtained during an endoscopic ultrasound examination of the water-filled stomach. T, transducer.*

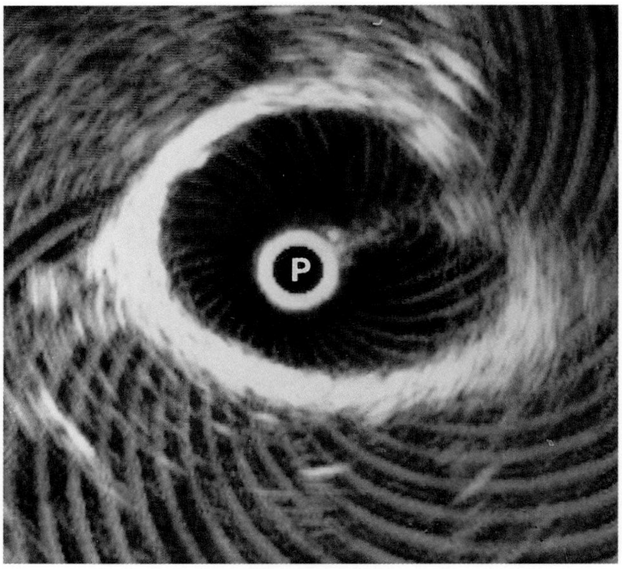

Figure 2.30 *Electrical interference artifacts, caused in this case by X-ray equipment located within the examination room. Artifacts are seen as white lines radiating from the ultrasound probe (P). Often, turning off unnecessary electrical equipment or using isolated wall outlets will eliminate these image-degrading artifacts.*

can avoid these artifacts. Because of the complex electronic circuitry of ultrasound systems, electrical interference may cause image artifacts and distortion with the appearance of electrical 'noise' seen as 'snow' or diagonal white lines on the image (Fig. 2.30). This interference may arise from electrical wiring of equipment in the examination room, e.g. video-endoscopes or various patient monitors. Often, when possible, turning off the equipment responsible for the interference or plugging the ultrasound system into a isolated electrical wall outlet will resolve this artifact. Another artifact is non-uniform rotational disformity (NURD), which occurs with mechanical transducers when the catheter binds in the narrow, sharply curved vessels or other lumina.

Acoustic coupling artifacts may result in image degradation, or, in the worst cases, a complete lack of image formation. When using rotating transducers housed in catheters, this results most commonly from air bubbles trapped within the distal chamber of the catheter because of improper preparation of the probe. It is imperative that proper care be exercised during the preparation of these catheters to avoid the frustrating situation of having the imaging catheter in the proper location within the patient but acquiring poor-quality images. This will add to the time and labor required to perform the examination, and may limit significantly the amount of diagnostic information obtainable.

FUTURE DEVELOPMENTS

A number of technical advances and the combination of various technologies has resulted in continued developments in endoluminal ultrasound scanners. By combining a high-frequency 20-MHz ultrasound catheter with simultaneous real-time pressure measurements, Miller et al[9] developed a method of quantitating the changes in esophageal wall motion while measuring the width of the muscularis propria in the esophageal body during swallowing. They correlated the changes in muscle thickness and lumen circumference with changes in luminal pressure and defined the sonographic appearance of the phases of swallowing based on manometrically defined pressure changes occurring within the esophageal lumen.

Endosonographically guided fine needle aspiration biopsy, although still a relatively new procedure, has become a valuable diagnostic test. Wiersema et al[10] demonstrated the utility of this method initially by performing endoscopic ultrasound followed by fine needle aspiration cytology on 56 consecutive patients with submucosal masses, gastric ulcers or surgical anastomoses suspected of malignancy but with previous negative findings on conventional forceps biopsy or brush cytology. For further discussion of the technique of fine needle aspiration biopsy, see Chapter 6.

Some echoendoscopes provide color and duplex Doppler capabilities. Real-time color flow imaging facilitates differentiation of blood vessels from other fluid-filled tubular structures. In addition, duplex Doppler waveforms can be used to better characterize bloodflow, including differentiating arteries from veins and obtaining flow velocity estimations or a variety of flow ratios.

Transcutaneous three-dimensional (3D) ultrasound has offered a unique method for depicting structures, particularly in obstetrical applications. The 3D reconstruction technique lends itself to endoluminal applications. Most investigations of 3D endoluminal ultrasound have involved intravascular applications, and the technique holds great potential for future uses.[11–14] A preliminary study by Kalimanis et al[15] evaluated the ability of 3D endoscopic ultrasound to evaluate the normal esophageal anatomy and pathologic conditions as compared with information obtained by conventional two-dimensional (2D) endoscopic ultrasound. An echogastroscope was withdrawn through the esophagus in a straight, slow and constant manner. Approximately 80 individual images were then digitized via off-line analysis and stored on an optical disk. The stored 2D images were then reconstructed with software that executed interpolation, boundary formation and surface rendering. Three-dimensional reconstruction offers a format in which a series of 2D images can be assessed and spatially related to each other more readily. In addition, the 3D format offers the advantage of displaying the profile of lesions in the optimal viewing plane, and allowing the viewing plane to be rotated to facilitate conventional or new image orientation displays. For more information on this subject, see Chapter 12.

Other combinations of high-frequency ultrasound catheters with varying diagnostic and therapeutic devices may make it possible to perform other types of procedures under real-time ultrasound guidance, e.g. use of a cytology brush for obtaining cytological specimens under ultrasound guidance (see Chapter 9). As previously mentioned, ultrasound catheters can be combined with manometry.[9] A prototype device with a cutting device has been fabricated so that cutting may be done under real-time ultrasound guidance (see Chapter 4) and a number of devices with dilation balloons around the transducer for dilation of strictures are currently under development.

REFERENCES

1. Bom NA, ten Hoff H, Lancee CT et al, Early and recent intraluminal ultrasound devices, *Int J Cardiac Imag* 1989; **4**:79–88.
2. Roelandt JRTC, Dimario C, De Feyer PJ et al, Intravascular ultrasound: instrumentation, promises and pitfalls. In: Hanrath P, Uebis R, Krebs W, eds. *Cardiovascular Imaging by Ultrasound* (Kluwer Academic Publishers: Dordrecht, 1993) 325–41.
3. Martin RW, Johnson CC, Design characteristics for intravascular ultrasonic catheters, *Int J Cardiac Imag* 1989; **4**:201–6.
4. Hoskins PR, McDicken WN. Techniques for the assessment of the imaging characteristics of intravascular ultrasound scanners, *Br J Radiol* 1994; **67**:695–700.
5. Kremkau FW, *Diagnostic Ultrasound: Principles and Instruments*, 4th edn (WB Saunders Company: Philadelphia, 1993).
6. McDicken WN, *Diagnostic Ultrasound: Principles and Use of Instruments*, 3rd edn (Churchill Livingstone: New York, 1991).
7. Hykes DL, Hedrick WR, Starchman DE, *Ultrasound Physics and Instrumentation*, 2nd edn (Mosby-Year Book: St Louis, 1991).
8. Fish P, *Physics and Instrumentation of Diagnostic Medical Ultrasound* (John Wiley & Sons: New York, 1990).
9. Miller LS, Liu JB, Colizzo FP et al, Correlation of high frequency esophageal ultrasonography and manometry in the study of esophageal motility, *Gastroenterology* 1995; **109**:832–7.
10. Wiersema MJ, Wiersema LM, Khusro Q, Cramer HM, Tao LC, Combined endosonography and fine-needle aspiration cytology in the evaluation of gastrointestinal lesions, *Gastrointest Endosc* 1994; **40**:199–206.
11. Klein HM, Gunther RW, Verlande M et al, 3D-surface reconstruction of intravascular ultrasound images using

personal computer hardware and a motorized catheter control, *Cardiovasc Intervent Radiol* 1992; **15**:97–101.

12. Franceschi D, Bondi JA, Rubin JR, A new approach for three-dimensional reconstruction of arterial ultrasonography, *J Vasc Surg* 1992; **15**:800–5.
13. Rosenfield K, Kaufman J, Pieczek A, Langevin RE Jr, Razvi S, Isner JM, Real-time three-dimensional reconstruction of intravascular ultrasound images of iliac arteries, *Am J Cardiol* 1992; **70**:412–15.
14. Ng KH, Evans JL, Vonesh MJ et al, Arterial imaging with a new forward-viewing intravascular ultrasound catheter, II: Three-dimensional reconstruction and display of data, *Circulation* 1994; **89**:718–23.
15. Kalimanis G, Garra BS, Tio TL et al, The feasibility of three-dimensional ultrasonography: a preliminary report, *Gastrointest Endosc* 1995; **41**:235–9.

Chapter 3 Intravascular ultrasound

Junbo Ge, Günter Görge, Dietrich Baumgart, Fengqi Liu, Michael Haude and Raimund Erbel

INTRODUCTION

In recent decades, coronary angiography has been considered to be a gold standard in the assessment of coronary morphology. Studies have shown that coronary angiography portrays only the contrast agent-filled lumen, giving little information on the vessel wall. Moreover, atherosclerotic lesions are frequently irregular and the vessels compensate in the presence of plaque formation in a remodeling fashion. Not surprisingly, considerable discrepancies exist between angiographic and pathologic examinations.[1–3] Novel diagnostic techniques open new windows to both coronary morphology and function and thus provide new information on the evaluation of coronary circulation. Intravascular ultrasound (IVUS), a new technique that images the vessel from inside, and supplies high-quality images of not only the lumen but also the vessel wall in high resolution, has given rise to great interest in the past few years.[4–10] It provides both the topography of the vessel wall and the characteristics of atherosclerotic lesions.[4–10] For quantitative assessment, accurate measurements of lesion size can be achieved.[7–10] Recently, IVUS has been extensively used in guiding and assessing the results of coronary interventions. More important is the use of it to clarify the underlying morphology of ambiguous lesions and coronary syndromes (myocardial bridging, coronary aneurysm, plaque rupture, thrombus formation, syndrome X, etc.). New insights into coronary atherosclerosis (according to the Stary classification) become clinically available. Tissue characterization and three-dimensional reconstruction seem to be possible.

HISTORY AND DEVELOPMENT OF INTRAVASCULAR ULTRASOUND

IVUS is a branch of intraluminal ultrasound. In 1955, Wild used a mechanically rotated transducer to localize a rectal tumor.[11] In 1956, Cieszynski built an ultrasonic catheter for intracardial investigation, and he was able to obtain ultrasonic reflections of soft tissues during model experiments.[12] In further experiments on dogs, he obtained good ultrasound reflections from the inner walls of the right and left ventricle as well as of the pulmonary artery. He noted that his method was harmless to the animals' health. One year later, Omoto used an intravenous probe with a guidewire tip to study cardiac structures,[13] and Ebina[14] described a miniature concave transducer for rotation inside a rubber cuff in the esophagus in 1964. In 1969, Bom initiated a program to develop two-dimensional, real-time invasive ultrasonic imaging using state-of-the-art technology.[15] A 32-element circular phased array with an outer diameter of 3.2 mm mounted at the tip of a 9 Fr catheter was constructed. With this transducer, real-time intraluminal images such as left ventricular cross-sections were recorded in the early 1970s. Generally speaking, today's transesophageal echocardiography and IVUS are used extensively in the fields of cardiology.

Because of the poor image quality and technical limitations of miniature ultrasound transducers, IVUS was used only as a research tool until the end of the 1980s. With the rapid development of interventional cardiology, it is necessary to seek a feasible method to guide coronary intervention and it is necessary to find a method to screen coronary artery disease. Today, there are two major types of IVUS catheter: the electronic multi-element system and the mechanically rotated system. The former was introduced by Hodgson et al, and consisted of a multi-element phased array with an integrated circuit for initial echo-data processing at the catheter tip.[16] With the improvement of the software, there has been great improvement of the image quality in the past few years. In combination with a balloon, IVUS can be used to guide percutaneous transluminal coronary balloon angioplasty (PTCA). The commercially available catheter is supplied by Endosonics (Rancho Cordova, CA, USA).

The mechanically rotated transducer consists of a single ultrasound crystal or in combination with a mirror which is driven by a motor outside in the catheter shaft to obtain a 360° display of the arterial cross-section. The commercially available catheters are Sonicath and the CVIS series (Clearview, Ultracross, etc.) manufactured by the Boston Scientific Corporation (Natick, MA, USA). The working frequencies range from 10 to 30 MHz. In very tortuous vessels or severely calcified lesions, mechanically rotated catheters may have non-uniform rotation and therefore result in image distortion.

The combination of imaging techniques with interventional devices is showing its advantages. Interventional procedures can be directly guided by ultrasound imaging. Yock et al developed a combination of an ultrasound catheter with an atherectomy catheter and demonstrated that the cutting process can be guided by IVUS imaging.[17] Erbel et al developed a vision-guided laser atherectomy technique which combined ultrasound and a laser catheter technique.[18] As mentioned above, Hodgson developed an electronic IVUS catheter and balloon catheter in 1989, and this is now used in clinical practice.[16]

Another development in the field of IVUS is the forward-viewing IVUS catheter which was developed by Evans and co-workers.[19,20] Currently, this is only a research tool. Recently Görge et al developed a steerable IVUS catheter which can be used to obtain an axial image, especially in the aortic arch.[21] In 1995, Serruys and Erbel first used a micro-motor ultrasound catheter for peripheral artery scanning. We believe that in the future we will need an IVUS catheter that is able to provide information not only on vessel morphology but also on the function (such as pressure and flow velocity) and that, in addition, can be used for intervention purposes.

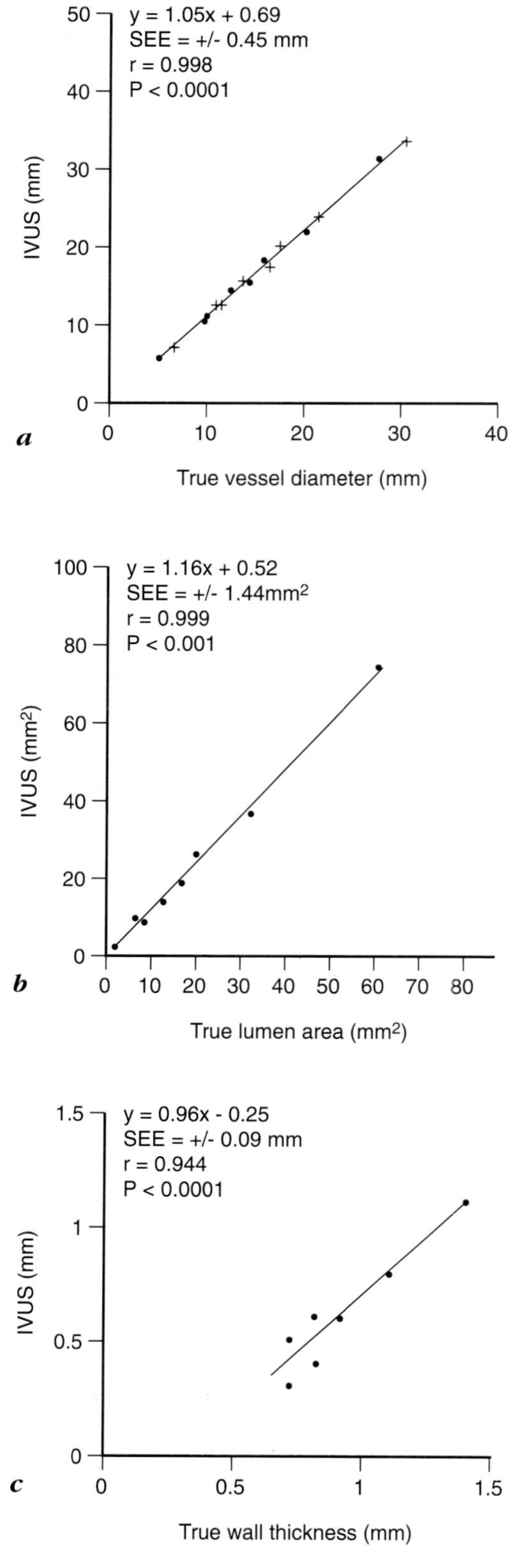

Figure 3.1 *Relationship between IVUS measurements and true vessel dimensions: (a) vessel diameter; (b) vessel area; (c) wall thickness. (From Ge et al[22] with permission.)*

VALIDATION OF IVUS

The following section addresses the accuracy and feasibility of IVUS in vitro and in vivo in assessing vessel morphology and dimensions.

EXPERIMENTAL STUDY

Quantative study

Phantom study

Before IVUS was used in clinical investigation, it had been validated in experimental studies both in

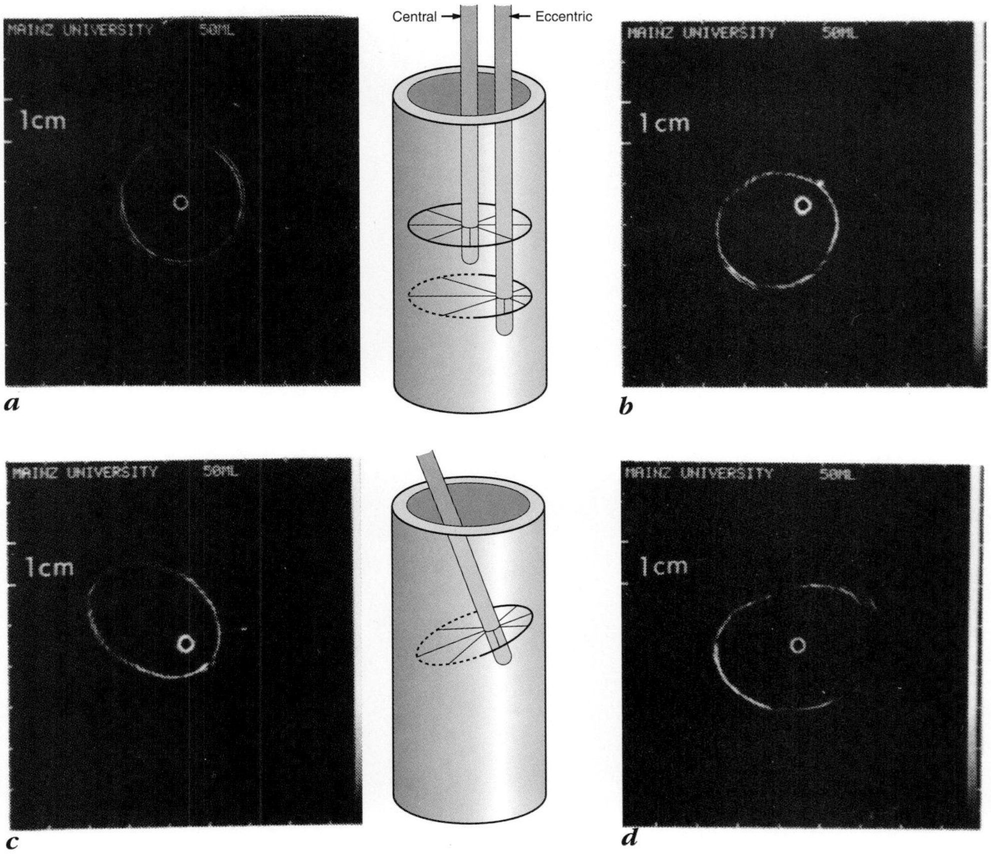

Figure 3.2 *The influence of the eccentricity and the angle between the transducer and the vessel wall on the IVUS images. (a) When the catheter is in the center of the vessel and the echo beam is perpendicular to the vessel wall. (b) The catheter is eccentric but the transducer is parallel to the long axis of the vessel wall. From 12 to 2 o'clock and from 6 to 7 o'clock, the echo beam is still perpendicular to the vessel wall. (c) Transducer eccentric; (d) Transducer concentric show that there are angles between transducers and the vessel walls. (From Ge et al[31] with permission.)*

vitro and in vivo. Studies using experimental models showed that IVUS can accurately portray the vessel size. In an experimental study using the plexiglass phantom model, close correlations between IVUS-derived measurements and true vessel dimensions were found (Fig. 3.1).[22,23] Studies also showed close correlations of luminal areas, luminal diameters and wall thickness between histologic measurements and ultrasound measurements using different systems.[22–25] Nevertheless, the vessel dimensions and the wall morphology are also influenced by the orientation of the echo beam with respect to the vessel wall (Fig. 3.2). An eccentric position of the IVUS transducer and angle between the transducer and the vessel wall may considerably affect the images and thus affect the measured dimensions. Moreover, the ultrasound velocity varies in different transmission media and at different media temperatures. Therefore, the IVUS-derived values are slightly different from the true vessel dimensions. In addition, the resolution of the IVUS system also affects the quantative measurement of the vessel dimensions. The axial resolution of the presently used 20–30-MHz IVUS catheter is 80–100 µm, and the lateral resolution depends on depth, averaging from 150 to 200 µm.[26,27]

Pathologic specimens

Similarly, IVUS is able to accurately measure the vessel area, lumen area and wall thickness in normal blood vessels.[10,22,28] In the case of atherosclerosis, Li et al found that IVUS can also accurately measure the lesion size[29] (Fig. 3.3). Di Mario et al reported, however, that the IVUS-derived plaque area was consistently larger than that obtained from histologic examinations.[24] Despite a good correlation between IVUS and histologic measurements, IVUS seems to overestimate plaque size. In another study, Mallery et al found that IVUS overestimates the mean intimal and total thickness by 0.3 mm and 0.7 mm compared to measurements in histologic sections ($P < 0.001$).[25] Similar results were reported by Finet et al in a recent study.[30] However, a good correlation exists between the IVUS and histologic measurements for the thickness of intima and media,[30] indicating that the IVUS so-called intima might not represent histologic intima.

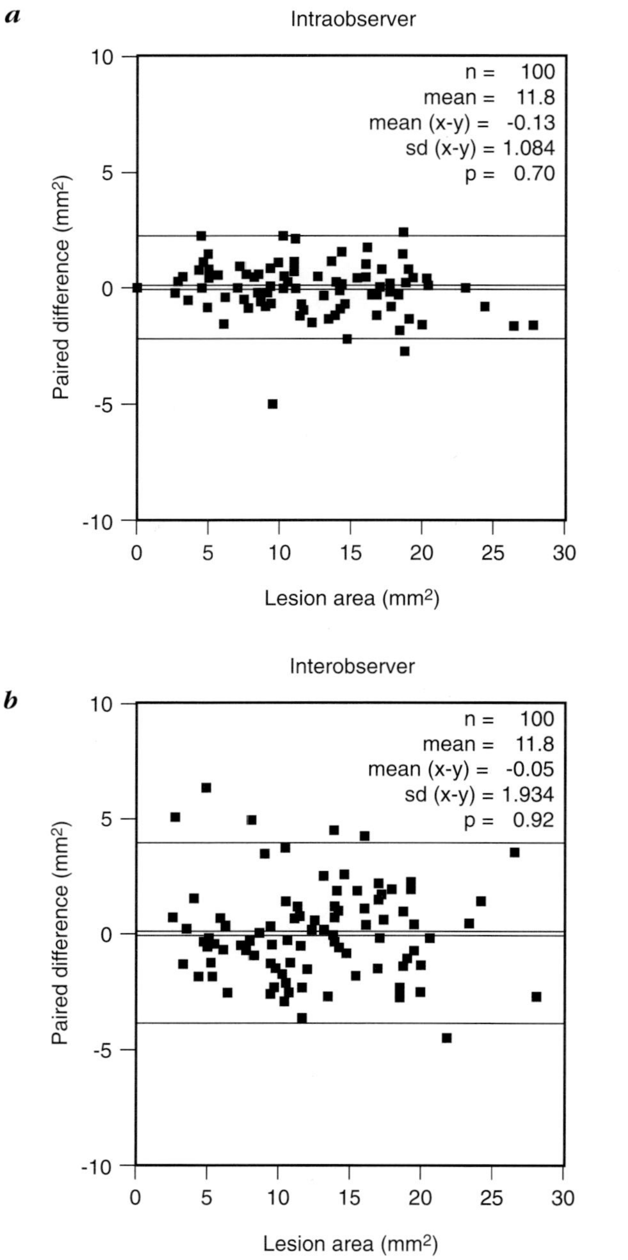

Figure 3.3 *(a) Intra- and (b) interobserver variability in lesion area measurements. The 95% confidence interval is indicated by the upper (mean + 2SD) and lower (mean – 2SD) vertical lines. (From Li et al[29] with permission.)*

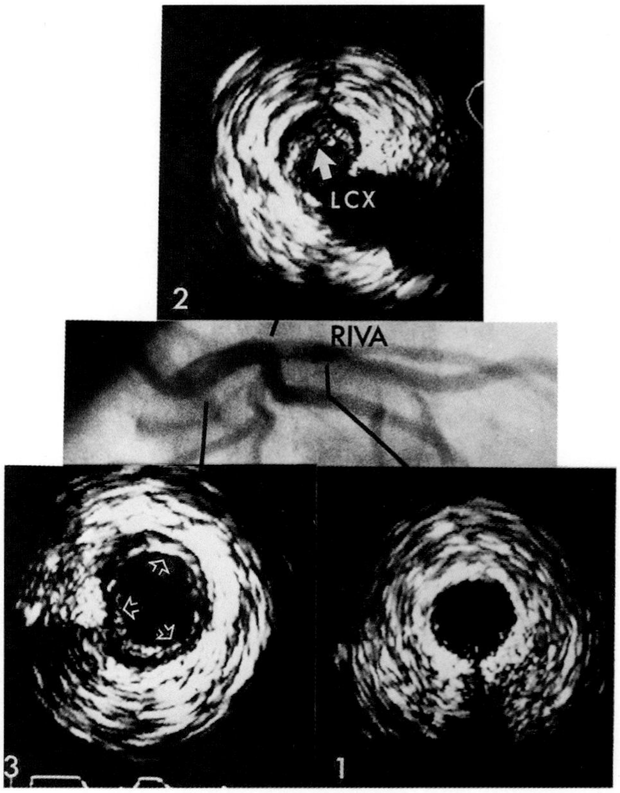

Figure 3.4 *Angiogram and IVUS images at corresponding sites of left coronary artery. No three-layer appearance is seen at the normal segment (position 1); an echolucent zone is clearly seen at the plaque segment (position 3). Position 2 indicates the origin of LCX and an eccentric plaque is clearly seen (arrow).*

Morphologic observation

IVUS images of the peripheral arteries showed a three-layered appearance in muscular arteries. These layers were considered to be histologic intima, media and adventitia.[10,23] However, a three-layered appearance was found using a 20-MHz IVUS catheter in segments of postmortem human aorta from which the intima had been removed, and the removed intima itself exhibited three layers.[31] Scanning of the human aorta using a transthoracic ultrasound transducer indicated that the double-line pattern is an artifact.[32] A more recent study using a 45-MHz transducer proposed that the middle echolucent layer in muscular arteries represents the histologic media.[33] The media in elastic arteries was isodense with other vessel layers, preventing ready identification of the outer intimal border.[34] This three-layered appearance is also frequently found in human coronary arteries, and the echolucent layer is interpreted as the histologic media. It is known that the intima thickens from a single layer at birth to a mean 60 μm from infancy to 5 years, 220 μm at 30 years, and 250 μm at 40 years.[35] The media retains a

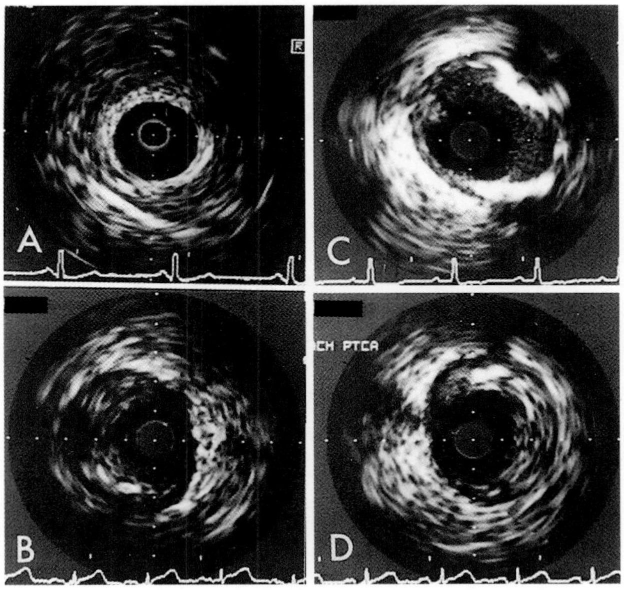

Figure 3.5 *(A) IVUS images of normal coronary artery, (B) lipid deposits in plaque, (C) calcium deposits in plaque, and (D) fibrous plaque.*

thickness of approximately 200 µm throughout life. It is also known that the media thins in the presence of atheromatous disease.[36,37] We cannot differentiate media from intima in normal coronary arteries with the presently used IVUS transducer. The echolucent layer cannot be histologic media (Fig. 3.4). Another explanation is that the resolution of current transducers may be inadequate to image intima less than 200 µm thick, so that the three-layered appearance cannot be seen in coronary arteries of transplanted hearts from younger donors (mean age 27 years), in contrast to older hearts.[38] The position of the transducer in the vessel and the angle between the ultrasound beam and the vessel wall also significantly affect the three-layer appearance. In an experiment using plastic cylinders, the three-layer appearance can only be imaged when the ultrasound beam is perpendicular to the vessel wall (Fig. 3.2).[31]

Commonly, atherosclerotic plaques are composed of different tissues. Nevertheless, we can still differentiate fibrous, lipid and calcified plaques according to the different degrees of echogenicity (Fig. 3.5). Lipid deposits are characterized by an echolucent core within the plaque (Fig. 3.5B). Calcium deposits are characterized by a bright echo reflection with an acoustic shadow cast behind (Fig. 3.5C). Fibrous plaque is characterized by an echodense reflection but without an acoustic shadow (Fig. 3.5D). The sensitivity and specificity vary for each plaque subtype (Table 3.1).[34] The identification of thrombi by IVUS is somewhat difficult, as their echogenicity is similar to that of sclerotic plaque. Thrombus formation may have a distinctive speckled echocardiographic appearance.[39] Figure 3.6 shows IVUS and pathologic images of a fresh mural thrombus: the

Table 3.1 The sensitivity and specificity of each plaque subtype (from Kearney and Erbel[34] with permission)

Study	*Tissue*	*Sensitivity, n/n(%)*	*Specificity, n/n(%)*
Potkin *et al.* [77]*	Lipid	7/9(78)	100/103(97)
	Fibrous	81/84(96)	26/28(93)
	Calcific	19/19(100)	93/93(100)
Siegel *et al.* [78]*	Thrombus	8/14(57)	51/57(90)
Suárez de Lezo *et al.* [56]†	Focal calcium	(56)	(76)
DiMario *et al.* [66]*	Lipid plaque	32/36(89)	62/64(97)
	Fibrous plaque	32/48(67)	52/52(100)
	Calcific	35/36(97)	63/64(98)
Peters *et al.* [79]*	Lipid pools	18/35(51)	67/69(97)
	Calcific	20/26(77)	78/78(100)
Rasheed *et al.* [80]†	'Soft'	15/16(94)	18/24(75)
	'Mixed'	10/16(63)	22/24(92)
	'Calcific'	7/8(88)	32/33(97)

*Histology study.
†Atherectomy study.

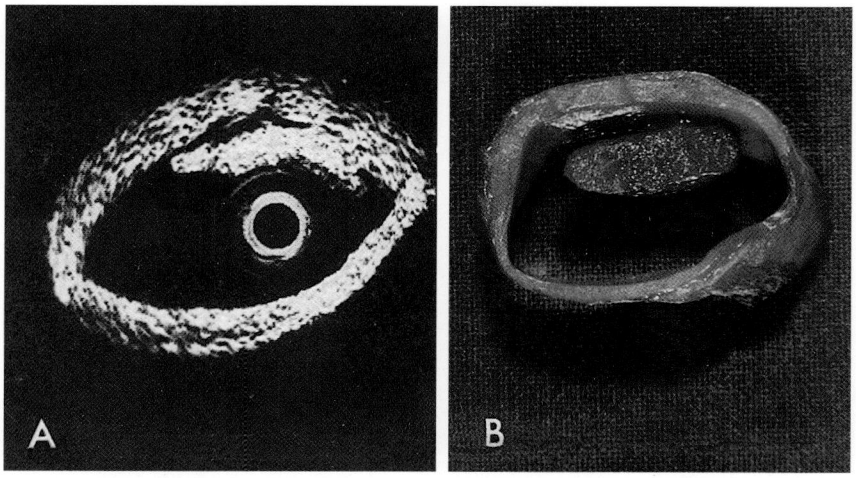

Figure 3.6 *In vitro IVUS examination of a fresh thrombus: (A) IVUS cross-sectional image of the vessel and a mural thrombus; (B) histologic specimen of the corresponding section.*

IVUS image shows bright, homogeneous reflections but without 'shadowing'; this was considered to be thrombi. Siegel et al compared IVUS and angioscopy with histologic examinations and found good agreement between histology and both angioscopy and IVUS for thrombus identification.[40]

IN VIVO HUMAN OBSERVATION

Quantitative study

The ultrasound velocity increases as the transmit medium temperature increases. The integrated measurement system of the IVUS device is based on the velocity of ultrasound in blood at 37°C of 1540 m/s. Goss et al reported sound velocities in blood of 1551 m/s at 20–25°C and 1565 m/s at 35–40°C which are dependent on hematocrit.[41] The difficulty of predicting the velocity in the human heart and vessels can explain in part the differences obtained by IVUS from true dimensions. In addition, coronary arteries pulsate during the cardiac cycle, which may result in area variations of the vessel during different phases of the cardiac cycle and beat-to-beat variation of the vessel lumen (Fig. 3.7).[8] As mentioned above, the eccentricity and angle between the transducer and the vessel wall also affect the IVUS-measured vessel dimensions. Fortunately, the diameter of the human coronary artery is not very large and the guidewire used for advancing the IVUS catheter may keep the IVUS transducer parallel to the vessel wall, so that coaxial images are obtained. In order to avoid false measurements, only images (segments) where the transducer is located centrally

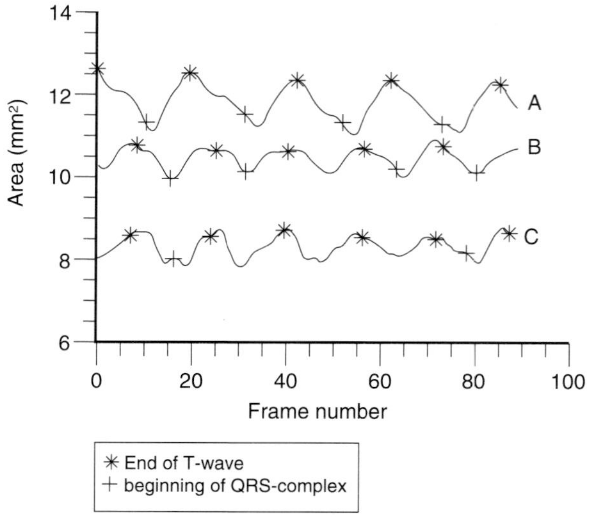

Figure 3.7 *Pulsatile variation in the cross-sectional area of the left main coronary artery (A), proximal left anterior descending artery (LAD) (B) and of the mid-LAD (C) in 90 consecutive frames of IVUS images (From Ge et al[8] with permission.)*

should be used. Good correlations still exist between IVUS and angiographic measurements[8,42] in normal vessels in corresponding segments and phase (Fig. 3.8). We evaluated the inter- and intraobserver variability of 30 IVUS images and found that good correlations exists between intraobserver measurements (r = 0.99, SEE = ±0.16 mm for lumen diameter, and r = 0.99, SEE = ±1.39 mm^2 for lumen area) and interobserver measurements (r = 0.99, SEE = ±0.17 mm for lumen diameter, and r = 0.98, SEE =

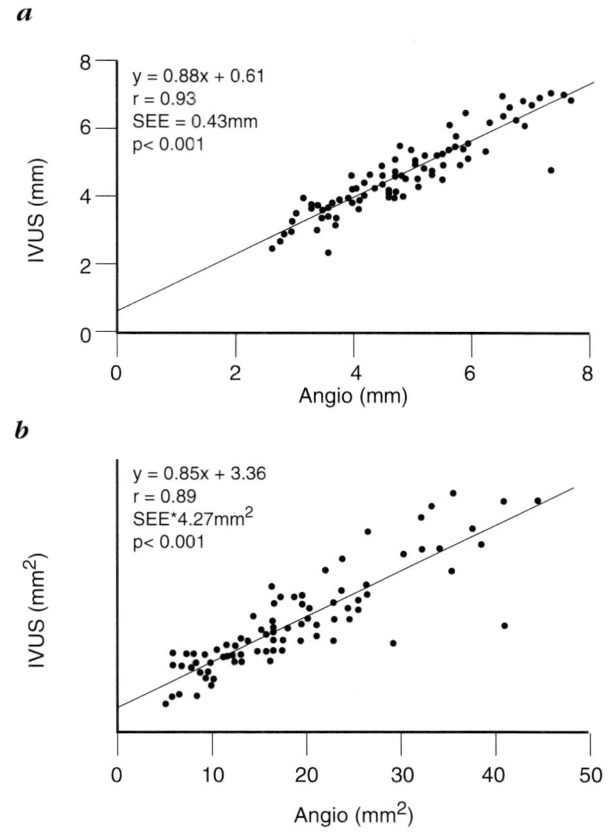

Figure 3.8 *Relationship between angiographic (angio) and IVUS measurements (IVUS) of lumen dimensions at normal sites: (a) lumen diameter; (b) lumen area. (From Ge et al[8] with permission.)*

±1.81 mm^2 for lumen area).[8] In the presence of atherosclerosis, the correlations between IVUS- and orthogonal angiography-measured lumen areas were poor in both the reference segments and intervention segments.[4] The underlying reason for this poor correlation in diseased vessels may be that the atherosclerotic lesions are frequently irregular or eccentric, and thus the angiography-derived lumen area may be different from the true lumen area. Coronary arteries enlarge in the presence of atherosclerosis to compensate for the lumen narrowing. However, it cannot be predicted whether or not the reference segment is normal by coronary angiography. IVUS, on the other hand, is able to assess this compensatory process by accurately providing the cross-sectional images of the vessel. This may also explain some of the discrepancies between IVUS and angiographic measurements.

Morphologic observation

As mentioned above, coronary angiography portrays only the contour of the vessel lumen, and gives little information on the vessel wall.[1–3] Coronary arteries enlarge in the presence of atherosclerosis and, moreover, plaques are frequently eccentric, irregular and diffuse. Therefore, considerable discrepancies exist between angiographic and pathologic observations.[1–3] Coronary angiography is not able to detect the early stage of atherosclerosis[8,9] and is not able to diagnose the severity of stenosis precisely.[8,9] We have found that coronary angiography cannot detect a lesion if the area percentage stenosis does not exceed 45% in the case of coronary arterial remodeling.[43] Thus, in the presence of atherosclerosis, there are inevitable differences between angiographic and IVUS examinations, and IVUS provides more accurate morphologic information on both the wall and the lumen. In addition, IVUS is able to provide functional information on the coronary artery in combination with intracoronary Doppler flow mapping. In the near future it will also be possible to evaluate by combining IVUS, Doppler and pressure measurement.

An understanding of plaque composition is very important for selecting intracoronary interventional procedures. However, the plaque echogenicity in vivo might be different from that in vitro. Thus, the plaque echogenicity and histopathologic results were compared in order to characterize the tissue type of the plaque. Rasheed et al examined the histologic samples obtained during directional atherectomy in comparison to IVUS imaging and found that IVUS has a high sensitivity and specificity in differentiating plaque types.[42] This evalua-

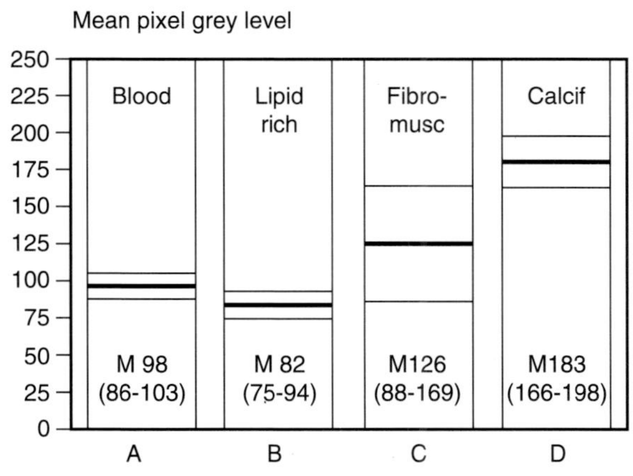

Figure 3.9 *Backscatter intensity of blood (A), lipid (B), fibrous tissue (C), and calcium deposits (D). (From Peters et al[45] with permission.)*

tion is inevitably subjective to some extent. Preliminary studies in analyzing ultrasonic radiofrequency signals reflected from the arterial wall in comparison with histologic examination showed that the integrated backscatter is 4.2 dB in normal vessel walls, 19.0 ± 5.3 dB in fat, 44.5 ± 5.9 dB in fibrous tissue, and 66.7 ± 9.1 dB in calcium deposits.[44] By analysis of the radiofrequency signal, tissue characterization might be possible in the near future in vivo using IVUS. Another possible way of differentiating the tissue character is to calculate the pixel gray levels of the plaques by analyzing the backscatter amplitude. However, the absolute backscatter intensity is influenced by differences in transducers, instrument gain settings and attenuation along the ultrasound pathway, which makes clinical application difficult. By analysis of values relative to materials with known ultrasound characteristics, such as blood or saline, these problems may be resolved (Fig. 3.9).[45]

PLAQUE CHARACTERISTICS

Coronary artery atherosclerosis is a long-term, slowly progressing disease. It only becomes coronary heart disease when the atherosclerotic disease results in

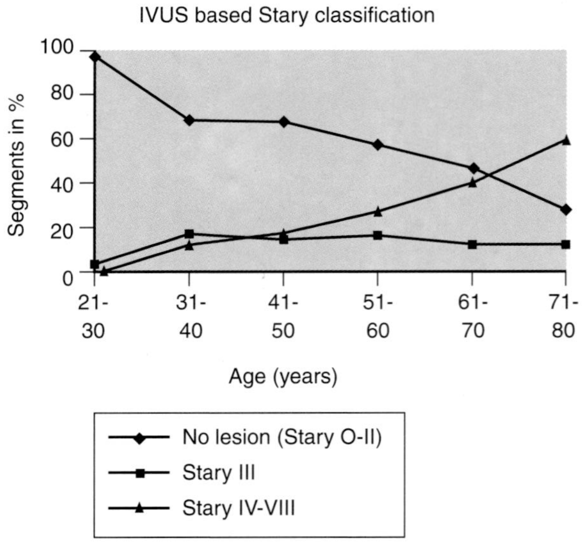

Figure 3.10 *Distribution of atherosclerotic lesions in 812 segments of 49 patients with angiographically normal angiograms. As age increases, the percentage of advanced lesions also increases. Accordingly, the percentages of normal segments and early lesions decrease.*

Table 3.2 Classification of atherosclerotic lesions based on pathologic observation[46–48]

Types	*Description*
Type I (initial lesion)	Lipoprotein accumulation in intima; lipid in macrophages. These changes are discernible only microscopically or chemically; no tissue damage is visible
Type II (fatty streak) IIa (progression-prone; co-localized with adaptive thickening) IIb (progression-resistant)	Lipoprotein accumulation in intima; lipid in macrophages and smooth muscle cells; quantities large enough to be visible to the unaided eye but still no tissue damage
Type III (pre-atheroma)	All type IIa changes plus multiple deposits of pooled extracellular lipid; macroscopic evidence of tissue damage or disorder
Type IV (atheroma)	All type IIa changes plus confluent mass of extracellular lipid (lipid core) with massive structural damage to intima
Type Va (fibroatheroma)	All type IV changes plus development of marked collagen layers and smooth muscle cell increase above lipid core
Vb (calcific lesion)	Any advanced lesion type composed predominantly of calcium; substantial structural deformity
Vc (fibrotic lesion)	Any advanced lesion type composed predominantly of collagen; lipid may be absent
Type VI (complicated lesion) VIa (fissure, erosion) VIb (hematoma, hemorrhage) VIc (thrombus)	All type IV and V changes plus a thrombotic deposit and/or hematoma and/or erosion or fissure

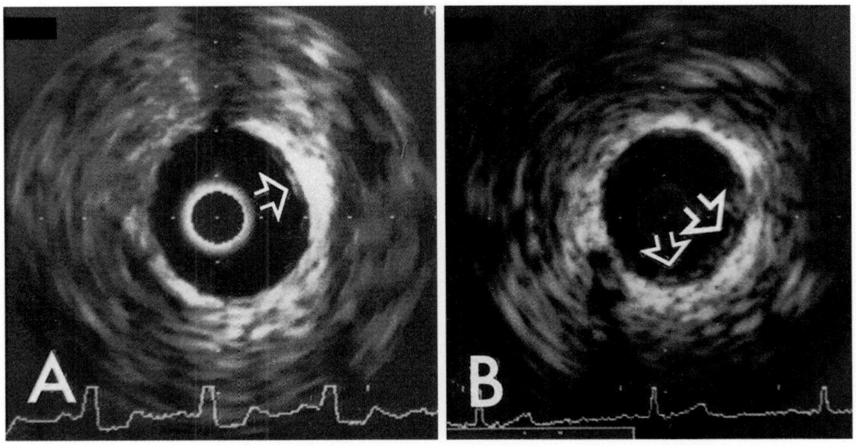

Figure 3.11 *IVUS images of normal or early stage of atherosclerosis. (A) A mild intimal thickening exists between 12 and 3 o'clock which presents a three-layer appearance. An obvious intimal thickening is seen between 4 and 9 o'clock. (B) A mild intimal thickening is seen between 5 and 7 o'clock.*

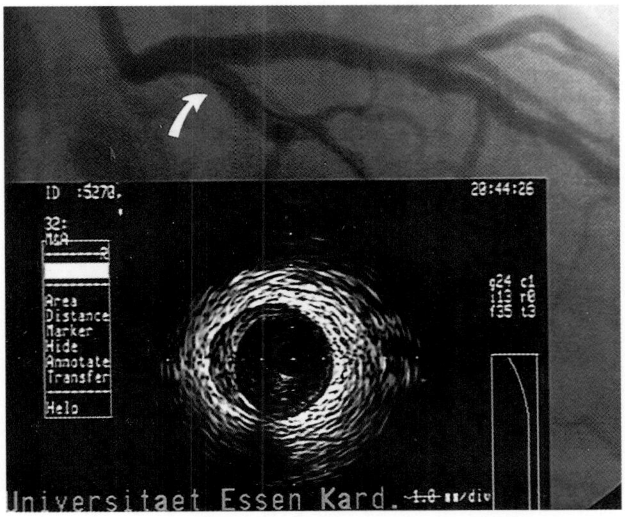

Figure 3.12 *An early stage of atherosclerosis (pre-atheroma) is seen in the IVUS image without lumen reduction angiographically (arrow).*

severe coronary lumen reduction which affects the coronary perfusion and cannot be compensated. Contrast coronary angiography is not able to detect the early stage of atherosclerosis. Based on early pathologic observations by Stary,[46,47] the Committee on Vascular Lesions of the Council on Atherosclerosis (American Heart Association) recently classified the atherosclerotic process into six stages (Table 3.2).[48] IVUS is able to provide high-resolution images of the vessel lumen and wall by imaging the vessel from inside. It is therefore, possible to stage the atherosclerotic process. Erbel et al evaluated 812 segments in 49 patients who had normal angiograms with IVUS and found 440/812 segments (54%) with plaque formation.[49] Early signs of atherosclerosis are mainly seen in young people. The percentage of advanced lesions increases as the patient's age increases. Even in angiographically normal coronary arteries advanced atherosclerotic lesions are found, explaining the potential risk of acute coronary syndromes in this group of patients (Fig. 3.10).[49,50]

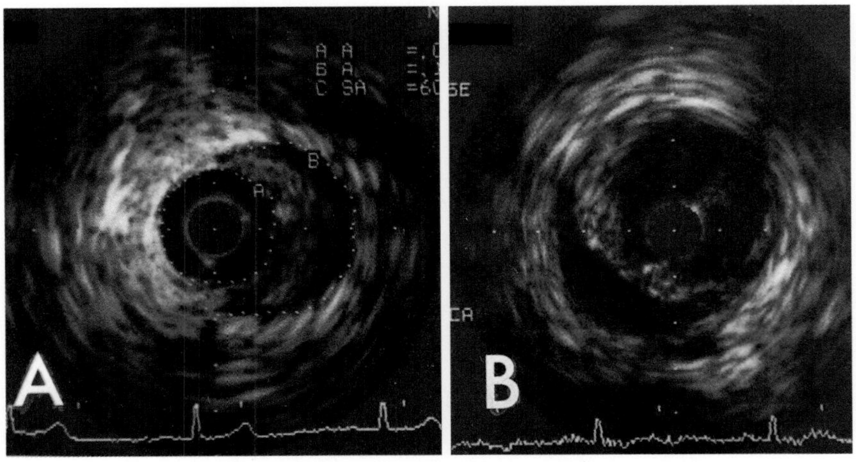

Figure 3.13 *(A) Advanced stage of atherosclerosis (stage IV) which is characterized by a large lipid core (echolucent zone on IVUS). (B) Stage V, which is characterized by a large lipid core and a thin fibrous cap. Both lesions are rather unstable and are referred to as 'plaque at risk', as they can rupture under high wall shear stress or as a result of inflammation of the cap.*

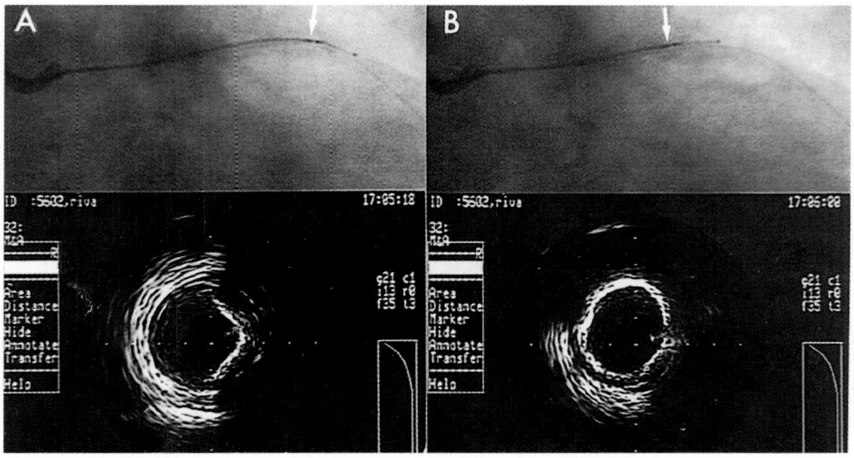

Figure 3.14 *Stage Vb (previously Stary VII) lesion; plaque with severe calcification, which is characterized by bright echoes with acoustic shadowing behind (from 6 to 12 o'clock).*

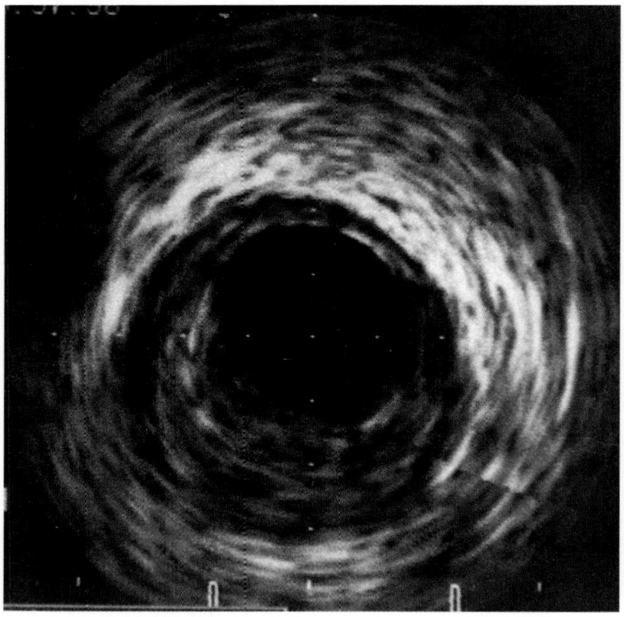

Figure 3.15 *Stage Vc (previously Stary VIII) lesion; fibrotic plaque, which presents on IVUS bright echoes without acoustic shadowing. It is considered to be the result of several episodes of plaque reorganization.*

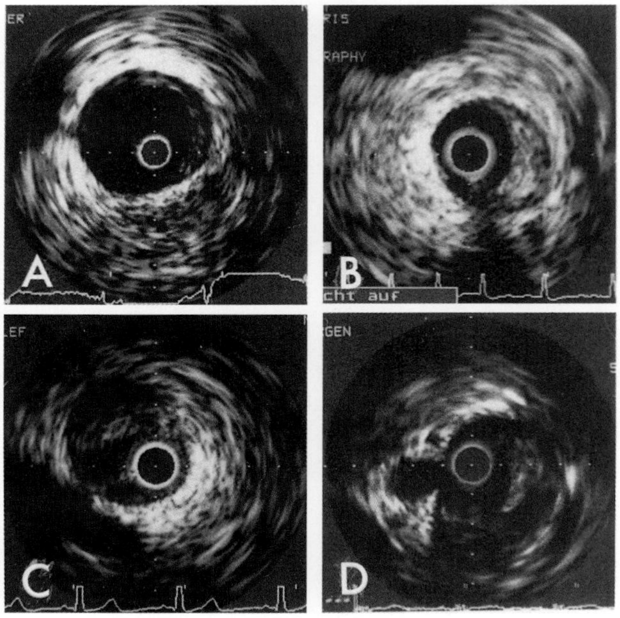

Figure 3.16 *Atherosclerotic process in different stages. (A) and (B) indicate early stages of atherosclerosis (stages II and III). (C) indicates plaque at risk with a lipid core and a thin cap (stage Va). (D) shows plaque rupture (stage VIa).*

By IVUS, type I and II lesions cannot be differentiated from true, normal coronary arteries. They present with a circular lumen with smooth wall or slight intimal thickening, with a so-called 'three-layer appearance' (Fig. 3.11).

Type III lesions present with not only eccentric or concentric intimal thickening, but also echolucent areas in the thickened intima (Fig. 3.12).

Type IV lesions present with concentric or eccentric plaque formation with a lipid core, which appears as an echolucent area within the plaque (Fig. 3.13A). Angiographically, type I–IV lesions do not cause lumen reduction because of the vessel compensation.

Type Va lesions present with a lipid core with a thin, fibrous cap over it (Fig. 3.13B). Sometimes, focal

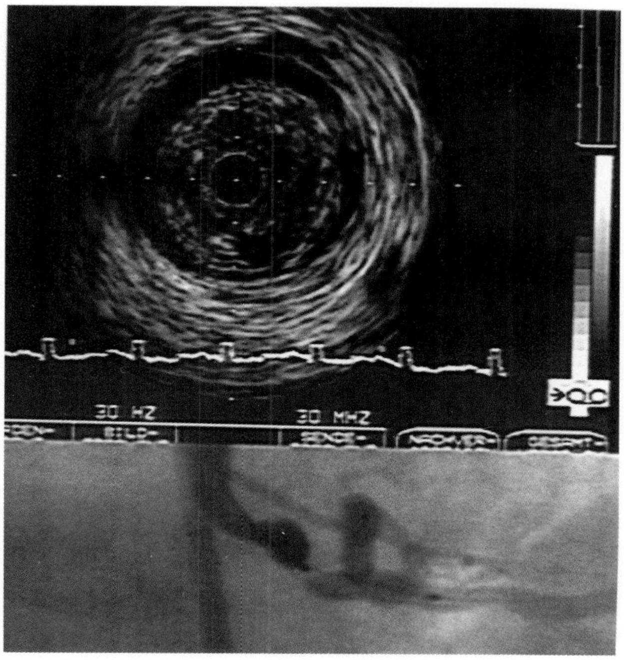

Figure 3.17 *Stage VIc (mural thrombus), which is characterized by speckled reflection and undulation (rain worm movement) mass in the lumen.*

calcium deposits exist in different types of lesions. Type IV and V lesions are described as 'plaques at risk'.[51] Type Vb lesions present mainly with calcium deposits, which are characterized by bright echoes and acoustic shadowing behind (Fig. 3.14). Type Vc lesions present with plaques with echodense reflections but without acoustic shadowing (Fig. 3.15). Focal calcium deposits may exist.

Type VI includes three subgroups. VIa presents with plaque fissure or rupture. IVUS shows an emptied plaque with a thin, fibrous cap (Fig. 3.16D). The emptied plaque cavity could be filled when injecting contrast agent. By coronary angiography, it is sometimes misdiagnosed as coronary aneurysm, because the emptied cavity is filled with contrast agent. IVUS is able to differentiate coronary aneurysm from plaque rupture.[52] Ruptured plaques may result in unstable angina, acute myocardial infarction and sudden death. They may also heal, subsequently, with thrombus formation followed by plaque reorganization[53] showing a 'layering effect'.[54] This may explain the 'layering effect' in plaques previously observed in pathologic studies. VIb is hemotoma or hemorrhage pathologically. It is normally difficult to identify this subtype by IVUS, because hemotoma or hemorrhage presents with an echolucent area within the plaque; the lipid core also presents with an echolucent area within the plaque. The difference between hematoma or hemorrhage and lipid core may be that the former is more in the wall, while the latter is more in the plaque. Until now, it has been difficult to differentiate these two situations when hematoma exists in plaque. However, it is easy to identify plaque hemorrhage, when a connection exists between the lumen and the hemorrhage, by injecting contrast agent during IVUS. VIc is thrombus formation. Fresh thrombus can be rather easily identified by IVUS, because it usually presents with a speckled undulating mass in the lumen (Fig. 3.17). Old thrombus is, however, usually to be differentiated from plaque when it is covered with fibrotic tissue (plaque reorganization). It normally presents with a 'layered appearance'.[54]

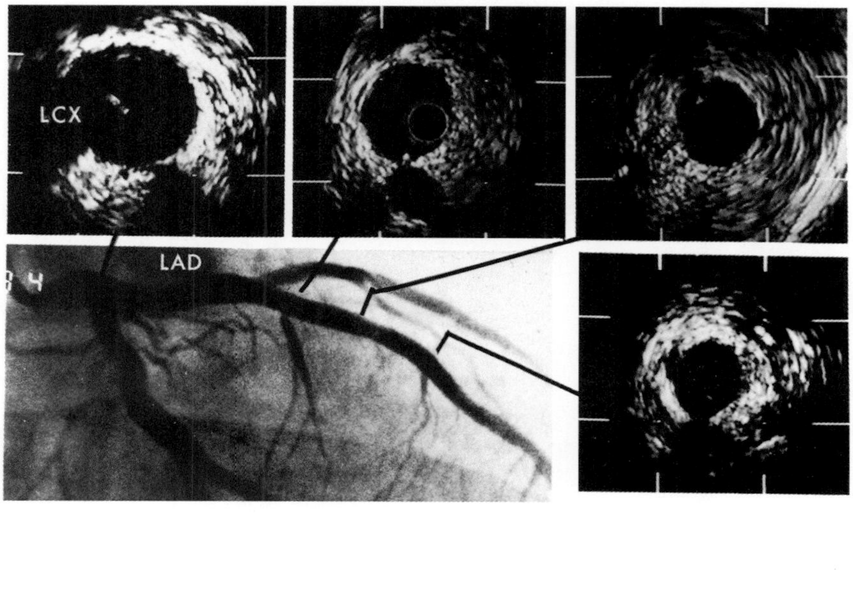

Figure 3.18 *IVUS imaging of a normal coronary artery. The normal arterial wall has a monolayer appearance.*

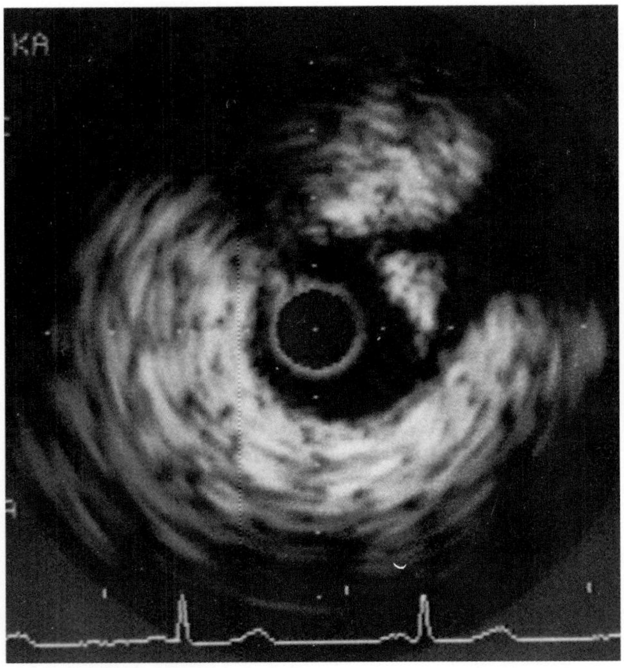

Figure 3.19 *A small eccentric plaque with calcification which is characterized by an acoustic shadow behind (2–3 o'clock).*

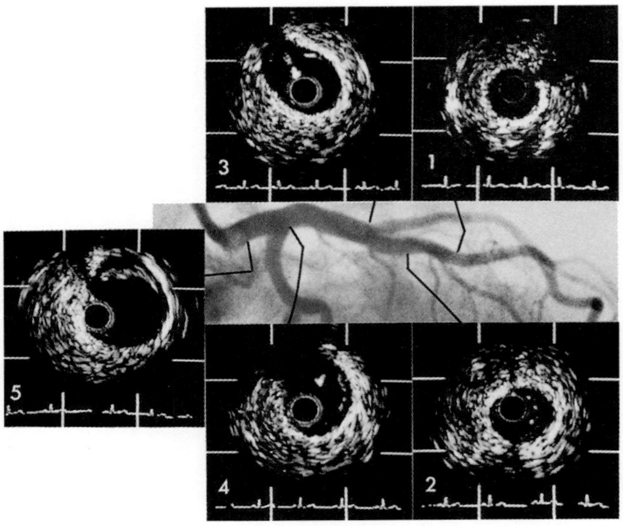

Figure 3.20 *Angiogram and IVUS images at corresponding sites of the left coronary artery. No abnormalities were documented by angiography while IVUS showed plaque formation in the left main coronary artery. (From Ge et al[8] with permission.)*

NORMAL CORONARY ARTERIES

Coronary arteries taper from proximal to distal in their course. With the use of intracoronary ultrasound imaging, we have evaluated 55 consecutive patients (28 men, 27 women) who underwent diagnostic coronary angiography for suspected ischemic heart disease and were found to have angiographically normal coronary arteries. The patients ranged in age from 42 to 70 years.[8]

MORPHOLOGIC OBSERVATIONS

A total of 413 sites in the 55 patients were analyzed. The lumen of the normal coronary segment portrayed by IVUS was circular or elliptical with a smooth surface (Fig. 3.18). Among the 413 sites examined, atherosclerotic plaques were identified by IVUS in 72 (17%) sites in 25 (45%) patients. The plaque area was 5.55 ± 3.56 mm^2 (2–26 mm^2), and comprised 28.8 ± 9.6% (13–70%) of the coronary cross-sectional area. In 24/72 (33%) sites of nine patients, calcific deposits were detected (Fig. 3.19). Most of the plaques (84%)

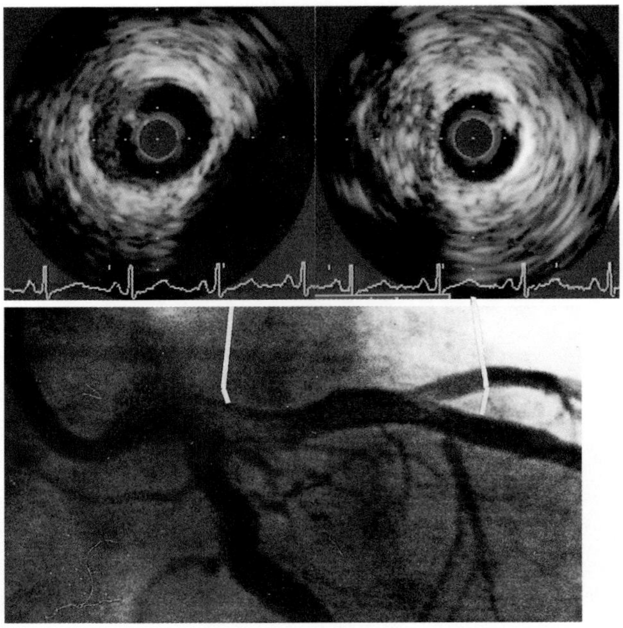

Figure 3.21 *Angiogram and IVUS images at corresponding sites of left coronary artery. No abnormalities are detected by angiography. An eccentric plaque in the left main coronary artery is clearly visualized by intracoronary ultrasound.*

Table 3.3 Cross-sectional areas of normal LCA during cardiac cycle

	Maximum area (mm²)	*Minimum area (mm²)*	*End-diastole (mm²)*	*Pulsation (%)*
LMCA	18.33 ± 8.18	16.49 ± 6.77[a]	17.33 ± 7.98[a]	10.2 ± 4.0
Range	9.74–36.02	8.83–29.95	9.12–30.71	
Proximal LAD	14.01 ± 5.54	12.95 ± 5.08[a]	13.56 ± 5.85[b]	8.3 ± 4.7
Range	6.91–26.21	6.34–23.61	6.42–26.10	
Mid-LAD	10.70 ± 4.47	9.78 ± 4.24[a]	9.75 ± 4.67[a]	9.8 ± 4.0
Range	4.78–22.74	4.49–21.47	4.53–22.01	

[a]$P < 0.001$, [b]$P < 0.005$. The values are mean ± standard deviation.

were eccentric. In all patients, no obvious stenoses were documented by coronary angiography. Because of the remodeling process in the development of atherosclerosis, the early stage of plaque formation cannot be detected by coronary angiography (Figs 3.20 and 3.21).

DIMENSIONAL CORRELATION WITH ANGIOGRAPHY

In the 341 normal sites, the lumen diameter ranged from 2.7 to 7.6 mm measured by IVUS, and from 2.6 to 7.3 mm measured by angiography. Linear regression of the lumen dimensions of 100 randomly selected sites was performed. Close correlations can be achieved (see Fig. 3.8).

NORMAL VALUES OF LEFT CORONARY ARTERY

Of the 30 patients without IVUS-detected plaques in the left coronary artery (LCA), 16 patients (8 male, 8 female, ranging in age from 42 to 68 years; 53.6 ± 7.4 years) free of risk factors for coronary artery disease, including systemic hypertension, cigarette smoking, hypercholesterolemia and diabetes mellitus, were adjudged to be truly normal subjects following their negative IVUS examination. The cross-sectional areas of the LMCA, proximal LAD, and mid-LAD at end-diastole (at the beginning of QRS complex) were: 17.33 ± 7.98 mm² (range 9.12–30.71), 13.56 ± 5.85 mm² (range 6.42–26.10), and 9.75 ± 4.67 mm² (range 4.53–22.01), respectively (Table 3.3). Significant differences were found between the maximum areas and the end-diastolic areas.

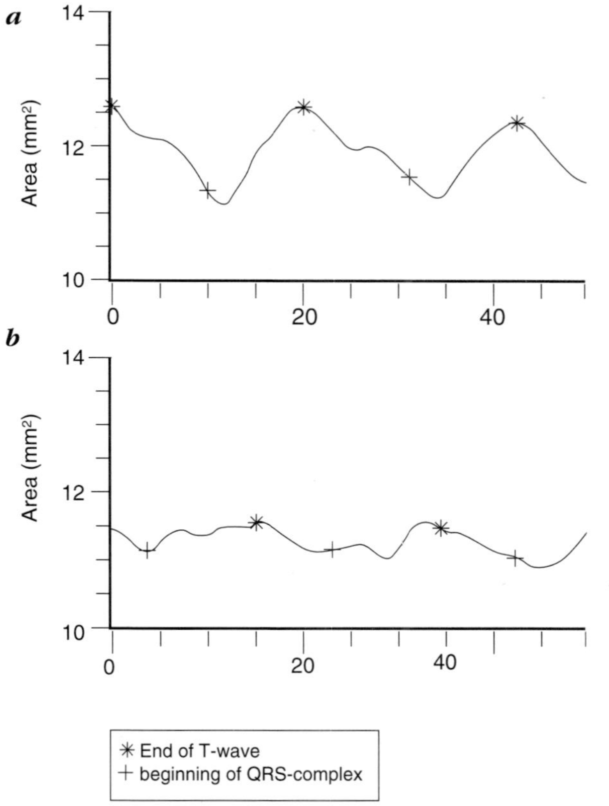

Figure 3.22 *Comparison of the pulsatile variation of the cross-sectional area of a normal (a) coronary artery and a coronary artery with an eccentric plaque (b).*

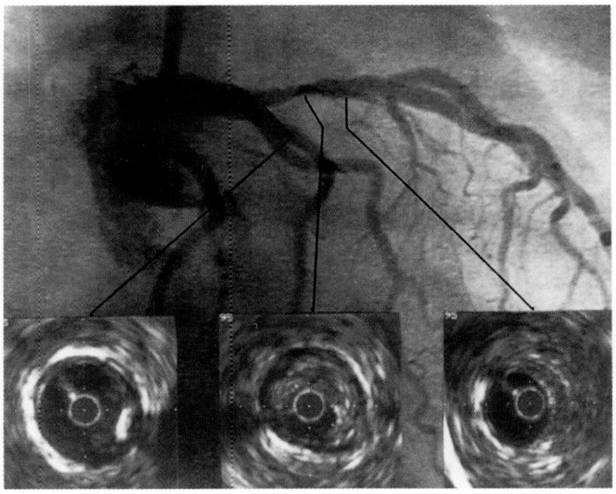

Figure 3.23 *Angiographic view in RAO projection of the left anterior descending coronary artery with an intermediate-type stenosis just distal to a large diagonal side-branch. Stenosis severity by quantitative coronary angiography is only 53%. In contrast, stenosis severity by IVUS amounts to 84% (central IVUS picture). Furthermore, the IVUS examination reveals atherosclerotic involvement proximal and distal to the lesion site.*

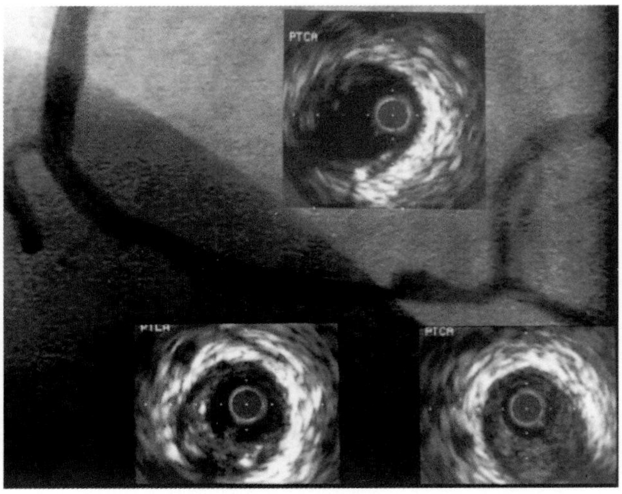

Figure 3.24 *Distal right coronary artery (RCA) with aneurysmatic widening of the coronary artery just proximal to the branching point of the RCA at the crux cordis. Given the IVUS examination, the angiographic picture is misleading. IVUS clearly identifies the lesion as an ulcerated plaque that has been washed out in the course of degeneration. Due to heavy atherosclerotic involvement of the RCA proximally and distally, such a lesion appears as an aneurysm-like structure. Without IVUS, a clear delineation between true and false aneurysms is not possible.*

PULSATILE VARIATION OF THE CROSS-SECTIONAL LUMEN AREA

The pulsatile variations during the cardiac cycle of the normal patients were 10.2 ± 4.0% in the LMCA, 8.3 ± 4.7% in the proximal LAD, and 9.8 ± 4.0% in the mid-LAD. The cross-sectional area changes on 90 consecutive frames incorporating three to five cardiac cycles of the LMCA (A), the proximal LAD (B) and the mid-LAD (C) are shown in Fig. 3.7. The pulsatile variation of 11 patients with plaques was 5.8 ± 3.1%, significantly decreased compared to the normal group ($P < 0.001$) (Fig. 3.22).

AMBIGUOUS LESIONS

Ambiguous lesions are intermediate lesions with unclear stenosis severity judged by coronary angiography. Sometimes the angiographic picture disagrees with the overall clinical picture and the symptoms of the patients. Furthermore, ambiguous lesions relate to unclear morphologic structures that cannot readily be identified by angiography, including ostial lesions and branching vessels. A third category of ambiguous lesions consists of unclear filling defects of haziness of either spontaneous or interventional origin.

INTERMEDIATE LESIONS WITH UNCLEAR STENOSIS SEVERITY

With the use of biplane angiography and multiple projections, it is possible to obtain an angiogram perpendicular to the maximal thickness of the plaque. As mentioned above, good correlation between angiography and IVUS exists concerning the vessel dimensions in normal coronary arteries. However, in diseased coronary arteries, large discrepancies exist between IVUS and angiography.[4] The angiographically 'normal' reference segment is

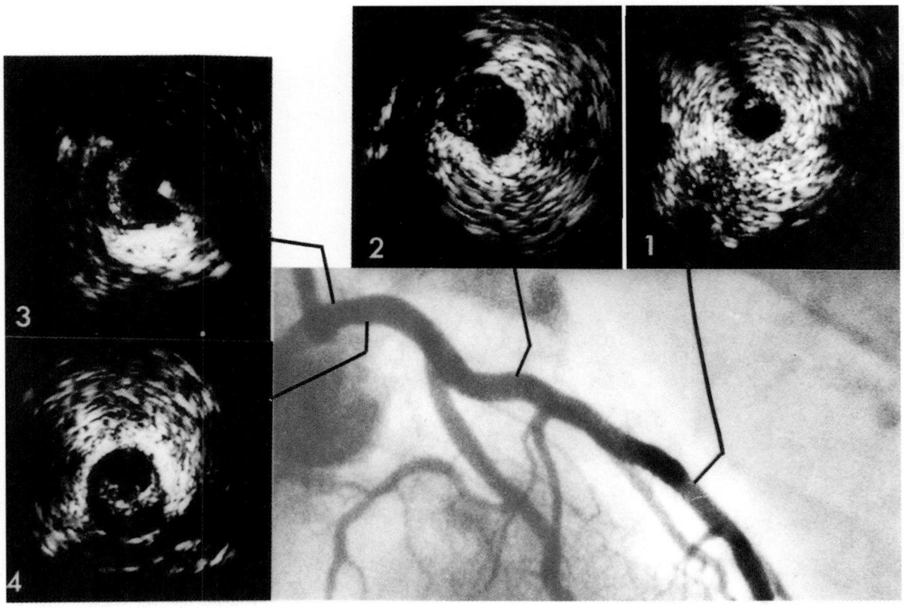

Figure 3.25 *A patient with chest pain comes for diagnostic angiography. No severe lumen reduction is noticed by angiogram, apart from a pressure drop when the catheter was positioned in the left ostium. IVUS shows a severe ostial stenosis (3,4).*

frequently diseased due to plaque involvement.[4,8] Thus, the vessel cross-sectional area of the reference segment measured by angiography might be smaller than that measured by IVUS. These methodological limitations of coronary angiography result in underestimation of the severity of stenosis (Fig. 3.23). In contrast, IVUS directly visualizes the plaque size as well as the eccentricity of the plaque from inside the vessel (Fig. 3.24).

OSTIAL LESIONS

The severity of ostial lesions is normally difficult to assess. First, the mostly rectangular branching of the major coronary arteries from the aorta causes a turbulent flow at the site of the ostia during contrast injection. Such turbulent flow may itself lead to a number of flow-mediated phenomena which hamper the assessment of coronary lesions located adjacent to the ostium. Second, the coronary diagnostic catheter cannot always be positioned in such a way as to provide optimal conditions for contrast medium injection. On the other hand, the catheter may be positioned only adjacent to the coronary ostium without sufficient back-up. In this case, a cloud of contrast medium will blur the picture during contrast injection making the correct diagnosis, especially in the ostial region, difficult. In addition, the catheter may be positioned to some extent within the coronary artery without necessarily causing a significant drop in perfusion pressure. In this case, the luminogram of the first part of the right coronary artery or the left main stem will be governed by the shape of the catheter partially masking the actual coronary lesion. Again, under these circumstances, correct diagnosis can be obtained using IVUS (Fig. 3.25).

VESSEL TORTUOSITY

Vessel tortuosity may be a projection-dependent phenomenon. Whereas in one projection the vessel seems to be extremely tortuous due to foreshortening of the specific projection, usually the rectangular projection will render a clear picture of the lesion site. Such vessel tortuosity may obscure the true severity of the lesion, particularly in type B2 or type C lesions. Vessel tortuosity is also a sign usually encountered in severe and extensive coronary artery disease and a typical sign of long lasting arterial hypertension.

Independent of the nature of the tortuosity, however, the phenomenon makes the estimation of the severity of stenosis extremely difficult from the angiographic image. With additional IVUS examination, the perception of the stenosis becomes much clearer. However, care has to be taken when analyzing the IVUS images. The tortuosity leads inevitably to eccentric positions of the IVUS catheter, giving rise to distorted IVUS images and tangential cross-sections which underestimate stenosis severity. A special problem is the non-uniform rotation which is quite often seen in tortuous vessels due to increased friction during catheter–transducer rotation. Nevertheless, the assessment of plaque burden at the site of the stenosis is far more accurate than with conventional angiography.

UNCLEAR SPONTANEOUS OR POSTINTERVENTIONAL HAZINESS

Haziness is an angiographic phenomenon describing uneven distribution of the contrast in a segment of the coronary angiogram, and is also called a 'ground glass' appearance. Haziness is a rather ambiguous phenomenon, as it does not correlate with any particular pathophysiologic entity. Basically, luminal haziness documents significant flow disturbances causing areas of high and low flow in which contrast medium is unequally distributed. Some of the pathologic findings in the coronary arteries that may also cause some degree of haziness have been mentioned above. Usually, we are concerned with the phenomenon of haziness postinterventionally, when a minor dissection has occurred. These types of dissection are usually of a benign nature, with little propensity to cause acute or subacute vessel closure. In these cases the haziness is caused by turbulent flow due to small intimal tears which are inherent to conventional balloon angioplasty. Nevertheless, as haziness is such a poorly defined entity and largely dependent on the subjective view of the operator, sometimes IVUS may detect major dissections. Based on our experience, the combination of haziness and a suboptimal contrast medium run-off should require subsequent IVUS examination in order to assess the type of dissection properly and to prevent adverse events.

Haziness can sometimes also be encountered during diagnostic angiography. In these cases, interpretation of the findings might be difficult, as no obvious manipulation has preceded the examination. Again, all obstacles that may disturb laminar coronary flow can be responsible. Commonly, spontaneous dissection, or spontaneous plaque ruptures as well as spontaneous thrombus formation, are encountered (Fig. 3.26).

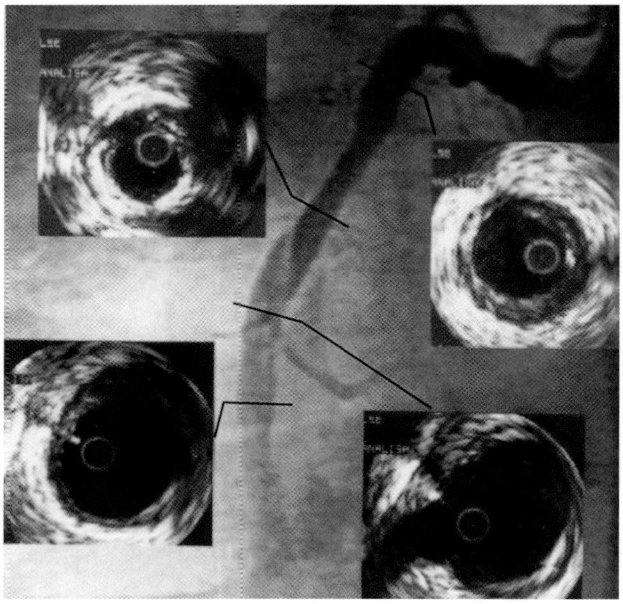

Figure 3.26 *RCA with no severe coronary stenosis. No previous interventional procedure was performed. However, in the mid-part of the RCA the angiographic picture resembles that of a spontaneous dissection. As the patient was symptomatic with angina pectoris under moderate exercise, IVUS examination was performed for further clarification of the lesion. Although angiography showed only minor irregularities of the proximal RCA, IVUS revealed concentric as well as eccentric atherosclerotic plaque along the entire RCA. The degree of atherosclerotic involvement varied significantly. As a consequence, drastic caliber changes occurred, resulting in turbulent flow. Such flow-related phenomena mimicked the picture of a spontaneous dissection in angiography. IVUS helped to find the right diagnosis. No intervention was performed.*

CORONARY SYNDROMES

MYOCARDIAL BRIDGING

A typical systolic compression (concentric or eccentric) with delayed relaxation was found in the bridge segment.[55,56] This compression can be enhanced by intracoronary application of nitroglycerin. Furthermore, a high percentage of plaque formation is found in the segment proximal to the bridge but not within the bridge segment (Fig. 3.27). With computer-assisted automated contour detection, pulsatile variation during the cardiac cycle of the normal segment and bridge segment can be quantified.[55] This shows that the pulsatile variation of the normal segment is 9 ± 7%, while the shape change in the bridge segment is 40 ± 25% (Fig. 3.28). Moreover, the maximal lumen of the bridge segment is seen in mid-diastole rather than in end-systole. Recently, a new

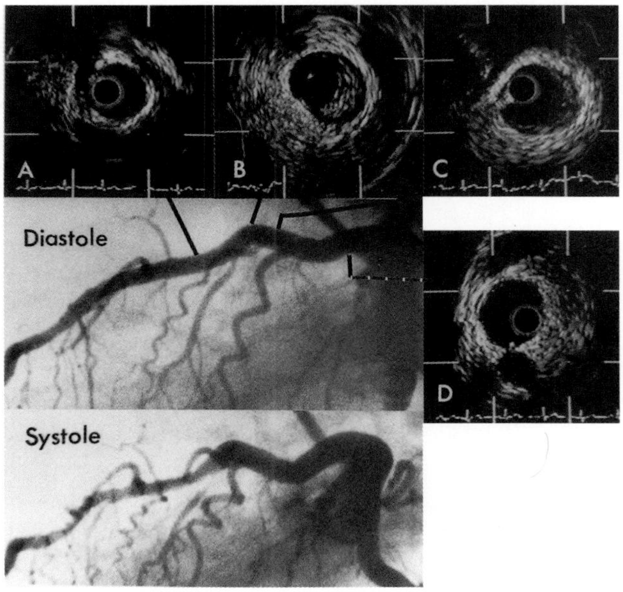

Figure 3.27 *IVUS appearance of the myocardial bridge segment and the LAD. An eccentric plaque formation is visualized in the segment proximal to the bridge (B). No abnormality was documented on angiography. (From Ge et al[55] with permission.)*

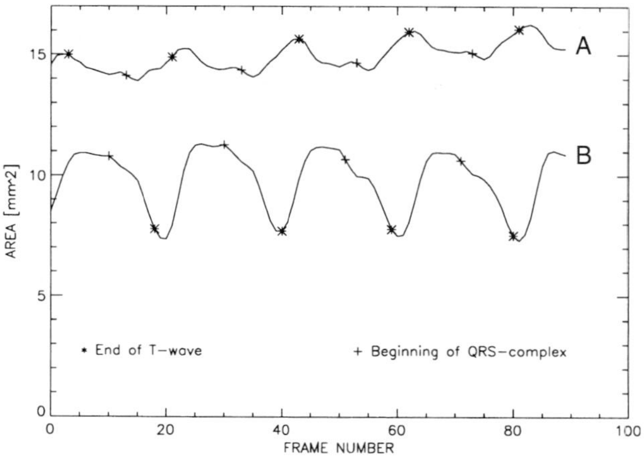

Figure 3.28 *Computer-analyzed cross-sectional area variation of the myocardial bridge during the cardiac cycle: (A) area variation at a normal segment proximal to the bridge segment; (B) area variation of the bridge segment during the cardiac cycle.*

and specific phenomenon has been described by our group in patients with myocardial bridging using IVUS (Fig. 3.29). When this phenomenon exists, myocardial bridging can be diagnosed.

A combined IVUS and double-tip intracoronary pressure measurement indicates that a pressure gradient between the proximal and distal coronary bridging segments exists.[57] A characteristic coronary pressure 'sucking effect' in the bridge segment and a backflow during systole, particularly after nitroglycerin, were found. This indicates that the high incidence of plaque formation in the segment proximal to the bridge might be caused by high wall stress. It explains in part the reason for a myocardial bridging segment distally for 'preventing' atherosclerosis as demonstrated by IVUS[55] and by pathologic examinations, because of the low pressure in the bridge segment and the segment distally.[58]

CORONARY ANEURYSM

Coronary aneurysm is defined as a local coronary artery enlargement with a diameter 1.5 to 2 times larger than that of the adjacent proximal reference

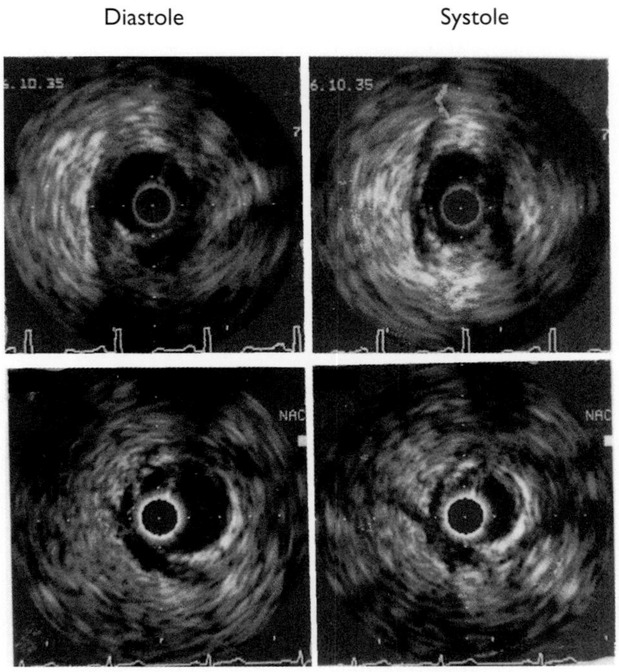

Figure 3.29 *Characteristic appearance of the bridge segment during diastole and systole. A specific 'half moon' phenomenon is seen around the bridge segment.*

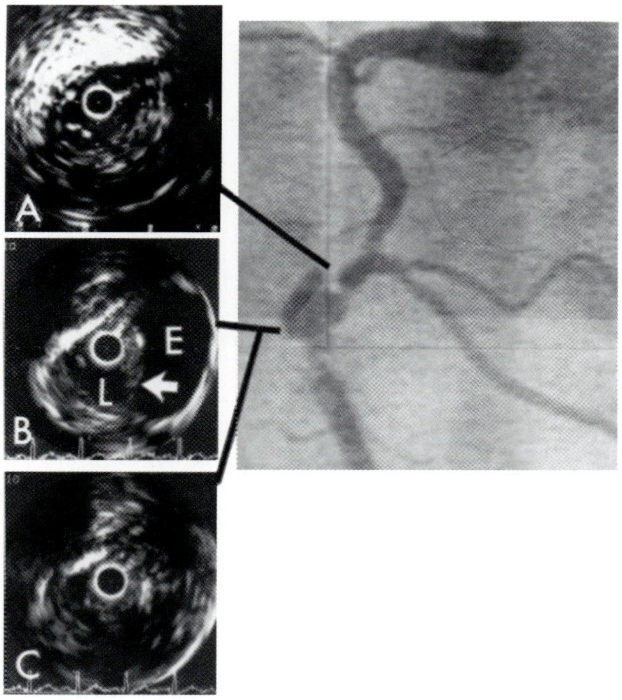

Figure 3.30 *Angiogram and IVUS images of the RCA from a patient. A huge eccentric plaque was found in the proximal reference segment (position A). IVUS showed an emptied plaque (E) at the angiographic aneurysm segment. The emptied plaque is filled with contrast medium when it is injected intracoronarily (position C). Positions B and C indicate the same position before (B) and during (C) the injection of contrast medium. L, lumen. Arrow indicates fibrous cap of the plaque.*

segment.[59,60] An understanding of this syndrome is important because serious complications such as rupture, thrombosis or embolization and even myocardial infarction may occur. As pointed out above, the reference segment is often not normal. Some of the complications may result from pseudoaneurysm (plaque rupture, see below), because coronary angiography is not able to differentiate true aneurysms and pseudoaneurysms, as the arterial wall is not visualized. Recently, this has been confirmed by Gerrand et al, who reported that IVUS identified a pseudoaneurysm following percutaneous transluminal coronary balloon angioplasty (PTCA) which was misdiagnosed as a true aneurysm angiographically.[61] We observed plaque ruptures in 15% of our patients with angiographically defined aneurysms.[52] The ruptured and emptied plaques were misinterpreted using coronary angiography[52] (Fig. 3.30).

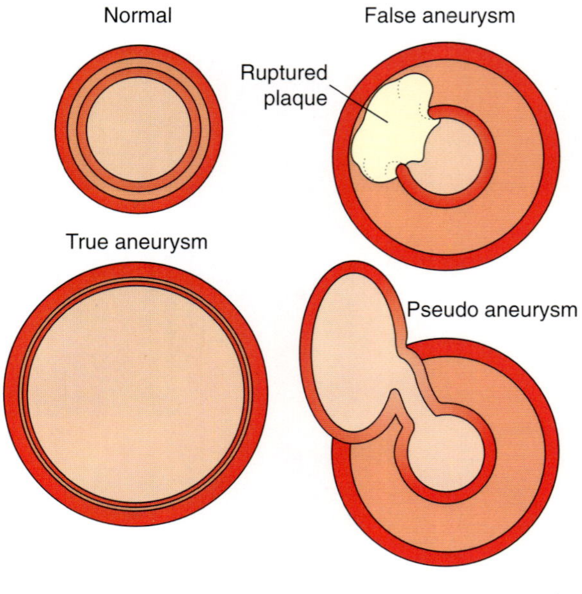

Figure 3.31 *Differentiation of true and false aneurysms by use of IVUS.*

Using IVUS, we proposed the morphologic criteria for differentiation of true and false (plaque rupture) coronary aneurysm shown in Fig. 3.31.

PLAQUE RUPTURE

Pathologic studies have shown that plaque disruption may lead to thrombus formation and can contribute to acute coronary syndromes such as unstable angina, myocardial infarction and sudden death.[62–64] Analysis of coronary arteries in patients who died of ischemic heart disease showed a morphology consistent with previously healed fissures with various stages of thrombus and thrombus organization, suggesting that most fissures probably reseal and incorporate thrombus at the same time but do not produce clinical symptoms.[62] With the use of IVUS, this process can be demonstrated in vivo[65] (Fig. 3.32). Even plaque at risk can be detected with a large lipid core and a thin, fibrous cap.[65] We found that plaques will rupture (plaque at risk) when the fibrous cap is thinner than 0.5 mm and the lipid core/plaque ratio is greater than 20%.[65]

SYNDROME X

For decades, patients with chest pain but with normal coronary angiograms were considered as having

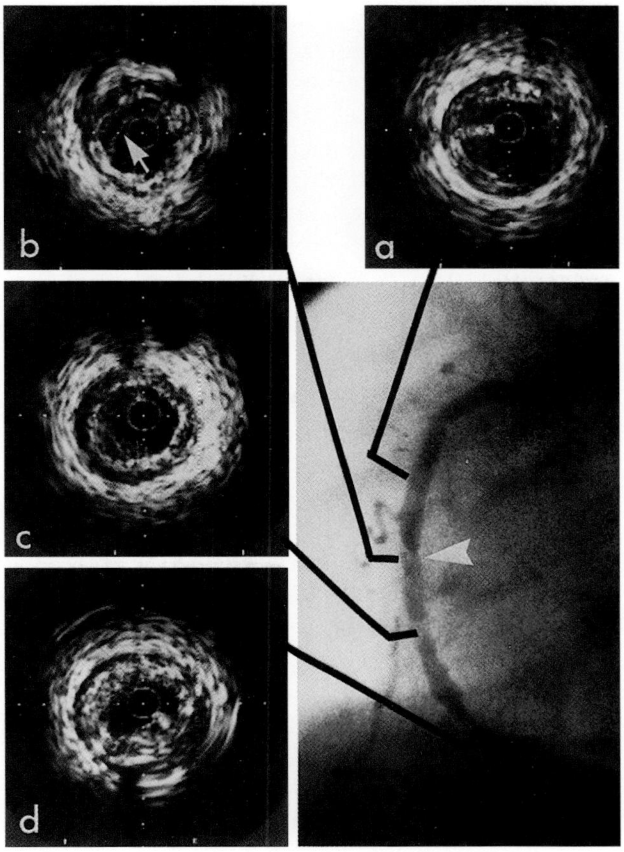

Figure 3.32 *A patient with plaque rupture in the RCA which healed 10 days after, was demonstrated by IVUS.*

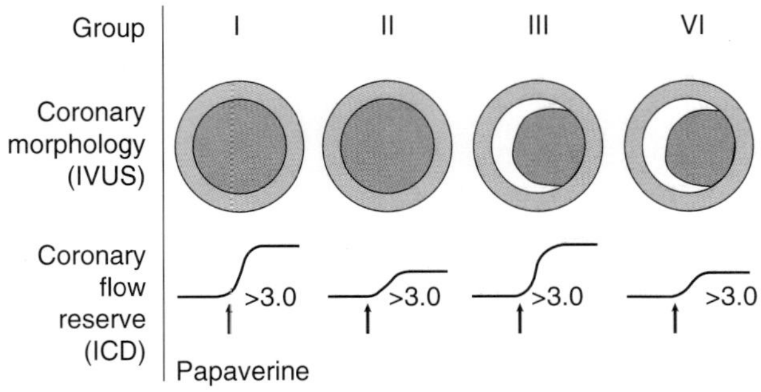

Figure 3.33 *Interpretation of patients with angiographically normal coronary arteries. Only patients with IVUS normal coronary artery but with reduced coronary flow reserve can be considered as having syndrome X (Group II).*

syndrome X. In a group of 55 patients with chest pain and normal coronary angiograms, we found plaque formation in 45%.[52] Most of the plaques (84%) were eccentric and not calcified.[52] Based on the detection of plaque formation by IVUS and reduction of coronary flow reserve by intracoronary Doppler, Erbel et al divided these patients into four groups.[66] Only patients without plaque formation and reduced coronary flow reserve can be considered as having syndrome X (Fig. 3.33). IVUS provides morphological evidence of early signs of atherosclerosis in a large proportion of the patients who were previously considered as having syndrome X. These studies demonstrated that angiography cannot detect the early signs of atherosclerosis and has the large discrepancy in results in patients with syndrome X.[43]

IVUS IN CORONARY INTERVENTIONS

Apart from the diagnostic use in coronary artery disease, the main use of IVUS in cardiology is in coronary interventions. Briefly, its importance can be summarized as follows: (1) assessment of the severity of stenosis; (2) assessment of the plaque morphology and characteristics in order to assist in the selection of appropriate devices; (3) evaluation of the mechanisms of the effects of different devices; (4) guidance of coronary interventions such as further cutting or stenting; (5) evaluation of the result of intervention; and (6) elucidation of the mechanism of restenosis.

For eccentric lesions with huge plaque masses, directional atherectomy should be the optimum procedure. For severe calcified lesions, especially superficial calcification, rotational atherectomy should be selected for elastic plaque or restenotic lesions or dissection after intervention. Stenting is an ideal procedure to prevent restenosis and acute vessel reocclusion. As mentioned above, IVUS is able to identify stable and unstable plaques. If unstable plaques exist, Reo Pro is recommended.

PERCUTANEOUS TRANSLUMINAL CORONARY BALLOON ANGIOPLASTY

Since its introduction by Grüntzig in the late 1970s, percutaneous transluminal coronary balloon angioplasty (PTCA) has had great clinical impact.[67,68] It is today's most commonly used intervention in cardiology and exceeds the number of bypass grafts in many countries. Although acute complications such as flow-limiting coronary artery dissections, acute myocardial infarctions or vessel perforation may occur, PTCA is surprisingly safe if performed by experienced operators.

Mechanisms of PTCA

Despite its widespread use, the mechanisms of PTCA are not well understood. The main reason is that the target of PTCA, the vessel wall and the underlying plaque, cannot be imaged by angiography directly.[69,70] Angiography is a silhouette method and is thus not able to provide sufficient information about the vessel wall. The pioneers of angioplasty in peripheral vessels and the coronary arteries, Dotter, Judkins and Grüntzig, suggested plaque compression or plaque remodeling as the major effect leading to luminal enlargement.[68,71] However, the composition of most coronary plaques, with high amounts of fibrotic or calcified lesions, makes this unlikely to be the predominant mechanism. The reason for the propagation of the compression and remodeling theory was that most of the animal models were based on a lipid-rich diet, leading to relatively soft, lipid-rich plaques with little fibrotic or calcified material.

Postmortem studies have had a tremendous impact on our knowledge and understanding of the PTCA mechanisms. Waller et al showed that fissures, plaque fracture and dissections are the main mechanisms of lumen enlargement after PTCA.[72] Düber et al and Jungbluth et al showed in postmortem cases that most of the PTCA-induced dissections in eccentric lesions occurred at the plaque–vessel conjunction, a region with high shear stress.[73,74] Nevertheless, it is unclear whether postmortem studies in patients who died due to complications after PTCA are representative of the effects of PTCA in all patients.

Definition of prognostic factors and role of IVUS

Because of these fundamental limitations, it is not surprising that a large number of studies have identified a wide range of clinical, anatomic and procedural factors influencing both the acute and the long-term outcome after PTCA.[75–77] One can speculate that a technique providing better evaluation of the acute effects of PTCA on the vessel wall and the underlying plaque would be very helpful in assessing and optimizing the effect of PTCA.[78–80]

In ex vivo studies, Gussenhoven and co-workers evaluated the effects of PTCA on vessel segments by high-frequency IVUS.[81–84] In this experimental study in 250 coronary segments, fissures and dissections were the main mechanisms of luminal enlargement. However, IVUS depicted only 60% of all dissections identified by histology, mainly due to the limitations of IVUS in radial and axial resolution even under optimal ex vivo settings. In almost every case the most severe damage to vessel walls after PTCA was found at the narrowest spot of the vessel segments.

IVUS after PTCA in patients

In clinical studies, various groups have reported findings obtained by IVUS after PTCA. These studies were in concordance concerning the feasibility and the relative safety of the procedure.[85–87] In order to obtain comparable data, the morphologic findings after PTCA were classified with regard to the presence or absence of calcifications, dissections, and symmetry of the lesion. Furthermore, various mechanisms of luminal enlargement after PTCA were identified, such as plaque compression, overextension of the entire vessel segment, subintimal or submedial dissections, and stretching of the disease-free segment of the vessel wall. While in the beginning the IVUS procedures were usually performed predominantly after PTCA, newer studies show the effect of PTCA before and after intervention.[88,89] While some groups just graded the effect of injury as 'superficial' or 'deep', others tried more detailed classifications. Honye et al proposed types A to E1/E2.[85]

Type A:	Radial fissure to intima
Type B:	Radial fissure to media
Type C:	Circular dissection beyond plaque <180°
Type D:	Circular dissection >180°
Type E1:	Concentric lesion, no fissures or flaps
Type E2:	Eccentric lesion, no fissures or flaps

Initially surprising was the fact that even in angiographically successful cases the residual area stenosis after PTCA was in the order of 60%.

Based on the results of Waller et al, Düber Jungbluth et al, Gerber et al described the effects of IVUS after PTCA using a classification of seven subtypes[72–74,86] (Fig. 3.34). The majority of patients had eccentric lesions, and dissections were found in approximately two-thirds of all patients after PTCA (Figs 3.35 and 3.36).

Plaque	Type	Mechanism	
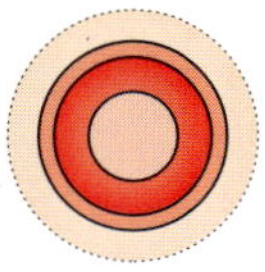 Concentric	1	Vessel stretching and/or plaque compression	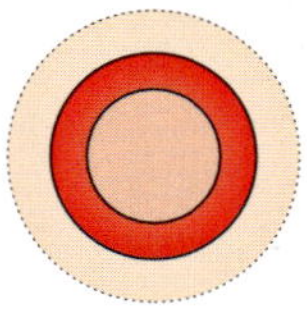
	2	Superficial tear	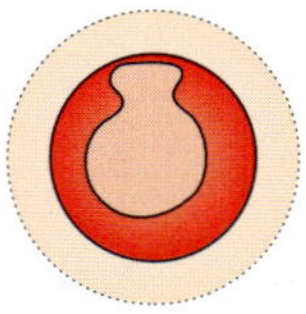
	3	Deep tear	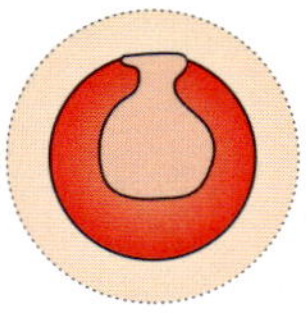
	4a	Subintimal dissection with flap	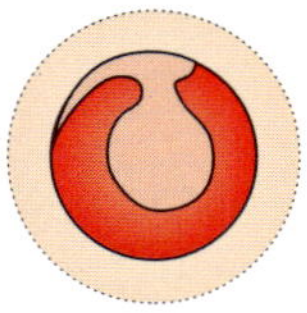
	4b	Submedial dissection with flap	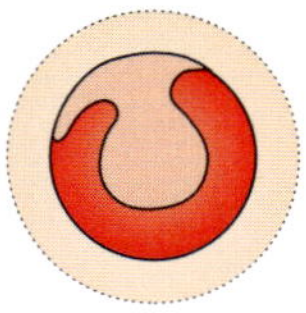

Plaque	Type	Mechanism	
Concentric or eccentric	5	Circular dissection	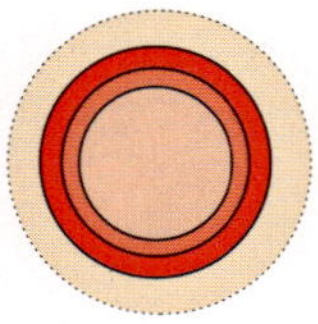
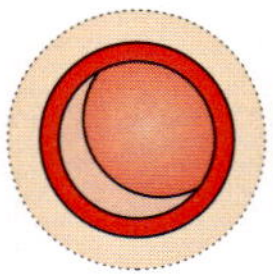	6	Stretching of plaque-free wall	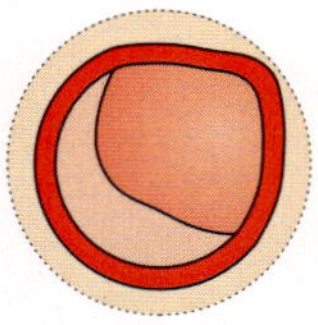
	7a	Subintimal dissection with flap	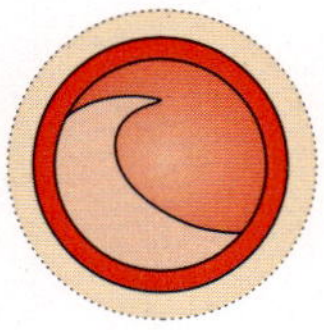
	7b	Submedial dissection with flap	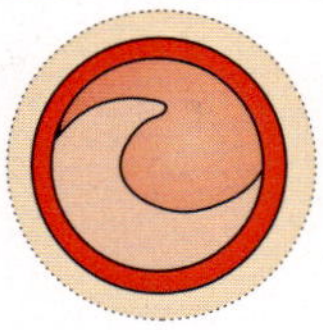

Figure 3.34 *Classification of morphologic effects of PTCA assessed by IVUS proposed by Gerber et al. Types 1–4 indicate concentric plaques; types 6 and 7 indicate eccentric plaques.*

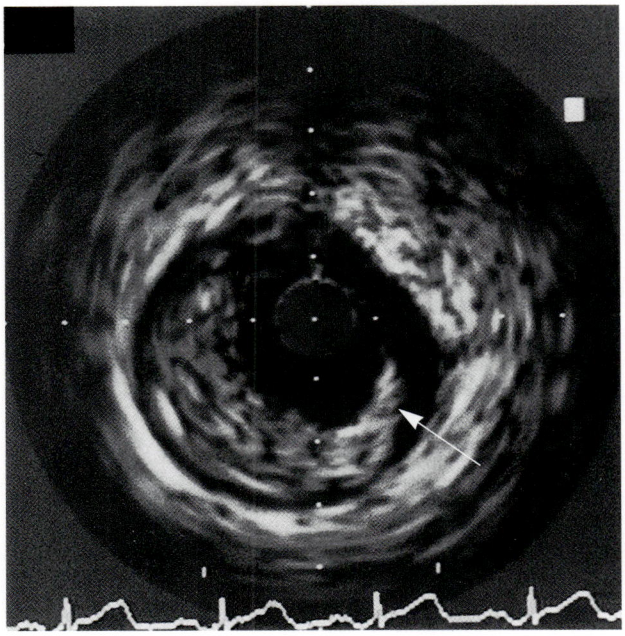

Figure 3.35 *IVUS image after PTCA in an eccentric plaque. A dissection (arrow) is clearly visualized beyond the media (type 7b).*

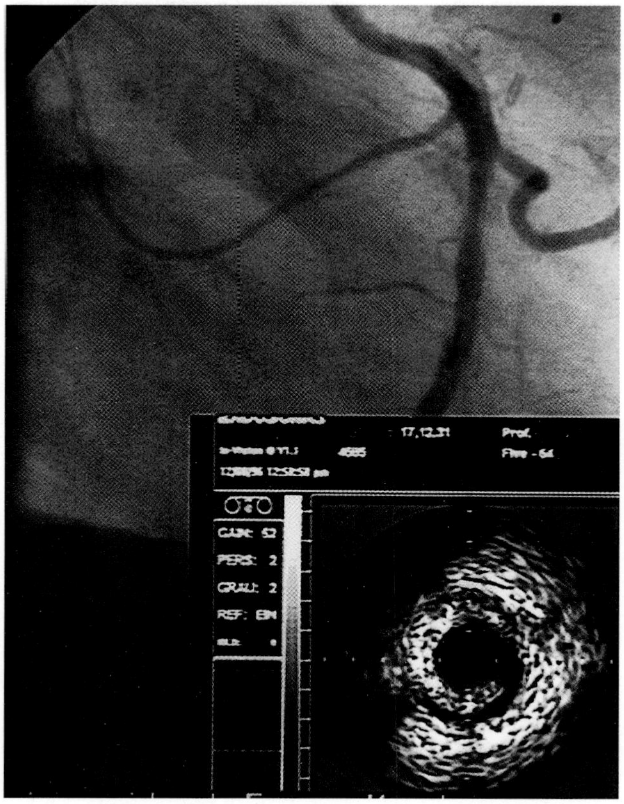

Figure 3.36 *Angiogram and IVUS image of RCA after PTCA. IVUS shows a type 7b dissection but the angiogram shows an optimal result after PTCA.*

Type 1:	Concentric lesion, no trauma
Type 2:	Concentric lesion, superficial fissures
Type 3:	Concentric lesion, deep radial fissures
Type 4:	Concentric lesion, deep dissection with flap extending to (4a) or beyond (4b) the media
Type 5:	Concentric or eccentric lesion with 'circular' dissection, without flap
Type 6:	Overextension of disease-free wall in eccentric lesions
Type 7:	Dissection with flap in eccentric lesions, and extension to (7a) or beyond (7b) the media

Thus, post-PTCA IVUS examinations proved to be effective in showing the effects of PTCA not only on luminal diameters, but also on vessel wall morphology. However, these studies also showed the relative imperfection of present PTCA interventions in terms of residual area stenosis, leaving in many patients a large plaque burden.

Comparison of angiography and IVUS for morphology and luminal dimensions

In patients after PTCA, comparison to quantative coronary angiography (QCA) and to visually assessed angiography-based morphologic classifications showed that the correlation of luminal dimensions between QCA and IVUS and detection of dissections is very poor.

Nakamura et al showed that the differences between QCA and IVUS are more pronounced in more deeply injured vessels in comparison to vessels with only minor vessel wall injuries seen by IVUS. Additionally, IVUS also revealed more dissections than angiography, but probably fewer than expected from ex vivo studies with histology as the gold standard.[24,90]

Serial IVUS studies before and after PTCA

Recently, studies assessing coronary artery lesions before and after PTCA had provided even more insight into the mechanisms of PTCA. Di Mario et al and Baptista et al showed that an increase in total vessel area accounted for over 40% of luminal enlargement.[88,89] Plaque compression was found more frequently in concentric than in eccentric lesions. Kimura et al, using SURE (serial ultrasound analysis of restenosis), also showed that vessel area increases and plaque area decreases acutely after PTCA.[91] All studies addressing the question of post-PTCA IVUS have shown that, even in angiographically successful interventions, the residual area of stenosis is in the range of 55–65%. The question is whether IVUS-guided interventions can improve the outcome of PTCA by reducing the residual plaque burden.

Hodgson et al, for the CLOUT study, reported an increase in post-PTCA luminal diameters when balloon size was determined from the mean value of the IVUS-estimated reference lumen and vessel measurements. This resulted in an upsizing of the balloon diameters in comparison to those selected on the basis of QCA. Complication rates were unchanged in comparison to other studies.[92]

CORONARY STENT

A very effective method for the management of complications during interventions, to prevent recoil after PTCA and to increase minimal luminal diameter in elective procedures, is the use of coronary artery

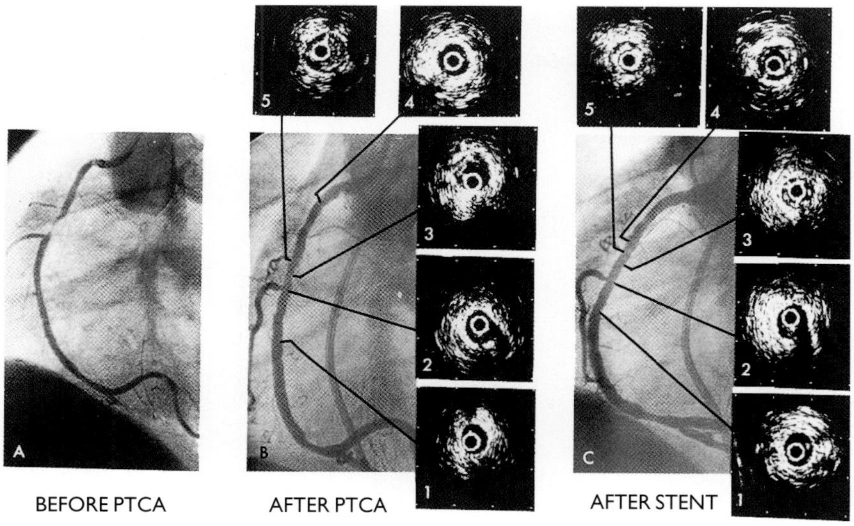

Figure 3.37 *Angiographically successful stent implantation (implantation pressure 6 atm) in 1992. IVUS was performed before and after stent implantation. IVUS shows a 'gap' between stent struts and the vessel wall.*

stents.[93–95] Stenting as an adjunct to recanalization or dilation of vessels was suggested by Dotter in 1969.[96] Puel, from Sigwart's group in Lausanne, implanted the first coronary artery stent in a patient, and Sigwart was the first to report on a larger series of patients with coronary artery stents.[93] However, the acceptability of coronary artery stenting for uses other than bail-out indications in patients with symptomatic dissections was questionable, because patients suffered from a high subacute stent thrombosis rate.[97,98] To limit subacute thrombotic events, patients were treated with elaborated regimes of heparin, warfarin, and aspirin, which resulted in high rates of bleeding complications and prolonged hospitalization.[99]

Role of IVUS in stenting

The reason for these complications was mainly incomplete stent expansion. Because most stents are almost radiolucent, complete stent expansion cannot be assessed by angiography techniques in sufficient detail.[100] Therefore, IVUS seems to be the ideal adjunct to angiography in patients after stenting, and the first studies were done mainly in the peripheral circulation.[101,102] Although many workers observed incomplete stent expansion and asymmetric stent geometry,[103] no negative consequences were reported for patients with stents in their peripheral circulation.[104] It was Colombo who pointed out the logical consequences of incomplete stent expansion seen by IVUS in the coronary circulation. He inaugurated the high-pressure coronary artery stent deployment and proved its effectiveness.[105–107] As a consequence, high-pressure coronary artery stent deployment is now the standard procedure and provided a breakthrough in coronary artery stenting (Figs 3.37 and 3.38). When it is used in conjunction with

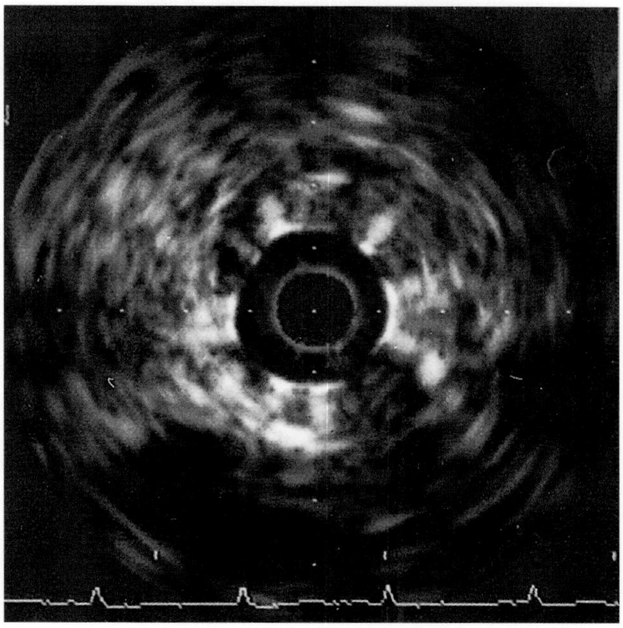

Figure 3.38 *IVUS image of a Palmaz–Schatz stent after high-pressure implantation. The stent struts are characterized by bright echoes with acoustic reverberation. Stent struts are optimally expanded.*

ticlopidine, subacute thrombosis and bleeding complications can be reduced to 1% or even less.[108,109]

Serial IVUS images during stent implantation have confirmed the value of high-pressure stent deployment, requiring sometimes 20 atm or more to achieve complete stent expansion.[106,108–110] In comparison to conventional techniques, this approach led to an almost 100% increase of the post-procedural coronary minimal luminal areas.[111] The overestimation of luminal dimensions by QCA found after low-pressure coronary artery stent deployment was caused by contrast filling of gaps between the outer stent border and the inner luminal margin (Fig. 3.37). With the use of high-pressure stent deployment, this systematic overestimation can be avoided.[20,112]

IVUS can more precisely than angiography reveal the action of coronary artery stents in attaching dissection membranes and ensure that the entire length of the dissection is covered by the stent. In a recent study, IVUS revealed incomplete or suboptimal stent expansion in 80% of cases, and even after the application of high-pressure stent deployment, forty per cent of patients still had abnormal IVUS findings.[113] It is unclear whether the prognosis of these patients is different from those of patients with symmetric stent expansion. However, beneficial results with high-pressure stent deployment, but without IVUS, have been reported. Nevertheless, IVUS-guided implantation results in larger luminal diameters in comparison to angiographically guided stent implantation.[108,109,114]

The consequences of IVUS-guided stent deployment for long-term prognosis are not clear and will be addressed in ongoing trials. IVUS will most likely have a place in the future in all complicated stent deployments (long lesions, diffuse disease, inconclusive angiographic results, very proximal or side-branch implantation) and during follow-up studies to reveal the amount of intimal hyperplasia within the stent.

IVUS in stent restenosis

Stent restenosis and the assessment of PTCA in stent restenosis can be best evaluated by IVUS. The main process of stent restenosis is intimal hyperplasia within the stent and in the adjacent coronary artery segments (Fig. 3.39). Stent recoil plays no significant role, at least not in stents of the Palmaz–Schatz type.[115,116]

Preliminary results show that PTCA in stent restenosis does not achieve the initial luminal dimensions in all patients.[117–119] In these cases, IVUS may help to guide other interventions instead of, or as adjuncts to, PTCA.

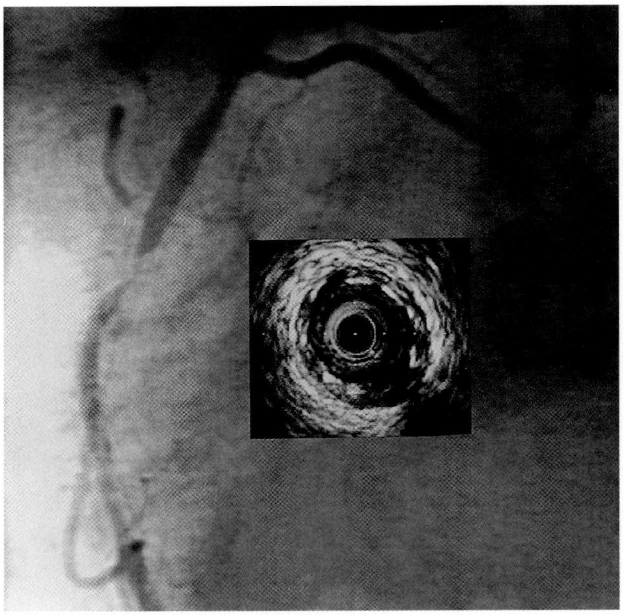

Figure 3.39 *Angiographic restenosis after stenting. IVUS shows that the stent was optimally expanded. The reason for restenosis is intimal hyperplasia, and coronary angiography is not able to address the question of whether restenosis is due to recoil or intimal hyperplasia.*

ROTATIONAL ATHERECTOMY

High-frequency rotational angioplasty (HFRA), also called high-speed rotational atherectomy, ablates and pulverizes non-compliant coronary plaque material by high-frequency rotation of a diamond-coated burr. It is usually used for coronary recanalization in total or subtotal occlusion and subsequently combined with other interventional procedures to achieve optimal results. Because the maximum burr size used is 2.5 mm in diameter, this is sometimes not enough for proximal epicardial coronary arteries. Recently it has usually been used for debulking of the plaque material with subsequent PTCA and stenting. Studies have shown that the mechanism of PTCA mainly involves plaque breaks or dissections, especially in calcified plaques, to create a wider lumen.[85,120,121] HFRA, however, is by pulverizing plaque materials to create a wide lumen.[122]

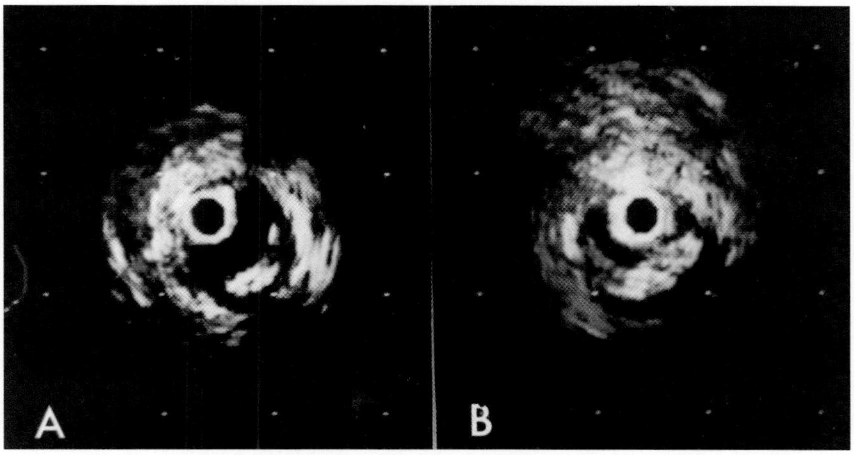

Figure 3.40 *IVUS images of two patients with superficial calcification of the plaques. Dissection is seen at the edge of the calcified plaque after PTCA.*

Morphologic observations

Coronary angiography is usually not able to detect the effects of coronary interventions. We compared a group of patients who underwent PTCA and HFRA using IVUS in comparison with angiography and found patients with HFRA only seldom have intimal dissections. The postintervention consequences of the plaques are closely related to their characters.[123] IVUS studies have shown that the vessel lumen after HRFA is usually circular and symmetric, and has a smooth surface without intimal dissection.[123,124] In severe calcified lesions, PTCA normally results in intimal dissection at the junction of calcium and fibrotic plaque, as described by Fitzgerald.[125] Figure 3.40 shows typical examples of post-PTCA dissection in calcified plaques. Even in severe superficial plaque, PTCA only creates small breaks in the plaque surface to increase the lumen, which presents a normal angiographically hazy appearance. In patients who have undergone HFRA, after subsequent PTCA the incidence of intimal dissection increases. One possible reason might be the damage to the integrity of the intima by HFRA. Therefore, PTCA should be carried out under lower pressure post-HFRA. Figure 3.41 shows a patient after HFRA and subsequent PTCA. A large intimal dissection is seen by IVUS which is not detected by coronary angiography. Figure 3.42 shows another patient after HFRA and subsequent PTCA. Coronary angiography shows haziness in the intervention segment. IVUS demonstrated plaque breaks (tear) in the intervention segment.

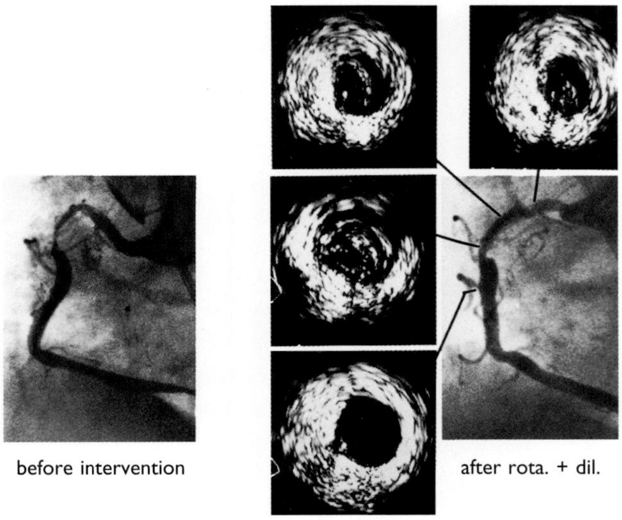

Figure 3.41 *Coronary angiograms before (left) and after (right) interventions. After HFRA and subsequent PTCA, a big intimal dissection is seen on IVUS which is not detected by coronary angiography.*

Decision-making

Coronary angiography, a contour technique, provides only the silhouette of the lumen, and gives little information on the wall or the plaque characteristics. It is not a sensible method for the detection of calcium deposits and cannot distinguish between superficial and deep calcification. Figure 3.43 shows a patient with unstable angina who presented for coronary intervention. Contrast coronary angiography shows a subtotal stenosis of the ostium of the left circumflex

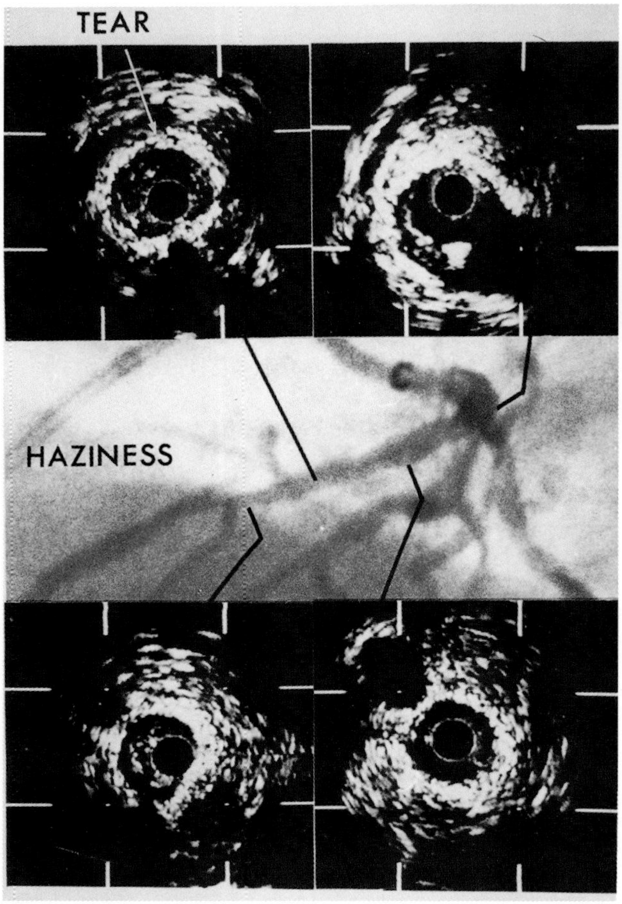

Figure 3.42 *Angiographic haziness in a patient after HFRA and subsequent PTCA. IVUS visualized multiple tears of the plaque which explain the angiographic haziness.*

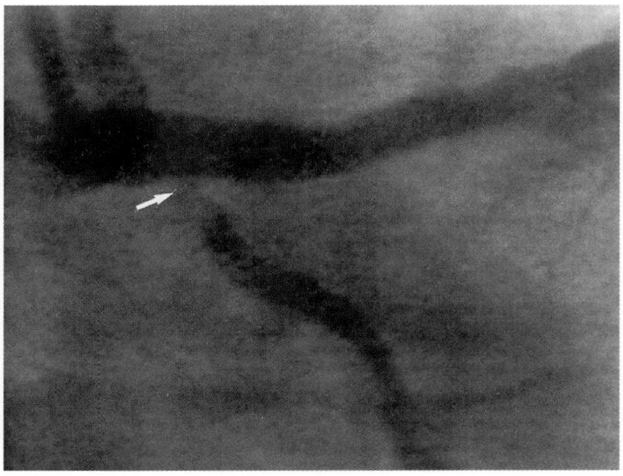

Figure 3.43 *A patient with unstable angina who presented for diagnostic angiography. Coronary angiography shows a subtotal occlusion of the ostium of the left circumflex coronary artery which needs intervention.*

which is suitable for directional coronary atherectomy. IVUS was performed before coronary intervention. A severe circular calcified plaque with severe stenosis is visualized (Fig. 3.44A). The patient developed severe chest pain during the IVUS examination because of the severe stenosis. Based on the IVUS images, HFRA was selected for debulking the plaque. After rotablation with 1.25-mm and 1.75-mm burrs, IVUS shows that the superficial calcium was partly ablated, leaving a good lumen but still a significant stenosis (Fig. 3.44B). Excellent results were achieved

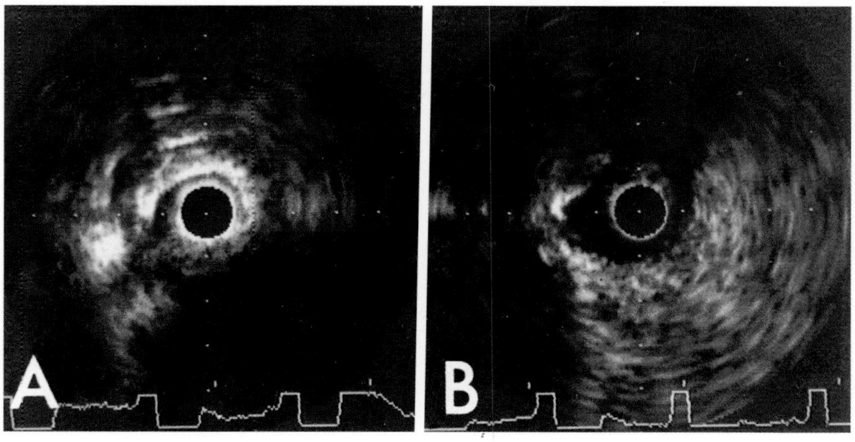

Figure 3.44 *IVUS images of the patient shown in Fig. 3.42 before (A) and after (B) HFRA. A severe superficial calcification of the plaque was found. Based on the IVUS finding, HFRA was performed using 1.25-mm and 1.75-mm burrs. (B) shows an optimal plaque debulking after HFRA.*

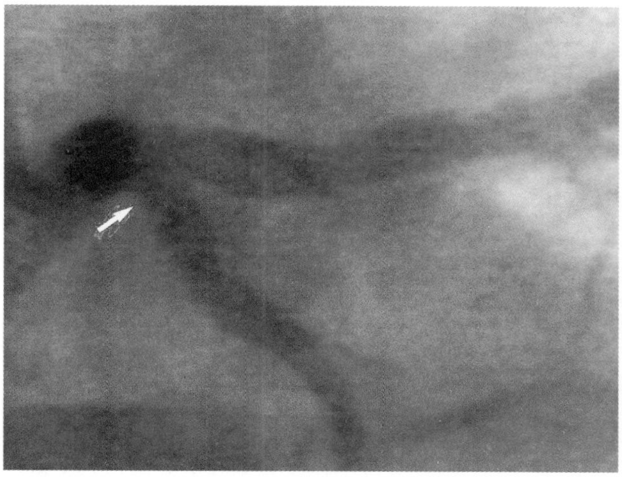

Figure 3.45 *The same patient as shown in Figs 3.43 and 3.44. After HFRA, subsequent stenting was performed with an excellent result.*

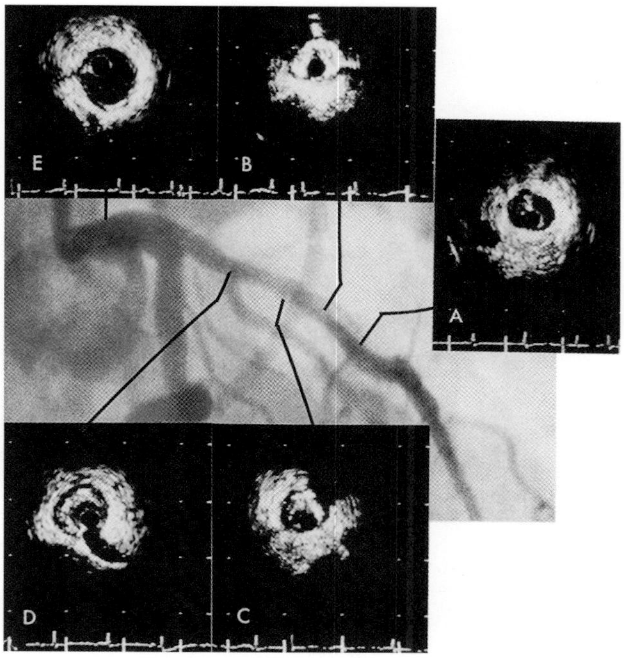

Figure 3.46 *A severe calcified stenosis of the LAD. After PTCA, IVUS shows that only two small cracks (B) were made by the balloon. No adequate improvement of the vessel lumen. HFRA should have been better in this situation.*

with subsequent PTCA and stenting (Fig. 3.45). If it had only been based on coronary angiography, directional coronary atherectomy could not have obtained an optimal result, because of the severe superficial calcification.

Figure 3.46 shows a patient after PTCA with suboptimal result. IVUS was performed after intervention and shows that only a small crack occurred in the middle of the severely calcified plaque. The superficial calcium deposit shows no change. The widened lumen is created by small cracks without substantial improvement of the vessel lumen. In the case of deep calcification with soft plaque over it (Fig. 3.47), HFRA might be of little help. An optimal result was achieved with PTCA alone (Fig. 3.47).

Therefore, it is very important to perform IVUS not only after intervention, for evaluating the results of coronary interventions, but also before intervention, to guide the selection of proper interventional procedures.

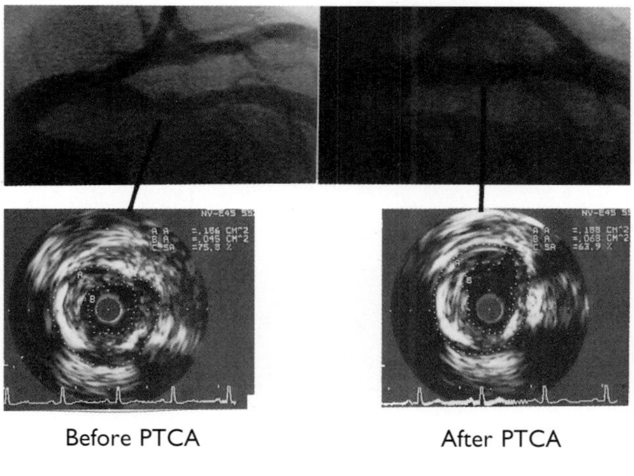

Figure 3.47 *Coronary angiograms and IVUS images of a patient with severe LAD stenosis. IVUS shows that only deep calcification exists. Conventional PTCA was performed with a good result.*

OTHERS

Directional atherectomy (DCA)

As mentioned above, IVUS is very useful in the guidance of DCA. Previous studies (CAVEAT, CCAT) using coronary angiography comparing PTCA and DCA with respect to success and restenosis have

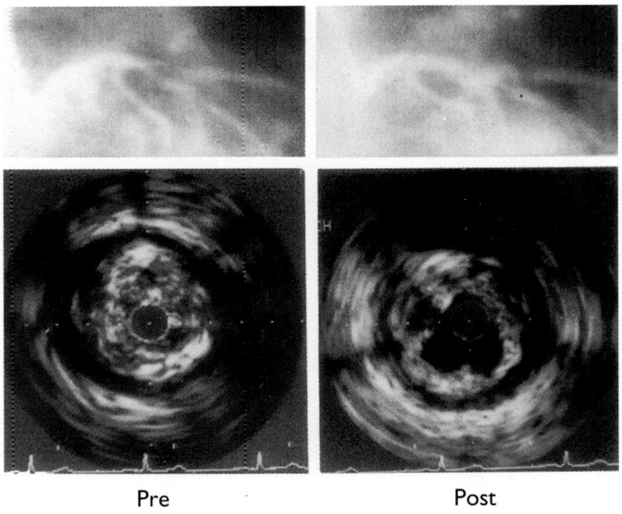

Figure 3.48 *Angiogram and IVUS image of a patient with restenosis of the LAD before and after directional coronary atherectomy. The angiogram shows a successful result (upper panel). IVUS shows that only several pieces of the plaque were cut. A severe residual plaque burden is still visualized.*

shown few differences.[126,127] However, as we know, coronary angiography tells us nothing concerning the residual plaque burden, because of the remodeling process. Figures 3.48 and 3.49 show the angiograms and IVUS images of a patient before and after angiography. Although the angiogram indicates successful atherectomy, IVUS shows a significant residual plaque burden. This might help to explain why there is such a high restenosis rate in patients after DCA, as the residual plaque burden is closely correlated with restenosis. Recent studies such as OARS (Optimal Atherectomy Restenosis Study) and BOAT (Balloon versus Optimal Atherectomy Trial) using IVUS guidance to remove maximal plaque burden demonstrated no increase in complications with aggressive debulking via IVUS guidance.[128,129]

Laser angioplasty

The importance of IVUS in laser angioplasty is not as great as in the interventional procedures mentioned above because of the implications of this technique. Laser angioplasty today is conventionally to ablate inorganic material by front-firing, UV laser light. The effect of laser angioplasty is concentric tracking over the guidewire. It would be ideal to use IVUS to guide this procedure. However, this technique is suitable to recanalize very tight lesions. Therefore, IVUS is frequently not able to cross the stenosis and has, hitherto, not played an important role in guidance of the procedure before intervention. Nevertheless, it is still useful in evaluating the result and mechanisms.[130,131] of laser angioplasty and to guide further interventional procedures (Fig. 3.50).

Ultrasound angioplasty

Ultrasound angioplasty is introduced as a new, alternative technique in interventional cardiology. The

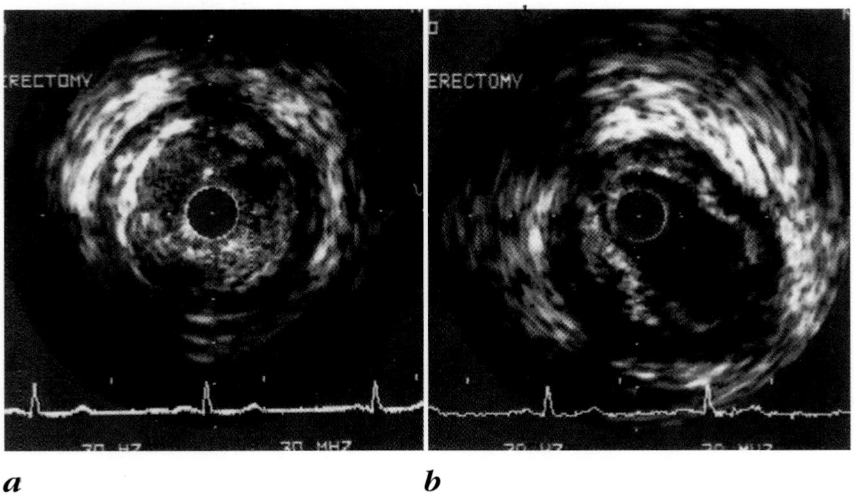

Figure 3.49 *IVUS images of a patient before (a) and after (b) directional coronary atherectomy. IVUS shows a huge residual plaque burden even though the angiogram shows a successful intervention.*

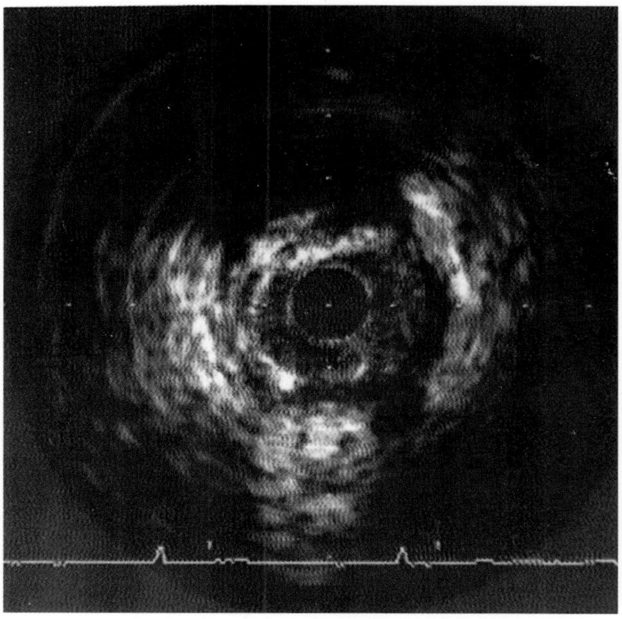

Figure 3.50 *IVUS image of a patient with chronic occlusion of the LAD after successful recanalization with a laser guidewire, and additional excimer laser angioplasty. Multiple breaks with an uneven surface can be visualized.*

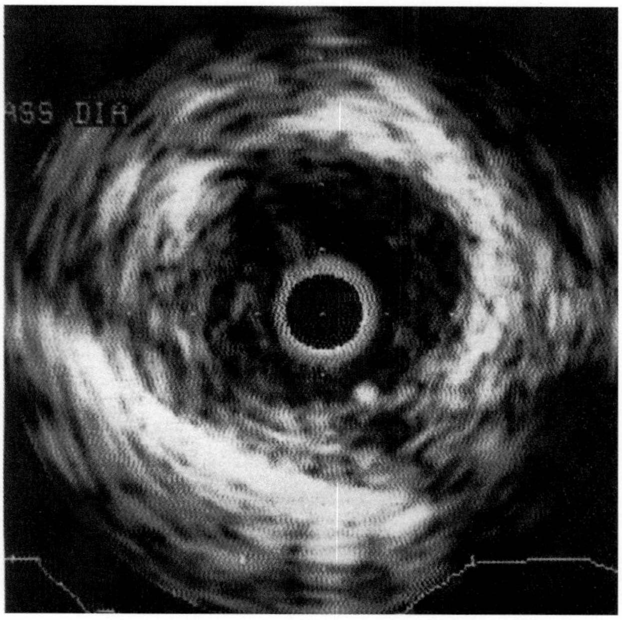

Figure 3.51 *IVUS images of a patient after successful ultrasound angioplasty of a vein graft occlusion. There is an irregular borderline between lumen and plaque. Ultrasound angioplasty was unable to eliminate these organized structures, which are probably composed of fibroblasts and interconnective matrix. On the other hand, it apparently shows a different appearance of this approach in comparison to other interventional procedures.*

Seigel group and the Rosenschein group contributed to the development of the technique and the initial use of it.[132,133] It is claimed that this technique is suitable in heavily calcified lesions to soften the plaque, and suitable in total vessel occlusion. Figure 3.51 shows a patient with severe coronary artery disease after ultrasound angioplasty.

BYPASS GRAFT

NORMAL VEIN GRAFT

A vein graft segment with a regular lumen and without obvious intimal thickening is considered ultrasonically normal. The typical appearance of a normal vein graft is of a thin-walled vessel on real-time IVUS imaging. The vessel wall gives a relatively homogeneous echogenic image with an absence of echo reflectance within the vessel lumen. In normal vein grafts, the three-layer appearance is rare. If there is a typical three-layer structure in IVUS imaging, it may imply the existence of intimal thickening, as suggested by histologic studies.[134] There is no obvious pulsatile variation during the cardiac cycle. Extravascular structures (possibly pericardium) can be commonly visualized as highly echogenic tissues. Figures 3.52 and 3.53 are examples of IVUS images of the normal saphenous vein. There is no intimal thickening or plaque formation.

DISEASED VEIN GRAFT

A segment showing eccentric or concentric atherosclerotic plaque is considered diseased. IVUS can show the pathologic changes of chronically implanted vein graft morphology, including intimal proliferation and atherosclerosis. The atherosclerosis in vein grafts may have the same manifestations as

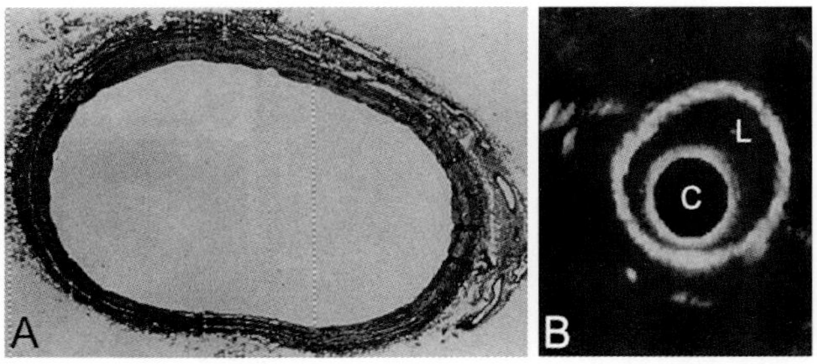

Figure 3.52 *Comparison between IVUS and histologic findings. Histologic cross-sectional view (A) of a freshly harvested saphenous vein (stained with Verhoeff–van Gieson stain, magnification ×6.25). A normal thin-walled vein with a widely patent lumen is demonstrated. The dark black fibers represent elastin, which accounts for the bright echogenic appearance on IVUS imaging (B). Note the absence of echo reflectance within the vessel lumen (From Willard et al[134] with permission.) C, IVUS catheter, L, vessel lumen.*

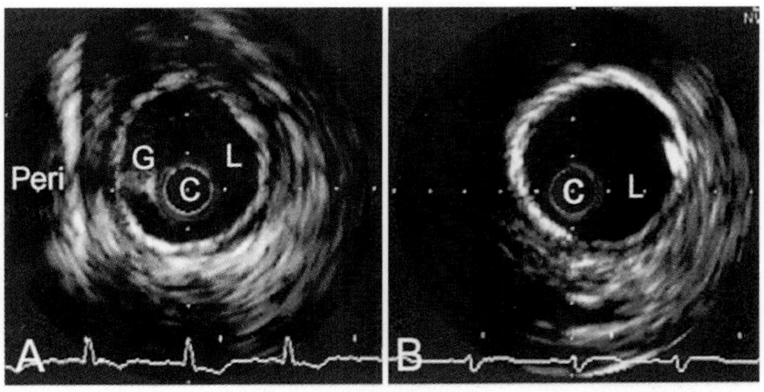

Figure 3.53 *These two cross-sectional images from one saphenous vein graft were found to be normal by angiography. The bypass operation was performed 4 years ago. (A) Large vessel with a regular lumen free of plaque. The vein wall is echogenically strong although it is not thick. The vessel wall cannot be divided into three layers with IVUS imaging. (B) The vein wall is very strongly echogenic from 7 o'clock to 3 o'clock. C, IVUS catheter; L, lumen; G, guidewire; Peri, assumed to be the pericardium.*

seen in the development of coronary artery atherosclerosis. Atheromatous tissue can be characterized according to the following four categories:

1. Soft plaque, when the echo reflectance of the atheroma is lower than that of the adventitia, including: (a) loose and cellular fibrous tissue—medium or low echo reflections in the atheroma; (b) lipid—extremely low echo reflectance or an echolucent space that is usually surrounded by echodense regions or fibrous cap (see below).
2. Fibrous plaque, when the echo reflectance of the plaque is as strong as that of the adventitia, including: (a) fibrous cap—intense ultrasound reflectance at the lumen surface of the atheroma with 'softer' echoes behind, indicating densely packed tissue high in collagen content; (b) dense fibrous tissue—highly echogenic intense ultrasound reflectance without deep acoustic shadows.
3. Calcium deposit—intense echo reflections with clearly defined acoustic shadows.
4. Thrombus—speckled low and medium echo reflectance at the surface of the atheroma plaque, conclusively identified when mobility of the thrombus is present.

In the subgroup of patients undergoing vein graft angioplasty, IVUS shows that soft plaques are

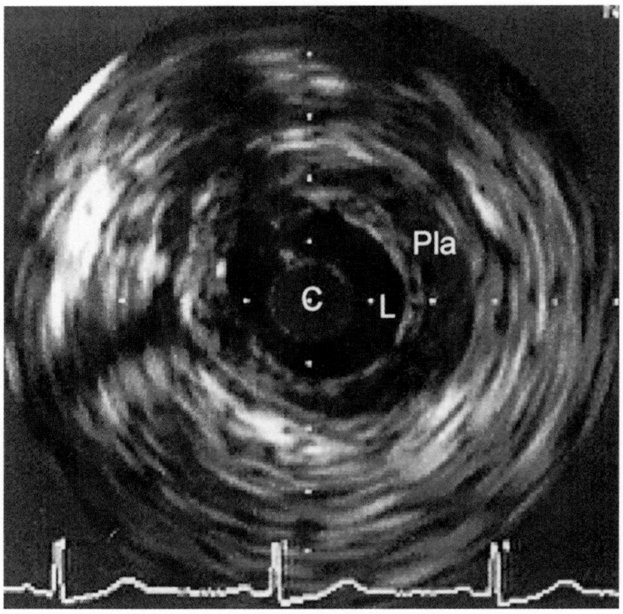

Figure 3.54 *IVUS imaging shows a diseased saphenous vein graft with a small eccentric soft plaque (Pla) occupying less than 20% of the lumen. The soft plaque is characterized by an echo signal intensity lower than that of the adventitia. In this image the plaque is homogeneous, without calcium deposits. C, IVUS catheter; L, lumen.*

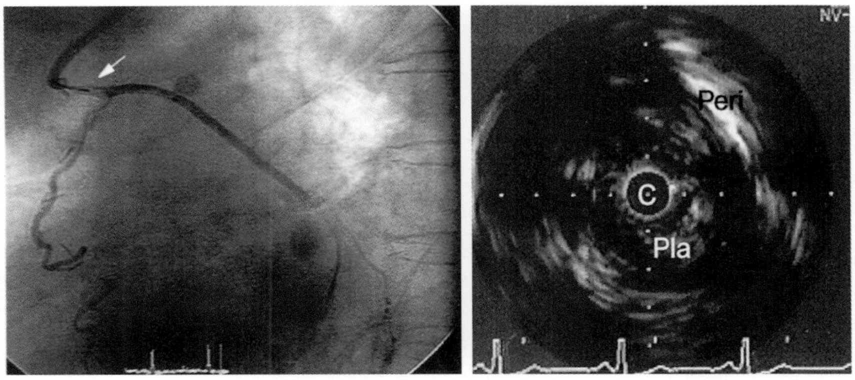

Figure 3.55 *This is an advanced plaque in venous grafts (8 years after bypass operation). The lesion is concentric with soft and fibrous compositions. C, IVUS catheter; L, lumen; Pla, plaque.*

common but calcified plaques are infrequent. Plaque ulceration or rupture is frequently detected, often complicated by thrombosis. In such circumstances, prompt intervention is indicated. IVUS can provide exact information on the lesion and guide appropriate angioplastic approaches. Figures 3.54 to 3.57 illustrate the manifestations and clinical uses of IVUS imaging in the case of diseased saphenous vein grafts. The abnormalities of saphenous vein grafts demonstrated by IVUS are: intimal thickening; early plaque formation (Fig. 3.54); advanced plaques (Fig. 3.55); special manifestations such as spontaneous plaque rupture (Fig. 3.56); and rupture complicated by thrombus (Fig. 3.57).

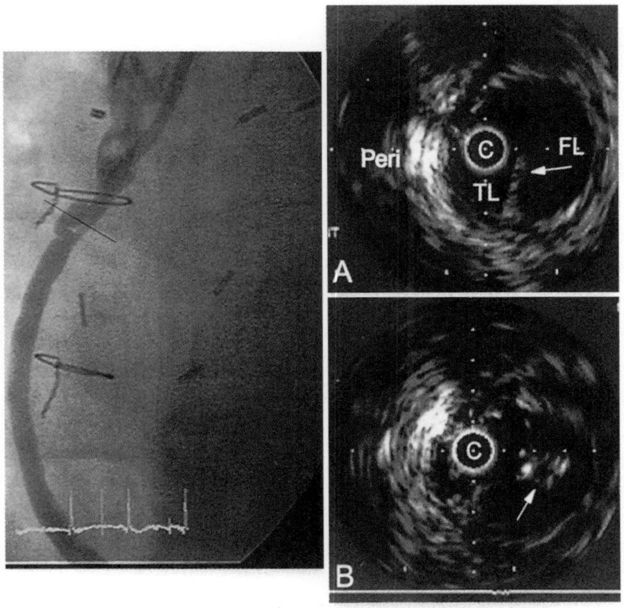

Figure 3.56 *This is a case of spontaneous plaque rupture in a saphenous vein bypass to the right coronary artery. The patient had the bypass 4 years ago and he recently suffered from unstable angina. Angiography indicated an ambiguous lesion in the proximal segment of the vein graft. IVUS images demonstrated a spontaneous plaque rupture. (A) A large vein graft with plaque formation: the plaque has a rupture and most of the content within the plaque has been washed away, leaving a thin plaque cap (arrow) and a huge false lumen (FL). (B) The image during contrast medium injection into the bypass. Contrast medium appears in the false lumen (arrow). C, IVUS catheter; TL, true lumen; FL, false lumen; Peri, pericardium.*

TRANSPLANT

Although the survival after heart transplantation has improved over the last decade,[135] rejection and infection are still thought to influence early survival. Nevertheless, the major cause of late death is the development of cardiac allograft vasculopathy, which is manifested as an accelerated form of coronary atherosclerosis.[136] The incidence of this vasculopathy has been reported to range from 5% to 25% at 1 year and from 50% to 60% at 5 years, resulting in up to 30% of late allograft failures.[137,138] The absence of afferent autonomic innervation results in allograft recipients being unable to experience classic symptoms of ischemia; as a result, the onset of allograft vasculopathy is frequently silent. Coronary angiography is not able to detect the early signs of vasculopathy. Moreover, there is no method available for the assessment of coronary perfusion.

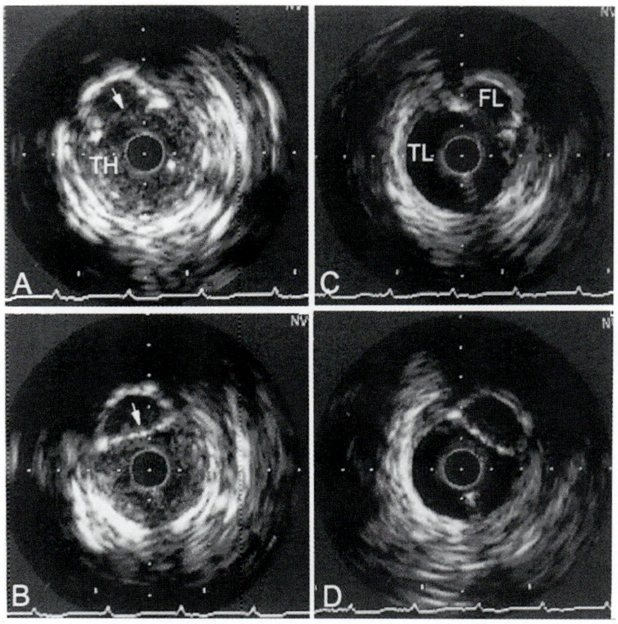

Figure 3.57 *The serial images illustrate a case of spontaneous plaque rupture complicated by thrombosis in the vein grafts and subsequently treated with balloon angioplasty. The patient had saphenous vein bypass grafts 15 years ago. He had angina pectoris in the grade between CCS III and VI. Angiography found a high-grade stenosis in the middle segment of the vein graft to the right coronary artery. IVUS shows a high-grade obstructive lesion. Furthermore, careful study of the images shows that there is a small, eccentric, ruptured plaque. The small plaque has a thin cap and a false lumen (FL). (A) and (B) are images before intervention. (C) and (D) are images after 4-mm balloon dilation. (A) shows a wide opening of the plaque into the vessel lumen (arrow). A bloodflow signal is seen in the false lumen (FL). At both sides of the opening there are calcium deposits. Around the IVUS catheter (C) is speckled material, which is assumed to be thrombus (TH). In the false lumen some speckled reflection can be seen. (B) Shows the image of the same lesion at a site slightly proximal to the opening. The plaque is the same shape but with a complete cap (arrow) on the surface side towards the lumen. No opening can be detected in the cap from this section. (C) The image after 4-mm balloon dilation at the same section as in (A). The speckled materials are almost all gone, which indicates that this is most probably a case of thrombosis after plaque rupture. Both the false lumen and the true lumen are free of thrombus. (D) The image at the same section of (B). The thin cap of the plaque is still the same as seen in (B), suggesting a cap with dense fibrous tissue. TL, true lumen; FL, false lumen; TH, thrombus.*

Whether the coronary atherosclerotic process is the continuation of the preexisting atherosclerotic lesions from the donor or a new onset which occurs after operation in the recipients remains unknown. Combining IVUS and Doppler flow mapping may provide detailed information concerning coronary morphology and function in evaluation of heart transplantation.

ALLOGRAFT CORONARY VASCULOPATHY

The Stanford group has studied patients serially after heart transplantation with coronary angiography and IVUS and found that intimal thickness was significantly increased at over baseline 1 year (Table 3.4). Based on the intimal thickness and vessel circumference involved, they classified the lesion severity as follows: class 0 = no measurable intimal layer by ultrasound; class 1 (minimal) = an intimal layer <0.3 mm thick involving <180° of the vessel circumference; class 2 (mild) = an intimal layer <0.3 mm thick involving >180° of the vessel circumference; class 3 (moderate) = an intimal layer of 0.3–0.5 mm or an intimal layer >0.5 mm thick involving <180° of the vessel circumference; and class 4 (severe) = >0.5 mm of intimal thickening involving >180° of the vessel circumference or an intimal layer >1 mm at

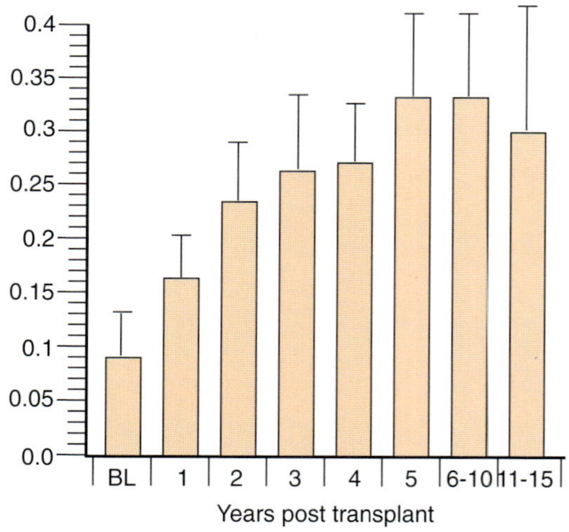

Figure 3.58 *Bar graphs showing the correlation of mean intimal thickness with time after transplantation. Data are expressed as mean ± SEM. BL, baseline (<2 months after transplantation). (From Rickenbacher et al[139] with permission.)*

Table 3.4 IVUS variables (from Richenbacher et al,[139] with permission)

Years after transplantation	*Pts (no.)*	*Intimal thickness (mm)*	*Intimal index*	*Stanford class*	*Ecc*	*Calc*
Baseline (< 2 mo)	50	0.09 ± 0.02*	0.07 ± 0.01*	1.5 ± 0.02*	18%	8%
1	52	0.16 ± 0.02†	0.14 ± 0.02	2.3 ± 0.2	44%	2%
2	47	0.23 ± 0.03	0.17 ± 0.02	2.5 ± 0.2	43%	9%
3	33	0.26 ± 0.04	0.20 ± 0.03	2.7 ± 0.2	39%	6%
4	34	0.27 ± 0.03	0.21 ± 0.03	2.5 ± 0.2†	35%	12%
5	35	0.33 ± 0.04	0.24 ± 0.03	3.2 ± 0.2	51%	6%†
6 to 10	42	0.33 ± 0.04	0.25 ± 0.03	3.0 ± 0.2	38%	24%
11 to 15	11	0.30 ± 0.06	0.27 ± 0.05	2.8 ± 0.3	27%	46%

*$P < 0.01$, †$P < 0.05$ versus value in succeeding year. Data are expressed as mean value ± SEM or percent of studies. Calc = studies showing calcification; Ecc = studies showing eccentric lesions; Pts = patients; Stanford class = Stanford classification of lesion severity.

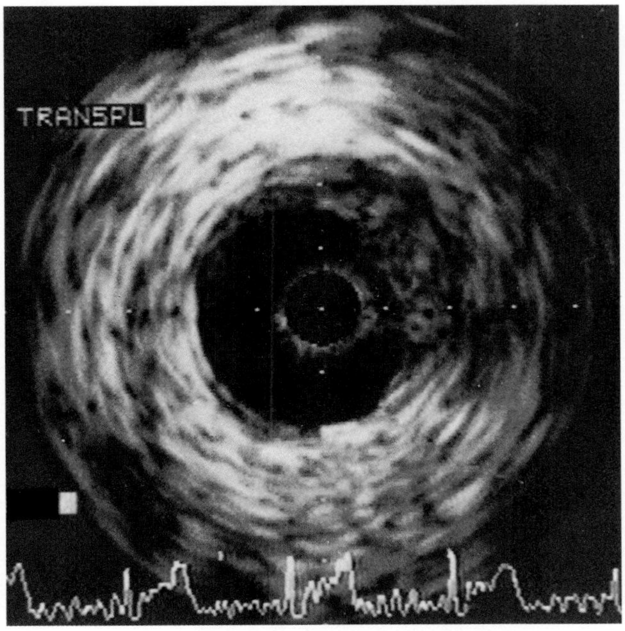

Figure 3.59 *Plaque formation in a patient 1 month after heart transplantation.*

any point of the vessel circumference.[139] They reported that the most striking progression of disease occurred during the first 2 years after transplantation (Fig. 3.58). In a serial examination in 21 patients involving IVUS of all the three vessels (a total of 63 coronary arteries), we found plaque formation in 18 vessels (Fig. 3.59) although all the coronary arteries presented normal coronary angiograms.[140] Intracoronary flow mapping using Doppler FloWire was available in 56 vessels; coronary flow reserve was found to be reduced in 34 vessels (61%). Reports indicate that decreased coronary flow reserve might be an early sign of rejection. In a serial follow-up study, we found that coronary flow reserve can be normalized after transplantation.

TRANSPLANTED CORONARY DISEASES

Transplanted coronary diseases are the coronary disorders deriving from the pre-existing coronary diseases of the donor, such as pre-existing atherosclerosis, coronary dysfunction and myocardial bridging. The Stanford group reported that only 22% of the patients studied during the first 2 months after transplantation had no evidence of intimal thickening and that 26% already had class 3 and 4 changes.[139] Plaque formation was also found in a patient 3 months after heart transplantation from a 19-year-old donor (Fig. 3.60). Whether the plaque formed after transplantation is not known.

However, pre-existing atherosclerotic lesions might be reversible. In a patient who had urgent heart transplantation grafted with an atherosclerotic donor heart due to severe congestive heart failure caused by idiopathic dilated cardiomyopathy, we have demonstrated plaque regression 5 years after heart transplantation (Figs 3.61 and 3.62).[141] Moreover, myocardial

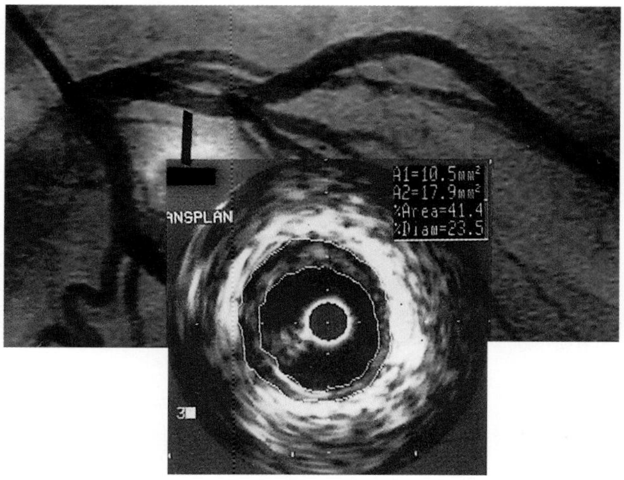

Figure 3.60 *Coronary angiogram and IVUS image of a patient 2 months after heart transplantation. Concentric intimal thickening produces a lumen area narrowing of 41% and a diameter narrowing of 23%. Coronary angiography does not show any abnormality of the vessel.*

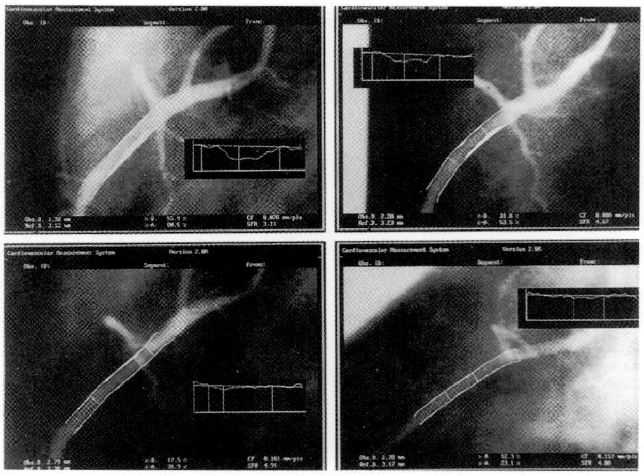

Figure 3.61 *Serial quantitative angiographic evaluation of an allograft atherosclerotic lesion 1 year (top left), 2 years (top right), 3 years (bottom left) and 5 years (bottom right) after urgent cardiac transplantation. (From Haude et al[141] with permission.)*

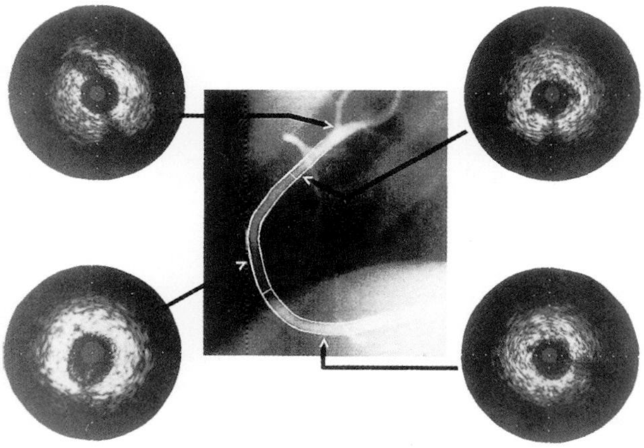

Figure 3.62 *Coronary angiogram and IVUS images 5 years after heart transplantation of the same patients as Figs. 3.4. IVUS shows a class 4 intimal thickening in the proximal segment without luminal narrowing. Coronary angiogram shows atherosclerosis regression in comparison to the examination performed serially. (From Haude et al[141] with permission.)*

bridging was found in two of the 22 patients (9%) in our center. Both of them presented with a typical 'finger tip' flow velocity profile in the segment proximal to the bridge. All the patients showed normal or nearly normal coronary angiograms.

FOLLOW-UP OF THE CORONARY ARTERY MORPHOLOGY AND FUNCTION IN TRANSPLANTED HEARTS

As pointed out above, coronary angiography frequently underestimates coronary artery disease and does not allow us to define early signs of atherosclerosis, especially in transplanted hearts.[142] In addition, it provides little information concerning coronary function. The combination of IVUS and Doppler flow mapping offers detailed information on coronary morphology and function. It has been shown that IVUS does not accelerate the progression of angiographically quantifiable coronary artery disease in cardiac transplant recipients.[143] Therefore, it is necessary to use IVUS and Doppler to detect the early allograft vasculopathy, so that the clinical management can be guided. Coronary arteries should be studied before transplantation to rule out coronary artery disease in the future. In a patient 2 months after transplantation from a 14-year-old donor, reduced coronary flow reserve was found in all three coronary arteries. Whether this reduced coronary flow reserve may normalize like plaque regression

Table 3.5 Limitations of three-dimensional reconstruction of intracoronary ultrasound images (from Roelandt et al,[150] with permission)

Related to image quality
Poor definition of the intimal border (blood echogenicity)
Poor definition of the plaque-media border (absence of hypoechoic media)
Shadowing by calcium
Noncoaxial position of the catheter tip (elliptical distortion)
Nonuniform rotation of the transducer
Related to acquisition
Vessel curvatures may induce distortion of the reconstructed image
Catheter tip position shifts in the lumen
Twisting of the catheter during pull-back induces mismatch between orientation of sequential two-dimensional images
Luminal area may change throughout the cardiac cycle

Table 3.6 Clinical applications of three-dimensional reconstruction of intracoronary ultrasound images (from Roelandt et al,[150] with permission)

Quantification of vascular dimensions
Luminal and plaque volumes
Study of restenosis and progression-regression
Interventional guidance
Selection of interventional device type and size
Avoidance of atherectomy in presence of extensive calcification
Dimensions and type of stent to be developed
Guidance of interventional procedures
Assessment of persistent plaque burden and direction of atherotome cuts
Optimize stent deployment to ensure symmetrical and uniform stent inflation
Comprehensive evaluation of interventional mechanisms and complications
Examination of complex spiral dissections for bailout stenting

remains unknown. Serial studies should be performed in order to answer this question.

FUTURE DIRECTION

TISSUE CHARACTERIZATION

Even though IVUS offers detailed information on the morphology of the atherosclerotic lesions,[144] it is sometimes difficult to differentiate the tissue characters, e.g. thrombus from soft plaque. Frimerman et al recently demonstrated that IVUS can differentiate thrombi with different compositions.[145] They concluded that platelet-rich thrombi are echolucent, and that the main echogenic reflectance of thrombi originates from red blood cells.[145] Lee et al indicated that thrombus presents a fine, homogeneous speckled pattern or a smooth pedunculated appearance, whereas plaque is an intrinsic component of the arterial wall and a more heterogeneous reflector of echo signals.[146] All these signs are unspecific. Fitzgerald et al, as well as our group, are now trying to differentiate tissue character by analyzing radiofrequency signals, this is not influenced by gain settings of the IVUS machine, and might have a promising future.[147]

THREE-DIMENSIONAL RECONSTRUCTION

IVUS provides information on the vessel wall in cross-section. In order to better understand the spatial orientation of the plaques and to quantify the plaque volumes, it is essential to reconstruct the IVUS images in three dimensions. Although the basic principle of three-dimensional reconstruction is known and studies have been done over the last several years,[148–150] some of the technical problems remain unsolved (Table 3.5).[150] These are mainly related to pulsation of the artery, catheter rotation and spatial orientation. If the limitations can be overcome, three-dimensional reconstruction will be able to help us to study the progression and regression of atherosclerosis (Table 3.6).[150] See Chapter 12 for more information about three-dimensional endoluminal ultrasound.

SAFETY OF INTRAVASCULAR ULTRASOUND

As the use of IVUS in coronary diagnosis has increased, cardiologists have encountered the challenge of several complications of advancing a catheter into the coronary artery. Like other interventional coronary catheters, IVUS catheters may also induce the common complications such as coronary spasm, coronary dissection, acute coronary closure, thrombus formation, arrhythmia and myocardial infarction. In a multicenter study of 2207 intracoronary examinations, 7.8% led to complications during interventional procedures of which 3.9% were judged to be not related to IVUS imaging.[151] In 229 consecutive IVUS procedures, we found an incidence of 4.8%.[152]

CORONARY SPASM

Coronary spasm is the most frequent complication during IVUS examination. In the above-mentioned multicenter IVUS study, the overall incidence of coronary spasm was found in 2.9%.[151] In our center, we found that the incidence of coronary spasm is lower if intracoronary nitroglycerin and heparin are given before the examination.[153] Fig. 3.63 shows an example of coronary spasm during IVUS examination, which is released after intracoronary administration of 0.2 mg nitroglycerin. In the presence of coronary spasm, the IVUS image mimics intimal thickening or plaque formation (Fig. 3.64). After the spasm was released, the intima presented a monolayer appearance (Fig. 3.65). Therefore, attention should be paid when interpreting the IVUS images. The operator must be sure that no spasm exists. Clinically, patients with coronary spasm may present ischemic ECG changes and experience angina pectoris. These manifestations improve when the spasm has released. Bory et al found that atherosclerotic plaque is always present at the site of focal vasospasm and that atherosclerosis plays an important role in the occurrence of vasospasm.[154]

ACUTE CORONARY CLOSURE

Acute closure of the coronary artery is a severe complication during the IVUS examination. In the

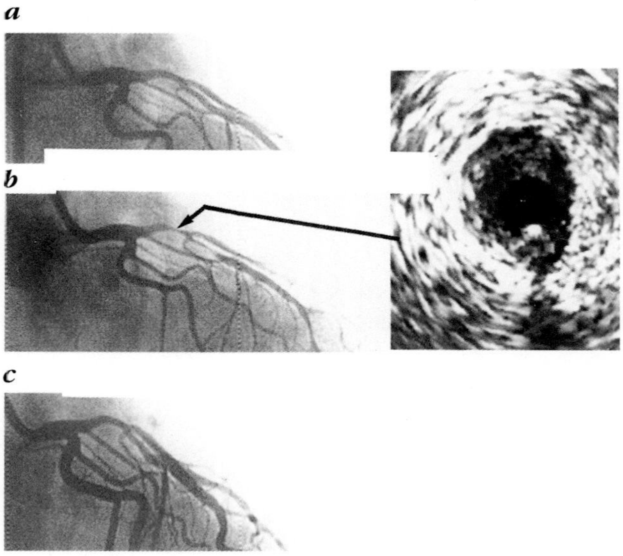

Figure 3.63 *Coronary artery spasm in LAD during IVUS imaging. Left panel shows the coronary angiogram before (a) and after (b) IVUS examination. After intracoronary administration of 0.2 mg nitroglycerin, the spasm released (c).*

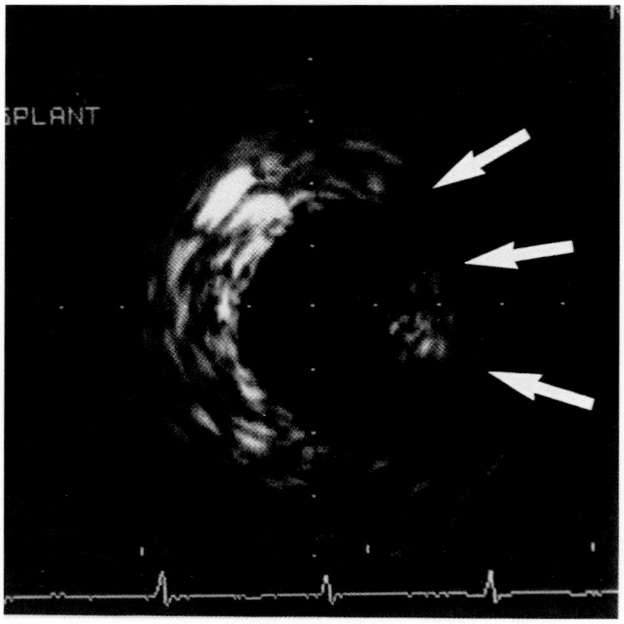

Figure 3.64 *IVUS image of a right coronary artery during spasm. A 'plaque' which causes a percentage stenosis of about 50% can be visualized.*

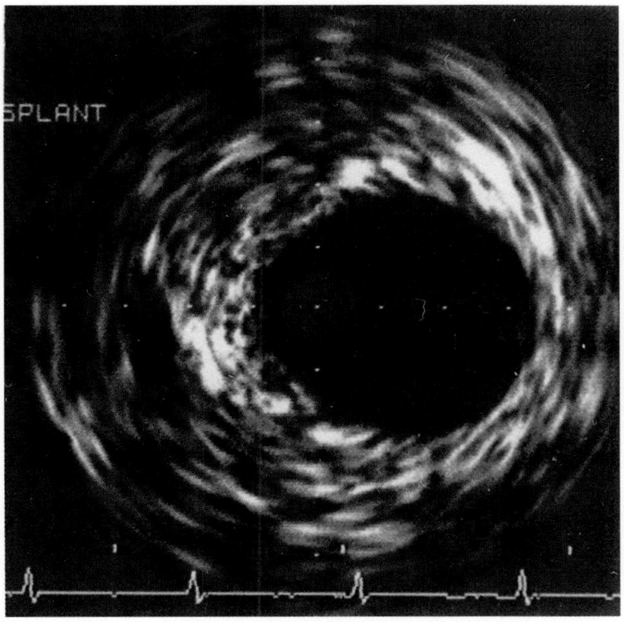

Figure 3.65 *IVUS image of the same cross-section as in Fig. 3.64 after intracoronary administration of nitroglycerin. No 'plaque' is visualized, indicating that the 'plaque' in Fig. 3.64 might actually be squeezed intima.*

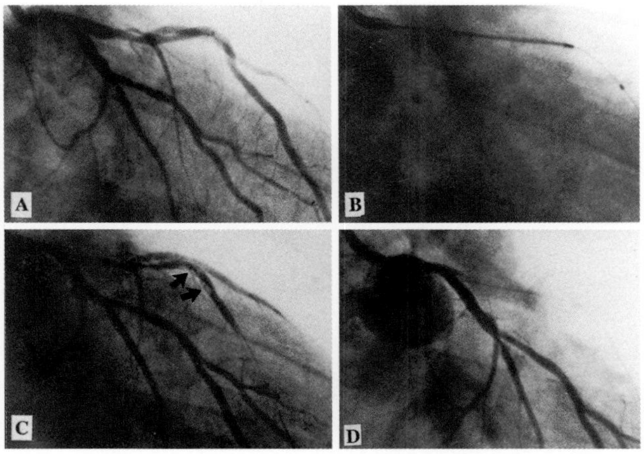

Figure 3.66 *Coronary angiogram of left coronary artery in RAO projection. (A) An 80% stenosis is seen in the proximal LAD. (B) The IVUS catheter is advanced into the LAD with a 0.014-inch guidewire in the distal segment. (C) Distal LAD is occluded with signs of intimal dissection and thrombus formation in the proximal LAD (arrows). (D) The whole LAD is occluded at the proximal part, with the guidewire positioned in the distal LAD. (From Ge et al[153] with permission.)*

multicenter registry, acute closure of the coronary artery was documented in 14/2207 patients (0.6%); 3/2207 (0.1%) were considered to be related to IVUS examination.[151] We studied 550 IVUS procedures in our center and found that 2/550 patients experienced acute closure of coronary arteries during the IVUS procedure.[153] Figure 3.66 shows an acute closure of the left anterior descending artery (LAD) during IVUS examination before coronary intervention by a 4.8-Fr monorail ultrasound catheter. After withdrawal of the IVUS catheter, it appeared that an intimal dissection and thrombus formation with subtotal occlusion of the proximal LAD was present (Fig. 3.66C), followed by a total occlusion (Fig. 3.66D). The occluded coronary artery was successfully recanalized by PTCA. However, thrombotic debris caused side-branch embolization (Fig. 3.67). Figure 3.68 shows a right coronary artery occlusion during IVUS examination. The cause was an intimal dissection of the distal segment by a 2.9-Fr over-the-wire ultrasound catheter sheath. The vessel was recanalized with an over-the-wire balloon catheter, but the two side-branches distal to the crux cordis still showed filling defects. The patient had a creatine kinase (CK) value of 432 U/l after he returned to the ward, compared with 50 u/l pre-examination. In the above-mentioned multicenter survey, all the acute closures were also successfully managed by PTCA or thrombolytic therapy.[151]

CORONARY DISSECTION AND THROMBUS FORMATION

Coronary dissection and thrombus formation may occur during IVUS examination. In our study mentioned above,[153] both patients with acute coronary closure had intimal dissection first, followed by thrombus formation which led to coronary occlusion. In the multicenter study, only one instance of dissection occurred and this was treated with PTCA. One patient with thrombus formation was successfully treated with thrombolysis. Although these complications are rare, they are serious, and great care should be taken during IVUS procedures to avoid them.

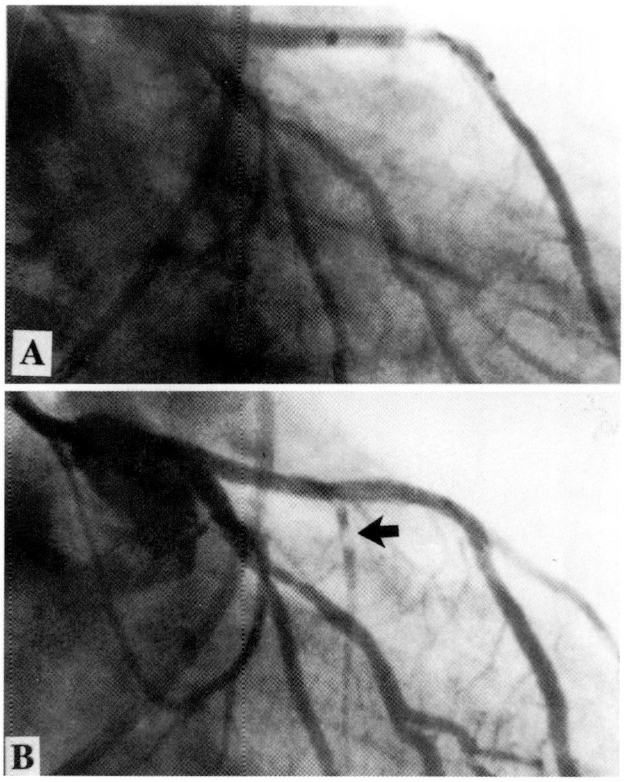

Figure 3.67 *The same patient as in Fig. 3.66. The vessel was successfully recanalized and dilated with a 3.0-mm continuous perfusion catheter. (A) The whole LAD is open with antegrade bloodflow of TIMI 3. (B) Residual thrombi can still be seen in the first septal branch (arrow). (From Ge et al[153] with permission.)*

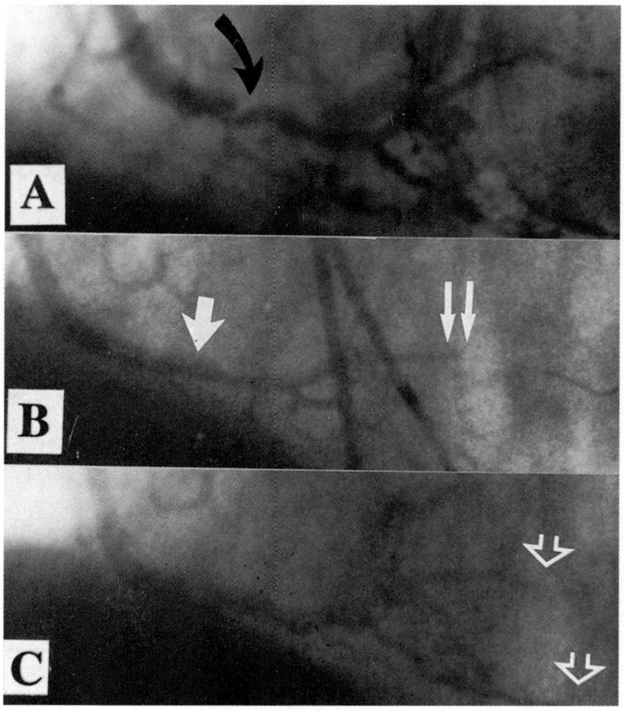

Figure 3.68 *Distal part of right coronary artery in LAO projection. A high-degree of stenosis is seen angiographically (A, arrow). (B) Intimal dissection (single white arrow) with the guidewire in the right coronary artery. (C) After recanalization and PTCA, the vessel is open but two small branches (open arrows) distal to the crus cordis retain contrast filling defects. (From Ge et al[153] with permission.)*

OTHER COMPLICATIONS

Apart from ischemic ECG changes caused by coronary spasm, the IVUS catheter may cause obstruction when crossing a severe stenosis and lead to ischemic changes. In this situation, patients normally present with angina pectoris in accordance with ST elevation. In the case of left main coronary artery stenosis, bradycardia or asystole may occur when the ultrasound catheter is placed in the left main coronary artery (Fig. 3.69). Extrasystoles and other arrhythmias such as ventricular tachycardia may also occur when the ultrasound catheter is advanced.

Because the presently used IVUS catheters are often monorail types, it is sometimes very difficult to guide the IVUS catheter into a tortuous coronary artery or an acute angle of the circumflex coronary artery. We have also found that, with the use of the Amplatz guiding catheter, non-uniform rotation of the mechanical rotating catheter often occurs because of the acute course of the catheter, and, moreover, guidewire shadowing artifacts are caused by every monorail IVUS catheter.

Another common complication during IVUS examination is guidewire winding (Fig. 3.70). This is due to the too-short monorail of the IVUS catheter. While the IVUS catheter is being pulled back and then advanced again, the soft guidewire could be advanced together with the ultrasound catheter, forming a loop just proximal to the monorail. While the IVUS is being pulled into the guiding catheter, the looped wire and IVUS catheter tip at the site of the monorail will be stacked at the tip of the guiding catheter (Fig. 3.70). This is more common when

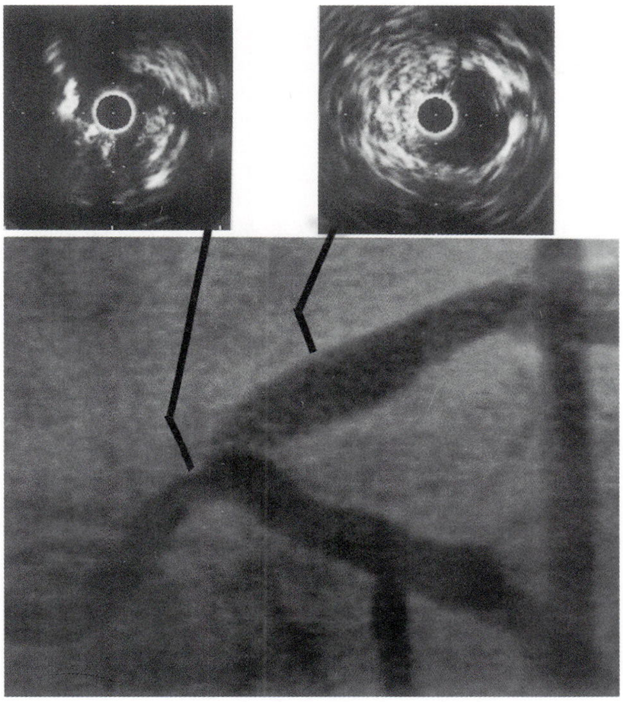

Figure 3.69 *A patient with left main coronary artery stenosis and ostium stenosis. Asystole occurred during IVUS examination.*

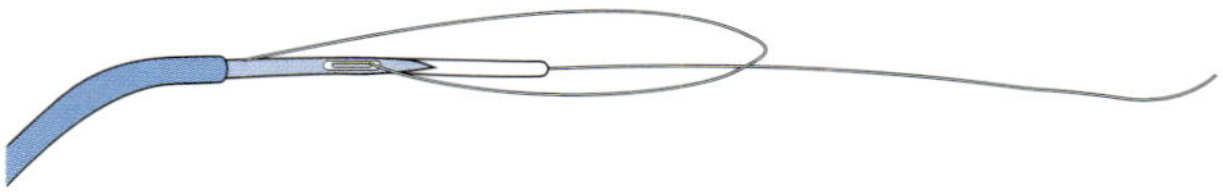

Figure 3.70 *Guidewire winding on the tip of the guiding catheter.*

using FloWire as guidewire, because the long distal part of the FloWire is very soft. Thus, when the coronary artery is repeatedly scanned, the IVUS catheter and FloWire should be withdrawn together and then advanced together again. When a normal floppy wire is used, it should be advanced as far as possible to the distal part of the target coronary artery to prevent this complication. When guidewire winding occurs, the whole system (guiding catheter, together with the IVUS catheter and guidewire) should be removed. Always avoid pulling the IVUS catheter with force!

IVUS is a useful tool in interventional cardiology today. Concerning the long-term effects of this procedure, no angiographically quantifiable changes in previously instrumented segments were found with regard to the acceleration atherosclerosis.[155] Therefore, the technique can be safely used for the evaluation of coronary artery disease, for diagnostic purposes and for follow-up studies.

REFERENCES

1. Vlodaver Z, Frech R, Van Tassel RA et al, Correlation of the antemortem coronary angiogram and the postmortem specimen, *Circulation* 1973; **47**:162–9.
2. Grodin CM, Dyrda I, Pasternac A et al, Discrepancies between cineangiographic and post-mortem finding in patients with coronary artery disease and recent myocardial revasculization, *Circulation* 1974; **49**:703–56.
3. Arnett EN, Isner JM, Redwood CR et al, Coronary artery narrowing in coronary heart disease: comparison of cineangiographic and necropsy findings, *Ann Intern Med* 1979; **91**:350–5.
4. Tobis JM, Mallery J, Mahon D et al, Intravascular ultrasound imaging of human coronary arteries in vivo, *Circulation* 1991; **83**:913–26.
5. Fitzgerald PJ, Ports TA, Yock PY, Contribution of localized calcium deposits to dissection after angioplasty, an observational study using intravascular ultrasound, *Circulation* 1992; **86**:64–70.
6. Honye J, Mahon DJ, Jain A et al, Morphological effects of coronary balloon angioplasty in vivo assessed by intravascular ultrasound, *Circulation* 1992; **85**:1012–25.
7. St Goar FG, Pinto FJ, Aldeerman EI et al, Intracoronary ultrasound in cardiac transplant recipients, in vivo evidence of 'angiographically silent' intimal thickening, *Circulation* 1992; **85**:979–87.
8. Ge J, Erbel R, Gerber T et al, Intravascular ultrasound imaging of angiographically normal coronary arteries: a prospective study in vivo, *Br Heart J* 1994; **71**:572–8.
9. Nissen SE, Gurley JC, Grines CL et al, Intravascular ultrasound assessment of lumen size and wall morphology in normal subjects and patients with coronary artery disease, *Circulation* 1991; **84**:1087–99.
10. Pokin BN, Bartorelli A, Gessert JM et al, Coronary artery imaging with intravascular high-frequency ultrasound, *Circulation* 1990; **81**:1575–85.
11. Wild JJ, Reid JM, Ultrasonic rectal endoscope for tumor location, *Am Inst Ultrason Med* 1955; **4**:59.
12. Cieszynski T, Intracardiac method for the investigation of

structure of the heart with the aid of ultrasonics, *Arch Immun Ter Dow* 1960; **8**:551–7.

13. Omoto R, Intracardiac scanning of the heart with the aid of ultrasonic intravenous probe, *Jpn Heart J* 1967; **8**:569–81.
14. Ebina T, Okla S, Tanaka M et al, The diagnostic application of ultrasound to the disease in mediastinal organs. Ultrasonotomography for the heart and great vessels, *Sci Rep Res Inst Tohoku Univ* 1965; **12**:199–212.
15. Bom N, Lancee CT, Van Egmond FC, An ultrasonic intracardiac scanner, *Ultrasonics* 1972; **10**:72–6.
16. Hodgson JMcB, Graham SP, Savakus AD et al, Clinical percutaneous imaging of coronary anatomy using an over-the-wire ultrasound catheter system, *Int J Card Imag* 1989; **4**:187–93.
17. Yock PG, Linker DT, White NW et al, Clinical applications of intravascular ultrasound imaging in atherectomy, *Int J Card Imag* 1989; **4** 117–25.
18. Erbel R, Roth T, Koch L, Ge J, Haude M, The precision guided directional laser atherectomy catheter: a new approach to percutaneous coronary revasculization, *J Am Coll Cardiol* 1995; **25**:268A.
19. Evans JL, Ng KH, Vonesh MJ et al, Arterial imaging with a new forward-viewing intravascular ultrasound catheter, I: initial studies, *Circulation* 1994; **89**:712–17.
20. Ng KH, Evans JL, Vonesh MJ et al, Arterial imaging with a new forward-viewing intravascular ultrasound catheter, II: Three-dimensional reconstruction and display of data, *Circulation* 1994; **89**:718–23.
21. Görge G, Ge J, Haude M, Baumgart D, Buck T, Erbel R, Initial experience with steerable intravascular ultrasound catheter in aorta and pulmonary artery, *Am J Card Imag* 1995; **9**:180–4.
22. Ge J, Erbel R, Seidel I et al, Experimental evaluation of the accuracy and safety of intraluminal ultrasound, *Z Kardiol* 1991; **80**:595–601.
23. Nishimura RA, Edwards WD, Warnes CA et al, Intravascular ultrasound imaging: in vitro validation and pathologic correlation, *J Am Coll Cardiol* 1990; **16**:145–54.
24. Di Mario C, The SHK, Madretsma S et al, Detection and characterization of vascular lesions by intravascular ultrasound: an in vitro study correlated with histology, *J Am Soc Echocardiogr* 1992; **5**:135–46.
25. Mallery JA, Tobis JM, Griffith J et al, Assessment of normal and atherosclerotic arterial wall thickness with an intravascular ultrasound catheter, *Am Heart J* 1990; **119**:1392–400.
26. Potkin BN, Keren G, Mintz GS et al, Arterial response to balloon coronary angioplasty: an intravascular ultrasound study, *J Am Coll Cardiol* 1992; **20**:942–51.
27. Dupouy P, Larrazet F, EI Ghalid A et al, Is intravascular ultrasound a new standard for coronary artery imaging? *J Interv Cardiol* 1993; **6**:321–30.
28. Pandian NG, Kreis A, Brockway B et al, Ultrasound angioscopy: feasibility and potential, *Echocardiography* 1989; **6**:1–7.
29. Li W, Gussenhoven WJ, Zhong Y et al, Validation of quantitative analysis of intravascular ultrasound images, *Int J Card Imag* 1991; **6**:247–53.
30. Finet G, Maurincomme E, Douek Ph et al, Three-layer appearance of the arterial wall in intravascular ultrasound imaging: artifact or reality? *Echocardiography* 1994; **11**:343–63.
31. Ge J, Erbel R, Görge G et al, Intravascular ultrasound imaging of arterial wall architecture, *Echocardiography* 1992; **9**:475–83.
32. Nolsoe CP, Engel U, Karstrup S et al, The aortic wall: an in vitro study of the double-line pattern in high-resolution US, *Radiology* 1990; **175**:387–90.
33. Lockwood G, Ryan L, Gotlieb A et al, In vitro high resolution intravascular imaging in muscular and elastic arteries, *J Am Coll Cardiol* 1992; **20**:153–60.
34. Kearney P, Erbel R, Imaging in the catheterization laboratory, *Curr Opin Cardiol* 1993; **8**:988–99.
35. Velican D, Velican C, Comparative study on age related changes and atherosclerosis involvement of the coronary arteries of male and female subjects up to 40 years of age, *Atherosclerosis* 1981; **38**:39–50.
36. Glagov V, Weisenberg E, Zarins CK et al, Compensatory enlargement of human atherosclerotic coronary arteriesm, *N Engl J Med* 1987; **316**:1371–5.
37. Gussenhoven EJ, Frietman PAV, The SHK et al, Assessment of medial thinning in atherosclerosis by intravascular ultrasound, *Am J Cardiol* 1991; **68**:1625–32.
38. Fitzgerald P, St Goar F, Connolly A et al, Intravascular ultrasound imaging of coronary arteries: is three layers the norm? *Circulation* 1992; **86**:154–8.
39. Pandian NG, Kreis A, Brockway B, Detection of intra-arterial thrombus by intravascular high frequency two-dimensional ultrasound in vitro and in vivo studies, *Am J Cardiol* 1990; **65**:1280–3.
40. Siegel RJ, Fishbein MC, Chae JS et al, Comparative studies of angioscopy and ultrasound for the evaluation of arterial disease, *Echocardiography* 1990; **7**:495–502.
41. Goss SA, Johnston RL, Dunn F, Comprehensive compilation of empirical ultrasonic properties of mammalian tissues, *J Acoust Soc Am* 1978; **64**:423–80.
42. Rasheed Q, Suneja R, Anderson J et al, Validation of intracoronary ultrasound defined plaque composition: correlation with histologic samples obtained during directional atherectomy, *J Am Coll Cardiol* 1993; **21**:193A.
43. Ge J, Erbel R, Zamorano J et al, Coronary artery remodeling in atherosclerotic disease: an intravascular ultrasonic study in vivo, *Coronary Art Dis* 1993; **4**:981–6.
44. Takano Y, Mizushige K, Morita H et al, Arterial wall tissue characterization by analysis of radio frequency signal using intravascular ultrasound, *Jpn J Med Ultrason* 1994; **21**:8–16.
45. Peters RJG, Kok WEM, van der Wal AC, Visser CA, Determinants of echodensity at the intima-media interface with intracoronary ultrasound imaging, *J Am Soc Echocardiogr* 1996; **9**:329–36.
46. Stary HC, Evolution and progression of atherosclerosis, *Atherosclerosis* 1989; **9**(Suppl I):19–32.
47. Stary HC, The sequence of cell and matrix changes in atherosclerotic lesions of coronary arteries in the first forty years of life, *Eur Heart J* 1990; **11**(Suppl E):3–19.
48. Stary HC, Chandler AB, Dinsmore RE et al, A definition of advanced types of atherosclerotic lesions and histological classification of atherosclerosis, *Circulation* 1995; **92**:1355–74.
49. Erbel R, Ge J, Jollet N, Görge G, Haude M, Intravascular ultrasound based Stary classification of coronary plaque formation, *J Am Coll Cardiol* 1996; **27**:40A.
50. Erbel R, Ge J, Görge G et al, Intravaskuläre Sonographie bei koronarer herzkrankheit, neu aspekte zur pathogenese, *Dtsch Med Wochenschr* 1995; **120**:847–54.

51. Ge J, Erbel R, Novel techniques of coronary artery imaging, *Curr Opin Cardiol* 1995; **10**:626–33.
52. Ge J, Liu F, Kearney P et al, Intravascular ultrasound approach to the diagnosis of coronary artery aneurysm, *Am Heart J* 1995; **130**:765–71.
53. Ge J, Haude M, Görge G, Liu F, Erbel R, Silent healing of spontaneous plaque disruption demonstrated by intracoronary ultrasound, *Eur Heart J* 1995; **16**:1149–51.
54. Kearney P, Erbel R, Rupprecht HJ et al, Differences in the morphology of unstable and stable coronary lesions and their impact on the mechanisms of angioplasty. An in vivo study with intravascular ultrasound, *Eur Heart J* 1996; **17**:721–30.
55. Ge J, Erbel R, Rupprecht HJ et al, Comparison of intravascular ultrasound and angiography in the assessment of myocardial bridging, *Circulation* 1994; **89**:1725–32.
56. Erbel R, Rupprecht HJ, Ge J, Gerber T, Görge G, Meyer J, Coronary artery shape and flow changes induced by myocardial bridging, *Echocardiography* 1993; **10**:71–7.
57. Ge J, Erbel R, Görge G, Haude M, Meyer J, High wall shear stress proximal to myocardial bridging and atherosclerosis: intracoronary ultrasound and pressure measurement, *Br Heart J* 1995; **73**:462–5.
58. Lee SS, Wu TL, The role of the mural coronary artery in prevention of coronary atherosclerosis, *Arch Pathol* 1972; **93**:32–5.
59. Daoud AS, Pankin D, Tulgan H, Florentin RA, Aneurysms of the coronary artery: report of ten cases and review of literature, *Am J Cardiol* 1963; **11**:228–37.
60. Befeler B, Aranda JM, Embi A, Mullin FL, El-Sharif N, Lazzara R, Coronary artery aneurysms: study of their etiology, clinical cause and effect on left ventricular function and prognosis, *Am J Med* 1977; **62**:597–607.
61. Gerrand TJ, Mintz GS, Popma JJ, Lewis SA, Vaughn NA, Leon MB, Intravascular ultrasound diagnosis of a coronary pseudoaneurysm following percutaneous transluminal coronary angioplasty, *Am Heart J* 1993; **125**:880–2.
62. Davies MJ, Bland MJ, Hangartner WR, Angelini A, Thomas AC, Factors influencing the presence or absence of acute coronary thrombi in sudden ischemic death, *Eur Heart J* 1989; **10**:203–8.
63. Fuster V, Stein B, Ambrose JA, Badimon JJ, Chesebro JH, Atherosclerotic plaque rupture and thrombosis: evolving concepts, *Circulation* 1990; **82**(Suppl II):47–59.
64. Ridolfi RL, Hutchins GM, The relationship between coronary artery lesions and myocardial infarcts: ulceration of atherosclerotic plaques precipitating coronary thrombosis, *Am Heart J* 1977; **93**:468–86
65.. Ge J, Liu F, Görge G, Haude M, von Birgelen C, Erbel R, Visualization of spontaneous plaque rupture by intracoronary ultrasound, *Eur Heart J* 1994; **15**:608.
66. Erbel R, Ge J, Bockisch A et al, Value of intracoronary ultrasound and Doppler in differentiation of angiographically normal coronary arteries: a prospective study in patients with angina pectoris, *Eur Heart J* 1996; **17**:880–9.
67. Grüntzig A, Perkutane dilatation von koronarstenosen—beschreibung eines neuen kathetersystems, *Klin Wochenschr* 1976; **54**:543.
68. Grüntzig A, Senning A, Siegenthaler WE, Nonoperative dilatation of coronary artery stenoses: percutaneous transluminal coronary angioplasty, *N Engl J Med* 1979; **301**:61–8.
69. Waller BF, 'Crackers, breakers, stretchers, drillers, scrapers, shavers, burners, welders, and melders'—the future treatment of atherosclerotic coronary artery disease? A clinical–morphological assessment, *J Am Coll Cardiol* 1989; **13**:969–87.
70. Waller BF, Pinkerton CA, Slack JD, Intravascular ultrasound: a histological study of vessels during life. The new 'gold standard' for vascular imaging, *Circulation* 1992; **85**:2305–10.
71. Dotter CT, Judkins MP, Transluminal treatment of arteriosclerotic obstruction: description of a new technique and a preliminary report on its application, *Circulation* 1964; **30**:654.
72. Waller BF, Morphologic correlates of coronary angiographic patterns at the site of percutaneous transluminal coronary angioplasty, *Clin Cardiol* 1988; **11**:817–22.
73. Düber C, Jungbluth A, Rumpelt H–J et al, Morphology of the coronary arteries after combined thrombolysis and percutaneous transluminal coronary angioplasty for acute myocardial infarction, *Am J Cardiol* 1986; **58**:698–703.
74. Jungbluth A, Düber C, Rumpelt HJ, Erbel R, Meyer J, Morphologic changes in a coronary artery after cardiac tamponade following percutaneous transluminal coronary angioplasty (PTCA), *Z Kardiol* 1988; **77**:125–9.
75. Serruys PW, Foley DP, Kirkeeide RL, King SB III, Restenosis revisited: insights provided by quantitative coronary angiography, *Am Heart J* 1993; **126**:1243–67.
76. Weintraub WS, Ghazzal ZM, Douglas JS Jr et al, Long-term clinical follow-up in patients with angiographic restudy after successful angioplasty, *Circulation* 1993; **87**:831–40.
77. Hirshfeld JW Jr, Schwartz JS, Jugo R et al, Restenosis after coronary angioplasty: a multivariate statistical model to relate lesion and procedure variables to restenosis, *J Am Coll Cardiol* 1991; **18**:647–56.
78. Coy KM, Maurer G, Siegel RJ, Intravascular ultrasound imaging: a current perspective, *J Am Coll Cardiol* 1991; **18**:1811–23.
79. Tobis JM, Mallery JA, Mahon D et al, Intravascular ultrasound imaging: a new method for guiding interventional vascular procedures, *Echocardiography* 1990; **7**:415–24.
80. Yock PG, Johnson EL, Linker DT, Intravascular ultrasound: development and clinical potential, *Am J Card Imag* 1988; **2**:185–93.
81. The SH, Gussenhoven EJ, Zhong Y et al, Effect of balloon angioplasty on femoral artery evaluated with intravascular ultrasound imaging, *Circulation* 1992; **86**:483–93.
82. van der Lugt A, Gussenhoven EJ, Stijnen T et al, Balloon angioplasty evaluated in vitro by intracoronary ultrasound: a validation with histology, *Eur Heart J* 1995; **16**:203.
83. Gussenhoven EJ, Essed CE, Lancee CT et al, Arterial wall characteristics determined by intravascular ultrasound imaging: an in vitro study, *J Am Coll Cardiol* 1989; **14**:947–52.
84. DiMario C, The SH, Madretsma S et al, Detection and characterization of vascular lesions by intravascular ultrasound: an in vitro study correlated with histology, *J Am Soc Echocardiogr* 1992; **5**:135–46.
85. Honye J, Mahon DJ, Jain A et al, Morphological effects of coronary balloon angioplasty in vivo assessed by intravascular ultrasound imaging, *Circulation* 1992; **85**:1012–25.
86. Gerber TC, Erbel R, Görge G, Ge J, Rupprecht HJ, Meyer

J, Classification of morphologic effects of percutaneous transluminal coronary angioplasty assessed by intravascular ultrasound, *Am J Cardiol* 1992; **70**:1546–54.

87. Jain SP, Jain A, Collins TJ, Ramee SR, White CJ, Predictors of restenosis: a morphometric and quantative evaluation by intravascular ultrasound, *Am Heart J* 1994; **128**:664–73.
88. DiMario C, Gil R, Camenzind et al, Quantative assessment with intracoronary ultrasound of the mechanisms of restenosis after percutaneous transluminal coronary angioplasty and directional coronary atherectomy, *Am J Cardiol* 1995; **75**:772–7.
89. Baptosta J, DiMario C, Ozaki Y et al, Impact of plaque morphology and composition on the mechanisms of lumen enlargement using intracoronary ultrasound and quantative angiography after balloon angioplasty, *Am J Cardiol* 1996; **77**:115–21.
90. Nakamura S, Mahon DJ, Maheswaran B, Gutfinger DE, Colombo A, Tobis JM, An explanation for discrepancy between angiographic and intravascular ultrasound measurements after percutaneous transluminal coronary angioplasty, *J Am Coll Cardiol* 1995; **25**:633–9.
91. Kimura T, Kaburagi S, Tashima Y, Nobuyoshi M, Mintz GS, Popma JJ, Geometric remodeling and intimal growth as mechanisms of restenosis: observations from serial ultrasound analysis of restenosis (SURE) trial, *Circulation* 1995; **92**(Suppl):1–76.
92. Hodgson JMcB, Stone GW, Linnemeier TJ, Sheehan HM, St Goar FG, Berry JL, Oversized balloons defined by intracoronary ultrasound results in dramatic improvements in angioplasty results: initial ultrasound analysis of the CLOUT pilot study, *Eur Heart J* 1995; **16**:487.
93. Sigwart U, Puel J, Mirkovitch V, Joffre F, Kappenberger L, Intravascular stents to prevent occlusion and restenosis after transluminal angioplasty, *N Engl J Med* 1987; **316**:701–6.
94. Fischman DL, Leon MB, Baim DS et al, A randomized comparison of coronary-stent placement and balloon angioplasty in the treatment of coronary artery disease. Stent Restenosis Study Investigators, *N Engl J Med* 1994; **331**:496–501.
95. Serruys PW, de-Jaegere P, Kiemeneij F et al, A comparison of balloon-expandable-stent implantation with balloon angioplasty in patients with coronary artery disease. Benestent Study Group, *N Engl J Med* 1994; **331**:489–95.
96. Dotter TC, Transluminally placed coilspring endarterial tube grafts: longterm patency in canine popliteal artery, *Invest Radiol* 1969; **4**:329–32.
97. Haude M, Erbel R, Straub U, Dietz U, Meyer J, Short and long term results after intracoronary stenting in human coronary arteries: monocentre experience with the balloon-expandable Palmaz–Schatz stent, *Br Heart J* 1991; **66**:337–45.
98. Haude M, Erbel R, Straub U, Dietz U, Schatz R, Meyer J, Results of intracoronary stents for management of coronary dissection after balloon angioplasty, *Am J Cardiol* 1991; **67**:691–6.
99. Haude M, Hafner G, Jablonka A et al, Guidance of anticoagulation after intracoronary implantation of Palmaz–Schatz stents by monitoring prothrombin and prothrombin fragment 1 + 2, *Am Heart J* 1995; **130**:228–38.
100. Schatz RA, A view of vascular stents, *Circulation* 1989; **79**:445–7.
101. Cavaye DM, Tabbara MR, Kopchok GE, Termin P, White RA, Intraluminal ultrasound assessment of vascular stent deployment, *Ann Vasc Surg* 1991; **5**:241–6.
102. Isner JM, Rosenfield K, Losordo DW et al, Percutaneous intravascular US as adjunct to catheter-based interventions: preliminary experience in patients with peripheral vascular disease, *Radiology* 1990; **175**:61–70.
103. Keren G, Bartorelli AL, Bonner RF, Douek PC, Leon MB, Intravascular ultrasound examination of coronary stents. In: Tobis JM, Yock JM, eds. *Intravascular Ultrasound Imaging*, 1st edn. (Churchill Livingstone: New York, Edinburgh, London, Tokyo), 1992) 219–30.
104. Görge G, Erbel R, Ge J, Gerber T, Haude M, Meyer J, Intravascular ultrasound after stent implantation: can stent recoil or compression occur? *Eur Heart J* 1992; **13**:308.
105. Goldberg SL, Colombo A, Nakamura S, Almagor Y, Maiello L, Tobis JM, Benefit of intracoronary ultrasound in the deployment of Palmaz–Schatz stents, *J Am Coll Cardiol* 1994; **24**:996–1003.
106. Colombo A, Hall P, Nakamura S et al, Intracoronary stenting without anticoagulation accomplished with intravascular ultrasound guidance, *Circulation* 1995; **91**:1676–88.
107. Nakamura S, Colombo A, Gaglione A et al, Intracoronary ultrasound observations during stent implantation, *Circulation* 1994; **89**:2026–34.
108. Morice MC, Zemour G, Benveniste E et al, Intracoronary stenting without coumadin: one month results of a French multicenter study, *Cathet Cardiovasc Diagn* 1995; **35**:1–7.
109. Morice MC, Breton C, Bunouf P et al, Coronary stenting without anticoagulation, without intravascular ultrasound. Results of the French registry, *Circulation* 1995; **92**(8): I-796.
110. Mudra H, Klauss V, Blasini R et al, Ultrasound guidance of Palmaz–Schatz intracoronary stenting with a combined intravascular ultrasound balloon catheter, *Circulation* 1994; **90**:1252–61.
111. Görge G, Haude M, Ge J et al, Intravascular ultrasound after low and high inflation pressure coronary artery stent implantation, *J Am Coll Cardiol* 1995; **26**:725–30.
112. Blasini R, Schühlen H, Mudra H et al, Angiographic overestimation of lumen size after coronary stent placement: impact of high pressure dilatation, *Circulation* 1995; **92**(8):I-223.
113. Serruys PW, di Mario C, Who was the thrombogenic: the stent or the doctor? *Circulation* 1995; **91**:1676–88.
114. Nunez BD, Foster-Smith K, Berger PB et al, Benefit of intravascular ultrasound guided high pressure inflations in patients with a 'perfect' angiographic result: the Mayor Clinic experience, *Circulation* 1995; **92**(8):I-545.
115. Ellis SG, Savage M, Fischman D et al, Restenosis after placement of Palmaz–Schatz stents in native coronary arteries: initial results of a multicenter experience, *Circulation* 1992; **86**:1836–44.
116. Painter JA, Mintz GS, Wong SC et al, Serial intravascular ultrasound studies fail to show evidence of chronic Palmaz–Schatz stent recoil, *Am J Cardiol* 1995; **75**:398–400.
117. Baim DS, Levine MJ, Leon MB, Levine S, Ellis SG, Schatz RA, management of restenosis within the Palmaz–Schatz coronary stent (the US multicenter experience), *Am J Cardiol* 1993; **71**:364–6.
118. Ikari Y, Yamaguchi T, Tamura T, Isshiki T, Saeki F, Hara K, Transluminal extraction atherectomy and adjunctive balloon angioplasty for restenosis after Palmaz–Schatz coronary stent implantation, *Cathet Cardiovasc Diagn* 1993; **30**:127–30.

119. Ikari Y, Hara K, Tamura T, Saeki F, Yamaguchi T, Luminal loss and site of restenosis after Palmaz–Schatz coronary stent implantation, *Am J Cardiol* 1995; **76**:117–20.
120. Block PC, Myler RK, Stertzer S, Fallon JT, Morphology after transluminal angioplasty in human beings, *N Engl J Med* 1981; **305**:382–5.
121. Mizuno K, Kurita A, Imazeki N, Pathological findings after percutaneous transluminal coronary angioplasty, *Br Heart J* 1984; **52**:588–90.
122. Erbel R, Zotz R, Stähr P, Dietz U, Rupprecht HJ, Meyer J, Percutaneous transluminal coronary rotational angioplasty. In: Topol EJ, Serruys PW, eds. *Current Review of Interventional Cardiology* (Philadelphia: Current Medicine, 1994) 10.2–10.25.
123. Ge J, Erbel R, Rupprecht HJ et al, Differentiation of the effects of balloon and high frequency rotational coronary angioplasty by intravascular ultrasound and angiography, *J Am Coll Cardiol* 1992; **19**:333A.
124. von Birgelen C, Umans VA, Di Mario C et al, Mechanisms of high-speed rotational atherectomy and adjunctive balloon angioplasty revisited by quantative coronary angiography: edge detection versus videodensitometry, *Am Heart J* 1995; **130**:405–12.
125. Fitzgerald PJ, Portss TA, Yoc PG, Contribution of localized calcium deposits to dissection after angioplasty, an observational study using intravascular ultrasound, *Circulation* 1992; **86**:64–70.
126. Topol EJ, Leya F, Pinkerton CA et al, A comparison of directional atherectomy with coronary angioplasty in patients with coronary artery disease, *N Engl J Med* 1993; **329**:221–7.
127. Adelman A, Cohen E, Kimball B et al, A comparison of directional coronary atherectomy with balloon angioplasty for lesions of the left anterior descending coronary artery, *N Engl J Med* 1993; **329**:228–33.
128. Dussaillant GR, Mintz GS, Popma JJ et al, Intravascular ultrasound, directional coronary atherectomy, and the optimal atherectomy restenosis study, *Coronary Art Dis* 1996; **7**:294–8.
129. Baim DS, Cutlip D, Ho KKL, Popma JJ, Senerchia C, Kuntz RE, Acute results of directional coronary atherectomy in the balloon versus optimal atherectomy trial (BOAT) pilot phase, *Coronary Art Dis* 1996; **7**:290–3.
130. Mintz GS, Kovach JA, Javier SP et al, Mechanisms of lumen enlargement after excimer laser coronary angioplasty: an intravascular ultrasound study, *Circulation* 1995; **92**:3408–14.
131. Honye J, Mahon DJ, Nakamura S et al, Intravascular ultrasound imaging after excimer laser angioplasty, *Cathet Cardiovasc Diagn* 1994; **32**:213–22.
132. Siegel RJ, Gunn J, Ahsan A et al, Use of therapeutic ultrasound in percutaneous coronary angioplasty: experimental in vitro studies and initial clinical experience, *Circulation* 1994; **89**:1587–92.
133. Rosenschein U, Bernstein JJ, DiSegni E, Kaplinski E, Bernheim J, Rozenzsajn LA, Experimental ultrasonic angioplasty: disruption of atherosclerotic plaques and thrombi in vitro and arterial recanalization in vivo, *J Am Coll Cardiol* 1990; **15**:711–17.
134. Willard JE, Netto D, Demian SE et al, Intravascular ultrasound imaging of saphenous vein grafts in vitro: comparison with histologic and quantative angiographic findings, *J Am Coll Cardiol* 1992; **19**:759–64.
135. Kriett JM, Kaye MP, The registry of the International Society for Heart and Lung Transplantation: Seventh Official Report—1990, *J Heart Lung Transplant* 1990; **9**:323–30.
136. Miller LW, Transplant coronary artery disease, *J Heart Lung Transplant* 1992; **3**:51–4.
137. Uretsky BF, Murali S, Reddy PS et al, Development of coronary artery disease in cardiac transplant patients receiving immunosuppressive therapy with cycloserine and prednisone, *Circulation* 1987; **76**:827–33.
138. Ventura HO, Smart FW, Stapleton DD, Toups T, Price HL, Cardiac allograft vasculopathy: current concepts, *J La State Med Soc* 1993; **145**:195–202.
139. Rickenbacher PR, Pinto FJ, Chenzbraun A et al, Incidence and severity of transplanted coronary artery disease early and up to 15 years after transplantation as detected by intravascular ultrasound, *J Am Coll Cardiol* 1995; **25**:171–7.
140. Ge J, Haude M, Caspari G et al, Detection of occult coronary artery disease in patients with heart transplantation, *Z Kardiol* 1996; **85**:II-66.
141. Haude M, Ge J, Machraoui A, Erbel R, Zerkowski HR, Regression of pre-existing coronary artery disease in a donor heart after cardiac transplantation, *Eur J Cardiothorac Surg* 1995; **9**:399–402.
142. Ventura HO, White CJ, Jain SP et al, Assessment of intracoronary morphology in cardiac transplant recipients by angioscopy and intravascular ultrasound, *Am J Cardiol* 1993; **72**:805–9.
143. Pinto FJ, St Goar FG, Gao SZ et al, Immediate and one year safety of intracoronary ultrasonic imaging, evaluation with serial quantitative angiography, *Circulation* 1993; **88**:1709–14.
144. Friedrich GJ, Moes NY, Mühlberger VA et al, Detection of intralesional calcium by intracoronary ultrasound depends on the histologic pattern, *Am Heart J* 1994; **128**:435–41.
145. Frimerman A, Miller HI, Hallman M, Laniado S, Keren G, Intravascular ultrasound characterization of thrombi of different composition, *Am J Cardiol* 1994; **73**:1053–7.
146. Lee DY, Eigler N, Fishbein MC, Bhambi B, Maurer G, Siegel RJ, Identification of intracoronary thrombus and determination of thrombectomy by intravascular ultrasound imaging, *Am J Cardiol* 1994; **73**:522–3.
147. Fitzgerald P, Yock PG, Tissue characterization by intraluminal ultrasound, Proceedings 7th Essen-Mayo-Mainz Symposium, Essen, 1995, 157.
148. Coy KM, Park JC, Fishbein MC et al, In vitro validation of three-dimensional intravascular ultrasound for evaluation of arterial injury after balloon angioplasty, *J Am Coll Cardiol* 1992; **20**:692–700.
149. Ge J, Koch L, Roth T et al, Three-dimensional reconstruction and quantification of intracoronary ultrasound images under guidance of biplane fluoroscopy, *Herz* 1995; **20**:263–76.
150. Roelandt JRTC, Di Mario C, Pandian N et al, Three-dimensional reconstruction of intracoronary ultrasound images Rationale, approaches, problems, and directions, *Circulation* 1994; **90**:1044–55.
151. Hausmann D, Erbel R, Alibelli-Chemarin MJ et al, The safety of intracoronary ultrasound. A multicenter survey of 2207 examinations, *Circulation* 1995; **91**:623–30.
152. Erbel R, Ge J, Gerber T, Görge G, Rupprecht HJ, Meyer J, Safety and limitations of intravascular ultrasound, *Circulation* 1992; **86**:I-195.

153. Ge J, Liu F, Kearney P, Görge G, Haude M, Erbel R, Acute coronary artery closure following intracoronary ultrasound examination, *Cathet Cardiovasc Diagn* 1995; **35**:232–5.
154. Bory M, Panagides D, Yvorra S, Colin R, Fourcade L, Bonnet JL, Intravascular ultrasound detection of atherosclerosis at the site of vasospasm in angiographically normal or mild narrowed coronary arteries, *Eur Heart J* 1995; **16**:250A.
155. Pinto FJ, St Goar FG, Gao SZ et al, Immediate and one-year safety of intracoronary ultrasonic imaging, evaluation with serial quantitative angiography, *Circulation* 1993; **88**:1709–14.

Chapter 4 Upper urinary tract

Demetrius H Bagley and Ji-Bin Liu

INTRODUCTION

Ultrasound has long been used for evaluation of the upper urinary tract. It remains the technique of preference for the initial evaluation of renal masses and for hydronephrosis.[1] It can be used to localize calculi for shock-wave lithotripsy.[2] The accuracy of ultrasound also carried it to the operating room to localize renal calculi intraoperatively for removal prior to the development of endourologic techniques.[3] Miniaturization of ultrasound probes has enabled them to be placed into the lumen of the ureter and upper collecting system. Techniques have been developed to use these devices in the upper urinary tract.[4–6] Through these studies, endoluminal sonography has become a valuable adjunct to endoscopy of the upper urinary tract.

The catheter-based transducers are an ideal size for introduction into the ureter, either directly or through a ureteroscope. The range of penetration of the transducers presently available is adequate for the ureter itself and the periureteral tissues, while the very high resolution is important for periureteral diagnosis. The findings from endoluminal sonography in the upper urinary tract have formed a valuable supplement to the information gained from endoluminal endoscopy and have been important in guiding several therapeutic procedures. Endoluminal sonography now has an established role in diagnosis and treatment within the upper urinary tract. This can be expected to expand as more specific instruments are developed for urologic applications.

INSTRUMENTATION

The standard catheter-based ultrasound probes, which have been used in other endoluminal vascular and nonvascular applications, can also be used for urologic purposes (Table 4.1). The probes range in size from 3.5 to 6.2 Fr (Microvasive, Boston Scientific Corporation, Natick, MA) (Fig. 4.1). The larger (6.2 Fr) catheters are available in two designs, one with a round tip and the other with a 'side-saddle' or over-the-guidewire design. Both of these can be passed through any portion of the ureter except the narrowest of strictures. They can be passed through a standard cystoscope or nephroscope into the ureter and can be advanced into the renal pelvis and upper infundibula. The over-the-guidewire design can be stabilized with a 0.025-inch (stiff) guidewire to be passed transurethrally through the bladder into the ureter.

Table 4.1 Endoluminal ultrasound probes used in the ureter.

Outside diameter (Fr)	*Length (cm)*	*Tip configuration*	*Frequency (MHz)*	*Recommended guidewire (inch)*
6.2	95	Round tip	20	N/A
6.2	95	Side-saddle	20	0.025
6.2	95	Round tip	12.5	N/A
6.2	95	Side-saddle	12.5	0.025
4.8	126	Over-the-wire	20	0.014
3.5	140	Rapid exchange	20	0.018

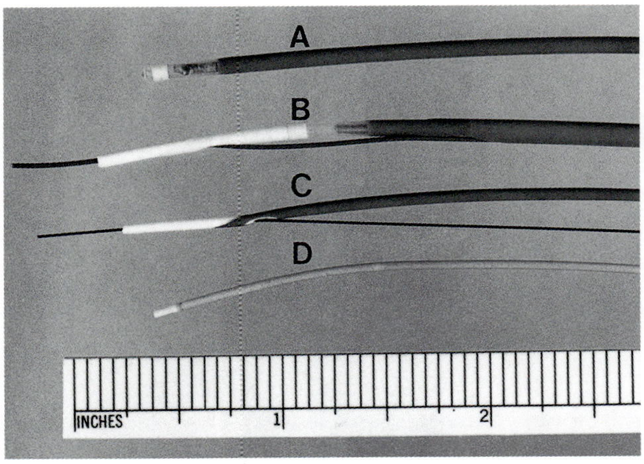

Figure 4.1 *Endoluminal ultrasound probes are available in sizes of 3.5 to 6.2 Fr. The largest probe is available either as a round-tip model or with a side-saddle design to be placed over a guidewire. (A) 6.2 Fr round tip. (B) 6.2 Fr side-saddle with wire. (C) 4.8 Fr over-the-wire design with guidewire. (D) 3.5 Fr catheter, rapid-exchange design.*

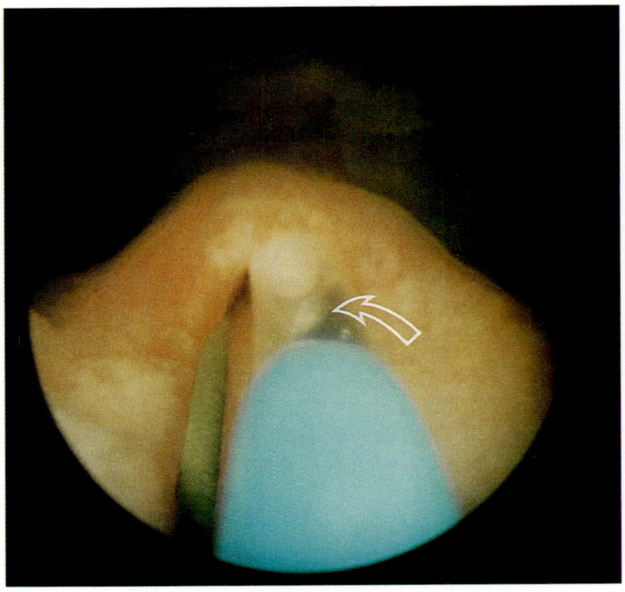

Figure 4.3 *The probe can be passed into the ureteral orifice either directly or over a guidewire. In the larger probes, the transducer (arrow) is visible cystoscopically through a window in the catheter itself.*

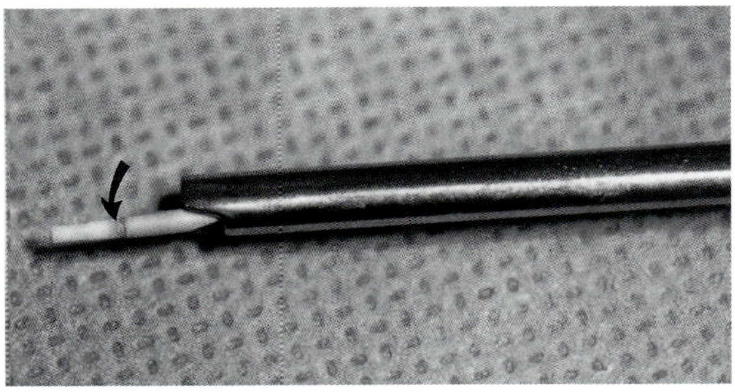

Figure 4.2 *The smaller probes can be passed through the working channel of some ureteroscopes, to be placed into the ureteral lumen under direct visualization. A 3.5 Fr probe (arrow) has been passed through the 5.4 Fr channel in a rigid ureteroscope.*

The smaller probes (3.5 and 4.8 Fr) can be passed through the working channel of many ureteroscopes (Fig. 4.2). These then have the advantage of being placed under direct visualization, which allows specific localization and orientation. The 4.8 Fr design can be passed over a 0.014-inch guidewire using the 'side-saddle' tip, while the 3.5 Fr probe uses a 0.018-inch guidewire. The single-crystal ultrasound transducers have been used at frequencies of 12.5 and 20 MHz. Both of these devices provide a cross-sectional image with penetration of 1.5–2 cm, which is adequate for visualization of most of the immediate periureteral structures. The transducers are attached to the special ultrasound unit (IVUS, Diasonics or Bruel & Kjaer 3535), which is equipped for real-time imaging as well as hard-copy and video recording.

The catheter must be filled with sterile water at the level of the transducer to provide an interface for ultrasound transmission. Since the catheter containing the transducer is packaged dry, water must be added. A 1-ml syringe fitted with a 27 gauge needle, supplied with the ultrasound probe, is first filled with water. The needle is then inserted through the tip of the catheter. It is inserted via the tip hole near the guidewire channel directly into the lumen in the 6.2 Fr catheter. In the smaller catheters, a special needle guide is provided to direct the needle into the lumen through the tip of the catheter. A full 1 ml of water is then injected into the lumen. Since there may be a bubble of air remaining at the tip, the catheter should be swung rapidly to allow centrifugal force to drive the water to the tip of the catheter. The transducer is then mounted on the ultrasound machine to confirm

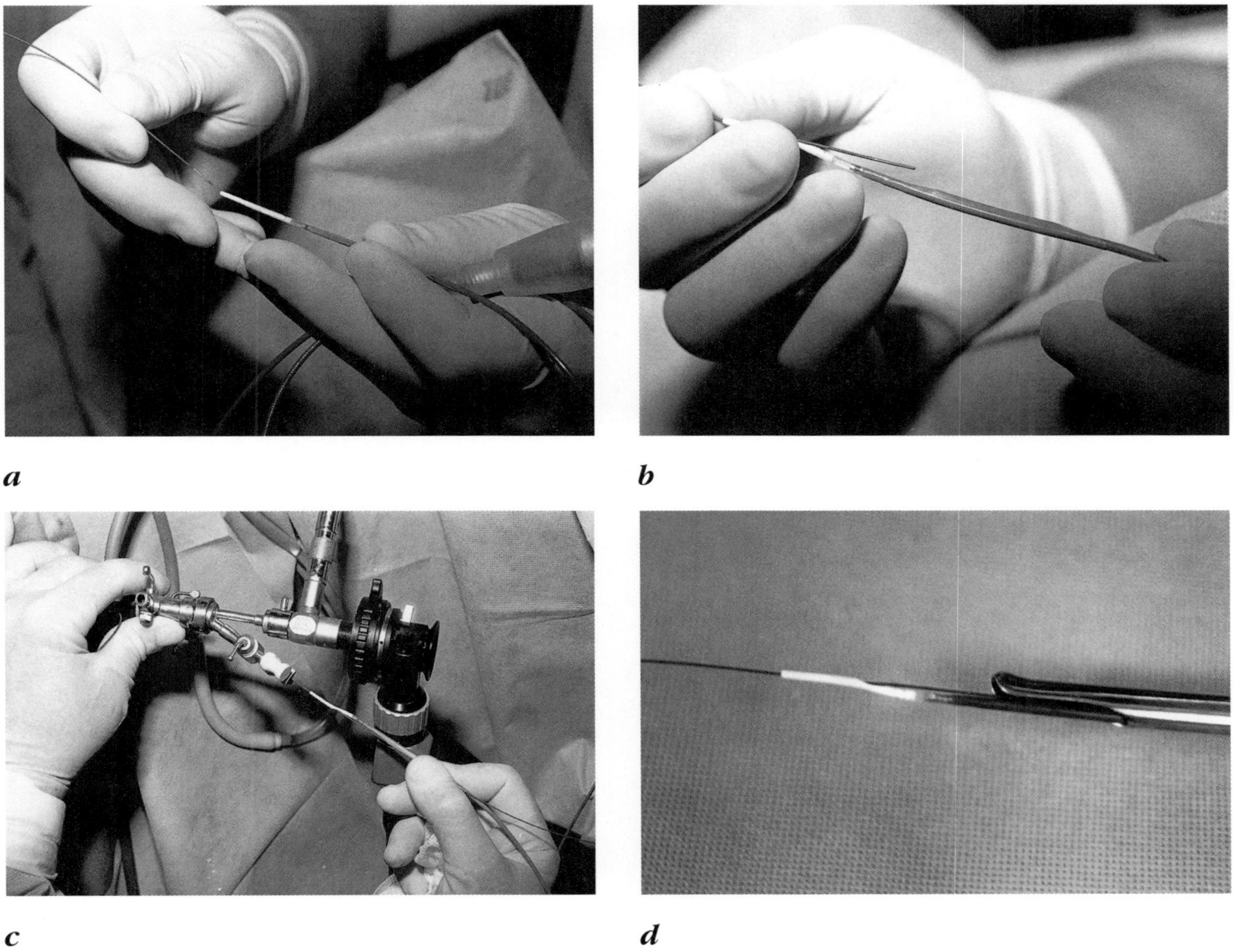

Figure 4.4 *The wire which has been passed cystoscopically into the ureteral orifice (a,b) is backloaded through the side-saddle (c) to direct the catheter into the working port (d). The catheter is thus stabilized with the wire enabling it to pass into the orifice.*

that there is good transmission of the ultrasound without interference from air within the catheter.

TECHNIQUES

Endoluminal ultrasound has been applied in the upper urinary tract along with intraluminal endoscopy. Both retrograde transurethral uretero-scopic approaches and percutaneous nephroscopic approaches have been employed. The choice of endoscope, approach and ultrasound probe depend upon the available access and, particularly, upon the diagnostic problem. The retrograde approach has generally been used unless there is a nephrostomy tract of adequate caliber in place.

The endoluminal ultrasound probes can be passed into the lumen of the ureter in a retrograde fashion using one of several techniques. The ultrasound catheters can be passed cystoscopically, using the working port to place the catheter just as with any other ureteral catheter. The round-tip probe (6.2 Fr) is easily passed through the working port into the ureter. Since there is a transparent segment at the level of the transducer, the point of visualization is easily seen as the catheter passes into the orifice (Fig.

4.3). However, it is lost to visual inspection within the ureter and its position can be determined only by fluoroscopy or recognition of the sonographic and anatomic findings. The catheter can be passed along the ureteral lumen until the area of interest is reached. Again, the position is confirmed fluoroscopically.

The catheters with the side-saddle or over-the-wire-design can be guided into the ureteral orifice with the guidewire. The appropriate size of wire is first passed cystoscopically. The wire is then backloaded through the tip of the catheter, which is advanced through the working port of the ureteroscope along the guidewire and into the orifice (Fig. 4.4). Again, the position can be checked fluoroscopically as the catheter advances into the ureter. This technique is particularly useful when there is any anticipated difficulty in passing the catheter, such as tortuosity or narrowing of the ureter. The shaft of the catheter is stabilized by the sheath of the cystoscope so that it can be advanced directly at the level of the ureteral orifice without kinking or coiling in the bladder.

An alternative technique is to place a guidewire into the ureteral orifice cystoscopically or ureteroscopically. The endoscope is then removed and the catheter can be threaded over the guidewire and advanced into the urethra, bladder and ureter with fluoroscopic monitoring alone. It is essential to follow the catheter as it advances, since it may coil within the bladder as the tip meets the resistance of the ureteral orifice. Since the catheter is stabilized only at the tip, it is much easier for the shaft to curl in the bladder or other-wise diverge from the path of the guidewire than for a similarly sized ureteral catheter to change direction.

For practical purposes, the technique of guidewire passage is limited to the 6.2 Fr catheters, since the smaller probe (4.8 Fr) accepts a 0.014-inch wire which is too flexible to provide sufficient stabilization in most cases. The 6.2 Fr catheter accepts a 0.025-inch wire, which should be of a stiff design. These same techniques of direct insertion or over-the-guidewire insertion can be used to pass the catheter nephroscopically or through a nephrostomy tract.

With the smaller ultrasound probes (<4.8 Fr), endoluminal sonography can be performed with the catheter passed directly through the working channel of the ureteroscope. The position of the probe can then be very accurately determined visually and confirmed fluoroscopically (Fig. 4.5). The location of any lesions and any other landmarks within the visual field can also be specifically determined.

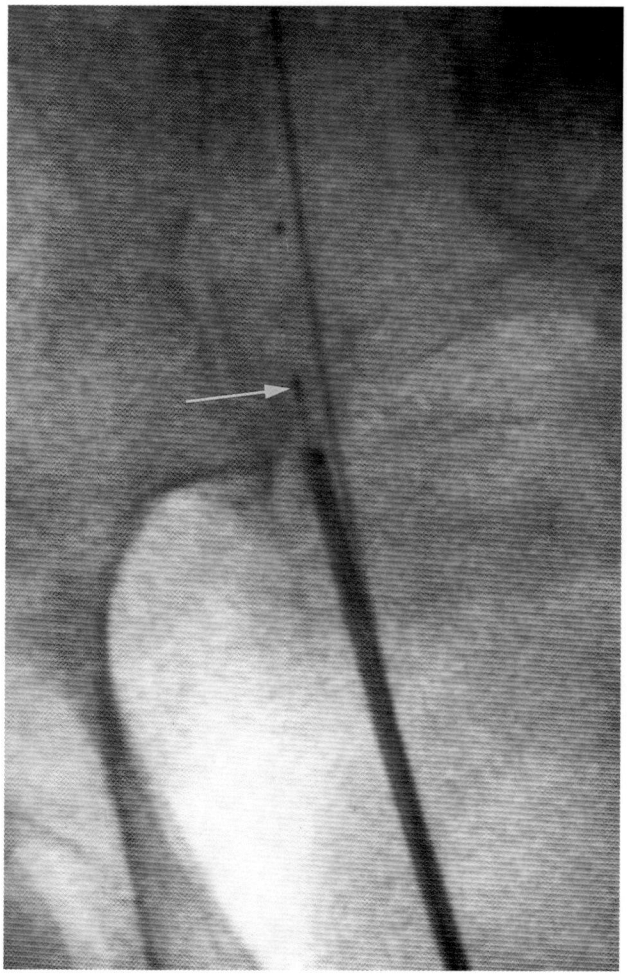

Figure 4.5 *The 3.5 Fr probe is also radio-opaque. It can be located with direct vision through the ureteroscope and can also be seen fluoroscopically. The transducer (arrow) in the probe is located at the tip of the ureteroscope.*

ORIENTATION

In our series, we have attempted to standardize the orientation of the image. It has been considered to be a cross-section viewed in a cephalad direction with the patient supine. It is then the image that would be obtained with the ultrasound catheter placed cystoscopically in a retrograde fashion. It is also the same orientation used for abdominal CT scan (Fig. 4.6).

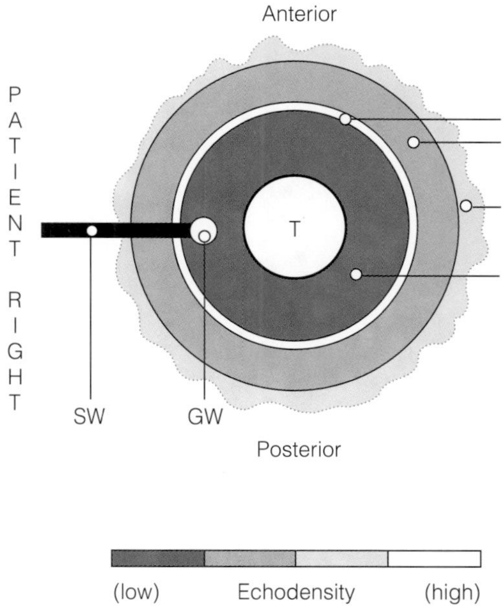

Figure 4.6 *The ultrasound image is oriented with the patient in the supine position and the ultrasound catheter placed in a retrograde fashion. Therefore, the upper portion of the image is anterior and the lower is posterior. The right side of the image represents the patient's left and the left side represents the patient's right. This is the same orientation used for abdominal CT scans. It can also be thought of as viewing from the urologist's position. The echodensity of the normal sonographic ureteral image is represented. GW, guidewire; SW, shadow; L, lumen; 1, mucosa; 2, muscularis; 3, adventitia; T, transducer (compare Fig. 4.15).*

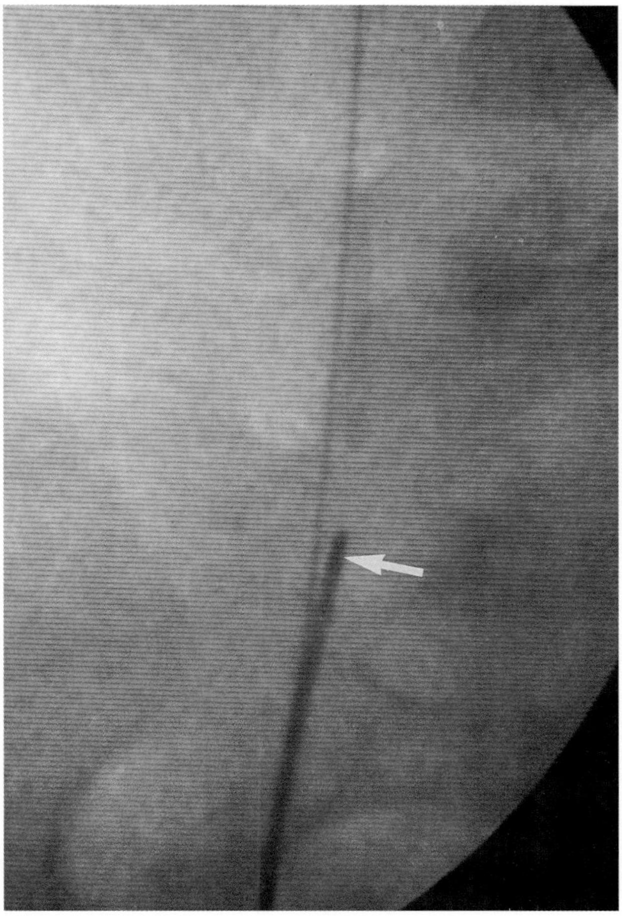

a

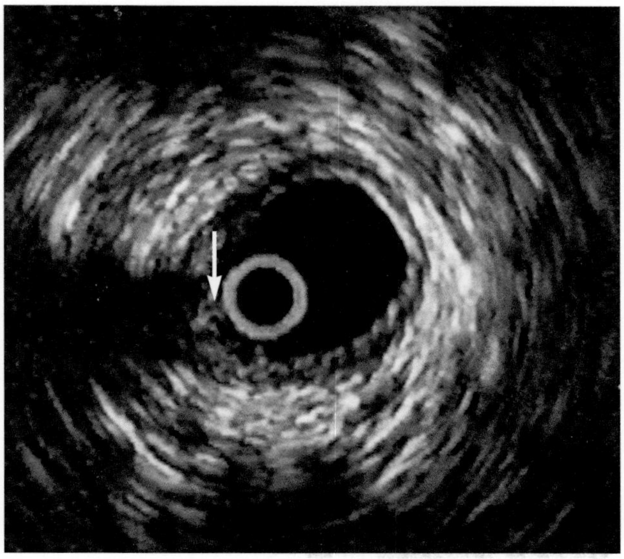

b

Figure 4.7 *Since the ultrasound image can be rotated during placement of the catheter, it can be justified on the viewing screen by relating the orientation of known landmarks, including the guidewire. Simultaneous fluoroscopy is particularly helpful in determining the position of the guidewire and, thereby, the appropriate orientation. In this example, the guidewire is located lateral to the ultrasound probe (arrow) in the left ureter (a). Therefore, the ultrasound image is oriented as indicated with the guidewire (arrow) located on the left in the image (b) .*

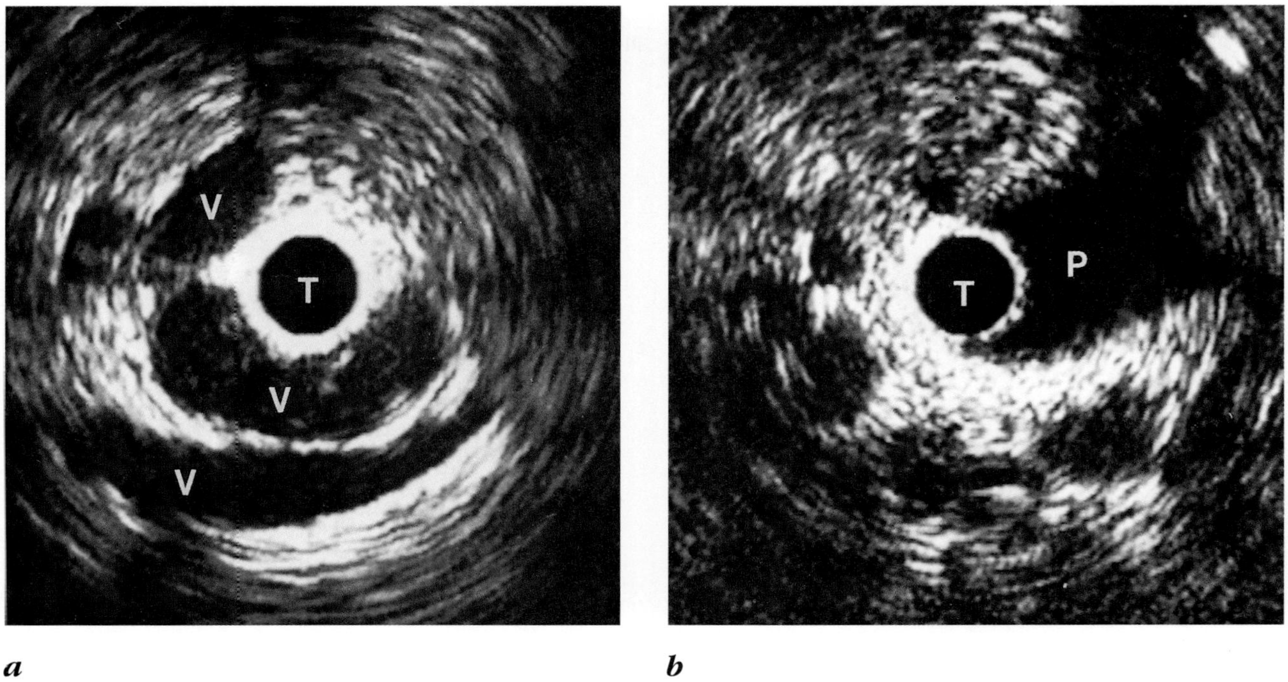

Figure 4.8 *(a) Endoluminal ultrasound of the ureteropelvic junction in an animal model demonstrates vessels (V) adjacent to the ureter containing the transducer (T). Their presence, location and size were confirmed by dissection. (b) The transducer (T) has been advanced into the renal pelvis (P).*

Since the image can be rotated by rotating the transducer, and the image on the screen can be justified to center or rotate the image, it is essential to have a reference point to determine rotational orientation at any specific level. A guidewire in the ureter adjacent to the probe can be seen both in the sonographic image and fluoroscopically for orientation (Fig. 4.7). It is quite easy to recognize the position of the wire when it is medial or lateral to the ultrasound probe. However, if it is directly anterior or posterior it may be very difficult to determine the appropriate orientation. An effort can then be made to change the position of the probe relative to the wire in order to orient it appropriately. Other landmarks, such as the ureteral orifice, the iliac vessels, psoas muscle or the renal pelvis, can be used to assist in orientation as well.

NORMAL ANATOMY

Normal endoluminal sonographic anatomy of the upper urinary tract can be well documented in patients studied with the techniques described. The initial studies were conducted in animals to determine the feasibility of endoureteral ultrasound and to delineate the anatomic images (Fig. 4.8). Similar findings have been confirmed in numerous patients with remotely located lesions and others with no abnormalities. It is important to be familiar with the normal anatomy in order to be able to recognize abnormal findings and also to aid in properly locating and orienting the probe within the ureter.

The normal ureteral anatomy demonstrated by endoluminal ultrasound is illustrated in Figs 4.9 to

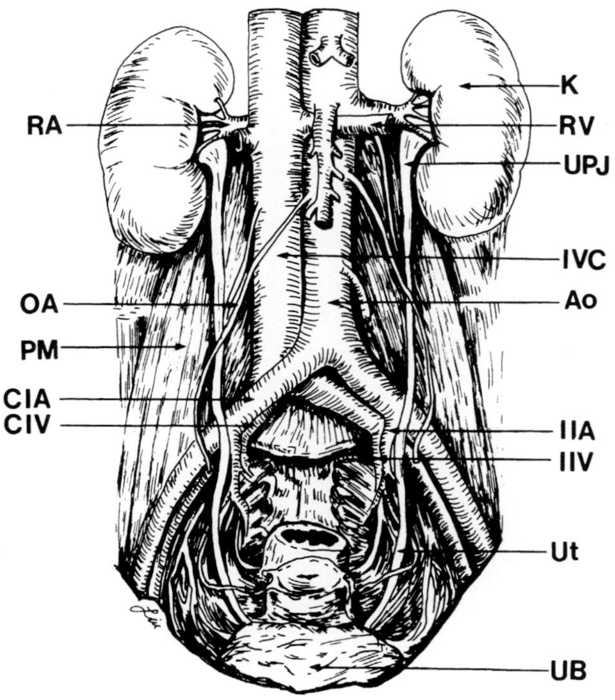

Figure 4.9 *The ureter passes adjacent to many strictures in its normal course from the kidney to the bladder. K, kidney; RV, renal vein; RA, renal artery; UPJ, ureteropelvic junction; IVC, inferior vena cava; OA, ovarian artery; Ao, aorta; PM, psoas muscle; CIA, common iliac artery; CIV, common iliac vein; IIA, internal iliac artery; IIV, internal iliac vein; Ut, ureter; UB, urinary bladder.*

4.20 as the probe is placed cystoscopically into the ureter and advanced proximally throughout the lumen to the renal pelvis and upper infundibulum. In its course between the bladder and the kidney, the ureter passes in close proximity to several normal structures which can be visualized with endoluminal ultrasound (Fig. 4.9). Recognition of these structures can provide orientation and guide ureteral procedures. As the ureter courses in a retrograde fashion from the level of the bladder, it first consists of an intravesical portion which is supported posteriorly by the muscle of the bladder. Anteriorly, the ureter is covered only with mucosa and is exposed to the limit of the bladder. It then courses through the wall of the bladder and exits to pass to the next constant landmark. At the pelvic brim, the ureter courses immediately anterior to the common iliac artery and vein. Just distal to that level it has been located medial to the external iliac vessels and anterior to the internal iliacs. Anteriorly, the peritoneum and its contents, specifically bowel, are situated. Proximally, the ureter passes anterior to the psoas muscle before it joins the pelvis. The blood supply of the ureter derives from the renal vessels and segmental branches along its entire length. Branches of these vessels lie adjacent to the infundibula as they course into the parenchyma. Both small arteries and veins lie within the adventitia along the entire ureter. The gonadal vessels, and even colonic vessels, may be in close proximity to the ureter along the course.

On endoluminal ultrasonography, the intravesical ureter is characterized by a cross-sectional pattern with the lumen of the bladder located anteriorly (Fig. 4.10). The ureteral lumen and the mucosa and muscularis of the ureter and bladder are evident, as is the bladder muscle posteriorly. Once the probe is passed more proximally, the bladder lumen is no longer seen and the intramural portion of the ureter is evident, but muscle surrounds the ureter circumferentially. The lumen and mucosa remain as described for the more distal portion. As the ultrasound probe exits the intramural ureter, it enters the distal ureter itself and here the characteristic image of the ureteral lumen, mucosa and muscularis surrounded by adventitia is evident. This is the image expected throughout most of the course of the ureter adjacent to other recognizable structures.

At the level of the iliac vessels, both the artery and vein can be seen, and often the bifurcation and branches of the iliac vessels are visible. Note that the lumen of the ureter is less than 2 mm from the lumen of the vessels (Figs 4.11, 4.12 and 4.13). The vein can be distinguished from the artery sonographically. In real time, the pulsations of the artery are quite visible. Slow-flowing venous blood is more echogenic than the arterial lumen (Fig. 4.12). Care should be taken in interpreting pulsations, since the arterial pulsations can also be transmitted through the vein or adjacent structure. The same criteria can be applied to smaller vessels. As they reach the range of 2 mm or less, the pulsations are even more important in distinguishing arteries from veins.

As the ureter ascends from the level of the iliac vessels, it lies on the surface of the psoas muscle. This can be recognized as one of the important landmarks sonographically (Fig. 4.14). Very frequently in this area, ureteral peristalsis is evident and is quite prominent. The lumen appears open sonographically and then, as the peristaltic wave passes, it closes (Fig. 4.15). Peristalsis can be seen

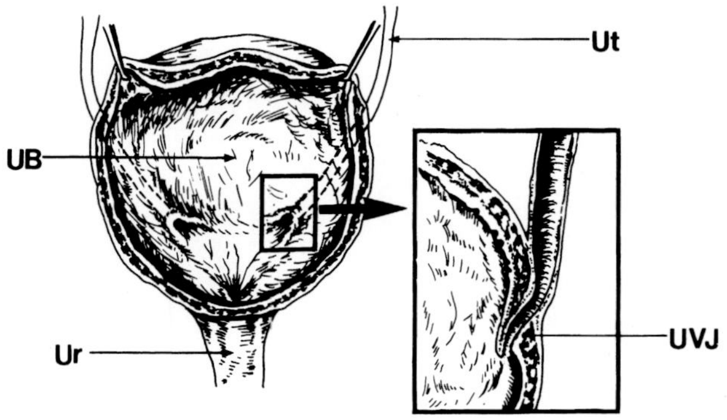

a

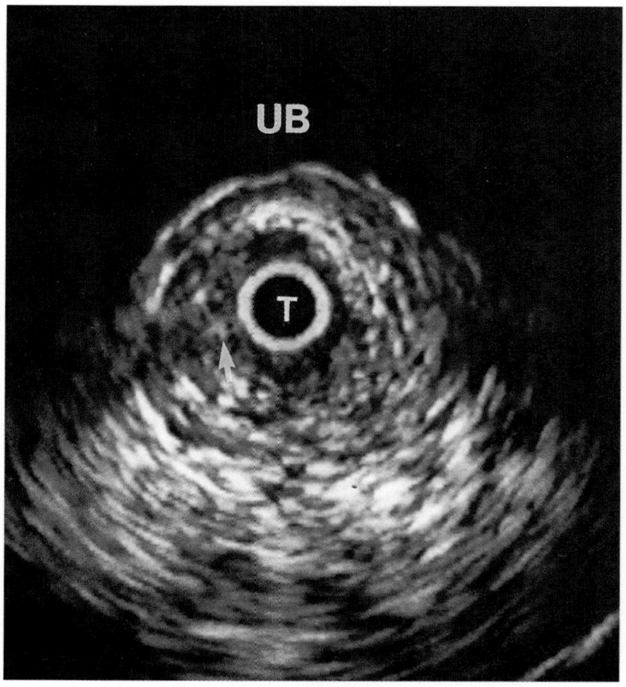

b

Figure 4.10 *(a) The ureter (Ut) courses through the wall of the bladder (UB) to form the ureterovesical junction (UVJ). Ur, urethra. (b) The transducer (T) is located within the intravesical ureter. A guidewire is located at 7 o'clock (arrow). The ureteral wall and the ureteral and bladder mucosa are located superiorly from 9 to 3 o'clock. The urine within the bladder (UB) is anechoic.*

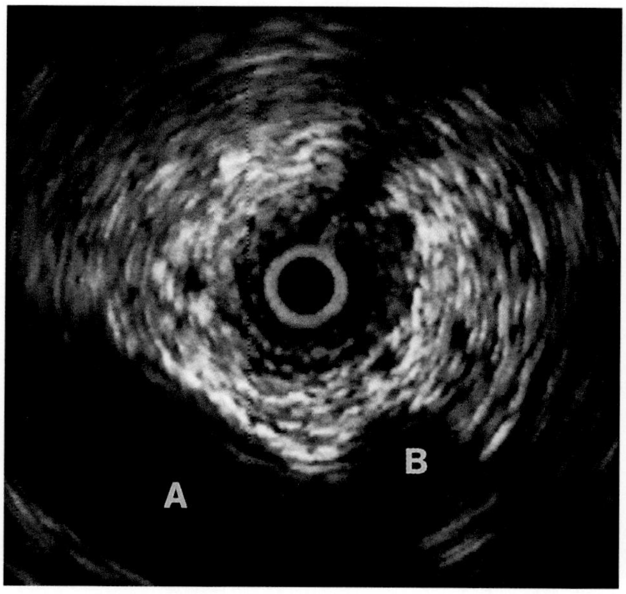

Figure 4.11 *The internal iliac artery (A) and a major branch (B) are shown.*

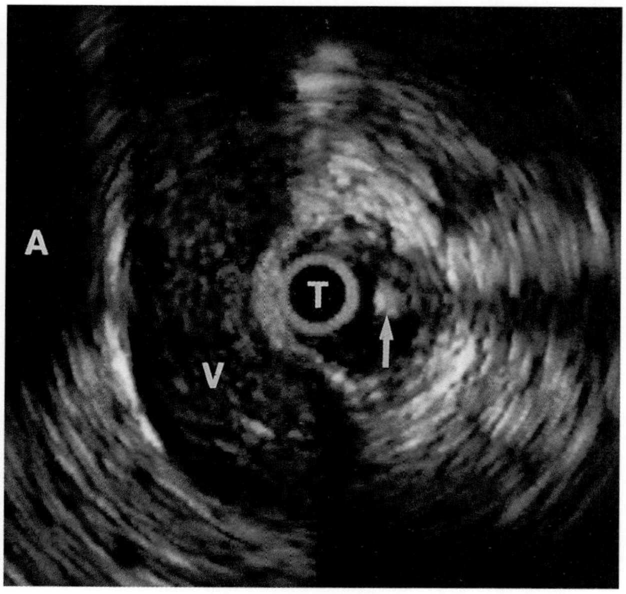

Figure 4.12 *At the level of the iliac vessels, the transducer (T) is located in the right ureter and the guidewire (arrow) is seen medially. Immediately adjacent to the ureter is the iliac vein (V) and further laterally is the artery (A).*

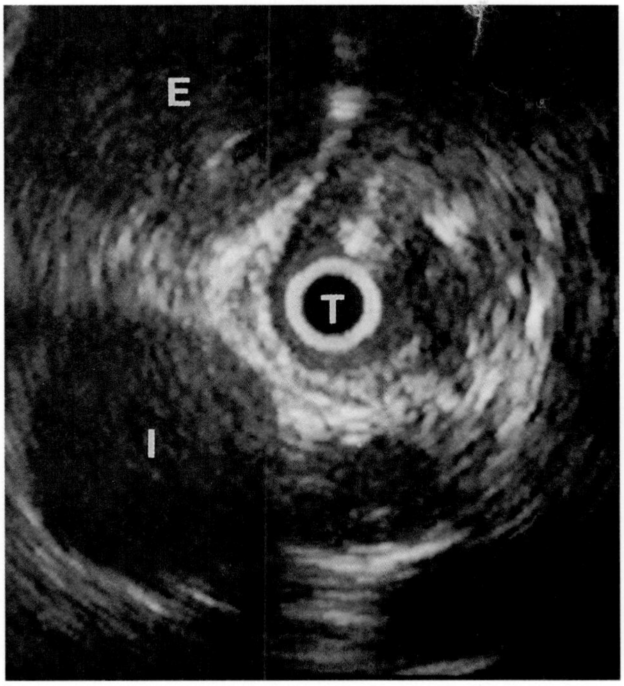

a

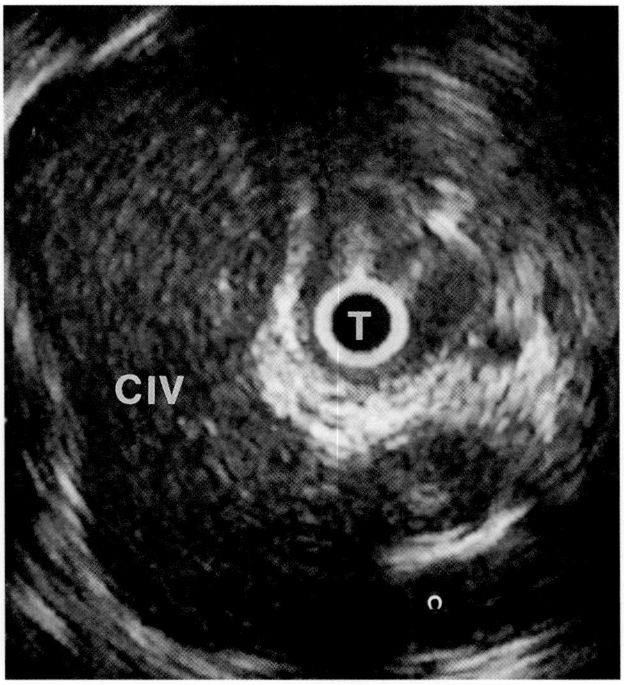

b

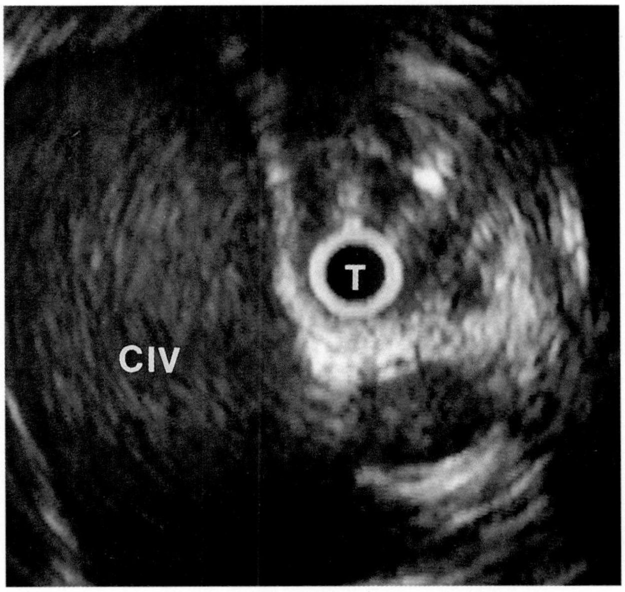

c

Figure 4.13 *As the transducer (T) is passed cephalad within the right ureter, the internal (I) and external (E) iliac veins (a) are shown joining at the bifurcation (b) to form the common iliac vein (CIV) (c).*

very well with real-time imaging. In this portion of the ureter, the gonadal vessels occasionally may be seen in close proximity (Fig. 4.16). The inferior vena cava may also be located near the ureter (Fig. 4.16).

The next major landmark as the probe passes cephalad is the ureteropelvic junction. Here there is usually an abrupt change in the diameter of the lumen as the ureter joins the renal pelvis (Fig. 4.17). The ureteral wall itself, including the mucosa and the muscularis, appears the same. Adjacent crossing vessels can be seen in less than 25% of patients with an apparently normal ureteropelvic junction.[6] Most of

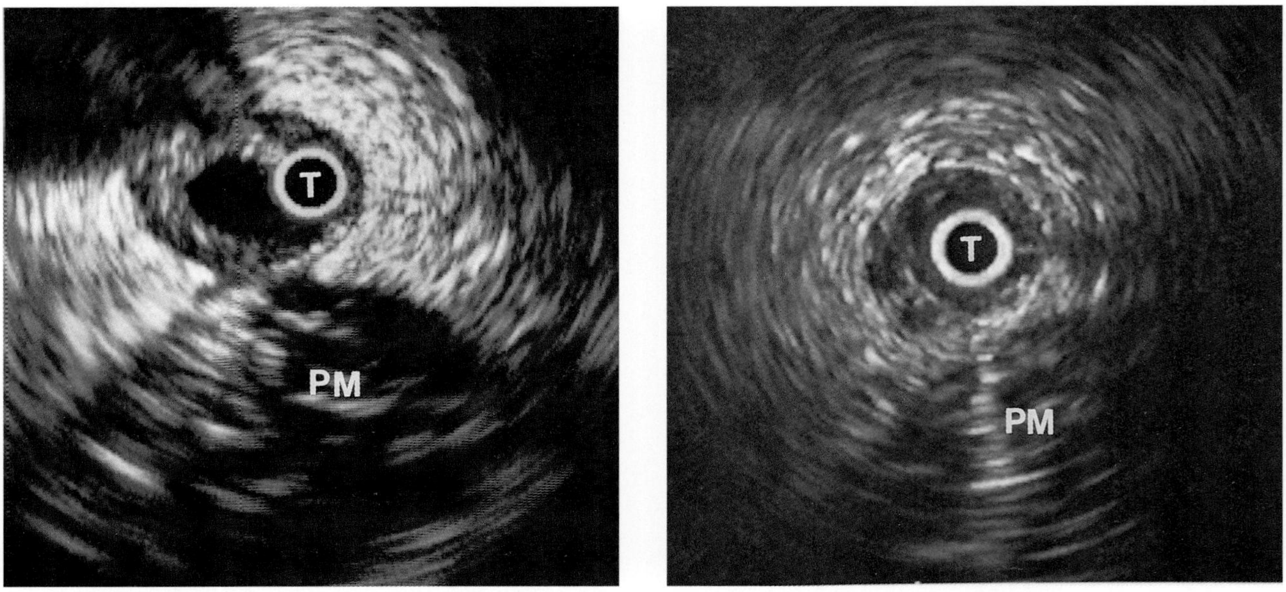

a *b*

Figure 4.14 *The psoas muscle (PM) is shown as the hypoechoic area inferior to the ureter containing the transducer (T) in two different patients (a,b).*

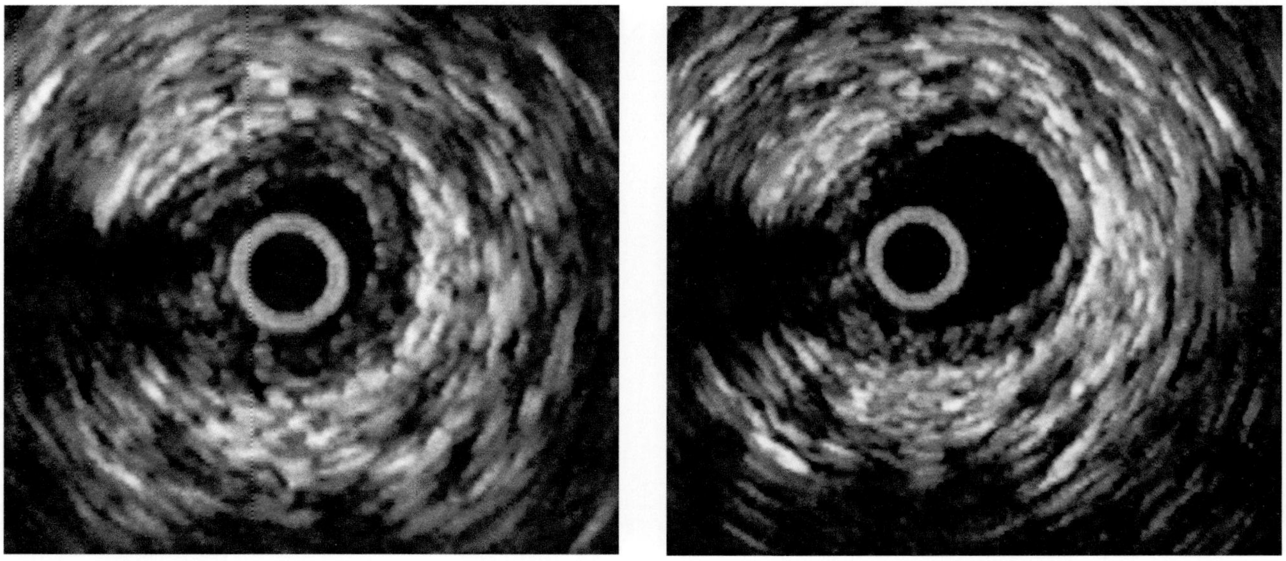

a *b*

Figure 4.15 *Ureteral peristalsis is often prominent in the lumbar ureter. The lumen opens (a–c) and then closes (d–f) with peristalsis.*

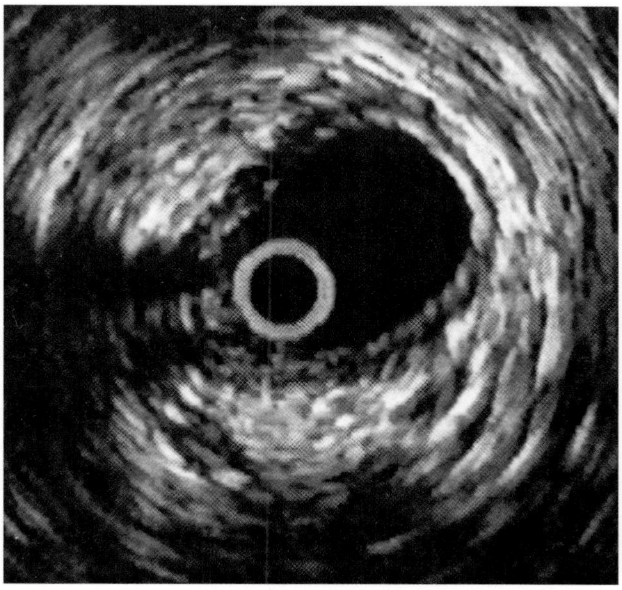

c

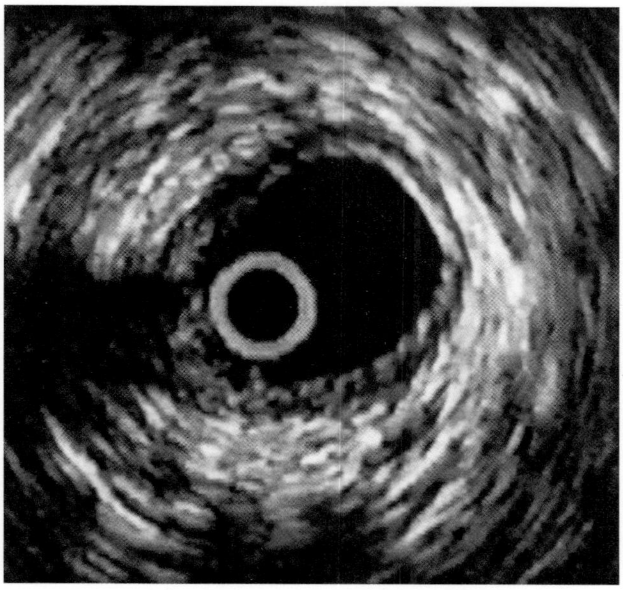

d

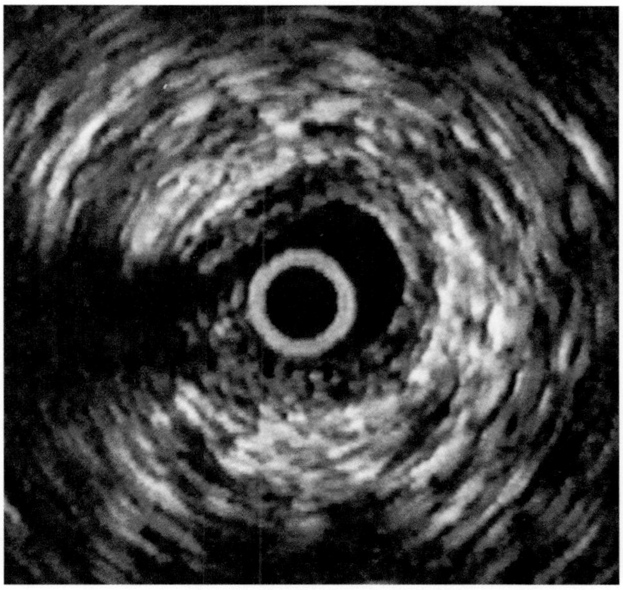

e

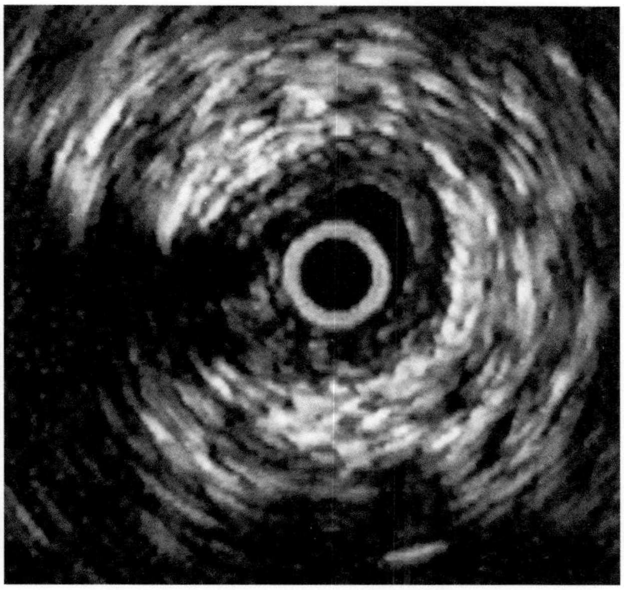

f

these vessels are 2 mm or less in diameter. Other minute periureteral vessels can be seen throughout the length of the ureter.

Within the renal pelvis, the sonolucent lumen reflects the extent of distension. At this level, quite large renal veins and arteries can be seen, usually anterior to the pelvis (Figs 4.18 and 4.19). In a normal situation, the major vessels enter the renal sinus anterior to the renal pelvis. They often branch at this level and in some cases the posterior branch of the renal artery may divide and course posterior to the renal pelvis.[7]

The ultrasound probe can also be inserted into the upper infundibulum. The mucosa is similar to that

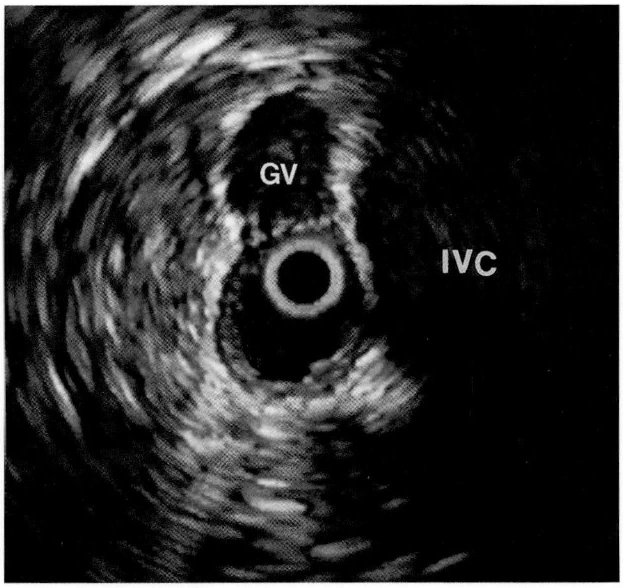

Figure 4.16 *The gonadal vein (GV) is located immediately superior to the ureter. The inferior vena cava (IVC) is located less than 2 mm medial to this right ureter and is seen on the right on this image.*

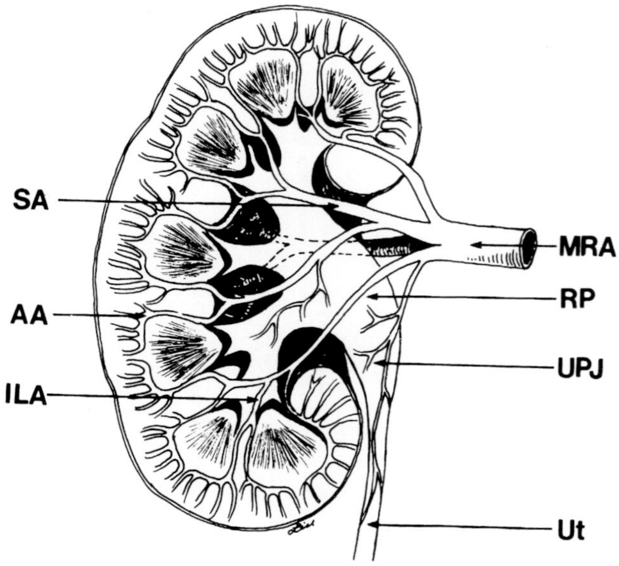

Figure 4.18 *The renal vessels lie adjacent to the renal pelvis (RP) in the renal sinus. This illustration indicates one example of the arterial supply. MRA, main renal artery; SA, segmental artery; AA, arcuate artery; ILA, interlobar artery; UPJ, ureteropelvic junction; Ut, ureter.*

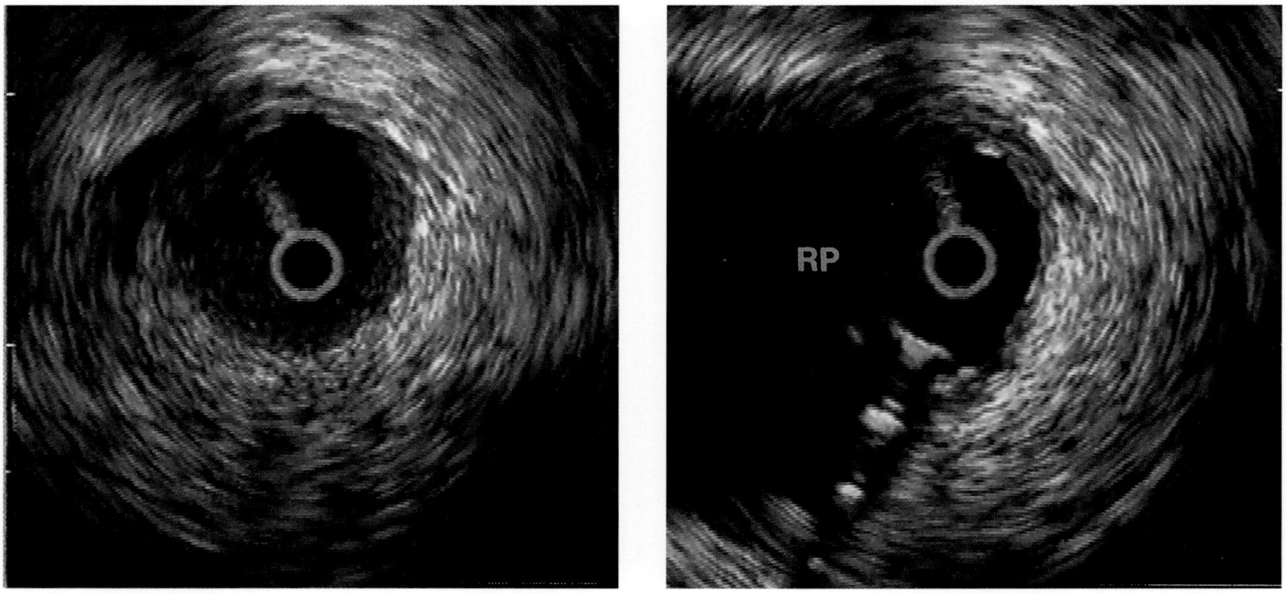

a *b*

Figure 4.17 *The larger lumen is easily recognized as the transducer is advanced from the ureter through the ureteropelvic junction (a) into the renal pelvis (RP) (b). This is an important sonographic landmark.*

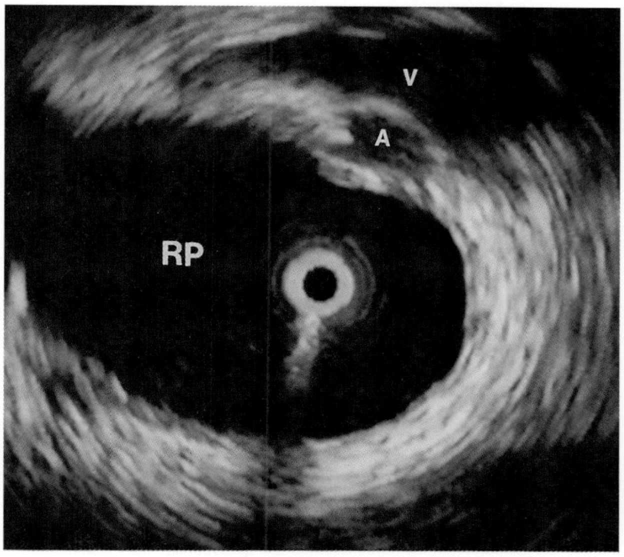

Figure 4.19 *With the transducer in the renal pelvis, the renal veins (V) and arteries (A) and their branches are visualized immediately adjacent to the pelvis (RP).*

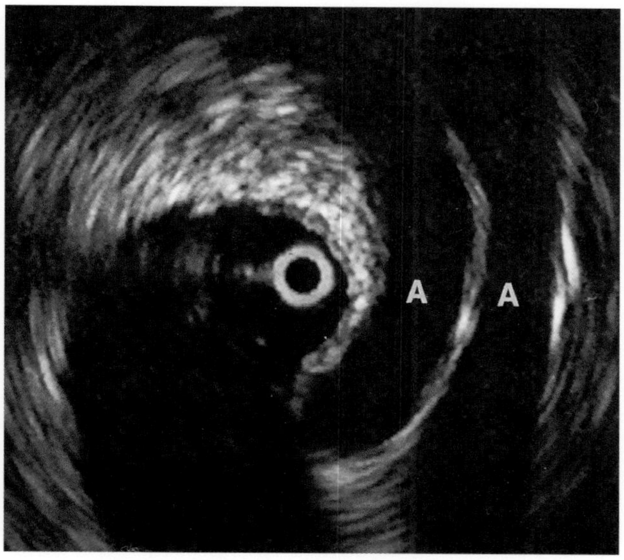

Figure 4.20 *As the probe is passed into an infundibulum, arteries (A) can be seen deep to the mucosa.*

seen in the ureter. Adjacent vasculature, both venous and arterial, is always seen along the infundibulum (Fig. 4.20). Occasionally, the papilla can also be seen at the level of the calyx. It appears as a hypoechoic prominence continuous with the underlying renal parenchyma.

NORMAL VARIANTS

Variations of normal anatomy are often seen and can be confused with abnormal findings. Prominent among these findings are mucosal edema, blood clots, air bubbles and the imaging alterations seen with guidewires.

Mucosal edema is seen as a thickening of the mucosa, which is usually diffuse and hypoechoic. On ultrasound it is also usually segmental and often not symmetrical (Fig. 4.21). This image is often seen after a ureteral catheter stent has been placed within the ureter and can usually be recognized endoscopically.

Another normal variant which can produce an echogenic mass is an intraluminal clot. The sonographic appearance of the clot can be quite variable and generally may not be easily distinguished from that of an intraluminal neoplasm (Fig. 4.22).

Air bubbles can be confused with calculi, since they are both hyperechoic and give an acoustic shadow (Fig. 4.23). However, air bubbles are always located superiorly within a fluid medium. Therefore, with the patient in the lithotomy position bubbles are always anterior, and when the patient is prone they will be posterior. Bubbles and freely moving calculi will move in opposite directions with a change in position of the patient. Submucosal calculi do not change position. The shadows produced by bubbles are usually poorly defined with some echoes or reverberation within the shadow areas ('dirty shadowing').

Lymph nodes can be seen adjacent to the ureter at any level, but are more common in the proximal and distal portions adjacent to the renal and iliac vessels. Lymph nodes are hypoechoic with a focus of echogenicity corresponding to the hilum, which may

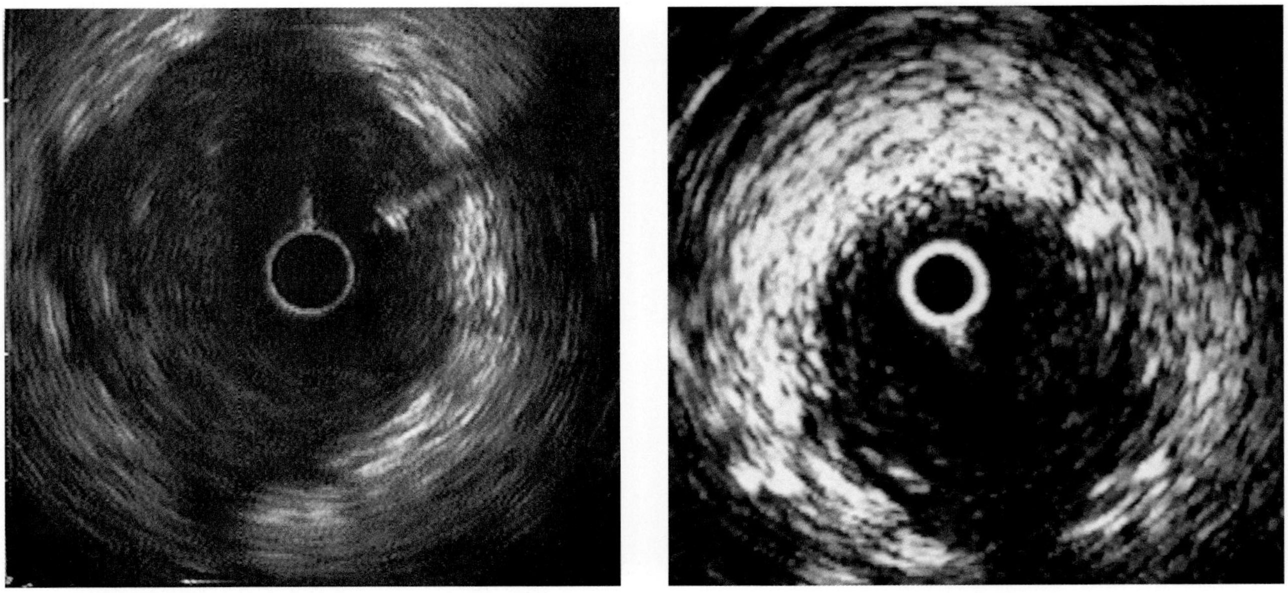

a ***b***

Figure 4.21 *Edema of the ureteral mucosa is seen as a hypoechoic thickening of this layer. It may be symmetrical (a) or localized (b).*

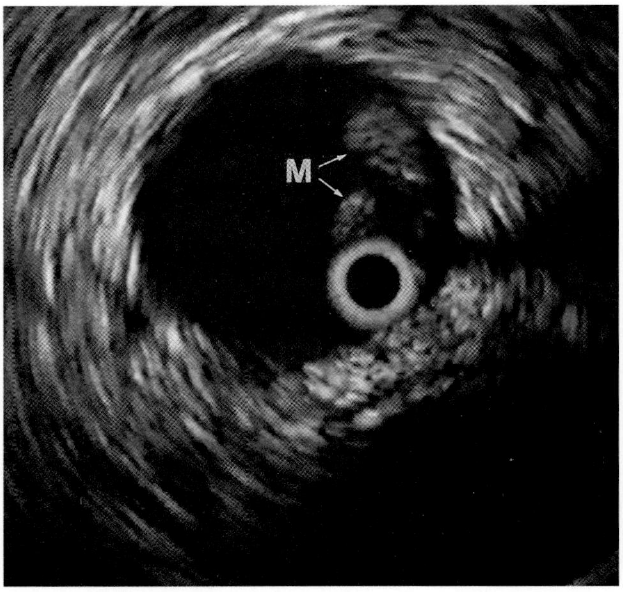

Figure 4.22 *A blood clot appears as a hypoechoic intraluminal mass (M). It can be confused with a neoplasm and may require endoscopic inspection for differentiation.*

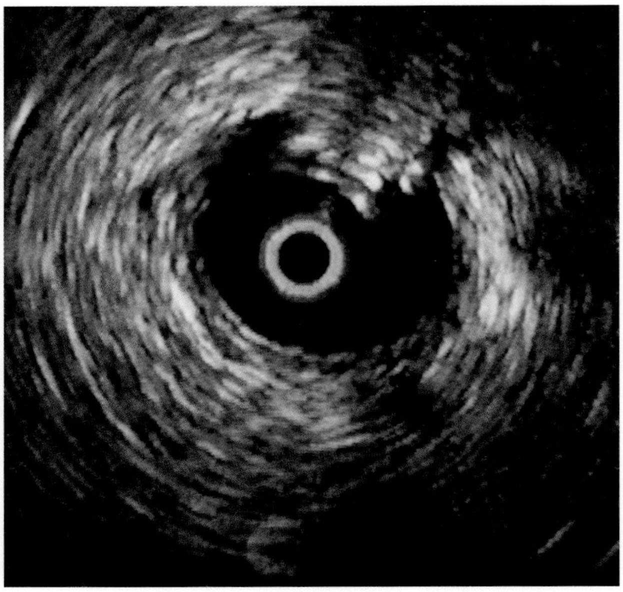

Figure 4.23 *Bubbles within the ureteral lumen are hyperechoic with irregular shadowing and typically extend into the lumen from the superior surface (12 to 2 o'clock). Bubbles can be confused with an intraluminal calculus.*

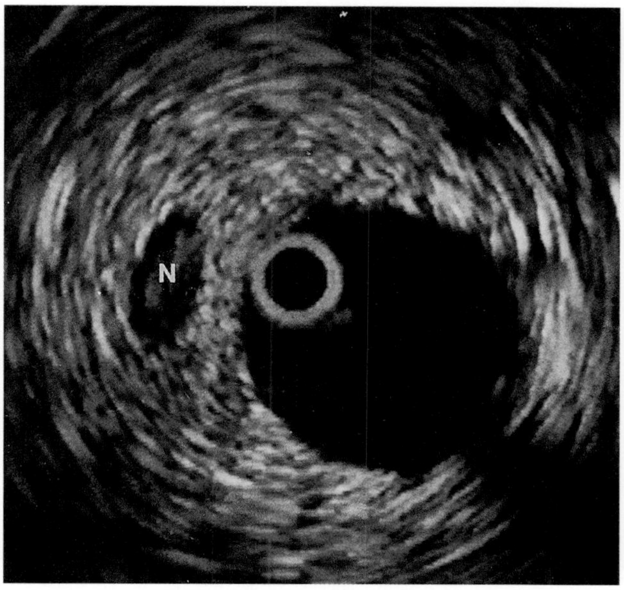

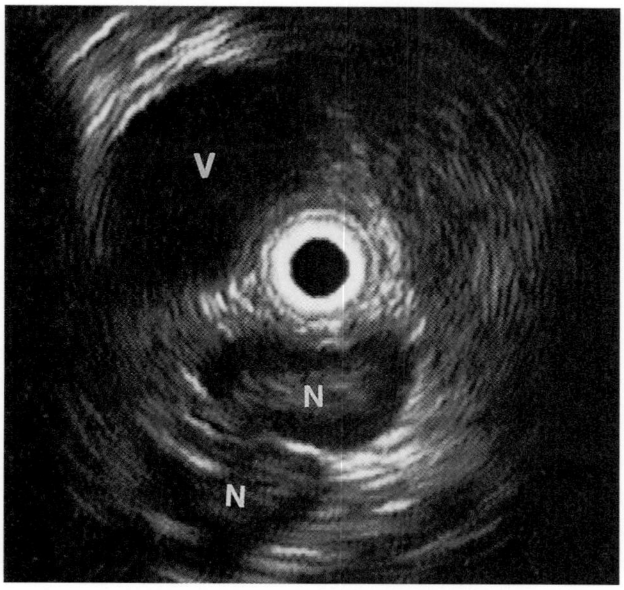

a *b*

Figure 4.24 *(a) A small lymph node (N) is located immediately adjacent to the ureter. It is hypoechoic with central echogenicity. Often the hilum can be located as an echogenic area peripherally. (b) Two lymph nodes (N) are located inferior to the ureter. They can be compared to the iliac vessel (V) located at 11 o'clock.*

be located centrally or peripherally, depending upon the specific view (Fig. 4.24).

The ureter often passes close to the bowel, which can be recognized as a hypoechoic structure which is mobile and characterized by peristalsis. It may contain liquid and gas. Therefore, it has a wide range of echogenicity (Fig. 4.25).

At the level of the kidney, cysts may be located within the range of the endoluminal ultrasound (Fig. 4.26). They appear as anechoic spheres, usually in the peripelvic tissue, and can vary widely in size and specific location.

Fluid may leak from the ureter during endoscopy, particularly after pressure irrigation or traumatization of the ureteral wall, such as with balloon dilation. If contrast is used in the irrigant, it can be visualized radiographically. Any fluid, however, can be seen sonographically. It appears as an anechoic area, usually immediately adjacent to the wall of the ureter itself. It can often be seen tracking both along the ureter and, more deeply, into the tissue distant from the ureteral lumen (Fig. 4.27).

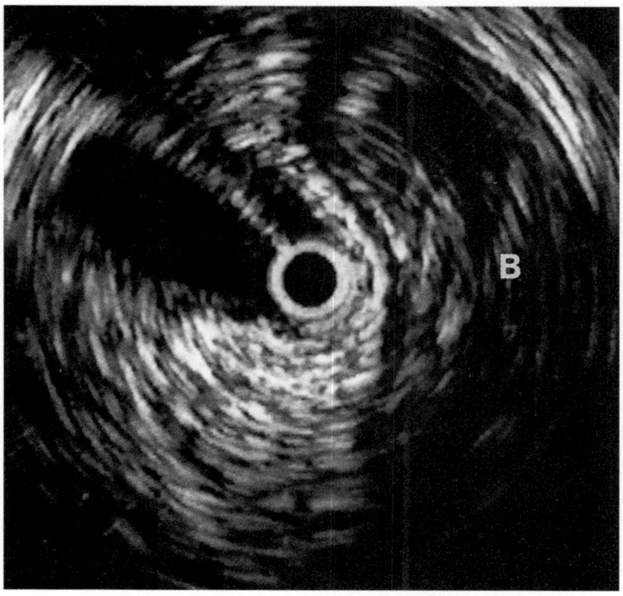

Figure 4.25 *A loop bowel (B) adjacent to the ureter shows a wide range of echogenicity.*

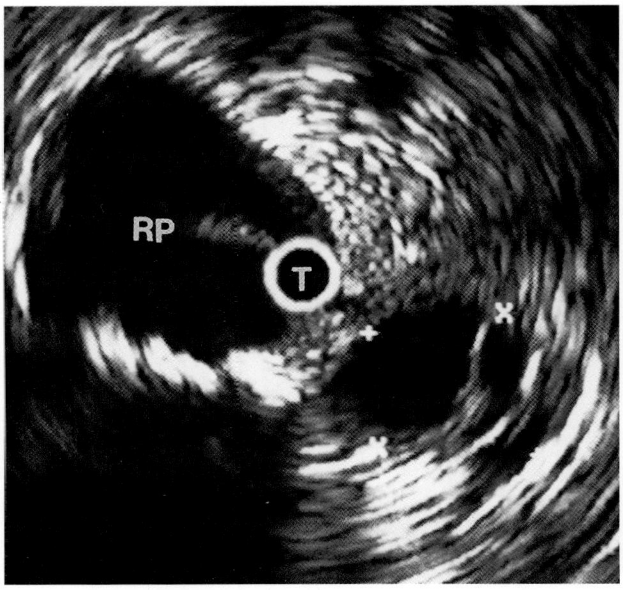

Figure 4.26 *The transducer (T) located within the renal pelvis (RP) also shows an anechoic area consistent with a peripelvic cyst (× and +).*

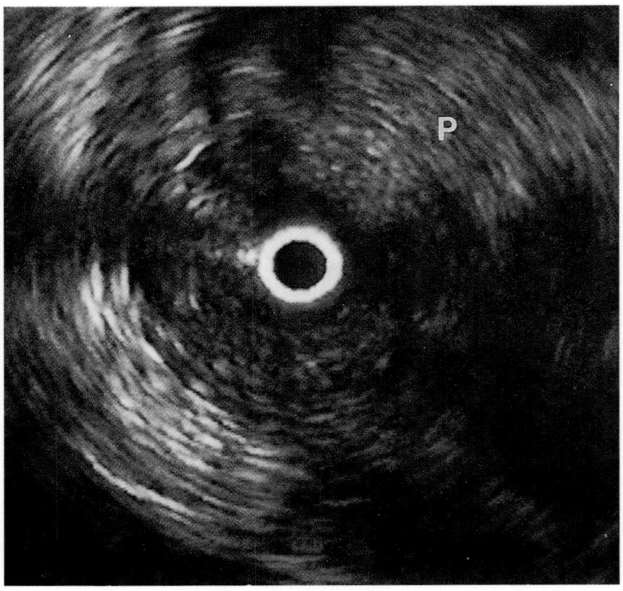

Figure 4.28 *Purulent (P) material within the urinary lumen gives a diffuse echogenic pattern which is characteristic on the real time imaging.*

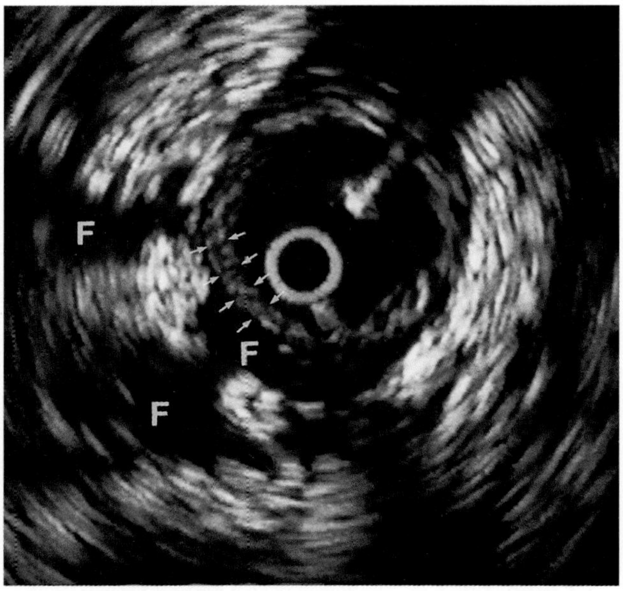

Figure 4.27 *Fluid (F) leaking out of the collecting system and located adjacent to the ureter produces irregular anechoic areas which usually outline the ureteral wall itself (arrow) and can also extend into the adventitia.*

Purulent material within the urinary lumen gives diffuse echogenicity. It is usually less echogenic than tissue but considerably more so than clear urine (Fig. 4.28). Echogenicity can be seen with any small particle in the lumen. It can be seen with very bloody urine and also after laser ablation or incision of tumor or normal tissue. With real-time imaging, the particles can be seen moving within the fluid medium.

A guidewire usually appears with a characteristic ultrasound image (Figs 4.11, 4.14, 4.15, 4.20 and 4.27). The wire is highly echogenic, with some ringing in a fluid medium and with an acoustic shadow in an echogenic medium. If the wire is quite closely applied to the transducer, it may not be very prominent. If it is also in the field with an image of a neoplasm, the deep portion of the neoplasm or the adjoining ureteral wall may be attenuated, giving the appearance (artifact) of a hypoechoic tumor invading into the ureteral wall itself. Thus, there may be the appearance of invasion when these two images coincide.

CLINICAL APPLICATIONS

The indications for the application of endoluminal ultrasound in clinical practice have grown as the techniques have developed. Important clinical settings have been defined and treatment has been directed in very specific ways to maximize efficiency and minimize risks. Two of the first indications, the submucosal calculus and the obstructed ureteropelvic junction, have remained important indications where endoluminal ultrasound has been able to provide valuable information. For other indications, such as urothelial neoplasms and strictures, endoluminal sonography is of less certain value. Their continued study is, however, important to determine both the value and the limitations of the techniques. The present applications can be considered individually.

SUBMUCOSAL CALCULUS

The submucosal urinary calculus was one of the first and most clearly important applications of endoluminal ultrasound in the upper urinary tract.[8] In this uncommon clinical entity, the patient typically has radiographic evidence of a calculus which is not detectable endoscopically. Simultaneous radiographs with endoscopy may indicate that the stones are located beyond the lumen of the ureter or renal pelvis, but the distance and exact location are often difficult to determine. Most of these patients have previously undergone lithotripsy, either endoscopic or external shock wave, but rarely submucosal migration can occur as a result of spontaneous forces of the urinary tract combined with prolonged impaction. The common presentation and indication for treatment in the initial series of patients was obstruction.

Patients identified with suspected submucosal calculi can be studied with contrast studies, both antegrade and retrograde, in an attempt to define the location of the calculus. They can also be examined endoscopically with simultaneous fluoroscopic or radiographic identification of the stone. With these techniques it is usually difficult to pinpoint the depth of the stone from the lumen.

Endoluminal ultrasound can be used to identify the location of the stone and its depth from the lumen very specifically (Figs 4.29, 4.30 and 4.31). Any of the ultrasound probes described can be employed. The

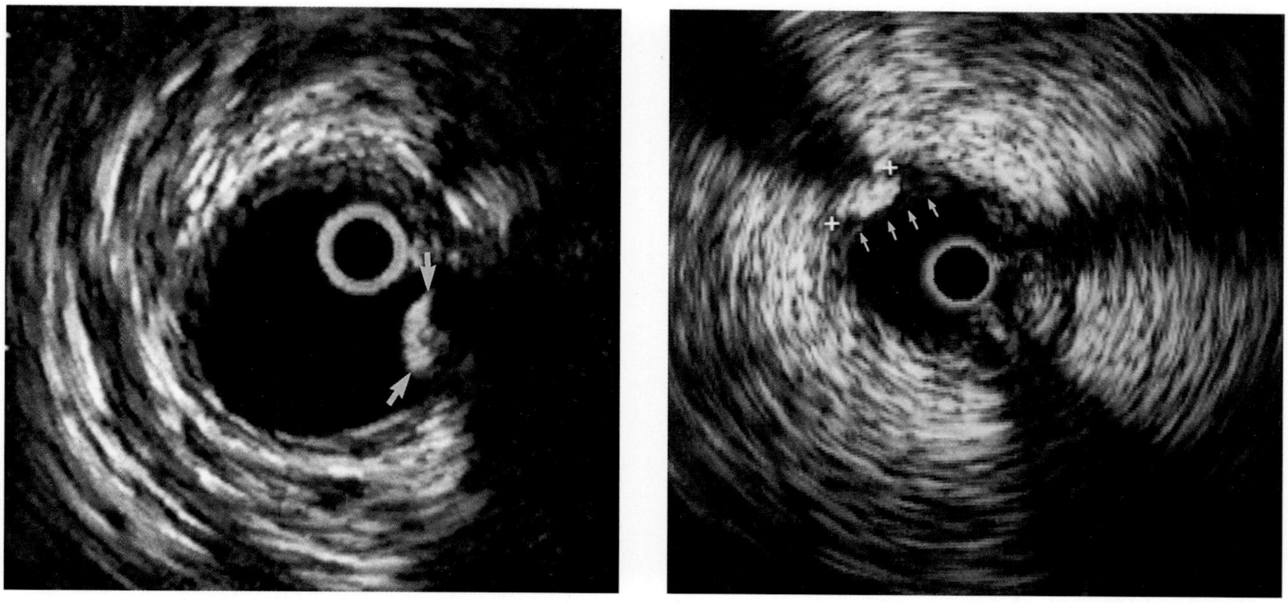

a *b*

Figure 4.29 *(a) An intraluminal calculus (arrows) is located at 4 o'clock in this ultrasound image. There is no evidence of ureteral mucosa covering the calculus. (b) A calculus (+ ···· +) at 11 o'clock is located within the submucosa with a mucosal covering (arrows).*

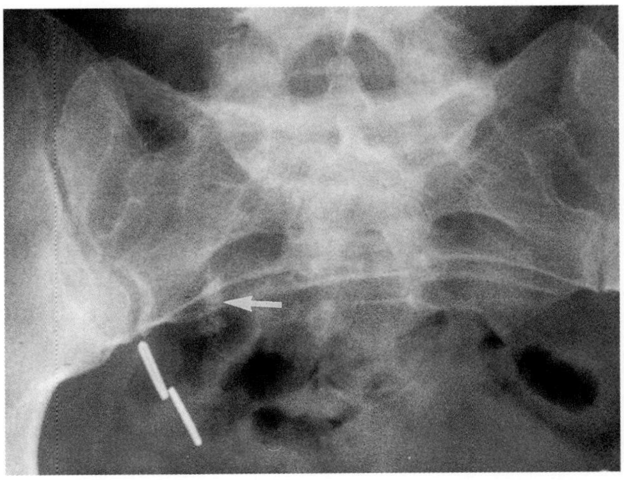

a

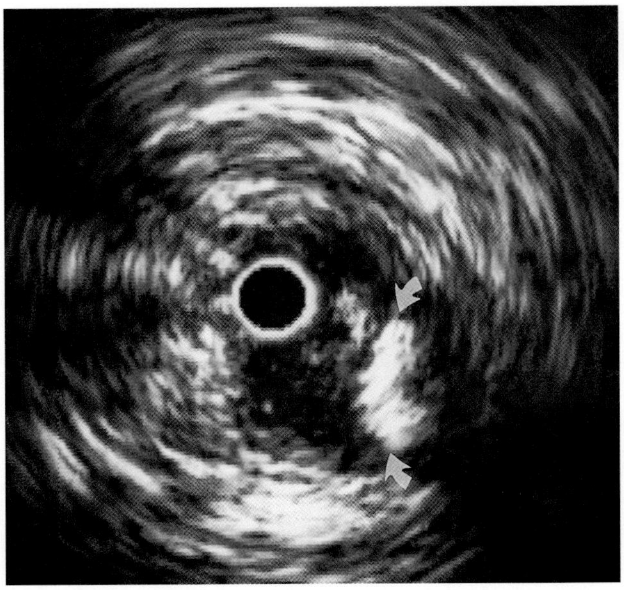

b

Figure 4.30 *(a) An abdominal radiogram demonstrates a calculus (arrows) which could not be seen within the ureteral lumen with ureteroscopy. (b) Endoluminal ultrasound of the same area shows the calculus (arrows) as a hyperechoic area within the submucosa with acoustic shadowing (3 to 4 o'clock).*

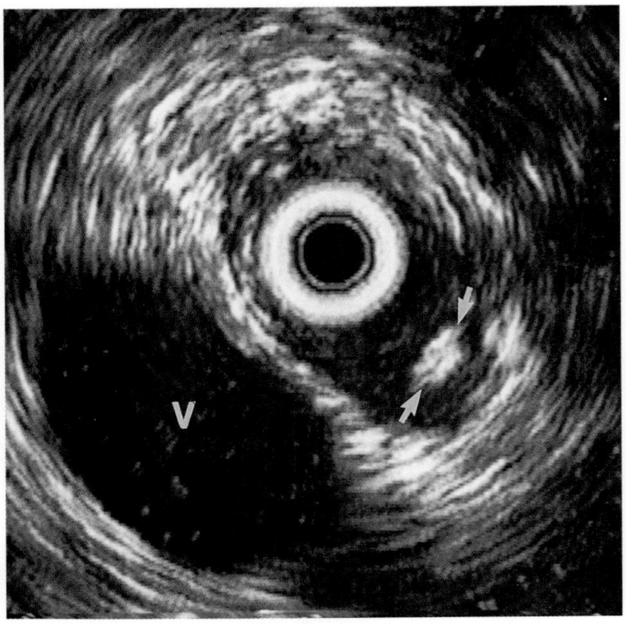

Figure 4.31 *A small calculus appears as a hyperechoic area in the submucosa at 4 o'clock with faint shadowing. The iliac vein (V) is located adjacent to the ureter at the same level.*

larger probes which are passed and localized radiographically can identify the stone and its exact distance from the ureteral or renal pelvic lumen. The rotational orientation is determined by comparing the position of a guidewire observed both fluoroscopically and sonographically simultaneously. A much more exact location can be obtained by passing the ultrasound probe through an endoscope. This can be done with the smaller probes passed through a ureteroscope or with the larger probe passed through a nephroscope. The exact relationship of the probe to a guidewire passed from the tip of the endoscope can then be determined visually.

Once the calculus has been specifically located with the ultrasound probe and endoscope, a decision can be made on attempting to remove it. Those located 3 mm or less from the surface tend to cause obstruction and can be removed. Solitary or few fragments can be removed relatively easily endoscopically. The mucosa is divided over the site of the calculus either with the tip of an endoscope or with a wire-pronged grasper. At the correct location, the calculus is invariably reached at the expected depth and can be grasped with the wire-pronged grasper for removal.

Multiple fragments located within the wall of the ureter (less than 3 mm of depth) are more problematic. The size and number of fragments can often be

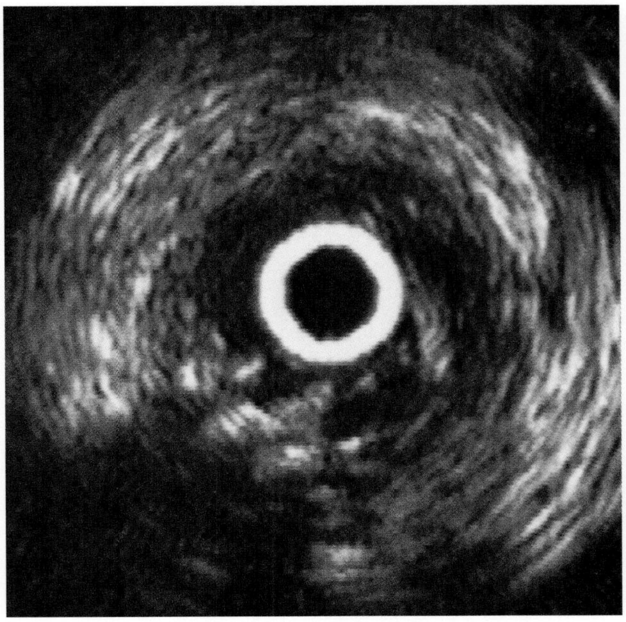

Figure 4.32 *Multiple small calculi with acoustic shadowing are located throughout the ureteral wall from 6 to 8 o'clock.*

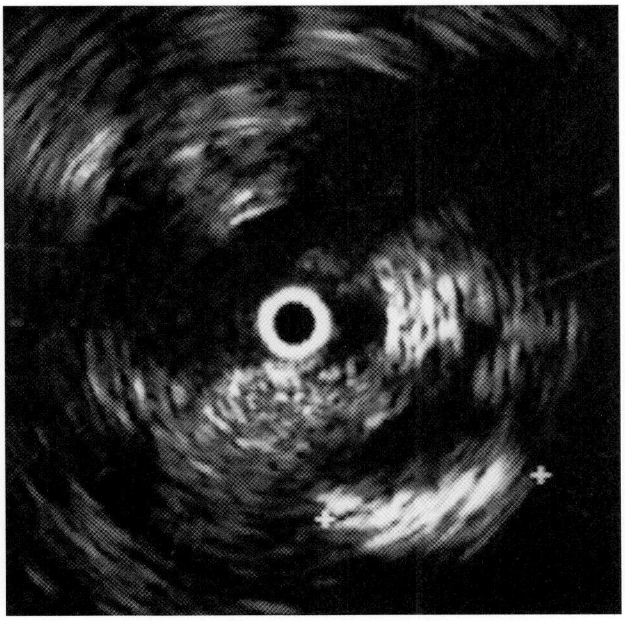

Figure 4.33 *A large calculus (+ ··· +) is located more than 4 mm from the ureteral lumen.*

seen with endoluminal ultrasound (Fig. 4.32). They may be too numerous or too small to remove. Patients may go on to form stricture as described for patients with submucosal stone granuloma formation.[9] This situation may require earlier surgical intervention if stricture formation is seen.

Stones which are 4 mm or more from the lumen of the ureter have rarely caused problems with obstruction or stricture. These calculi can be left in place without risk of later complications (Fig. 4.33). Others have made similar observations.[10]

Endoluminal ultrasound can also be used to determine the adequacy of stone removal. The stone-bearing area can be imaged before and after attempts at removal to determine the extent or adequacy of stone retrieval. This is particularly helpful when there are numerous small fragments, particularly when endoscopic visualization is suboptimal. Thus, endoluminal ultrasound can be used to guide therapy (Fig. 4.34) (Table 4.2).

Table 4.2 Submucosal calculi: treatment based on endoluminal ultrasound.

Depth from lumen	*Treatment*
1–3 mm Solitary calculus	Remove
1–3 mm Multiple fragments	Remove (Note: risk of strictures)
>4 mm	Leave in place

URETEROPELVIC JUNCTION OBSTRUCTION

Endoluminal sonography has been particularly valuable for visualization of the obstructed ureteropelvic junction. Since obstruction can be caused by one or more factors, including intrinsic narrowing, a crossing vessel or high insertion of the ureter at the pelvis, careful delineation of the anatomy of the

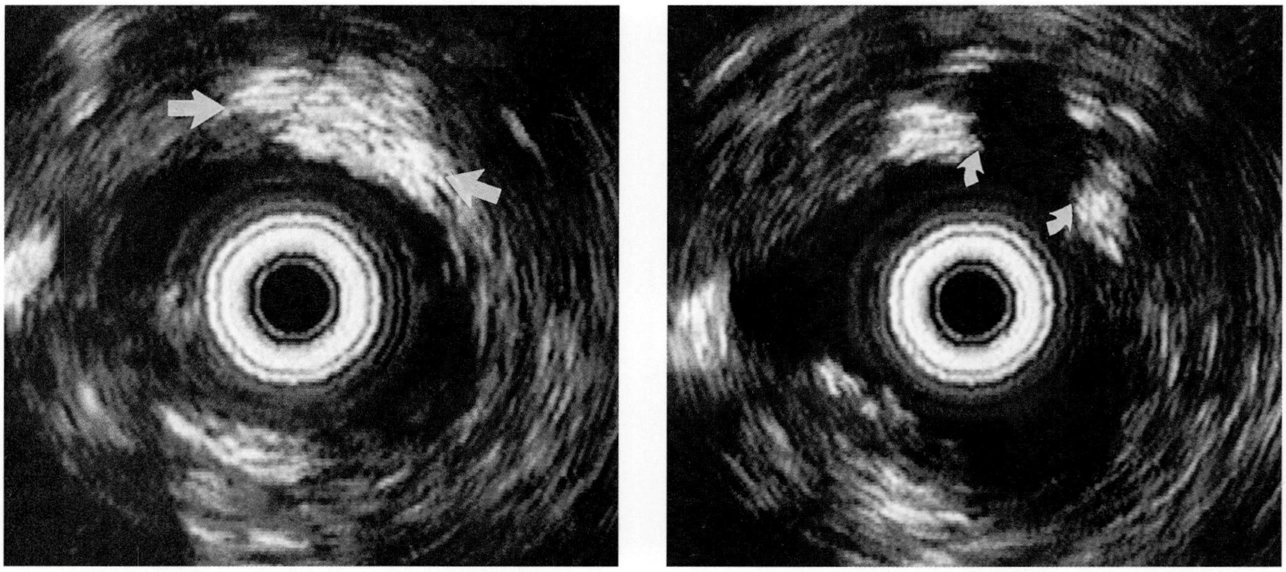

a *b*

Figure 4.34 *(a) A group of calculus fragments (arrows) is located immediately submucosally in the renal pelvis. The ultrasound probe has been placed through a nephroscope. (b) An ultrasonic lithotriptor probe has been passed to evacuate some of the fragments. The endoluminal ultrasound probe is again used to visualize the area, demonstrating subtotal removal of the calculi, with fragments remaining on both sides of a sonolucent defect (arrows).*

ureteropelvic junction is essential (Fig. 4.35). Endoluminal sonography is particularly well suited to detecting periureteral vessels, or a septum between the ureter and renal pelvis. It appears to be a valuable adjunct to the endoluminal incisional therapy of ureteropelvic junction obstruction.

Ureteropelvic junction obstruction is thought to have a congenital basis although symptoms can present decades later in life. Clinical presentation in the adult most commonly occurs during the second or third decade of life with intermittent flank pain. The pain is typically intermittent and can occur after ingestion of large volumes of fluid. It can be of varying severity and usually clears spontaneously after hours or days. The symptoms are only occasionally accompanied by hematuria and, more frequently, infection is present.

Complete evaluation of these patients includes radiographic imaging and functional studies. An excretory urogram is usually performed and can demonstrate hydronephrosis with prominent caliectasis. Classically, the ureter is not visualized. The presence of obstruction is more subtle, as there may be mild fullness of the collecting system but variable loss of parenchyma. The radionuclide scan can provide a more accurate indication of function, including the extent of obstruction. Determination of the split renal function with a radionuclide scan can indicate the contribution of each kidney. Evaluation of clearance of the radionuclide from the affected kidney can indicate the presence or absence of obstruction. In equivocal situations, a diuretic (such as furosemide) is administered to initiate a diuresis[11] and clearance is again followed. A more invasive but perhaps more accurate determination of obstruction is the irrigation flow study known as the Whitaker test.[12] Fluid is infused through a percutaneous nephrostomy tube into the pelvis of the affected kidney and the intrarenal pressure is simultaneously measured. Increasing pressure during irrigation indicates the presence of obstruction. Together these studies can usually define the presence of significant obstruction.

Many different options are available for the treatment of properly diagnosed ureteropelvic junction obstruction. Conventional therapy has been an open

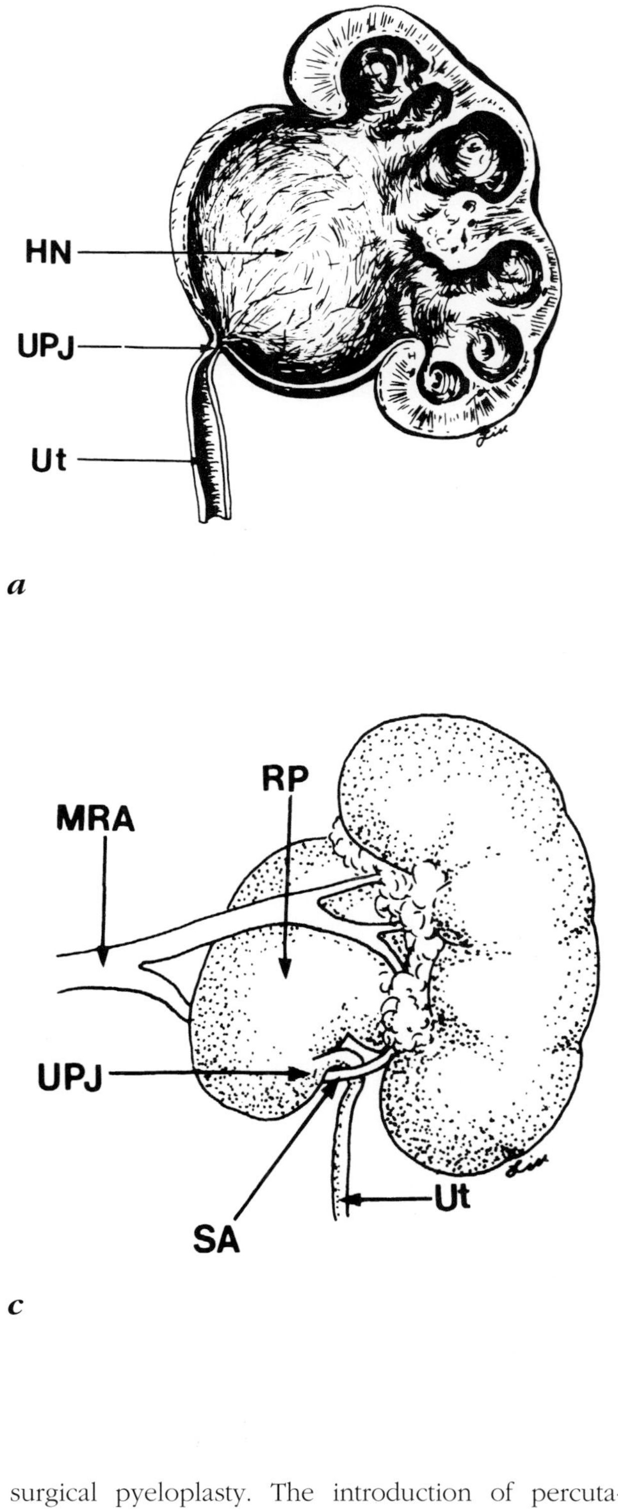

Figure 4.35 *The ureteropelvic junction may be obstructed by a narrow segment (a), a high insertion of the ureter into the pelvis (b) or a vessel adjacent to the ureter (c). UPJ, ureteropelvic junction; Ut, ureter; S, septum; MRA, main renal artery; SA, segmental artery; RP, renal pelvis; HN, hydronephrotic pelvis.*

surgical pyeloplasty. The introduction of percutaneous endopyelotomy has markedly changed the approach in treatment.[13–15] With this technique, a percutaneous nephrostomy is placed and, under direct visualization, the narrow ureteropelvic junction is incised with a cold knife. The full thickness of the ureter is incised to expose the periureteral fat, and a stent is subsequently placed for several weeks. The success for endopyelotomy, according to several reports, is approximately 80–85%.[13–15] This is probably less than can be achieved with an open pyeloplasty, although patients who have undergone the latter have rarely been studied with the rigorous criteria used for endopyelotomy.

Other approaches to incision of the ureteropelvic junction have included ureteroscopic techniques and electroincision with the wire applied with a balloon catheter. Since the ureteroscopic series are smaller, success has ranged from 83% to >90%.[16–18] The balloon incision devices (Acucise) have achieved a success of approximately 80%.[19,20]

An alternative technique has been described for balloon overdilation of the ureteropelvic junction up to diameters of approximately 1 cm. Although the initial report was encouraging, subsequent studies have not confirmed the high success rate.[21]

All of the incisional techniques carry with them the risk of damage to any periureteral vessels located at the site of the incision, although extensive bleeding has not been common in the reported series. Previous reports have suggested that crossing vessels occur in 25–32% of patients with ureteropelvic junction obstruction.[22,23] Other studies have confirmed a significant portion of patients with crossing vessels. In a study utilizing angiography, Van Cangh[24] found that 39% of patients with ureteropelvic junction obstruction had crossing arterial vessels at the level of the ureteropelvic junction.

The importance of vessels at the ureteropelvic junction may not be limited to their being a source of hemorrhage. In Van Cangh's[24] series, the success of the procedure could be related to the presence of crossing vessels (Table 4.3). When no vessels were present, the success of percutaneous endopyelotomy was 95%. However, when there were associated vessels, the success dropped to 39%. The presence of vessels was not the only factor affecting the results of endopyelotomy; but the presence of hydronephrosis was also a detrimental factor. In a smaller series, Bagley and Liu[18] noted that the presence of periureteral vessels at the ureteropelvic junction was detrimental to the success of endoluminal endopyelotomy, whether performed by percutaneous or ureteroscopic approaches. Moreover, in groups with small numbers there appeared to be a greater effect from vessels posterior to the ureteropelvic junction. In two patients with vessels on two sides of the ureter, rapid reobstruction developed (Fig. 4.36).

Endoluminal ultrasound offers an excellent and accurate technique for the identification of vessels crossing at the level of the ureteropelvic junction. The ultrasound probe can be passed using one of the many techniques described above to visualize the area in question. Orientation must be maintained with use of a guidewire adjacent to the catheter with simultaneous intermittent fluoroscopy. In this way, vessels adjacent to the ureteropelvic junction can be recognized and localized. Arteries can be differentiated from veins and the depth and size of the vessel can be accurately determined. The appropriate

Table 4.3 Success of endopyelotomy: effects of crossing vessels and hydronephrosis.

Hydronephrosis	*Crossing Vessel*	*Success (%)*
absent	absent	95
present	absent	77
absent	present	50
present	present	39

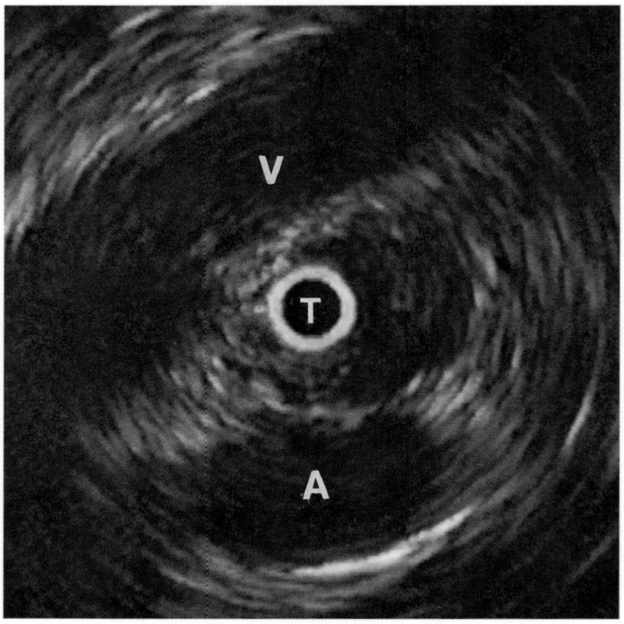

Figure 4.36 *Vessels are seen in two areas adjacent to the ureteropelvic junction in this patient with left ureteropelvic junction obstruction. One vessel (V) is crossing from the medial to anterolateral areas while another is located posterior to the ureter (A). T, transducer*

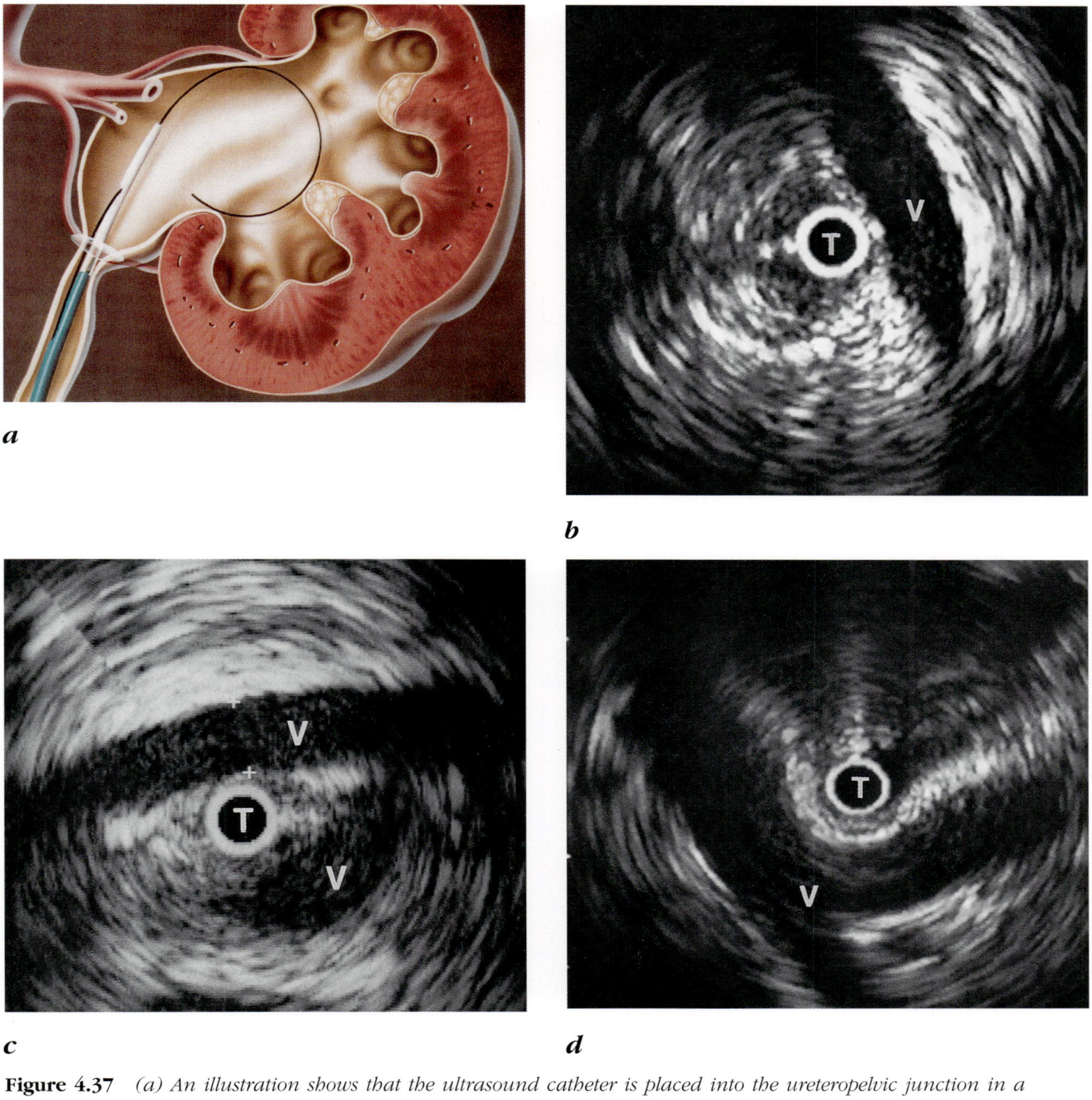

Figure 4.37 *(a) An illustration shows that the ultrasound catheter is placed into the ureteropelvic junction in a retrograde path through a guidewire. Crossing vessels (V) have been demonstrated in many patients. (b–d) The exact location, including the size of the vessel and its distance from the ureter, can be defined. The lumen of the vessel is usually located <1 mm from the lumen of the ureter containing the transducer (T). Arteries can be distinguished from veins with real-time ultrasonography.*

location for incision can then be determined. These findings have been demonstrated in many patients (Fig. 4.37).

There are other techniques to locate vessels at the ureteropelvic junction. Spiral CT scans can demonstrate arterial vessels as small as 1–2 mm. This is a rapid noninvasive technique but it has the obvious limitation of resolving smaller vessels, cost, and the need for contrast administration. Arteriography can also be used to evaluate vessels. It is more invasive and also requires the use of contrast but has excellent resolution for arterial vessels. Both techniques

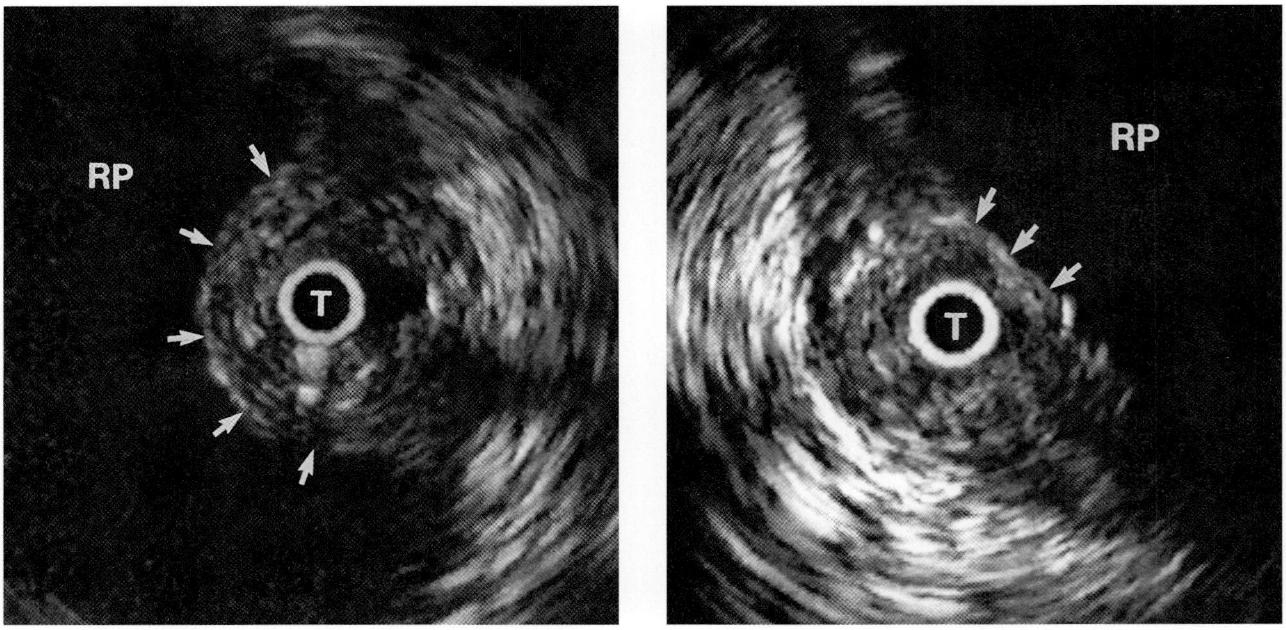

a *b*

Figure 4.38 *High insertion of the ureter into the renal pelvis occurs with a septum dividing the lumen of the pelvis and the ureter. This septum can be seen with endoluminal ultrasound. The thickness of the septum and the presence of vessels can also be determined. The transducer (T) is located within the ureter and the septum (arrows) separates it from the renal pelvis (RP).*

may fail to demonstrate smaller veins. In comparison, the ultrasound unit and catheter transducers are portable and can be used in the operating room at the time of the procedure. Thus, the image obtained by endoluminal ultrasound accurately represents the anatomy at the site of the endoscopic procedure which may have been affected by changes in volume of the collecting system and by positioning. In this way, ultrasound imaging may be more accurate than the techniques performed at an earlier time.

Endoluminal ultrasound has been particularly useful to demonstrate a septum located between the ureter and the renal pelvis in those patients with high insertion of the ureter into the renal pelvis (Fig. 4.38). This configuration can occasionally be demonstrated radiographically. If the entire course of the ureter is demonstrated, for example with a retrograde ureteropyelogram, the exact site of insertion may be demonstrated. However, it is often impossible to make the exact determination of the relationship of the ureter to the renal pelvis with contrast studies alone. Frequently, a streaming effect of contrast into the renal pelvis can mimic high insertion. In comparison, endoluminal sonography of the ureter can demonstrate the specific site of the ureteropelvic junction when the image is correlated with fluoroscopic appearance. We can consider a septum between the ureter and the renal pelvis as diagnostic of high insertion even when the radiographic studies are equivocal.

Crossing vessels can also be associated with a high insertion. These may be at the same level or may be a few to several millimeters lower along the ureter. It may be impossible to determine the importance of each factor in causing obstruction (Figs 4.39 and 4.40).

The sonographic image can also be used to direct the endoscopic incision, specifically the positioning of the incision. Sonographic imaging after cutting can be used to monitor the adequacy of the incision (Fig. 4.41).

Partial duplication of the renal pelvis is not infrequent. Obstruction can occur in one limb.[25] The same range of etiology can be considered in these patients

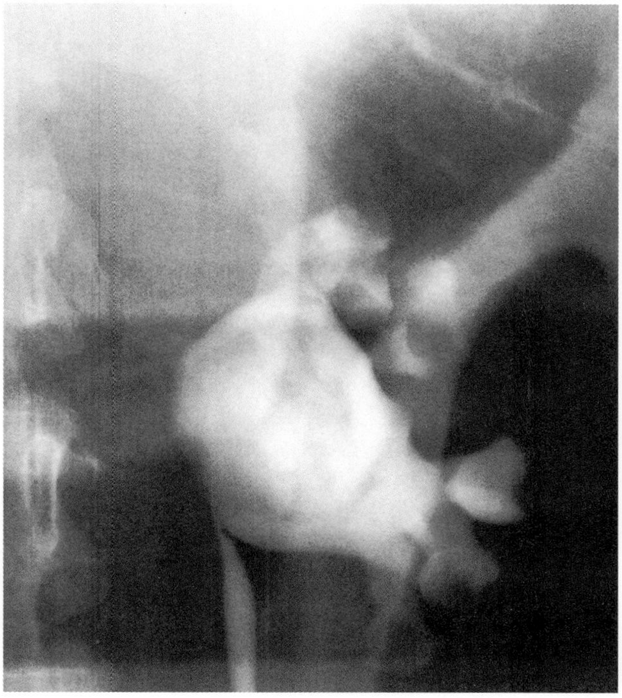

a

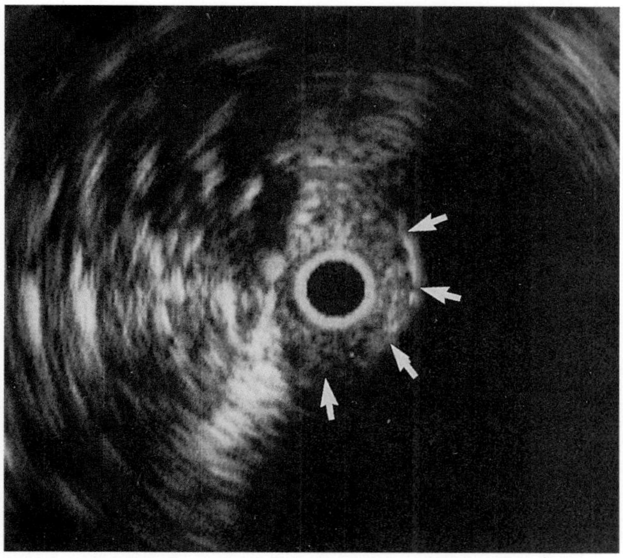

b

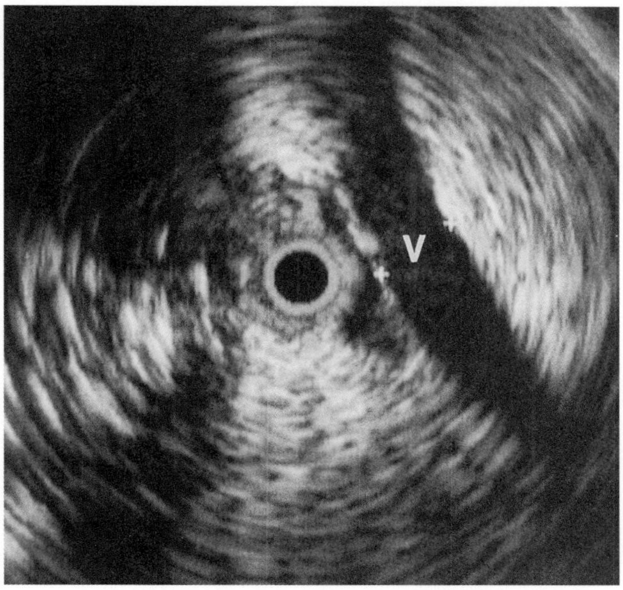

c

Figure 4.39 *Ureteropelvic junction obstruction with high insertion can also be associated with a crossing vessel. (a) A retrograde ureteropyelogram outlines the ureteropelvic junction obstruction and suggests high insertion of the ureter. (b) In the same patient, the septum (arrows) of high insertion is shown. (c) A crossing vessel (V) is shown with the transducer located a few millimeters distally in the ureter.*

as in those with the more conventional ureteropelvic junction obstruction. Specifically, the possibility of crossing vessels or stenoses must be entertained. Endoluminal ultrasound has been particularly valuable in these patients to demonstrate the presence of any adjacent vessels and also to demonstrate the distance between the lumens of each segment of the renal pelvis (Fig. 4.42). Thus, it can be used to guide incisional therapy.

INFUNDIBULAR OBSTRUCTION

Partial obstruction can occur in portions of the intrarenal collecting system. Infundibular obstruction has been defined previously, with crossing vessels demonstrated by arteriography. Vessels adjacent to the infundibula can also be demonstrated with endoluminal ultrasound. Normally, vessels are seen adjacent to the infundibula, but crossing vessels have

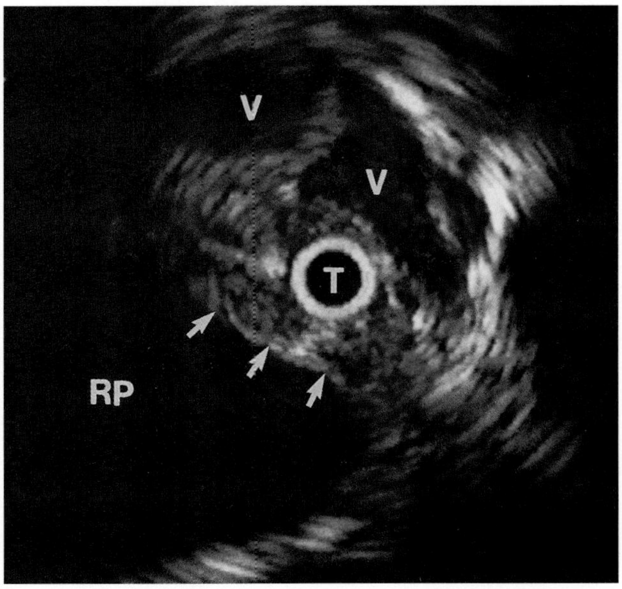

Figure 4.40 *The septum (arrows) of a high insertion separates the lumen of the ureter containing the transducer (T) from the renal pelvis (RP). Vessels (V) are located adjacent to the ureter at the same level.*

been demonstrated at the level of obstruction. The greatest value of this study seems to be in conjunction with endoscopy to rule out neoplasm as the source of obstruction (Fig. 4.43).

PERIURETERAL VESSELS

The same techniques can be used to demonstrate periureteral vessels throughout the distribution of the ureter. The findings can be used to diagnose filling defects, ureteral obstruction and notching found on contrast studies. It can also be used to locate periureteral vessels in order to relate them to intraluminal lesions requiring treatment. Endoluminal ultrasound provides information in these situations that is not available from other techniques, short of superselective venography.

Endoluminal ultrasound in the ureter has been particularly valuable in visualizing structures deep to the ureteral lumen. All of the ureter, including the adventitia, can be visualized. Adjacent structures such as lymph nodes, skeletal muscle and vessels can also

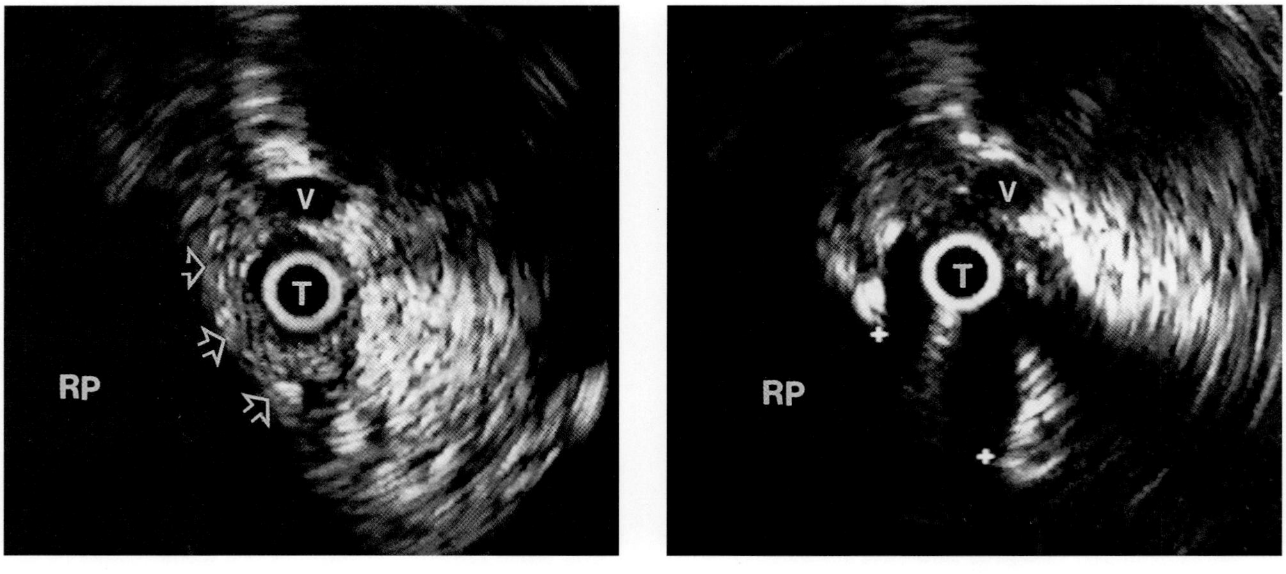

a ***b***

Figure 4.41 *(a) Endoluminal ultrasound of an obstructed ureteropelvic junction shows the septum (arrows) of a high insertion. (b) After ureteroscopic incision of the high insertion, the adequacy of the endopyelotomy (+···+) is demonstrated by ultrasound imaging at the same level. T, transducer; RP, renal pelvis; V, vessels.*

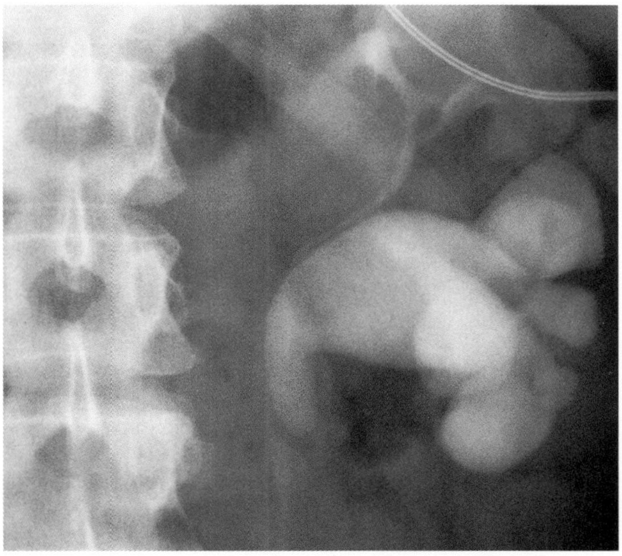

a

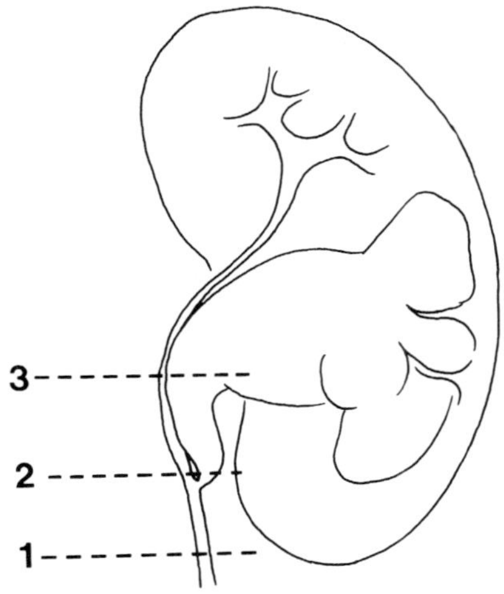

b

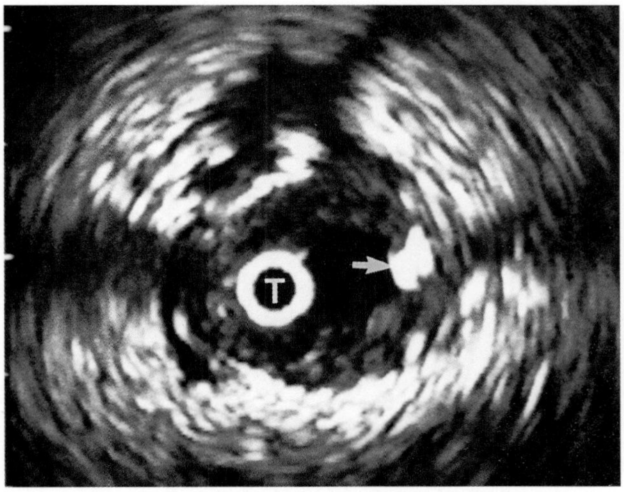

c

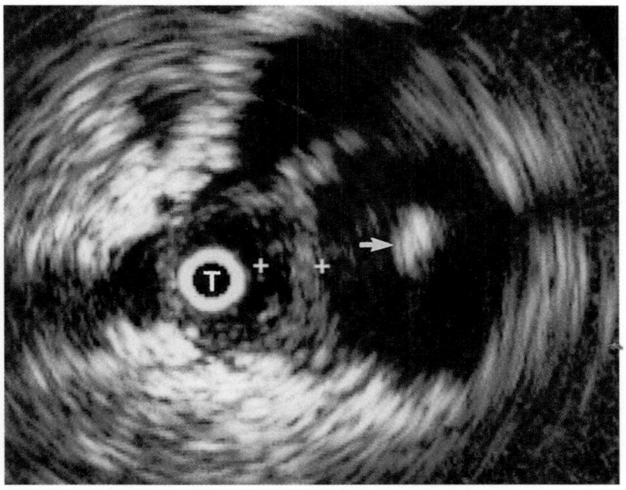

d

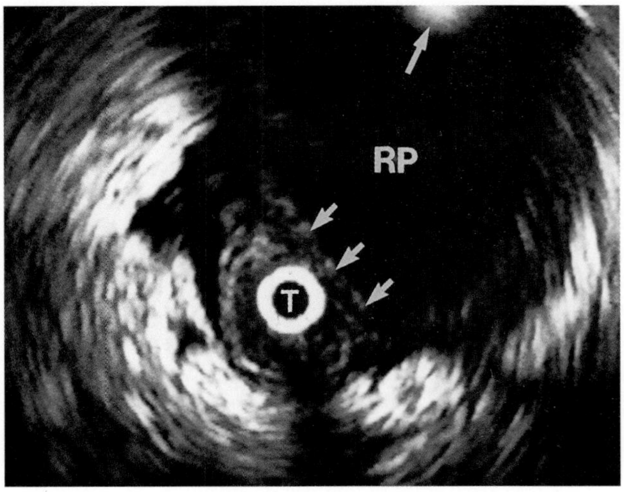

e

Figure 4.42 *(a) A retrograde ureteropyelogram demonstrates obstruction of the lower portion of a duplicated collecting system at its junction with the upper ureter at the level of the transverse process of L-3. (b) Schematic illustration of the collecting system in (a). (c) Ultrasound image at level 1 in (a) shows the transducer (T) in a single ureteral lumen. The guidewire (arrow) is also evident. (d) The ultrasound image at level 2 in (a) shows the transducer (T) in a lumen separated by a septum (+···+) from the dilated lumen of the ureter to the inferior collecting system. The guidewire (arrow) is evident in the dilated lumen. (e) Ultrasound image at level 3 in (a) shows the transducer (T) in the lumen separated by a septum (arrows) from the renal pelvis (RP) of the inferior collecting system. The guidewire (arrow) is evident in the distance in the renal pelvis.*

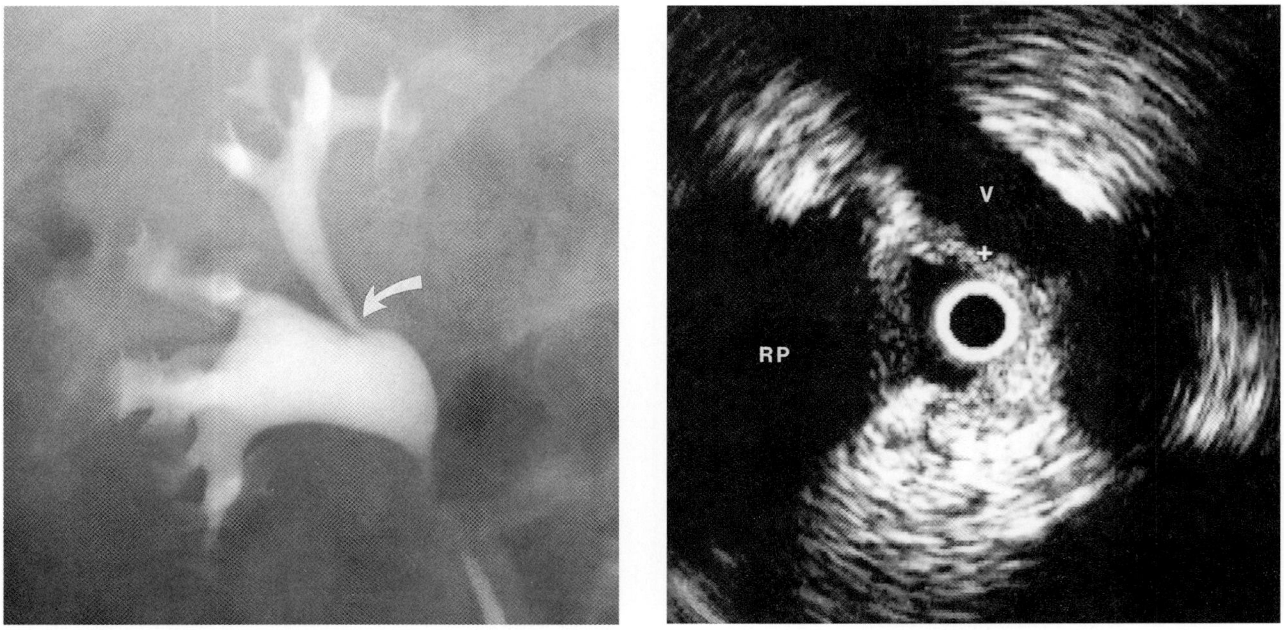

a *b*

Figure 4.43 *(a) Retrograde pyelogram demonstrates a narrowing of the right upper infundibulum (arrow). The patient had a previous excretory urogram which defined this as an increase in narrowing from previous studies. (b) Endoluminal ultrasound shows a vessel (V) immediately adjacent to the infundibulum at the point of obstruction. The renal pelvis (RP) is seen at the same level. The lumen was adequate both by ultrasonographic visualization and by endoscopic inspection.*

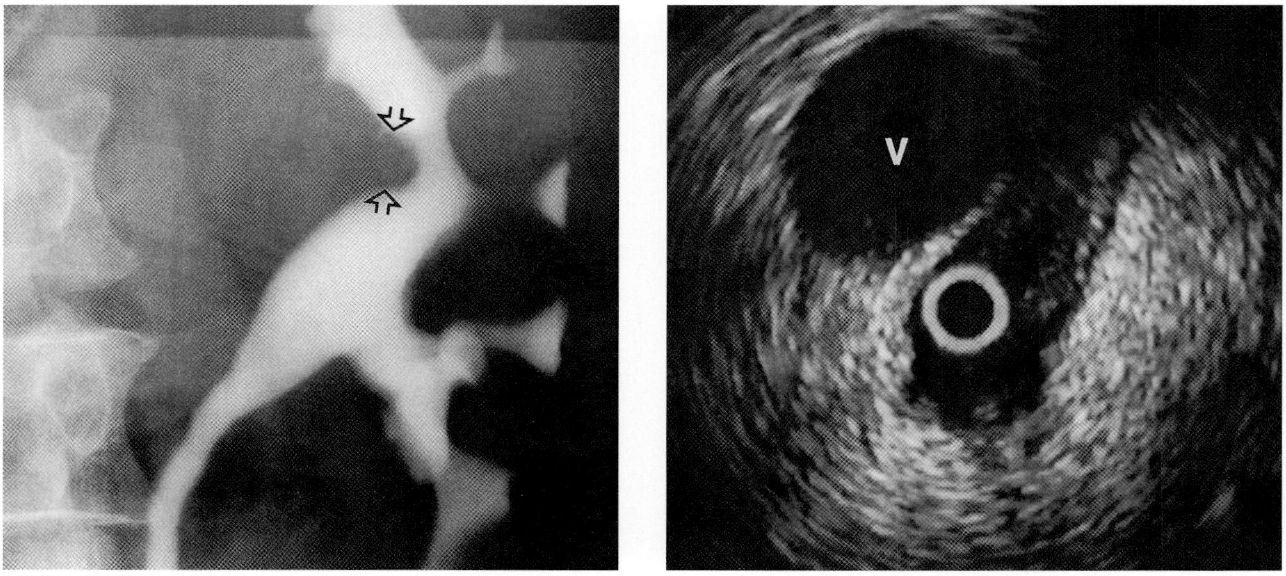

a *b*

Figure 4.44 *(a) A patient with microscopic hematuria was found on excretory urogram to have a renal pelvic filling defect (arrows). The same finding could be confirmed on retrograde ureteropyelography. (b) Endoluminal ultrasound demonstrated that the filling defect corresponded to a peripelvic vessel (V). The finding was confirmed endoscopically since an extrinsic mass was seen which became more prominent on emptying of the pelvis and less prominent with filling of the pelvis.*

be seen. Iliac vessels and the psoas muscle comprise significant landmarks facilitating orientation of endoluminal ultrasound within the ureter. In the same way, abnormal features, such as vessels in an abnormal position or periureteral scar and even periureteral foreign bodies, can be localized.

Some of the most important structures which can be seen adjacent to the ureter are vessels. These are important not only for orientation but also to guide treatment, both endoluminal and transmural. For example, the lumen of the ureter may be separated from the lumen of the iliac vein by less than 1 mm of tissue. Clearly, it is important to minimize trauma to the ureteral wall at this level during any intraluminal therapy. Similarly, transmural treatment such as incision of a stricture should be avoided at the level of a vessel.

Significant periureteral vasculature may be suspected from radiographic findings on the excretory urogram. Filling defects in the renal pelvis or elsewhere in the intrarenal collecting system may be discovered on excretory urography performed for microscopic hematuria or multiple other indications. Although a vascular impression on the renal pelvis is sometimes characteristic, it is often impossible to determine the cause of the filling defect and differentiate it from a neoplasm without endoscopic inspection (Fig. 4.44).

Endoluminal ultrasound can add a considerable level of certainty to endoscopic diagnosis of periureteral vessels which have been defined as filling defects. These may be relatively difficult to diagnose endoscopically, since only the impression of the vessel against the ureteral or renal pelvic wall is evident. The presence of an arterial impression is evident from visible pulsations and because the impression is more prominent as the urinary lumen empties and less prominent as it fills. These, however, are nonspecific findings and, in fact, the pulsations can be transmitted through a solid mass and any extraluminal impression will become less prominent, with distension of the urinary lumen. The specific visibility and resolution of endoluminal ultrasound, however, allow visualization of the periurinary mass and definition of a vascular lesion. Thus, ultrasound is extremely useful in evaluating solitary filling defects, notching along the ureter and sites of obstruction (Figs 4.45 and 4.46). It has also been particularly useful in evaluating the obstructed ureteropelvic junction and, therefore, the subject is considered separately.

In evaluation of periureteral vessels, the same techniques employed for ureteral endoluminal

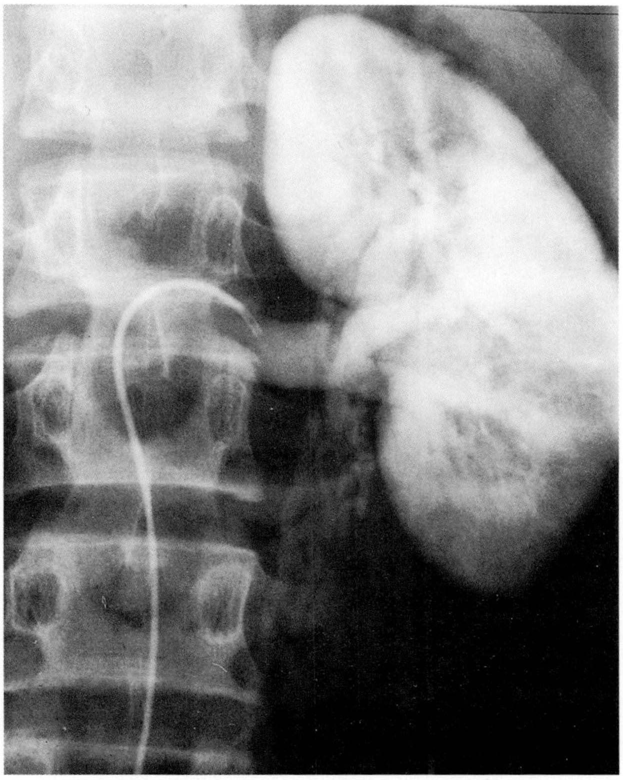

a

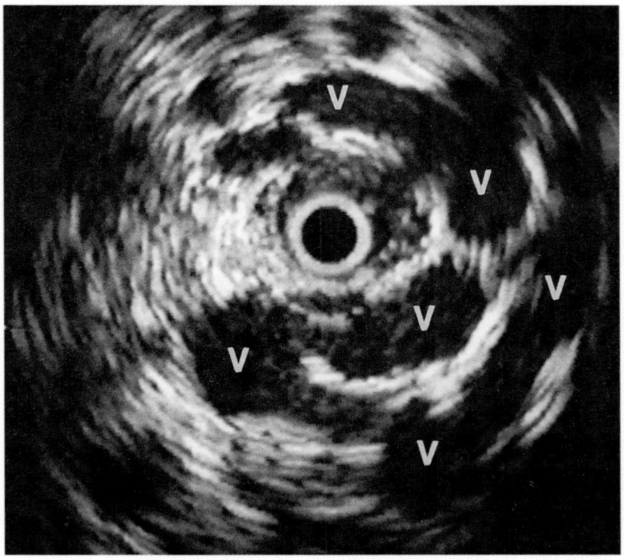

b

Figure 4.45 *A 17-year-old male with gross unilateral hematuria was found to have notching on the excretory urogram. (a) Renal venography demonstrated varices throughout the length of the ureter. (b) Endoluminal ultrasound demonstrated large veins (V) within the adventitia along the ureter corresponding to the vessels seen on venography.*

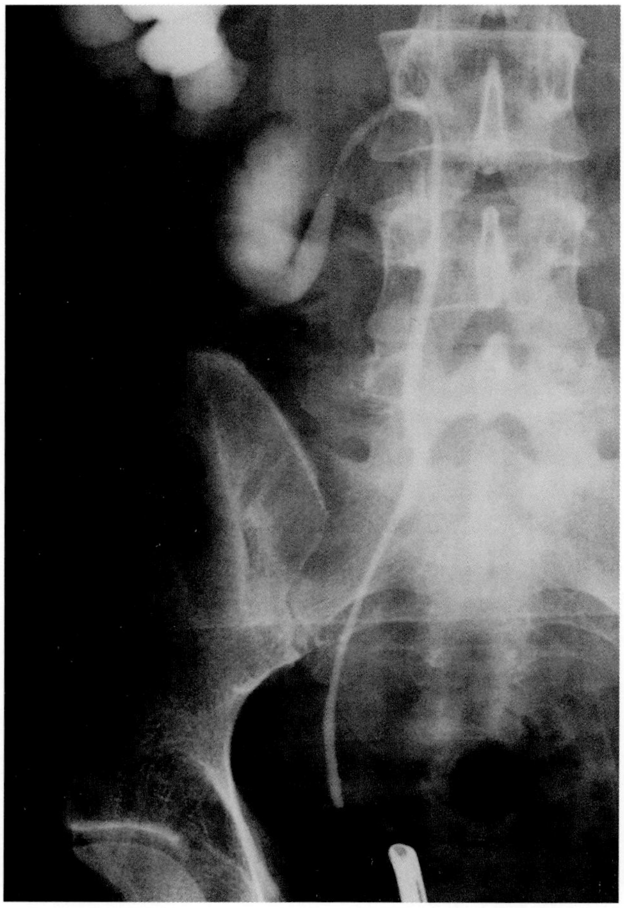

a

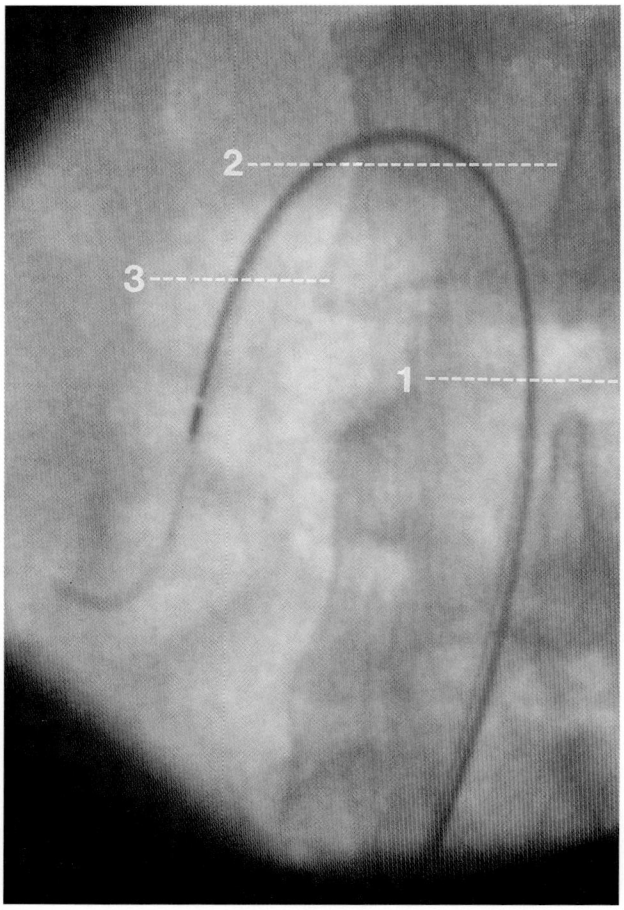

b

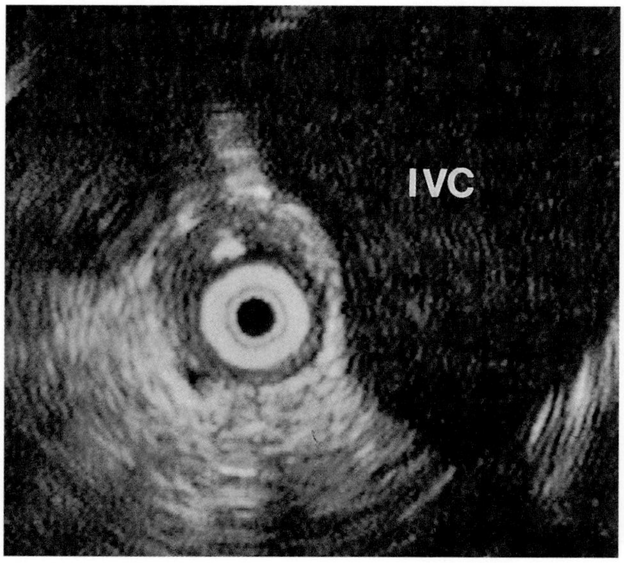

c

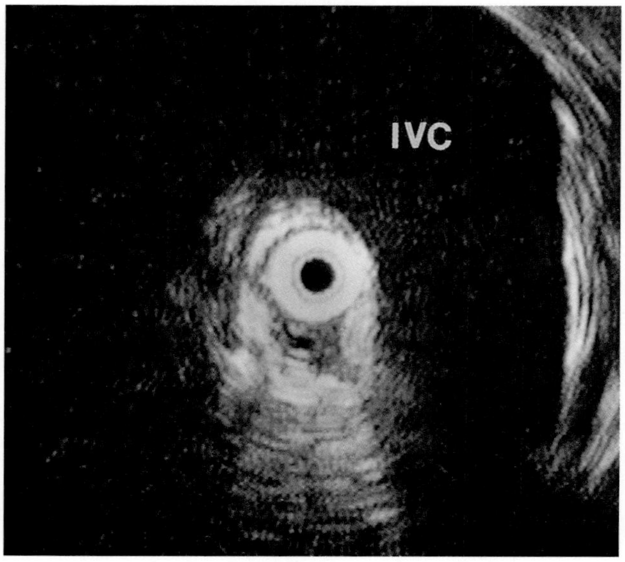

d

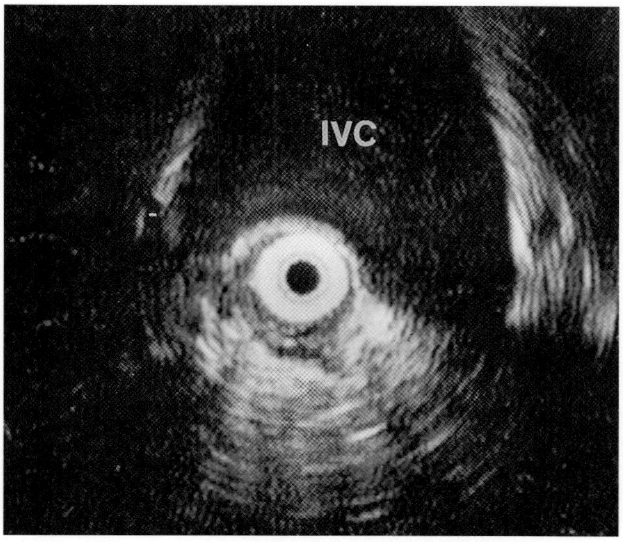

e

Figure 4.46 *(a) A patient with flank pain was found to have a retrocaval ureter on radiographic studies. (b) An ultrasound catheter (arrow) was passed to the level of the tortuosity. (c,d,e) Endoluminal ultrasound of the area demonstrated the inferior vena cava (IVC) coursing around the entire ureter as the transducer was advanced within the ureteral lumen. (c) is the sonographic image at level 1; (d) is the sonographic image at level 2, and (e) is the sonographic image at level 3 in (b).*

ultrasound in general are useful. The ultrasound transducer can be passed in either retrograde or antegrade fashion, depending upon the available access. It is then extremely important to localize the position of the transducer relative to the lesion in question. This requires simultaneous radiographic and ultrasonographic imaging. It can be helpful to position the probe through an endoscope for most accurate positioning. Direct imaging also gives the best orientation and can also be accomplished by simultaneous radiographic and sonographic imaging with a known landmark, such as a guidewire in the field of both images.

URETERAL STRICTURES

Ureteral strictures comprise another major potential application for endoluminal ultrasound. Since the stricture involves scarring of the ureter and possibly the adjacent periureteral tissue, it would appear to lend itself well to endoluminal sonographic evaluation. The depth, luminal extent and possibly the density of the stricture may be evaluated. Additionally, this information may be translated to permit ultrasound-guided incision of the stricture to find the depth and extent of incision as well as to avoid periureteral vessels.

Patients with ureteral stricture most frequently present with flank pain, although a decrease in renal function or otherwise asymptomatic presentation can occur. The radiographic findings include, by definition, a narrowing of the ureter. There may be evidence of obstruction with proximal dilation with hydroureter and hydronephrosis or there may be diminution of function even to the extent of nonfunction of the affected renal unit. The options in therapy for strictures include endoluminal dilation of the affected area, incision of the stricture (both with subsequent stenting) and surgical repair.[26–28] Since most patients are amenable to and choose endoluminal therapy, endoluminal ultrasound to guide this therapy is even more important.

Endoluminal sonography has demonstrated different patterns in patients with ureteral strictures. There is some suggestion that these can be related to the efficacy of incisional treatment. Sonographic findings in ureteral strictures have included isolated thickening of the mucosa only. Others have exhibited hyperechoic scarring limited to the ureteral wall or extending to the periureteral tissue or well beyond the ureter to include the entire periureteral tissue. There is evidence that those with mucosal thickening alone do well with treatment. On the contrary, scarring extending well into the periureteral tissue is a less promising finding. It should be stressed that these are preliminary findings and must be tempered by further experience (Fig. 4.47).

One of the most consistent findings has been the absence of peristalsis in the region of the stricture. Normally, the ureteral lumen can be demonstrated sonographically to enlarge and then contract as peristaltic waves pass. The area of the stricture remains tightly constricted around the lumen without the features of peristalsis.

Strictures can develop at other locations, particularly at surgical sites. One of the most common of these has been at the site of ureteral intestinal

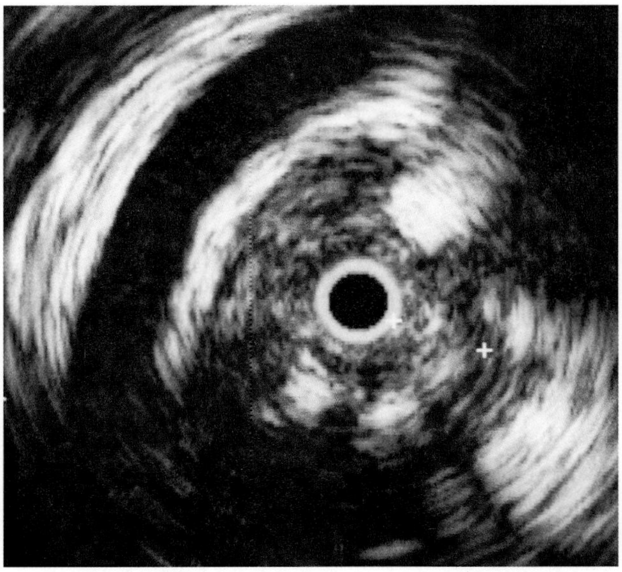

Figure 4.47 *Endoluminal ultrasound at the level of a ureteral stricture demonstrates hyperechogenicity of the wall (+···+). There was no shadowing from these areas and no calculus could be seen on radiographic study. These findings suggest scarring of the ureteral wall and the adventitia.*

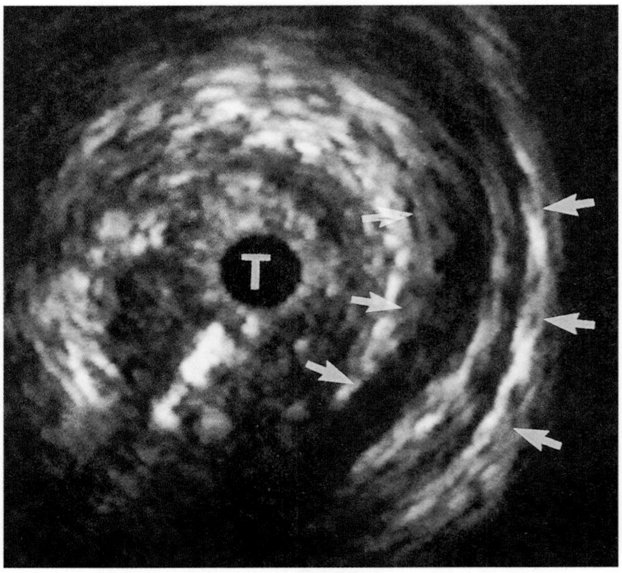

Figure 4.48 *Endoluminal ultrasound of a ureterocolonic anastomosis demonstrates the transducer (T) within the lumen surrounded by the ureteral mucosa (hypoechoic). This, in turn, is surrounded by the colonic structure (arrows). The guidewire is located at 7 o'clock.*

anastomoses performed for urinary diversion. These areas may become obstructed, and differential diagnosis then develops between recurrent tumor and benign stricture. In the presence of a benign stricture, there can be an option of endoluminal incisional treatment. Endoluminal ultrasound has been particularly useful in evaluating these patients, both in a search for neoplasm and to guide the endoluminal incision (Fig. 4.48).

Changes in technique may improve the accuracy of sonographic imaging, particularly of strictures. In some cases we have noted better visualization of the stricture with dilation of the ureter. This has been helpful in defining the area of restricted dilation, corresponding to the stricture, and also in giving a better image of the mucosa and the wall of the ureter. We have achieved this by placing the ultrasound probe through an endoscope and irrigating simultaneously. We can also do it by placing an open-end ureteral catheter over the guidewire used for placement of the ultrasound probe. After a side-arm irrigating adapter is placed on the distal end of the catheter, irrigant can be passed into the ureteral lumen. Care should be taken to avoid introducing air into the system, since these bubbles will interfere with the sonographic imaging.

NEOPLASMS

Upper tract urothelial tumors are uncommon, comprising less than 10% of urinary neoplasms. Transitional cell carcinoma (TCCa) is by far the most frequent of these, although benign lesions occur, including fibroepithelial polyps, inverted papillomas and hemangiomas.

The clinical presentation for any of the upper-tract lesions may be similar. Most commonly, hematuria, either gross or microscopic, is the first sign. Upon investigation, the lesion is usually seen as a filling defect with excretory urography. Cytology is frequently positive with a high-grade tumor and much less frequently with a low-grade papillary TCCa. Calculi presenting as filling defects can usually be

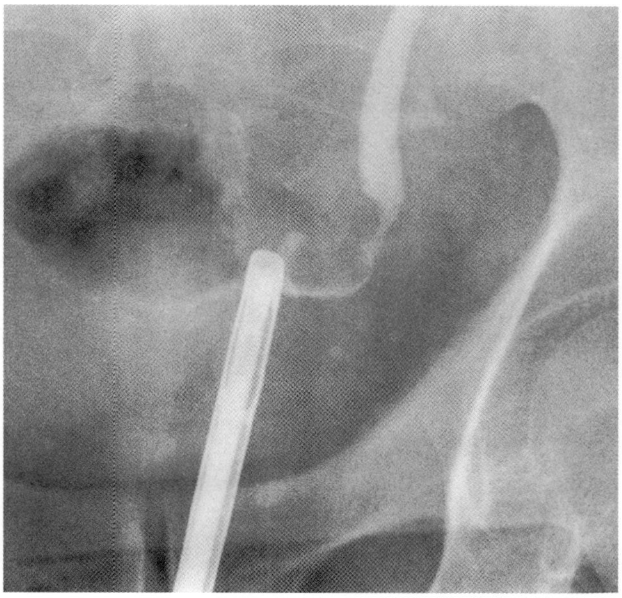

a

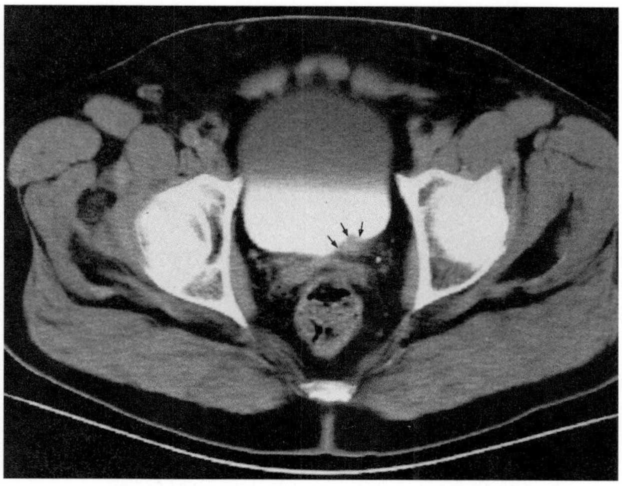

b

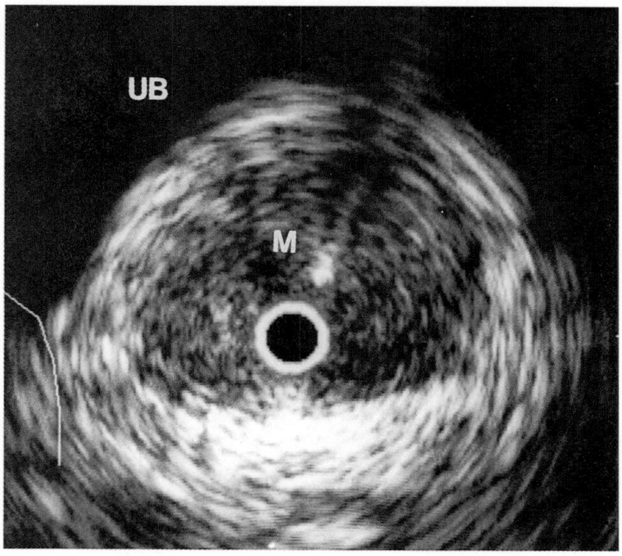

c

Figure 4.49 *(a) Gross hematuria led to an investigation of a patient defining a filling defect in the left distal ureter. (b) A soft-tissue mass was seen in this area on the CT scan (arrows). (c) Endoluminal ultrasound demonstrated a hypoechoic mass (M) filling the distal (intravesical) ureter. The guidewire is seen at 1 o'clock and the lumen of the bladder (UB) is visible peripherally from 9 o'clock to 3 o'clock. On endoscopy, a papillary tumor was biopsied and diagnosed as Grade II TCCa. Treatment was distal ureterectomy.*

distinguished on ultrasound or CT scan from soft-tissue lesions. A firm diagnosis of neoplasm may require direct ureteroscopic inspection and sampling.[29,30]

After the establishment of a diagnosis, appropriate treatment can be undertaken. The standard treatment has included nephroureterectomy, although low-grade distal ureteral lesions can be treated equally successfully with distal ureterectomy.[31,32] Endoscopic treatment was introduced initially for high-risk patients with a solitary kidney or compromised contralateral kidney.[33,34] In some instances, the indications have been extended for patients with bilateral kidneys, particularly those with unstable and potentially life-threatening medical illnesses. Both ureteroscopic and percutaneous approaches have been used.[35] The latter have been applied more frequently for large intrarenal lesions, while the ureteroscopic techniques are better suited to smaller lesions, within either the intrarenal collecting system or the ureter.

The characteristic endoluminal sonographic appearance of a low-grade TCCa is a hypoechoic area within the urinary lumen (Figs 4.49, 4.50 and

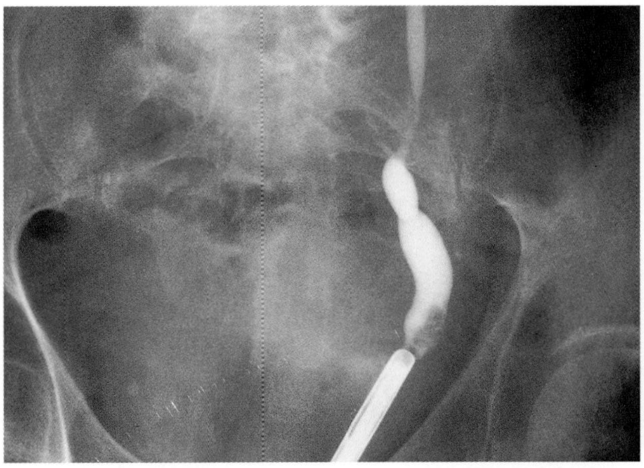

a

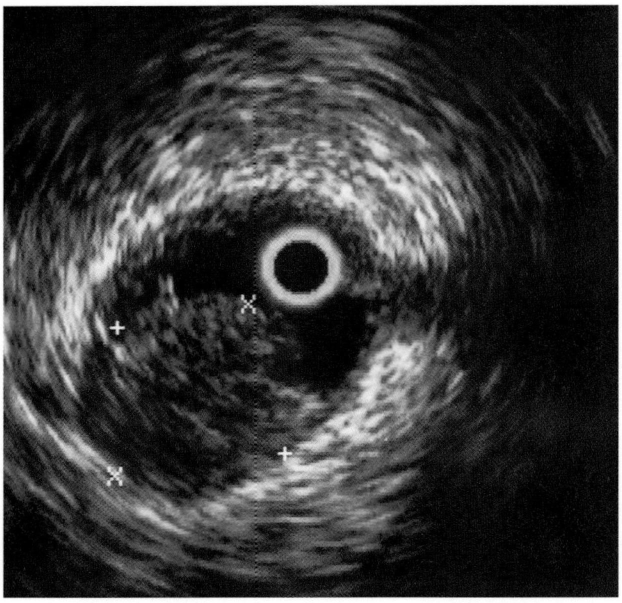

b

Figure 4.50 *(a) Retrograde pyelogram outlines a distal ureteral filling defect. (b) Endoluminal ultrasound demonstrates a hypoechoic mass (+···+) with an intact ureteral wall. This Grade I–II TCCa was treated with endoscopic resection.*

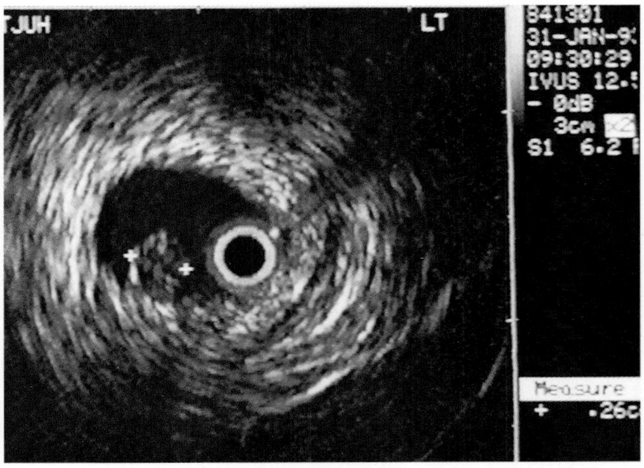

Figure 4.51 *A small (2.6-mm) intraluminal TCCa is seen as a hypoechoic lesion (+···+). The guidewire is located at 1 o'clock.*

4.51). Occasionally, the base itself can be visualized as well as areas of lumen adjacent to but free from tumor. In our series, bulging of the lumen has been observed without loss of definition of the wall of the ureter. In a small number of patients, there has been observed a loss of distinction between the tumor and the ureteral wall which has been interpreted as invasion (Fig. 4.52). Since the numbers have been small, it is impossible to evaluate fully the accuracy of this finding.

The endosonographic image is also useful in locating tumors relative to periureteral vessels. For instance, by endoscopic visualization alone, it is difficult to determine the exact level of the iliac vessels. Tumors located in this area which are to be treated endoscopically may be lying directly over the vessels or several millimeters away. With endosonographic imaging, it is possible to distinguish the specific location. With this information, it may be possible to resect the tumor endoscopically more deeply if it is not located directly over the iliac vessels (Fig. 4.53).

The same techniques can be used with lesions in the renal pelvis and upper infundibulum. It is usually not possible to place the ultrasound transducer into the mid-infundibular or lower infundibula. Transitional cell carcinoma within the intrarenal collecting system has the same endoscopic and sonographic appearance as tumors in other portions of the urinary tract (Fig. 4.54).

Fibroepithelial polyps have a different sonographic appearance. Both fibroepithelial polyps observed in this series were notably more echogenic than the transitional cell carcinomas (Fig. 4.55). This pattern might be expected from the histologic structure of these tumors, which consist of fibrous and epithelial

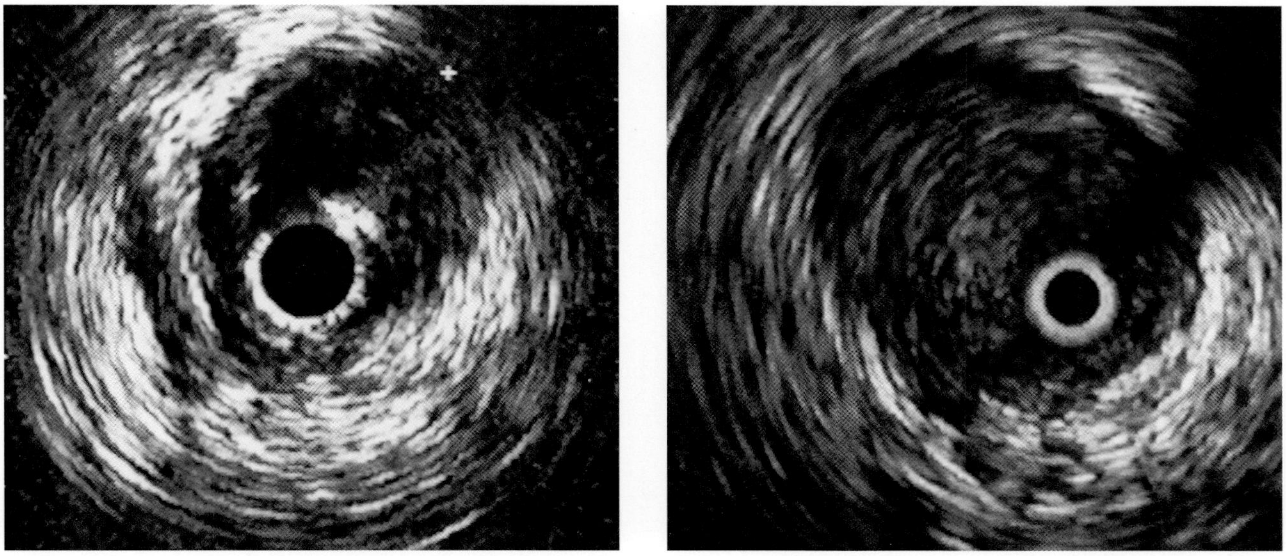

Figure 4.52 *Invasion of TCCa into the wall of the ureter can be seen with this technique. (a) Endoluminal ultrasound of a mid ureteral TCCa demonstrates loss of definition of the ureteral wall (12 to 3 o'clock). The intact mucosa is well seen from 6 to 12 o'clock. (b) Another invasive TCCa shows loss of the ureteral wall from 7 to 1 o'clock. The ureteral mucosa from 3 to 6 o'clock is well defined with a prominent hyperechoic adventitia. This definition is lost where the tumor is invasive.*

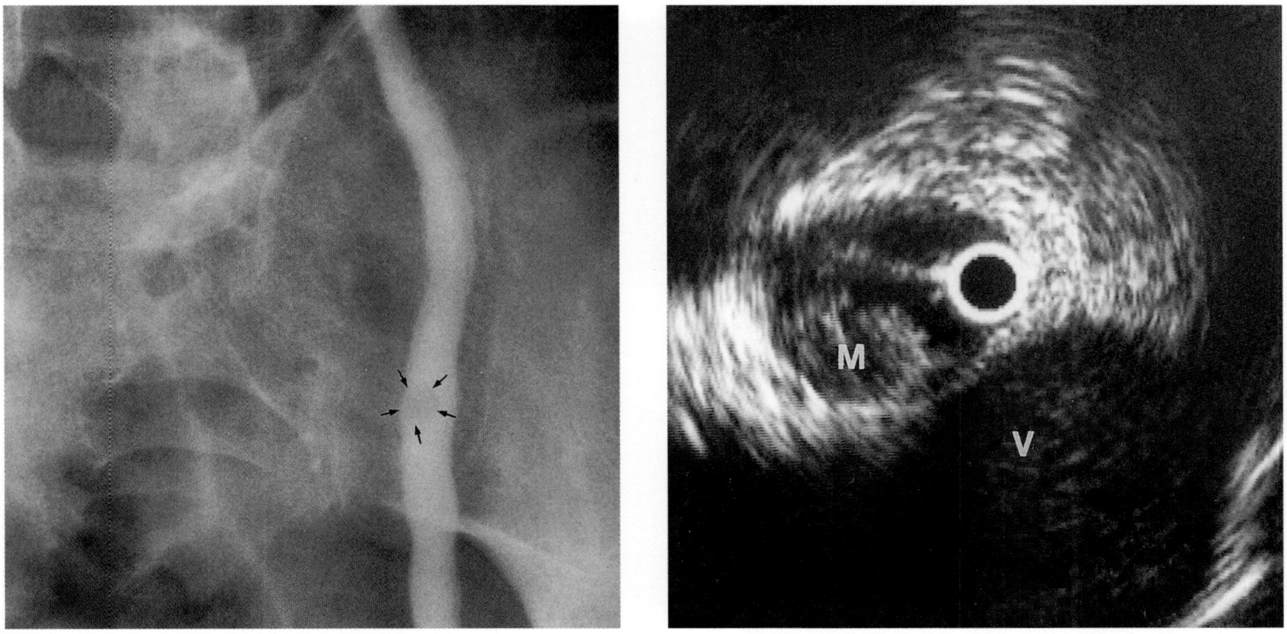

Figure 4.53 *(a) A filling defect (arrows) demonstrated in the ureter at the level of the iliac vessels by retrograde pyelogram was confirmed as a low-grade TCCa by endoscopic inspection and biopsy. (b) The endoluminal ultrasound demonstrates the typical hypoechoic mass (M) within the ureteral lumen. It can be seen to be located immediately adjacent to the iliac vessel (V). Suitable care must be taken in the endoscopic treatment of lesions at this level.*

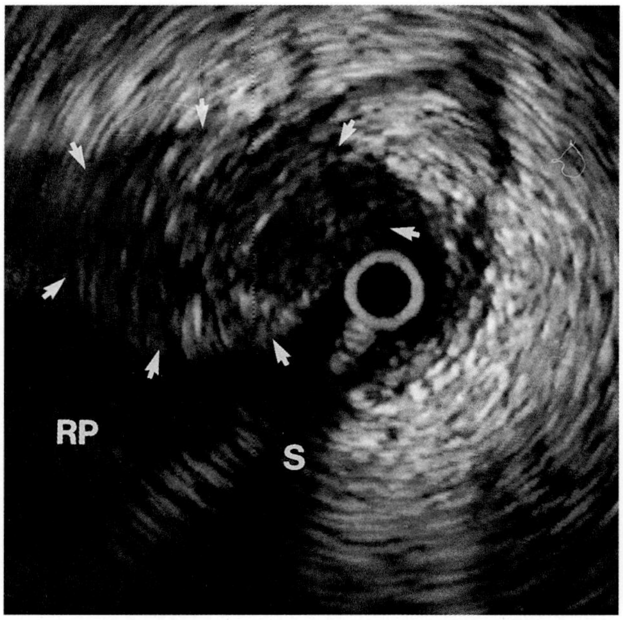

Figure 4.54 *Low-grade TCCa is located in the renal pelvis (RP). It is a typical hypoechoic mass (arrows) on endoluminal ultrasound. Shadowing (S) from the wire at 7 o'clock obscures the image of the tissue in that area and can obscure the base of the tumor or even mimic the findings of invasion.*

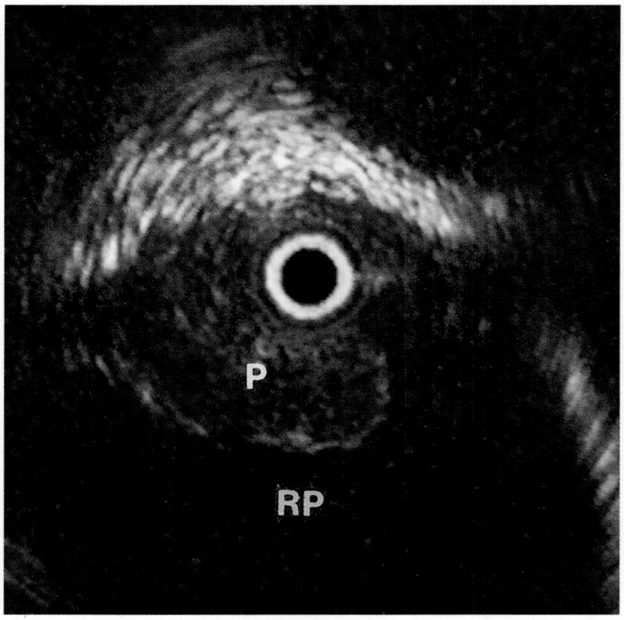

Figure 4.55 *Fibroepithelial polyp (P) appears on ultrasound as a central hypoechoic mass surrounded by an echogenic layer. The lesion in the renal pelvis (RP) extends from 5 o'clock to 9 o'clock in this endoluminal ultrasound image.*

components. In contrast, low-grade papillary transitional cell carcinomas appear as a uniform hypoechoic mass, as described above.

The sonographic image can also be used to assess the adequacy of treatment (Fig. 4.56). The image of the neoplasm obtained prior to treatment can be compared to that after treatment. The extent of tumor removal can then be assessed. It may be difficult in interpreting the second image, since blood clot can have the same appearance and bubbles produced during electrocoagulation or laser therapy can interfere with the image. Nevertheless, early studies indicate the potential for sonographic monitoring of tumor treatment.

OTHER APPLICATIONS

Endoluminal ultrasonography has been used in the upper urinary tract and in other individual cases, where the indications cannot be considered major but illustrate a major benefit of the technique. Two of these indications are a periureteral foreign body and an obliterated ureteral orifice. In each case, endoluminal ultrasonography was used for accurate localization of a structure and to guide therapy.

In the first case, a 30-year-old female had undergone a laparoscopic gynecologic procedure and suffered injury to a ureter with a subsequent stricture (Fig. 4.57). She was also found to have a clip lying immediately adjacent to the ureter. Upon ureteroscopic examination, the stricture was visualized but the adjacent clip could not be seen. Endoluminal sonography of this area demonstrated the location of the clip. The ureter was incised at this location and the clip and adjacent suture material were removed through the ureteral lumen. The patient recovered without recurrent stricture over the 9-month follow-up period.

The second patient, a 60-year-old male, had undergone endoscopic resection of a bladder tumor

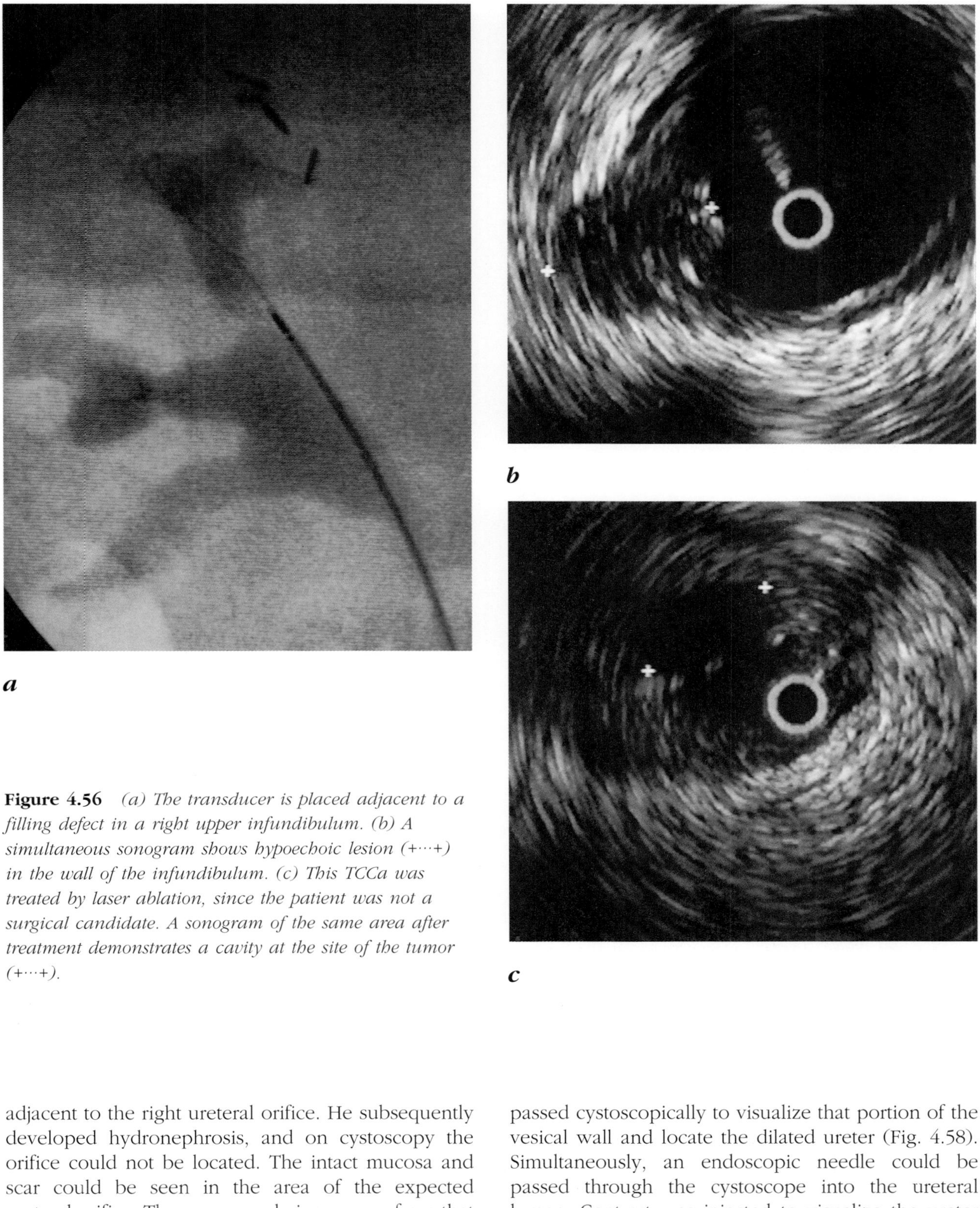

Figure 4.56 *(a) The transducer is placed adjacent to a filling defect in a right upper infundibulum. (b) A simultaneous sonogram shows hypoechoic lesion (+···+) in the wall of the infundibulum. (c) This TCCa was treated by laser ablation, since the patient was not a surgical candidate. A sonogram of the same area after treatment demonstrates a cavity at the site of the tumor (+···+).*

adjacent to the right ureteral orifice. He subsequently developed hydronephrosis, and on cystoscopy the orifice could not be located. The intact mucosa and scar could be seen in the area of the expected ureteral orifice. There was no drainage seen from that collecting system endoscopically or by renal scan. The patient refused percutaneous drainage or other percutaneous manipulation. A 6.2 Fr probe could be passed cystoscopically to visualize that portion of the vesical wall and locate the dilated ureter (Fig. 4.58). Simultaneously, an endoscopic needle could be passed through the cystoscope into the ureteral lumen. Contrast was injected to visualize the ureter fluoroscopically and a guidewire passed into the lumen. A new orifice was then created by incision of the tunnel and subsequent stenting. His ureter

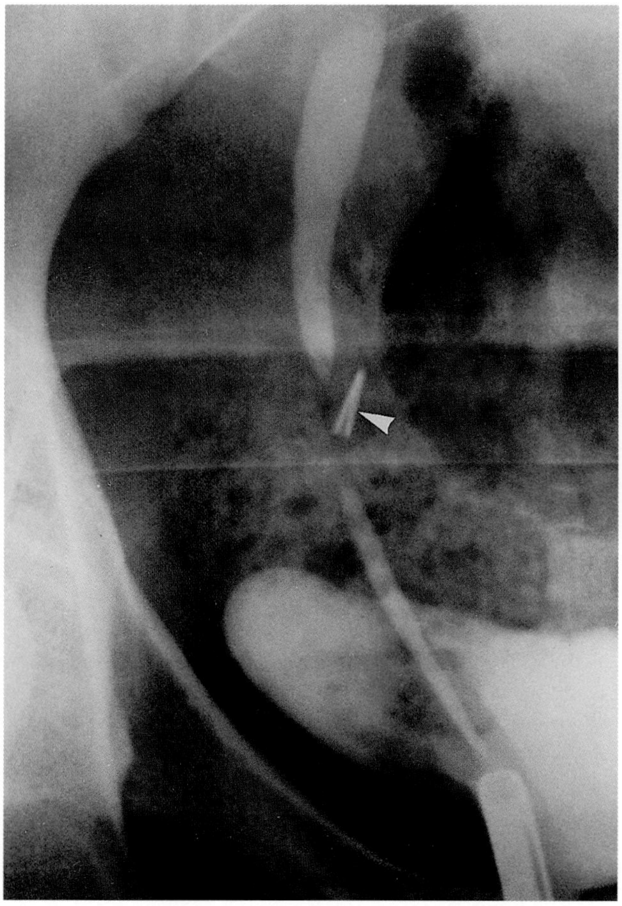

a

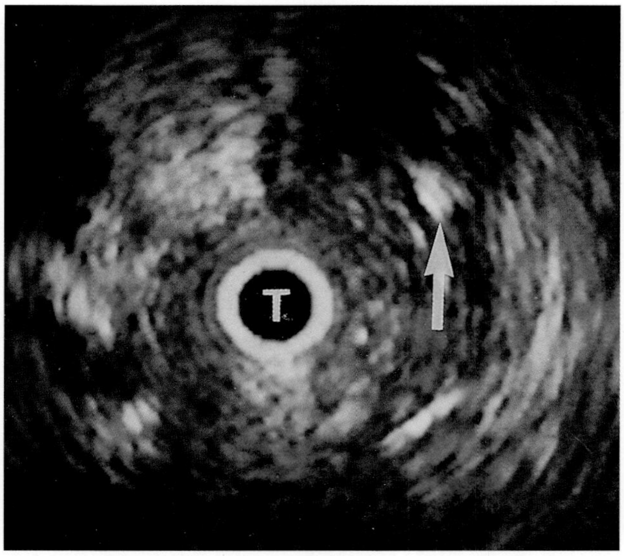

b

Figure 4.57 *(a) Retrograde ureterogram outlines a ureteral stricture adjacent to a surgical clip (arrowhead). (b) Endoluminal ultrasound demonstrates the area of ureteral stricture with an echogenic shadowing structure (arrow) adjacent to it. This is correlated with the clip seen radiographically. Endoluminal ultrasound imaging along with fluoroscopic monitoring guided incision of the ureter to allow removal of the clip and adjacent suture material with subsequent healing of the ureter without obstructive stricturing. T, transducer.*

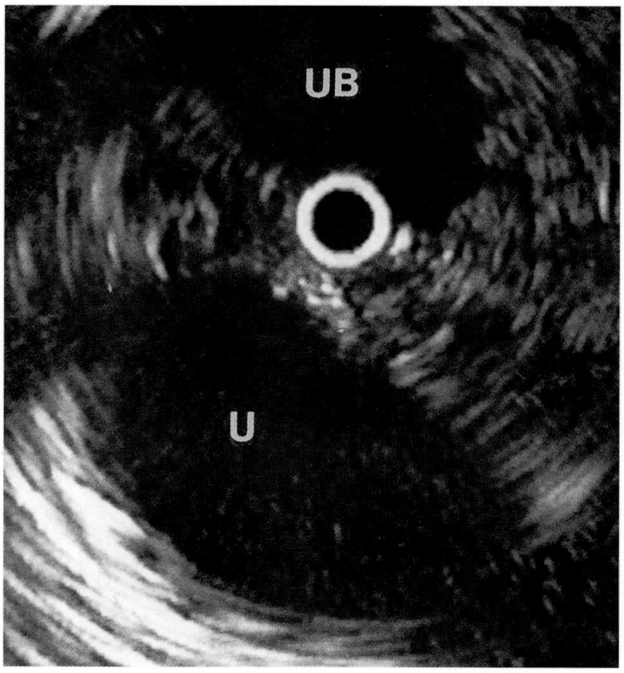

Figure 4.58 *The ultrasound transducer placed cystoscopically reveals the dilated blind-ending ureter (U) located posterior to the bladder lumen (UB).*

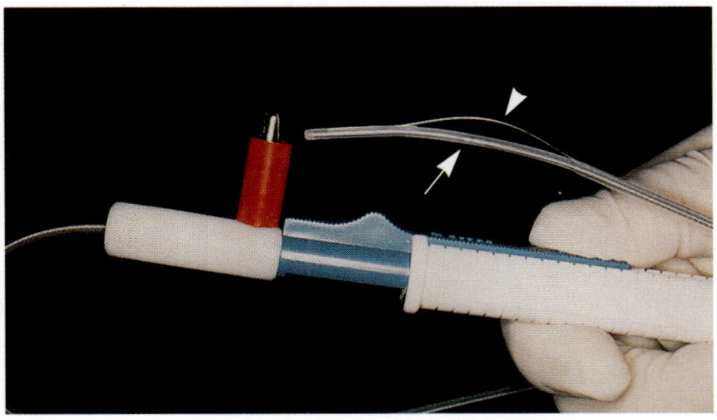

a

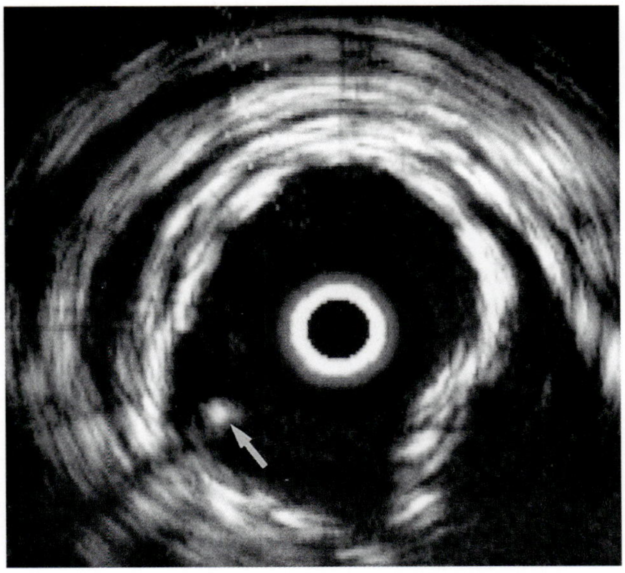

b

Figure 4.59 *(a) A double-lumen catheter contains a 20-MHz transducer (arrow) and an electrosurgical wire (arrowhead) for incision. (b) Sonographic image with this catheter in a phantom demonstrates the cutting wire (arrow).*

remains patent at 15 months of follow-up. Because of the limitations imposed by the patient's refusal to have a nephrostomy tube placed, contrast could not be introduced into the collecting system directly and endoscopic ureteroneocystostomy would not have been possible without the ultrasonic guidance.

These two cases illustrate the wide range of isolated indications that will develop with increasing experience with endoluminal sonography.

FUTURE OF ENDOLUMINAL SONOGRAPHY IN THE UPPER URINARY TRACT

The present applications and techniques for endoureteral ultrasonography represent only the infancy of an important technique. In the future, it can be expected that the indications will expand and the present applications will be refined.

Several major advances in endoluminal sonography can be expected. First, we can anticipate a decrease in size of the probes with continued improvement in resolution. The smaller-diameter probes can then be used simultaneously with endoscopy with more accurate localization by eliminating many of the questions related to the simultaneous radiographic localization of the probe and known landmarks. Smaller probes can also be passed through either the smaller working channels in the miniature ureteroscopes or through flexible ureteroscopes.

Another possible change is to develop transducers with different imaging characteristics. In addition to cross-sectional imaging, forward or even retrograde imaging may be possible. Thus, the optimal probe for visualization of the target area can be selected.

Another major advance will be endoluminal sonography combined with devices for treatment within the imaged area (Fig. 4.59). In this way, simultaneous imaging and treatment can be guided by the sonographic findings.

Application of these anticipated improvements can be expected in each treatment group. Several examples may illustrate the potential benefits. In patients with submucosal calculi, either simultaneous endoscopic visualization and sonographic visualization or ultrasound-guided division of the mucosa can enable direct, accurate incision of the tissue at the exact location of the calculus to permit its retrieval. Sonography can also be used to determine the adequacy of stone removal. Forward-viewing transducers can be used within the kidney to visualize areas relatively inaccessible to the side-imaging catheters.

Simultaneous imaging and treatment can benefit patients in several clinical groups. The patient with ureteropelvic junction obstruction and an adjacent vessel can benefit from very accurate incision guided by simultaneous endoscopic and sonographic visualization or from a sonographically guided cutting device. In the same way, a stricture may be cut more accurately when therapy is guided in real time by an endoluminal ultrasound image. Calculi which are visually obscured may be accessible to ultrasound-guided retrieval or lithotriptor devices.

CONCLUSION

The indications for and the use of endoluminal ultrasound within the upper urinary tract can be expected to grow with increasing experience; it has become an important technique which yields information not available through other techniques. It adds another dimension to endoluminal endoscopy, specifically imaging deep to the surface of the urinary lumen. Direct real-time imaging in combination with therapeutic procedures can be expected to improve their accuracy and, therefore, their safety and possibly efficacy.

REFERENCES

1. Neiman HL, The urinary system. In: Goldberg BB, ed., *Textbook of Abdominal Ultrasound* (Williams & Wilkins: Baltimore, 1993) 330–90.
2. Baumgartner BR, Steinberg HV, Ambrose SS, Walton KN, Bernardino ME, Sonographic evaluation of renal stones treated by extracorporeal shock wave lithotripsy, *AJR* 1987; **149:**131–5.
3. Cook JH III, Lytton B, Intraoperative localization of renal calculi during nephrolithotomy by ultrasound scanning, *J Urol* 1977; **117:**543–6.
4. Goldberg BB, Liu JB, Merton DA, Kurtz AB, Endoluminal US: experiments with nonvascular uses in animals, *Radiology* 1990; **175:**39–43.
5. Bagley DH, Liu JB, Goldberg BB, Use of endoluminal ultrasound of the ureter, *Semin Urol* 1992; **10**(3):194–8.
6. Bagley DH, Liu JB, Goldberg BB, Grasso M, Endopyelotomy: the importance of crossing vessels demonstrated by endoluminal ultrasound, *J Endourol* 1995; **9**:465–7.
7. Sampaio FJB, Favorito LA, Ureteropelvic junction stenosis: vascular, anatomical background for endopyelotomy, *J Urol* 1993; **150:**1787–91.
8. Grasso M, Goldberg BB, Liu JB, Bagley DH, Submucosal calculi: endoscopic and endoluminal ultrasonographic diagnosis and treatment options, *J Urol* 1995; **153:**1384–9.
9. Dretler SP, Young RH, Stone granuloma: a cause of ureteral stricture, *J Urol* 1993; **150:**1800–2.
10. Evans CP, Stoller ML, The fate of the iatrogenic retroperitoneal stone, *J Urol* 1993; **150:**827–9.
11. Conway JJ, 'Well-tempered' diuresis renography: its historical development, physiological and technical pitfalls, and standardized technique protocol, *Semin Nucl Med* 1992; **22:**74–84.
12. Whitaker RH, Clinical assessment of pelvic and ureteral function, *Urology* 1978; **12:**146–50.
13. Motola JA, Badlani GH, Smith AD, Results of 212 consecutive endopyelotomies: an 8 year follow up, *J Urol* 1993; **149:**453–6.
14. Kuenkel M, Korth K, Endopyelotomy: long term follow up of 143 patients, *J Endourol* 1990; **4:**109–16.
15. Gerber GS, Lyon ES, Endopyelotomy: patient selection results and complications, *Urology* 1994; **43:**2–10.
16. Meretyk I, Meretyk S, Clayman R, Endopyelotomy: comparison of ureteroscopic retrograde and antegrade percutaneous techniques, *J Urol* 1992; **148:**775–83.
17. Thomas R, Endopyelotomy for ureteropelvic junction obstruction and ureteral stricture disease: a comparison of antegrade and retrograde techniques, *Current Opin Urol* 1994; **4:**174–9.
18. Bagley DH, Liu JB, Intracavitary sonographic imaging of the ureteropelvic junction obstruction, *J Endourol* 1995; **10**:105–10.
19. Chandhoke PS, Clayman RV, Stone AM et al, Endopyelotomy and endoureterotomy with the Acucise ureteral cutting balloon device: preliminary experience, *J Endourol* 1993; **7**(1):45–51.
20. Hall SM, Babayan RK, Treatment of ureteral strictures and UPJ obstructions with the Acucise catheter: two year follow up, *J Urol* 1994; **151:**280A.
21. O'Flynn K, Hehir M, McKelvie G, Hussey J, Steyn J, Endo-balloon rupture in stenting for pelviureteric junction obstruction: techniques and early results. *Br J Urol* 1989; **64:**572–4.
22. Stephens FD, Ureterovascular hydronephrosis and the 'aberrant' renal vessels, *J Urol* 1982; **128:**984–7.
23. Clark WR, Malik RS, Ureteropelvic junction obstruction: observations on the classic type in adults, *J Urol* 1987; **138:**276–9.
24. Van Cangh PJ, Wilmont JF, Opromer RJ, Abi-Aad A, Wese FX, Lauge F, Long term results and late recurrence after endoureteropyelotomy: a critical analysis of prognostic factors, *J Urol* 1994; **151:**934–7.
25. Terai A, Terachi T, Machida S, Endopyelotomy: percutaneous surgery for ureteropelvic junction obstruction in a bifid pelvis: further experience, *J Urol* 1988; **139:**803–4.
26. Kramolowsky EV, Tucker RD, Nelson CMK, Management of benign ureteral strictures: open surgical repair or endoscopic dilation? *J Urol* 1989; **141:**285–6.
27. Netto NR Jr, Ferreira U, Lemos GC, Claro JFA, Endourological management of ureteral strictures, *J Urol* 1990; **144:**631–4.
28. Thomas RJ, Choosing the ideal candidate for ureteroscopic endoureterotomy, *J Urol* 1993; **149:**314A.
29. Bagley DH, Rivas D: Upper urinary tract filling defects: flexible ureteroscopic diagnosis, *J Urol* 1990; **143:**1196–200.
30. Streem SB, Pontes JE, Novick AC, Montie JE: Ureteropyeloscopy in the evaluation of upper tract filling defects, *J Urol* 1986; **136;**383–5.
31. Mazeman E: Tumours of the upper urinary tract calyces, renal pelvis and ureter, *Eur Urol* 1976; **2:**120–8.

32. Zincke H, Neves RJ: Feasibility of conservative surgery for transitional cell cancer of the upper urinary tract, *Urol Clin North Am* 1984; **11:**717–24.
33. Huffman JL, Bagley DH, Lyon ES, Morse MJ, Herr, HW, Whitmore Jr, WF: Endoscopic diagnosis and treatment of upper tract urothelial tumors—a preliminary report, *Cancer* 1985; **55:**1422–8.
34. Blute ML, Segura JW, Patterson DE, Benson Jr. RC, Zincke H: Impact of endourology on diagnosis and management of upper urinary tract urothelial cancer, *J Urol* 1989; **141:**1298–301.
35. Sweetser PM, Jarrett TW, Weiss GH, Smith AD, Treatment of transitional cell carcinoma involving the renal pelvis—percutaneous approach. In Smith AD (ed.) *Controversies in Endourology* (Philadelphia: WB Saunders Company, 1995) 193–200.

Chapter 5 Lower urinary tract

Michael B Chancellor and Ji-Bin Liu

INTRODUCTION

Since the 1980s, new electronic and acoustic technology has permitted the development of miniaturized intraluminal ultrasound systems to evaluate a variety of vascular and nonvascular lumina throughout the body. Successful acquisition of intraluminal ultrasound involves a combination of both ultrasound transducer and catheter technologies. During the past several years, miniature catheter-based ultrasound transducers have become commercially available and have been used in a variety of studies, in both animals and humans, to establish their efficacy.[1-10]

The application of endoluminal ultrasound in the lower urinary tract is an exciting area which has only recently undergone systematic examination. The study of endoluminal ultrasound in the lower urinary tract has been a fruitful collaboration between endourology and ultrasonography. In this chapter we will first briefly discuss the relevant anatomy of the lower urinary tract for endoluminal ultrasound. We will then discuss the specific techniques of endoluminal ultrasound for the lower urinary tract, and the indications for which endoluminal ultrasound has been found to be helpful, specifically, examination of bladder neoplasms, evaluation of urethral diverticulum and fistula, examination of the urethra after endoluminal stent insertion, and assessment of periurethral bulking agent injection for the treatment of stress urinary incontinence. Lastly, we will speculate on the future of endoluminal ultrasound in the lower urinary tract.

ANATOMY

URINARY BLADDER

The urinary bladder is a highly distensible hollow muscular sac, lined with transitional epithelium, which serves to store urine until it can be eliminated under socially acceptable conditions. The normal capacity of the bladder is 300–1000 ml. It is located deep in the bony pelvis immediately posterior to the symphysis pubis (Fig. 5.1).

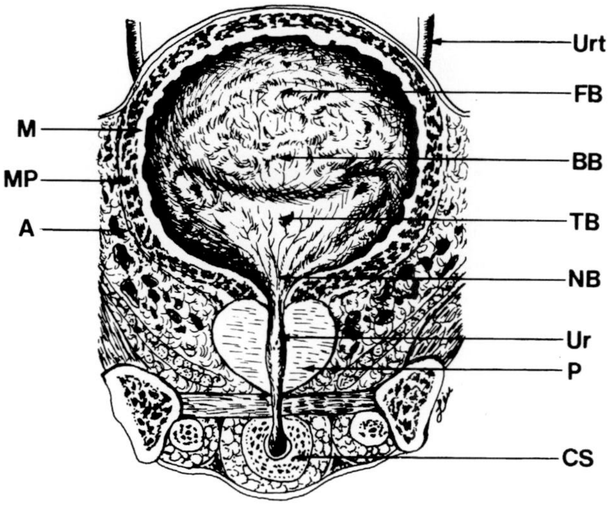

Figure 5.1 *Diagrammatic representation of the urinary bladder in frontal section. Urt, ureter; FB, fundus of bladder; BB, body of bladder; TB, trigone of bladder; NB, neck of bladder; Ur, urethra; P, prostate; CS, corpus spongiosum; M, mucosa; MP, muscular propria; A, adventitia.*

The bladder is regarded as having two anatomically distinct areas. One is the body of the bladder. It is composed of the lateral walls, dome, and floor of the sac to the point of the areas of insertion of the ureters. The musculature of the bladder body is composed of coarse bundles which do not form distinct layers, but rather freely intermingle without any specific circular or longitudinal orientation. At the area where the ureters enter the bladder, the muscular bundles become more organized, and from three identifiable layers at the level of the bladder outlet.

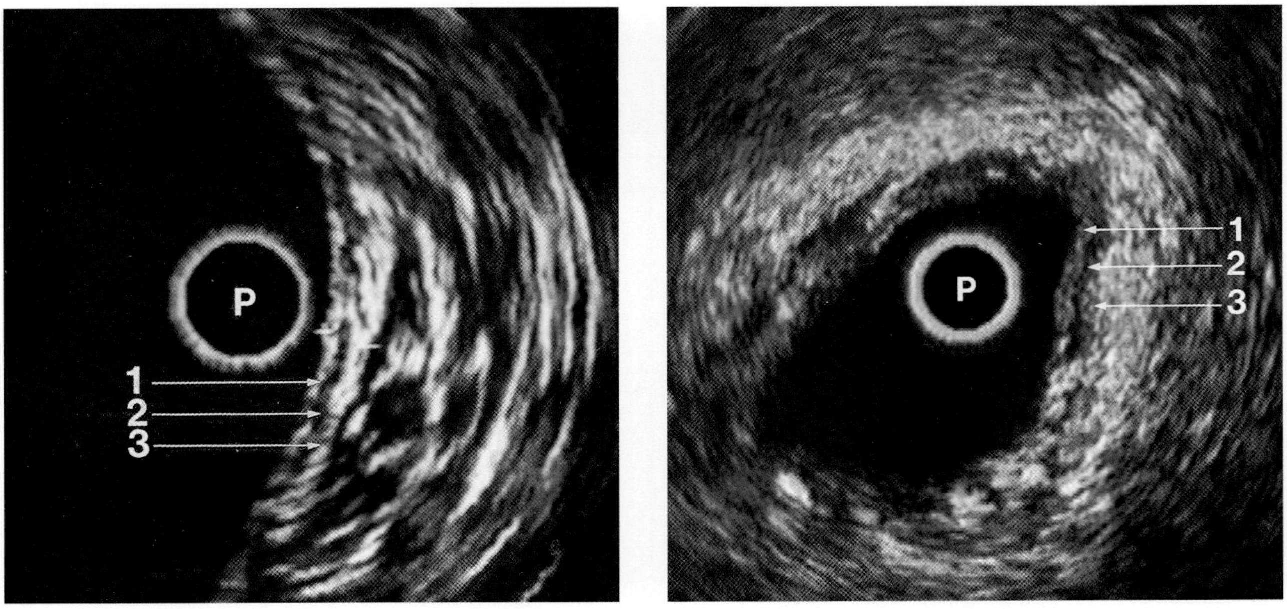

a *b*

Figure 5.2 *Endoluminal ultrasound images obtained from within the distended urinary bladder (a) and within the almost emptied urinary bladder (b). Three layers are noted. From the bladder lumen out, they are the hyperechoic mucosa (1), hypoechoic muscular propria (2), and hyperechoic adventitia (3). P, probe.*

The second distinct area of the bladder is that of the trigone. This is represented by the triangular area demarcated by the two ureteral orifices and the opening of the bladder into the urethra, the bladder neck (Fig. 5.1). The trigone region is felt to be composed of two muscular layers which lie on the detrusor muscle. Superficial trigonal musculature is a continuation of the ureteral musculature, while the deeper layer is fibromuscular and in continuity with Waldeyer's sheath, which supports the insertion of the ureter into the bladder. The trigone region is thicker and more rigid than the rest of the bladder wall and is separated from the anterior vaginal wall only by a thin layer of fat and loose connective tissue.

In the area of the bladder neck, the bladder body muscular bundles become organized into three distinct muscular layers. An outer longitudinal layer is best recognized anteriorly and may cross the area of the urachus, where posteriorly this layer fuses with the deep trigone and mixes with the muscle of the urethra and prostate in the male. A middle circular layer is especially prominent at the area of the vesical neck, but becomes less distinct proximally and distally. The inner longitudinal muscle layer seems to emanate in radial fashion from the bladder neck itself and extends distally into the urethra to form its inner longitudinal muscular layer.

On a sonogram, the fluid-distended bladder appears as a sonolucent structure with smooth and symmetrical walls. The measurement of the wall thickness is 2–6 mm depending on the degree of bladder filling. By using a high-frequency (12.5–20 MHz) catheter-based ultrasound probe, it is possible to visualize the layers of the bladder wall, including the hyperechoic mucosa/submucosa, hypoechoic muscular media, and hyperechoic adventitia (Fig. 5.2). The mucosa and submucosa are indistinguishable unless separated by edema.[11] The outer margin of the wall may be difficult to define, as it merges with the perivesical fat.

THE FEMALE URETHRA

The female urethra is a short muscular tube which acts as a conduit for drainage of urine from the body. It usually measures approximately 4 cm in length and is suspended from the symphysis pubis by

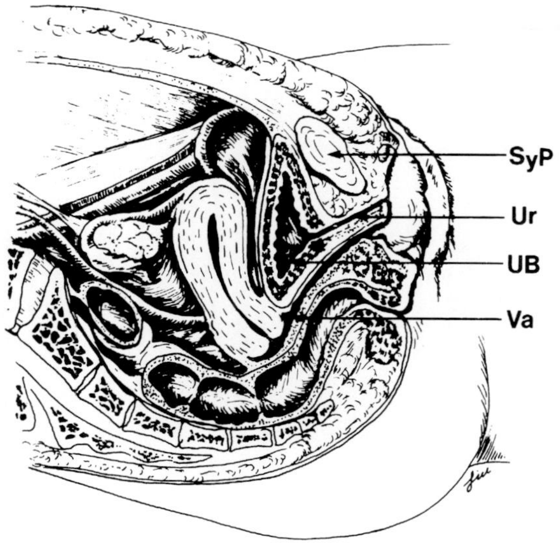

Figure 5.3 *A view of organs in the female pelvis and relationship of the urethra to surrounding structures. SyP, symphysis pubis; Ur, urethra; UB, urinary bladder; Va, vagina.*

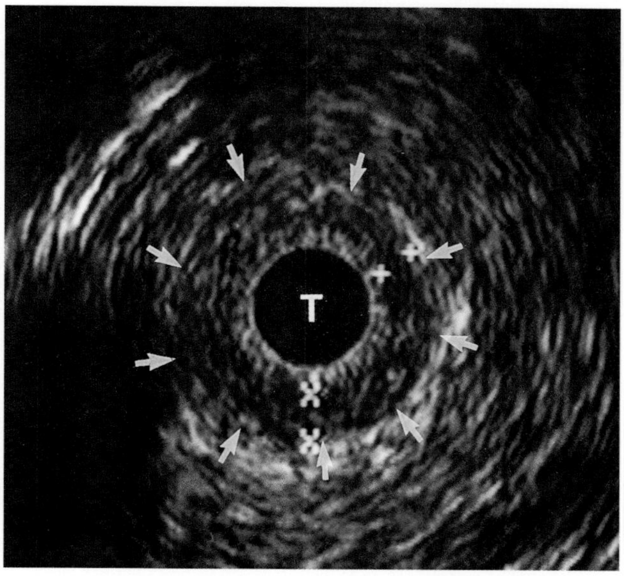

Figure 5.4 *Cross-sectional ultrasound image obtained from within the female urethra at the level of the urogenital diaphragm shows the hypoechoic sphincter urethrae muscle (arrows) and periurethral tissue. T, transducer.*

pubourethral ligaments. Additional support of the urethra is provided by the endopelvic fascia, which acts as a hammock to suspend the urethra and bladder from a tendinous arc attached to the pelvic sidewall (Fig. 5.3).

The urethra is composed of inner longitudinal and outer circular smooth muscular layers, which are lined by transitional epithelium proximally and squamous epithelium distally. On sonogram, the wall of the urethra appears as a hypoechoic structure. The muscular fibers are a direct extension of the bladder neck detrusor fibers. Striated muscle fibers surround the midurethral portion and act to provide voluntary sphincter function. At its exit from the bladder, the urethra is surrounded by a thickened region of bladder wall known as the internal sphincter. The external sphincter can be recognized as an oval-shaped, hypoechoic structure (Fig. 5.4).

THE MALE URETHRA

The male urethra is more complex than that of the female. It not only acts as a conduit and sphincter for

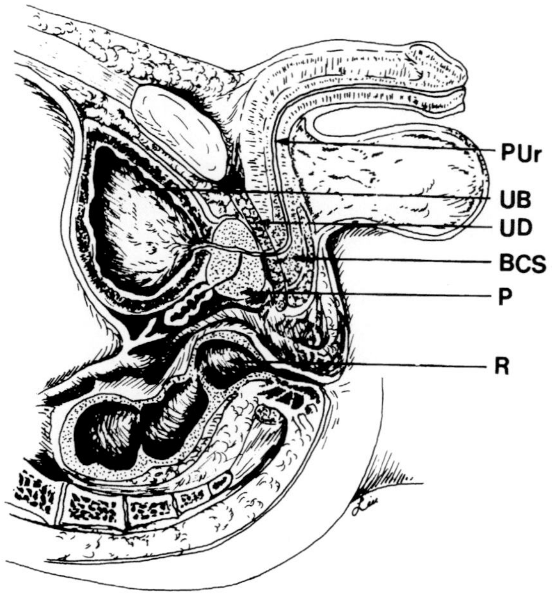

Figure 5.5 *A view of organs in the male pelvis and relationship of the urethra to surrounding structures. PUr, penis urethra; UB, urinary bladder; UD, urogenital diaphragm; BCS, bulb of corpus spongiosum; P, prostate; R, rectum.*

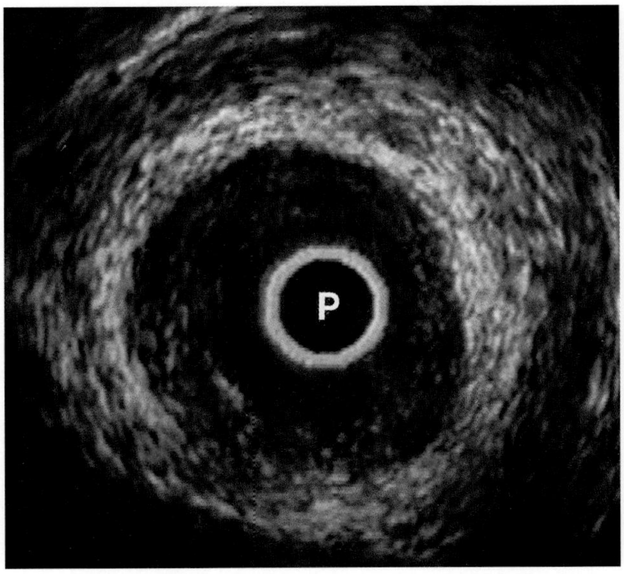

a

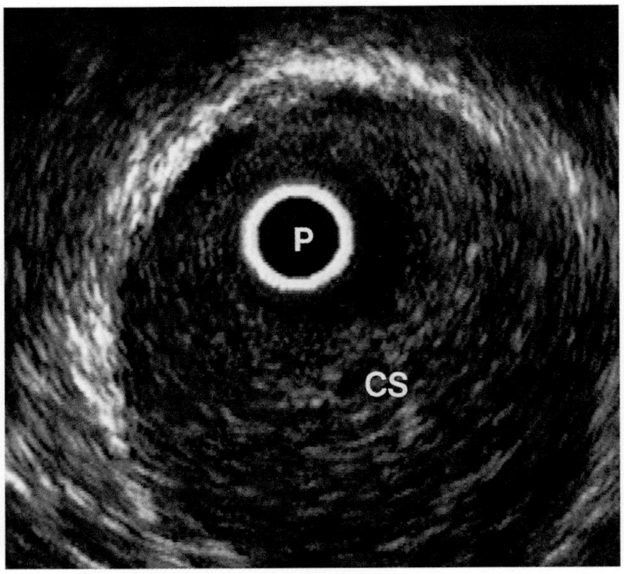

b

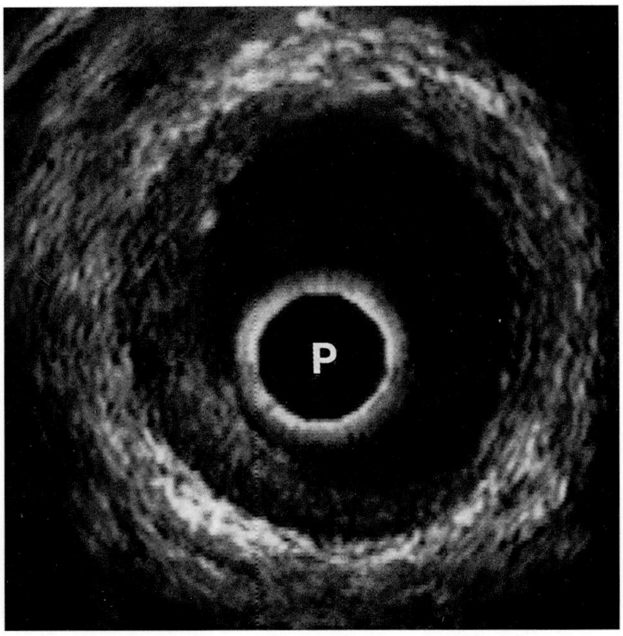

c

Figure 5.6 *(a) Endoluminal ultrasound imaging of the penile urethra obtained at the level of the urogenital diaphragm. (b) Hypoechoic corpus spongiosum (CS) at the level of the bulbous urethra. (c) Fossa navicularis of the urethra at the most distal portion of the penis. P, probe.*

the passage of urine from the bladder, but is also responsible for the delivery of semen from the genital tract. In the male, three distinct regions of the urethra are recognized. These include the prostatic, membranous and penile urethra (Fig. 5.5).

The prostatic urethra is that portion which traverses the prostate gland (Fig. 5.5). Approximately 3 cm in length, it contains the ejaculatory ducts and the remnant of the mullerian system in the male, the prostatic utricle. The 2 cm portion of the urethra which passes through the urogenital diaphragm is referred to as the membranous urethra. It is composed of both smooth and striated musculature, and provides voluntary continence, as the striated muscle component constitutes the external sphincter mechanism.

The penile urethra is the most distal portion, entering from the urogenital diaphragm to the urethral orifice (Fig. 5.6a). It is entirely contained within the corpus spongiosum. Its most proximal portion, the bulbous urethra, is the widest, and is surrounded by the bulbospongiosus muscle (Fig. 5.6b). Proximally, the urethra is lined with transitional epithelium, which becomes flattened and eventually terminates as stratified squamous epithelium at the most distal portion, where a slight dilation is known as the fossa navicularis (Fig. 5.6c).[12]

THE PROSTATE

The prostate is composed of both muscular and glandular elements. Its function is mainly to support insemination. The glandular components produce fluid which constitutes 15% of the normal ejaculate. The prostate is hormonally sensitive, and therefore does not reach significant size until puberty. In the adult male, the prostate reaches a diameter of 3–5 cm, and weighs approximately 30 g. The base of the prostate is firmly and circumferentially attached to the bladder neck. The apex of the prostate abuts the urogenital diaphragm, while its upper aspect is anchored to the posterior symphysis pubis by the paired puboprostatic ligaments.

Prostatic secretions are delivered through ductules into the prostatic portion of the urethra. The ejaculatory ducts of the seminal vesicles traverse the substance of the prostate to enter the prostatic urethra just proximal to the prostatic utricle and verumontanum, a small protuberance on the posterior aspect of the urethra.

Previously, the prostate was recognized to have five anatomic lobes: two lateral, one anterior, one median, and one posterior. This was based on its endoscopic appearance. More recent anatomic study has revealed that the prostate is composed mainly of two separate zones, the large peripheral zone and a central zone. A transition zone may comprise 5% of prostatic tissue in the normal male: however, with age the development of benign prostatic hyperplasia (BPH) in this area may constitute a significant amount of prostatic mass. It should be noted that while the transition zone is felt to be the site of the development of BPH, the peripheral zone is most likely to be the origin of adenocarcinoma (Fig. 5.7). With the use of high-frequency endourethral ultrasound, the preurethral portion of prostate can be clearly imaged, especially the central zone (Fig. 5.8). However, the penetration of the ultrasound beam may limit the evaluation of the peripheral zone of the prostate.

a

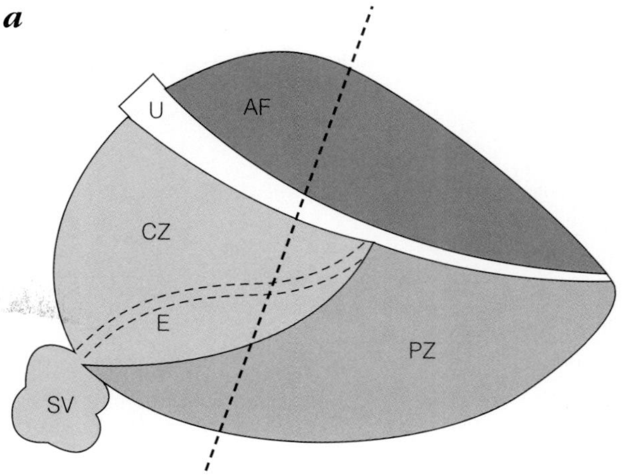

b

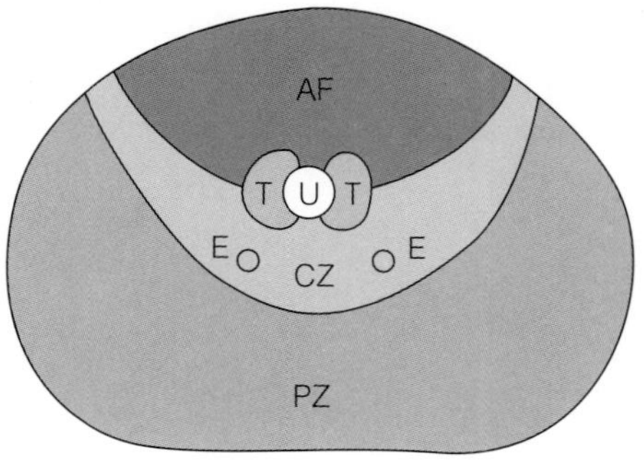

Figure 5.7 *The zonal anatomy of the prostate. (a) The midline longitudinal view. The dashed line corresponds to the axial plane in (b). (b) The axial sectional view. U, urethra; AF, fibromuscular stroma; CZ, central zone; PZ, peripheral zone; E, ejaculatory duct; SV, seminal vesicle; T, transition zone.*

REVIEW OF EARLY TRANSURETHRAL ULTRASOUND

Holm and Northeved[13] first described transurethral ultrasound in 1974. The technique has been primarily used to image bladder tumors and in attempts to improve staging accuracy. The scanner for transurethral ultrasound fits with the standard 24 Fr cystoscope sheath and consists of a motor that rotates a long rod connected at the opposite end to an interchangeable 3.5–10 MHz transducer. The instrument is

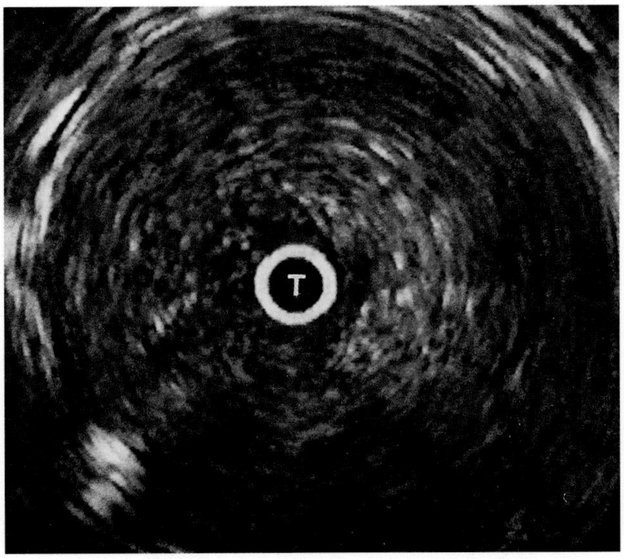

Figure 5.8 *Cross-sectional ultrasound image obtained from within the prostatic urethra demonstrates the relatively hypoechoic prostate. T, transducer.*

placed into the fluid-filled bladder and multiple transverse images may be obtained. With the use of these 3.5–10 MHz transurethral transducers, the bladder musculature appears as highly echogenic. Therefore, the layers of the bladder wall are difficult to distinguished.[14] The bladder neck and ureteral orifices provide landmarks in localizing abnormalities within the bladder. To facilitate complete scanning of the bladder wall, transducers are set at 60°, 90° or 135° and are rotated through 360° by a motorized probe. The procedure is best performed with the patient under anesthesia. Resnick and Kursh in 1988 reported their experiences on transurethral ultrasonography of the urinary bladder.[15]. They found that this technique is very useful in the staging of bladder tumors and also has a role in helping to monitor the depth of transurethral resection as a primary mode of treating those patients with bladder tumors. However, with this technique it is difficult to assess pelvic lymph nodes for metastatic deposits.

High-frequency ultrasound scanning within the lumen of the bladder allowed improved visualization but not distinct visualization of different bladder wall layers.[16] Therefore, the accurate staging of transitional cell carcinoma of the bladder was not possible.

More recently, transurethral ultrasound-guided laser-induced prostatectomy (TULIP) has been studied.[17] In this minimally invasive alternative to conventional prostatectomy, laser prostatectomy is guided by an incorporated ultrasound scanner that produces a 90° real-time sector scan from the 7.5 MHz transducer. Angular resolution is approximately 2 mm and depth of view may be set from 2–5 cm. This is the first report of a prostatectomy that has been completely done under ultrasound guidance.

TECHNICAL CONSIDERATIONS

The endoluminal ultrasound system described in this chapter is available commercially from Diasonics (IVUS®, Santa Clara, CA). The 12.5–20 MHz, 6.2–9 Fr catheter-based transducers are produced by Boston Scientific Corporation (Sonicath®, Natick, MA). For a more complete understanding of the imaging system and miniature transducers, see Chapters 1 and 2.

If the endoluminal ultrasound is to be done in the operating room to aid an endoscopic procedure, a complete cystourethroscopy is first performed. The ultrasound examination can be done through a working port of a cystoscope or by directly cannulating the urethra with the ultrasound probe after the cystoscope is removed. Endoluminal ultrasound used in conjunction with cystoscopy is helpful when visualizing a landmark, such as the verumontanum, is important in the area of the prostate and external sphincter and during endoscopic collagen injection for the treatment of stress urinary incontinence.

It is important to perform the endoluminal ultrasound study with the bladder partially distended for orientation and ultrasound examination of the bladder. After the cystoscope is removed, the urethra is catheterized using a well-lubricated endoluminal ultrasound probe. Orientation is established by placing the catheter into the bladder, utilizing suprapubic compression to identify the 12 o'clock position on the real-time ultrasound image (Fig. 5.9). Ultrasound examination can also be done without using a cystoscope.

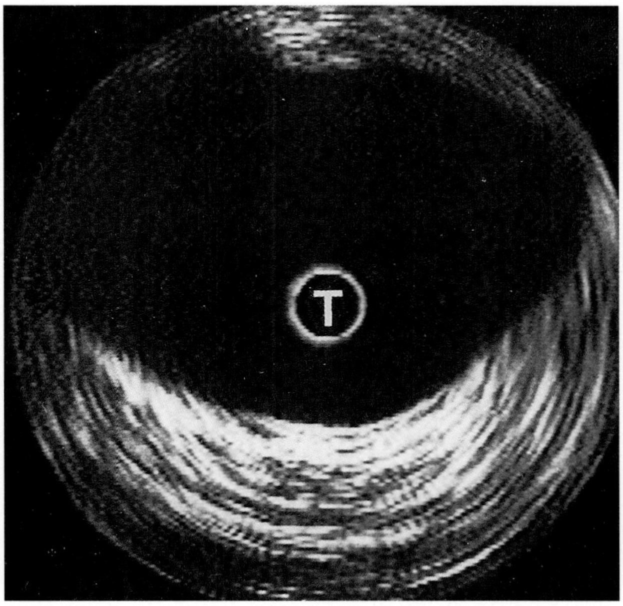

a

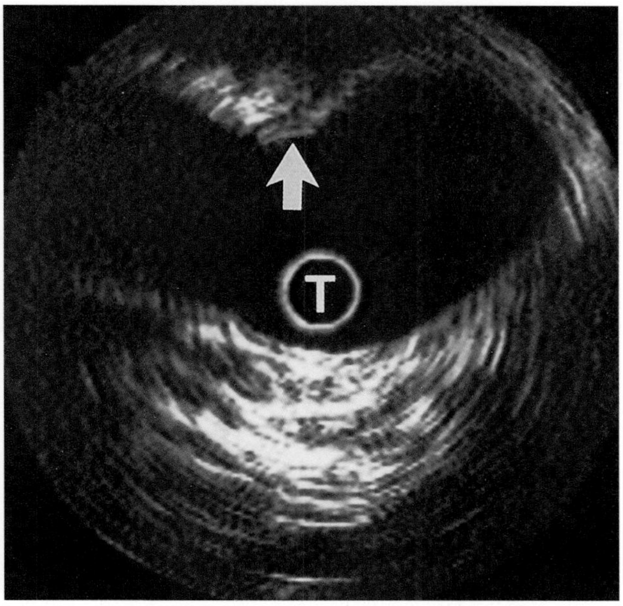

b

Figure 5.9 *(a) Cross-sectional intravesical ultrasound imaging of urine-filled bladder. Initial imaging without compression of anterior wall. (b) Cross-sectional imaging of urine-filled bladder after distortion of anterior wall (arrow) by pressure applied suprapubically in order to confirm proper orientation of catheter-based transducer (T). (Reproduced with permission from Goldberg BB et al.[3])*

In women, the ultrasound catheter is then withdrawn into the urethra, and a metallic instrument placed in the vagina, in order to confirm identification of the 6 o'clock position. This instrument is held up against the anterior vaginal wall and is identified as a bright reflector with distal acoustic shadowing (Fig. 5.10). Serial sections of the urethra are then examined using endoluminal ultrasound and correlated with prior radiographic images and urethroscopic findings.

In men, after orientation is established in the bladder, the ultrasound catheter is withdrawn into the prostatic urethra. A reference probe can be inserted in the rectum to identify the 6 o'clock position, but in men with enlarged prostate the depth of penetration with endoluminal ultrasound does not allow a clear visualization beyond the prostatic capsule. Distal to the membranous urethra, orientation can be reconfirmed by using a metallic instrument held against the perineum and the ventral aspect of the penis. Serial sections of the urethra are then examined using endoluminal ultrasound and correlated with prior radiographic images and urethroscopic findings. When the appropriate diagnosis is made intervention can then proceed.

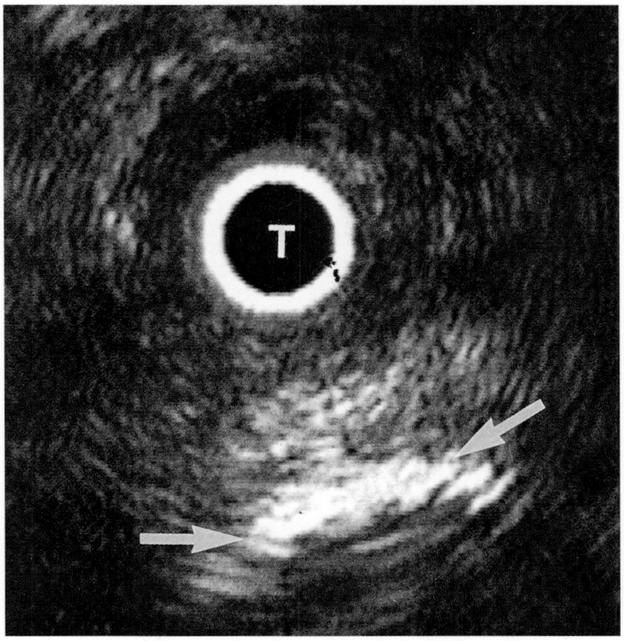

Figure 5.10 *Endoluminal ultrasound transducer (T) within the urethra was orientated by placing an instrument against the anterior vaginal wall to produce a bright reflector (arrows) with distal acoustic shadowing.*

CLINICAL APPLICATIONS

Endoluminal ultrasound adds the third dimension of depth to endoscopic procedures. Although a cystourethroscope allows for direct inspection of the urethral lumen and luminal surface, visual examination can provide little information regarding the wall of the urethra or adjacent structures. Prior to the initial clinical experience, animal studies were performed in dogs and pigs comparing endoluminal ultrasound visualization of the lower urinary tract with pathologic examination. In all cases, it was possible to obtain cross-sectional images from the various luming entered and to determine their wall thicknesses and sonographic textural patterns. To establish variability in four female dogs, multiple measurements were obtained of each structure. The average thickness of the proximal urethra was 1.3 mm (range 0.9–1.9 mm). The urinary bladder wall thickness varied according to the amount of urine but averaged 1.4 mm (range 0.9–2.3 mm). Close correlation was found between these measurements and the cross-sectional anatomic specimen. As the ultrasound probe is passed through the urethra, it has been possible to visualize various anatomic structures.[2,3,18].

A large number of normal and abnormal urethral endoluminal ultrasound examinations have been performed in women and men. There are some established uses, while others show great promise. These catheters are no more than 2–3 mm in diameter, so they can be easily passed into the urethra without the need for dilation. In addition to the normal urethra, prostate and bladder, the following conditions have been examined: benign and malignant tumors of the bladder and urethra, urethral strictures, BPH, detrusor-external sphincter dyssynergia and follow-up after sphincterotomy, laser prostatectomy, endoluminal stent placement in the prostatic urethra, urinary sphincter, and bulbous urethral stricture, urethral diverticulum and fistula, as well as foreign body localization in the periurethral area. Some of the documented indications for endoluminal ultrasound in the lower urinary tract include assessment of function and obstruction of endoluminal urethral stent prosthesis, diagnosis and localization of urethral diverticulum and fistulas, and as a visualization aid for periurethral bulking agent injection.

BLADDER NEOPLASMS

Animal studies have been conducted to demonstrate the feasibility and accuracy of high frequency endoluminal ultrasound in imaging bladder tumors. Six C57BL/6L female mice were used for this study. The MB49 tumor (DMBA-induced, C57B1) was instilled into the bladder of the mice. Following 3 weeks of growth, the bladders of tumor-bearing and control mice were imaged using a 20 MHz, 6.2 Fr catheter transducer inserted transrectally. Bladders of tumor implanted and control mice were identified by 20 MHz endoluminal ultrasound after distension with 0.15 ml of normal saline. When compared with the results of histologic analysis, transrectal ultrasound accurately identified tumor presence, size and location.[19] In a tumor-instilled mouse, ultrasound demonstrated thickening of the bladder wall which was confirmed both at gross inspection and following histologic examination as tumor. Microscopic examination showed the thickening to be secondary to an arc of high grade transitional cell carcinoma growing along the posterior wall, and tumors as shallow as 0.7 mm were identified. The tumor measured 15–20 cell layers thick and was superficial, being primarily confined by the muscularis mucosa (Fig. 5.11). In another tumor-instilled mouse, transvesical ultrasound demonstrated a 2.2 mm hypoechoic mass. Histologically, a polypoid mass, measuring 2.0 mm at maximum diameter, was evident at the base of the bladder (Fig. 5.12).[19]

In this study, the placement of a ultrasound catheter into the mouse rectum provided an accurate and noninvasive means of imaging the mouse bladder tumors. Correct determinations of the presence or absence of tumor and its location were made in all cases. No false negatives or false positives were encountered in this small series. Some investigators successfully used magnetic resonance imaging (MRI) to image and monitor murine bladder tumor implants.[20] Because MRI can be expensive and time consuming, transvesical ultrasound has advantages over MRI.

Clinically, accurate bladder tumor staging is required for proper management of patients with bladder carcinomas. Although conventional radiographic techniques, including CT and MRI, have reliably predicted extravesical tumor involvement, differentiation between superficial and muscle-invasive tumors has been poor because of the similar density of the tumor and the normal bladder detrusor.[21] Itzchak et al reported their experience of using transabdominal ultrasound in an attempt to improve the estimation of local bladder tumor involvement. Approximately 32% of these tumors were missed because of their small size (<0.5 cm) or their location at the bladder dome. Compared to pathologic

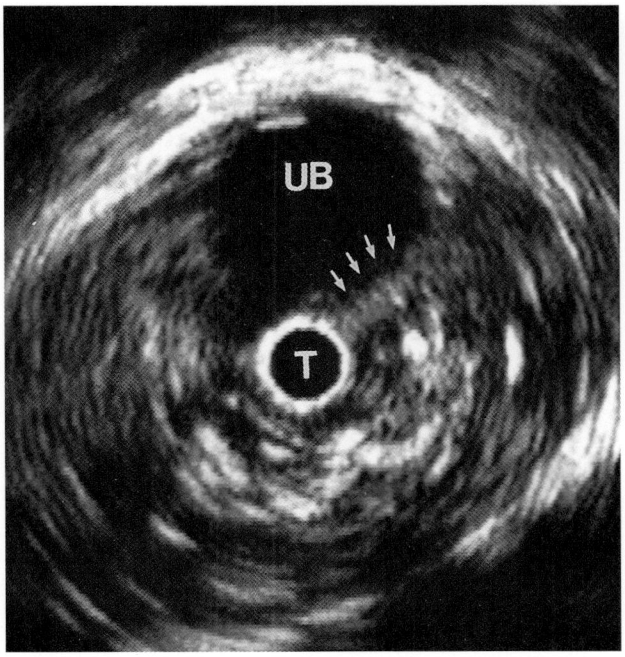

a

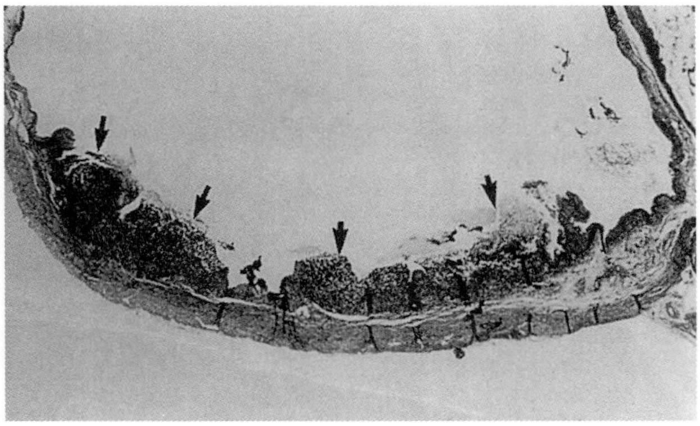

b

Figure 5.11 *(a) Transrectal ultrasound of a tumor-instilled mouse demonstrated a localized thickening of the bladder (UB) wall (arrows). T, transducer. (b) Photomicrograph of bladder wall from this region (arrows) shows 0.7 mm thick transitional cell carcinoma growing superficially without penetrating bladder musculature. ×20. (Reproduced with permission from Alexander AA et al.[19])*

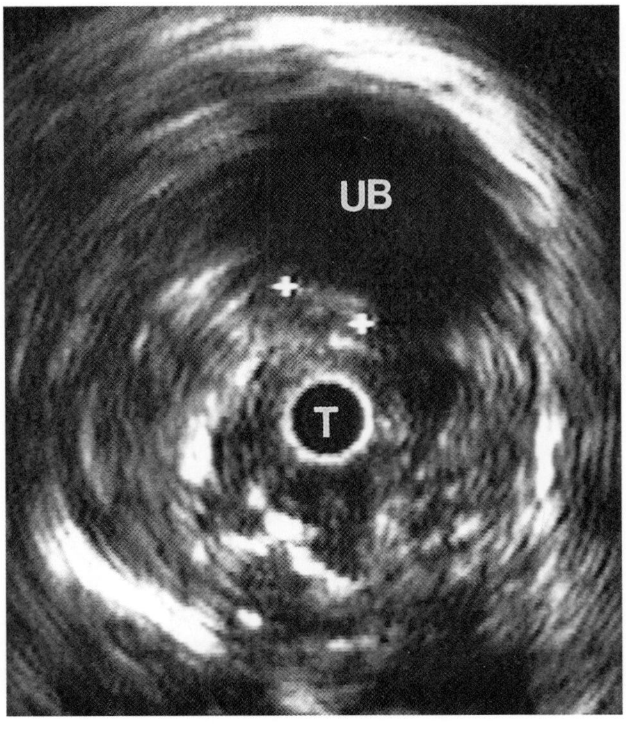

a

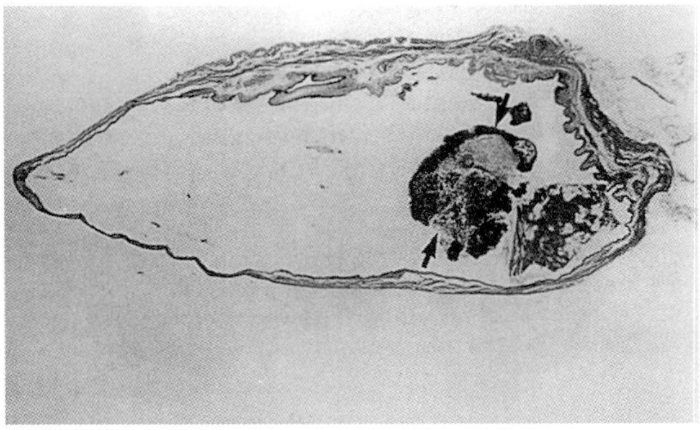

b

Figure 5.12 *(a) In another tumor-bearing mouse, transrectal ultrasound identified a 2.2 mm polypoid mass (+) protruding into the bladder cavity (UB). T, transducer. (b) Photomicrograph of bladder showing a 2.0 mm mass and fibromuscular stalk. ×20. (Reproduced with permission from Alexander AA et al.[19])*

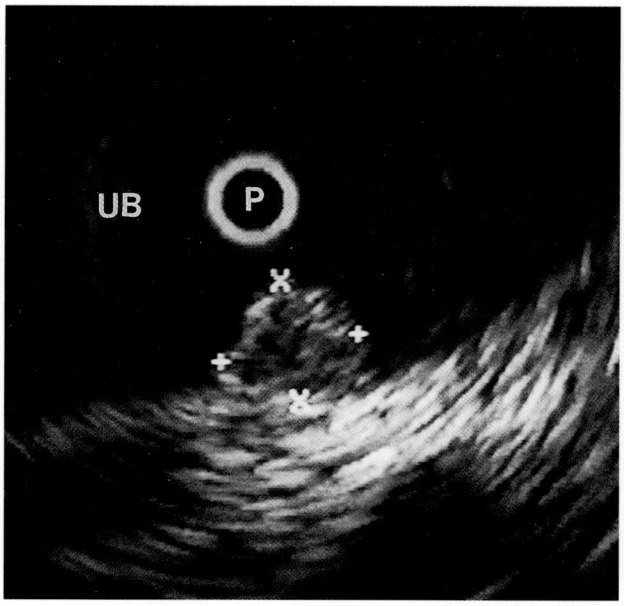

Figure 5.13 *Transurethral ultrasound demonstrates a hypoechoic mass (× and +) arising from the posterior wall of the bladder (UB). The mass has a narrow streak without any evidence of invasion.* P, *catheter-based probe.*

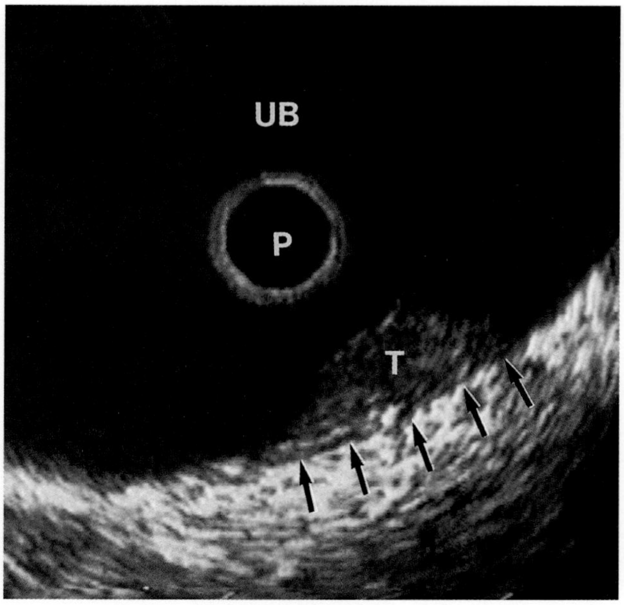

Figure 5.14 *Superficial, noninvasive tumor (T) is seen with a well-defined base. Note that the normal layers (arrows) of the bladder wall beneath the lesion are preserved. P, ultrasound probe; UB, urinary bladder.*

staging, it was found to be accurate in differentiating higher-stage disease, such as perivesical invasion, but less accurate in differentiating superficial from muscle-invasive lesions.[22] Other studies found that only 38%[23] and 45%[24] of tumors measuring less than 0.5 cm were detected by transabdominal ultrasound. Patient obesity, bladder wall inflammation and tumor location are factors related to the high false-negative rates. Since Holm and Northeved introduced intravesical ultrasound in 1974,[13] many researchers have reported their results and efficacy when using this technique with regard to the diagnosis and staging of bladder tumors.[25–34] Jaeger et al studied 571 patients with bladder carcinoma demonstrating that the total accuracy of intravesical sonography is 70% and the sensitivity for the detection of tumor infiltration is 90% when compared to pathology.[35]

Catheter-based endoluminal ultrasound combined with cystoscope ought to be ideally suited to overcome the inadequacies of transabdominal bladder ultrasound. First, very high frequency (20 MHz) transducers can produce an excellent resolution image; second, catheter-based transducers can pass through a working channel of a cystoscope under direct visualization to image lesions; and third, endoluminal ultrasound can be used to monitor tumor resection or laser ablation during endourologic procedures.

Generally, bladder tumors appear ultrasonically as hypoechogenic masses projecting into the cavity of the distended bladder. It is difficult to differentiate benign from malignant masses by means of their sonographic appearances. The tumor is always fixed to the bladder wall. Mobile masses may represent stones, blood clots or debris. Superficial, noninvasive tumors will have a well-defined base and produce no distortion of the bladder wall (Figs 5.13 and 5.14). Invasive tumors tend to have broader bases, with the normal layers of the bladder wall beneath the lesion poorly defined or interrupted, suggesting the presence of infiltration (Fig. 5.15).

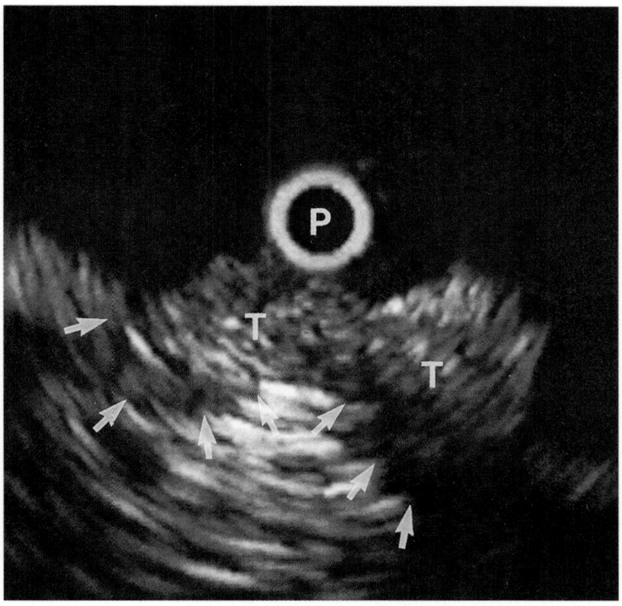

Figure 5.15 *An invasive bladder tumor (T) is seen with a broader tumor base (arrows) and the bladder wall is distorted and interrupted, suggesting the presence of infiltration. P, ultrasound probe.*

URETHRAL STENT

The self expandable wire-mesh endoluminal urethral stent, similar to an endovascular stent, is becoming available for use in the lower urinary tract. Indications for endoluminal urethral stents include BPH, detrusor-sphincter dyssynergia in patients with spinal cord injury, and recurrent bulbous urethral strictures.[36] A important issue associated with urethral stent insertion is the potential for epithelial hyperplasia within the lumen of the wire-mesh stent that may cause recurrent obstruction. The thickness of this neo-epithelial overgrowth is difficult to assess by conventional modalities but can be clearly delineated by endoluminal ultrasound.

The Urolume™ endourethral Wallstent® prosthesis (American Medical Systems, Minnetonka, MN) can be inserted using a 21 Fr cystoscopic insertion tool. Several stent lengths are manufactured, including lengths of 2, 2.5 and 3 cm. Transurethral endoluminal ultrasound can be used to assess the deployment of intraprostatic and intrasphincter urethral stents and to evaluate the regrowth of neo-urothelium in patients over time.[37] High-resolution transurethral ultrasound can precisely identify the proximal and distal margins of the stent and measure the stent diameter (Fig. 5.16). Follow-up examinations have shown the thickness of hyperplastic overgrowth to be approximately 1.5 mm, with a maximum thickness of 4.3 mm (Fig. 5.17). In addition, endoluminal ultrasound can be used to determine stent wire unraveling, breakage, stone formation, or scar capsule formation surrounding the stent. Thus, these catheter-based transducers can provide important information to the urologist regarding the long term follow-up of intraurethral stents.[38]

URETHRAL DIVERTICULUM

Perhaps the most compelling use of endoluminal ultrasound for lower urinary tract applications today is the examination of urethral diverticula. They are an uncommon cause of lower urinary tract symptomsand symptoms are often nonspecific, mimicking those of other illnesses.[39] The incidence of urethral diverticula has been reported to vary from 1% to 6% of adult women.[39–41] In these studies, the demographic data were obtained by screening asymptomatic women with positive-pressure urethrography. The traditional radiographic method for the imaging of urethral lesions, including diverticula, has been the voiding cystourethrogram (VCUG). The positive-pressure, double-balloon retrograde urethrogram is an alternative, less commonly performed, method, because it may be difficult, time-consuming and poorly tolerated by the patients. It is suspected that false-negative studies are relatively uncommon, but this is difficult to verify. Considering that the mere presence of a diverticulum does not necessarily demand surgical treatment, it is not easy to justify such an invasive, uncomfortable procedure for all cases.

Classically, physical examination reveals a tender anterior vaginal wall mass from which purulent urethral discharge is produced on palpation. If this is not evident, diagnosing the urethral diverticulum may be difficult. Traditional diagnostic imaging studies of the urethral diverticulum, including voiding cystourethrography, urethroscopy and positive-pressure double-balloon retrograde urethrography, may yield false-negative results.[42,43] Voiding cystourethrography has been used for screening, but has an overall

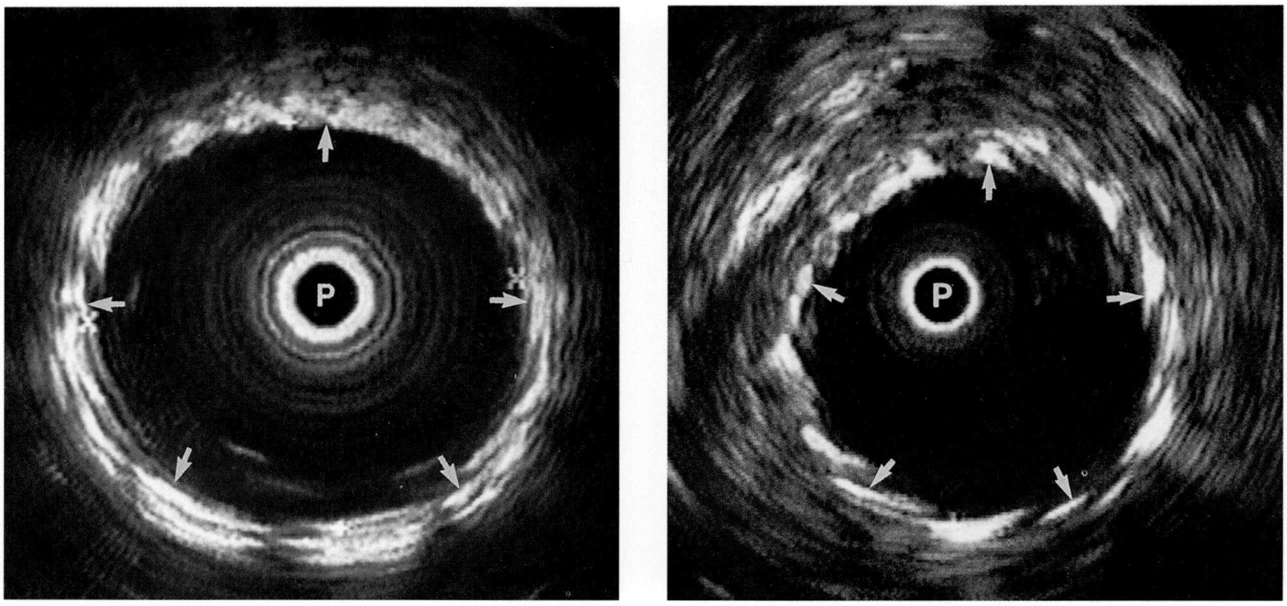

a *b*

Figure 5.16 *High resolution endoluminal ultrasound can precisely measure the diameter of the stent (arrows) in vitro (a) and in vivo (b). Note that the diameter of the stent is slightly smaller in vivo than that in vitro due to the tension of the urethral wall. P, ultrasound probe.*

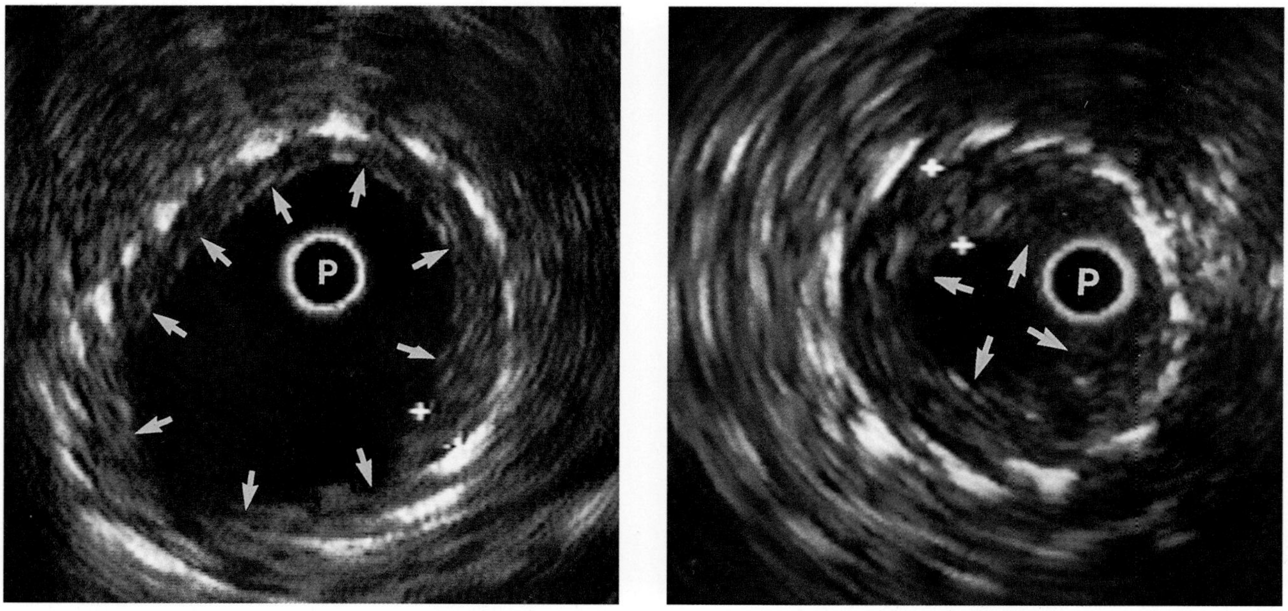

a *b*

Figure 5.17 *Follow-up examination of the urethral stent demonstrated the epithelial hyperplasia (arrows) within the opening of the wire-mesh stent. (a) 6 months follow-up; (b) 12 months follow-up. P, ultrasound probe.*

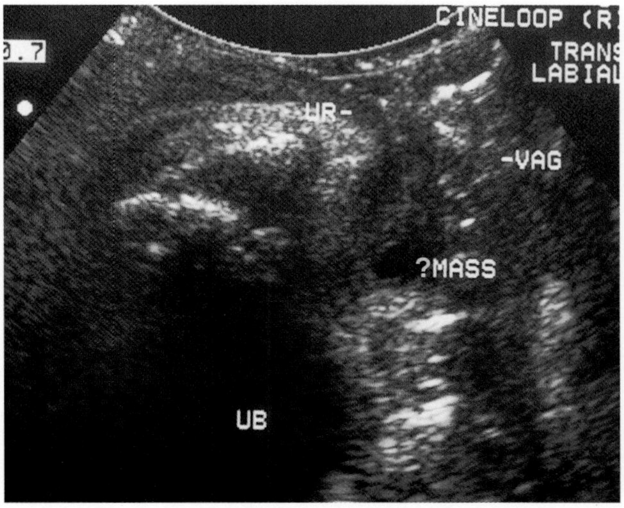

a

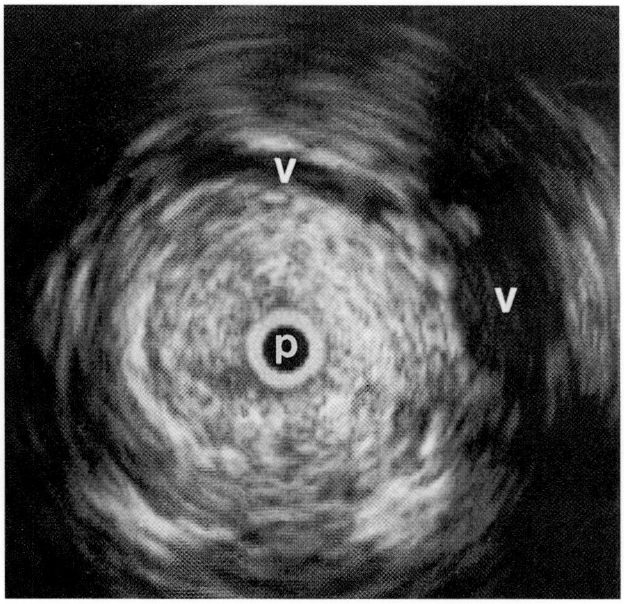

b

Figure 5.18 *(a) False positive transvaginal ultrasound of a urethral diverticulum. UB, urinary bladder; VAG, vagina; UR, urethra. (b) Intraoperative endoluminal ultrasound showing no evidence of a cystic mass at the region of the periurethra. The surgical result confirmed endoluminal ultrasound findings. P, probe; V, vessel.*

accuracy of only 65%.[41] In addition, the double balloon study is difficult to perform and poorly tolerated by many patients.[43,44]

Urethral diverticula have been studied on transabdominal sonography. In 1977, Lee and Keller[45] first described the sonographic appearance. Subsequent reports by other investigators have confirmed this appearance as a cystic structure at or below the bladder base and with or without septa and internal debris.[46,47] Because of its relative insensitivity for smaller lesions, transabdominal ultrasound has not been accepted as a screening test. Recently, transvaginal, transperineal and translabial ultrasound, as well as MRI have been described as alternatives for evaluating urethral diverticula.[48-52] These techniques seem to make the diagnosis of urethral diverticula easier than with transabdominal ultrasound. However, no radiographic modality has yet proven useful as an intraoperative adjunct during the surgical repair of urethral diverticula.

In our institution, patients with preoperative diagnoses of a urethral diverticulum were evaluated by intraoperative endoluminal ultrasound. Prior to surgery, patients underwent either a VCUG, a transvaginal ultrasonogram, or a double-balloon urethrogram. The results of preoperative radiographic evaluation and intraoperative endoluminal ultrasound were compared. In addition, continuous monitoring using the miniature ultrasound probes assisted in the surgical dissection of the diverticula.[53]

In certain patients, the definitive diagnosis of a urethral diverticulum could not be confirmed radiographically. In 12 patients, comparison of preoperative studies with intraoperative surgical and endoluminal ultrasound findings revealed two false-negative VUCGs and one false-positive VUCG, one false-negative transvaginal ultrasound, and one false-negative double-balloon urethrogram (Fig. 5.18). With endoluminal ultrasound, however, all diverticula were well visualized (Figs 5.19 and 5.20). This technique demonstrated improved imaging by enabling not only the identification of the size and orientation of the diverticular lumen, but also the extent of periurethral inflammation, debris within the diverticulum, wall thickness, and the distance between the diverticular wall and the urethral lumen

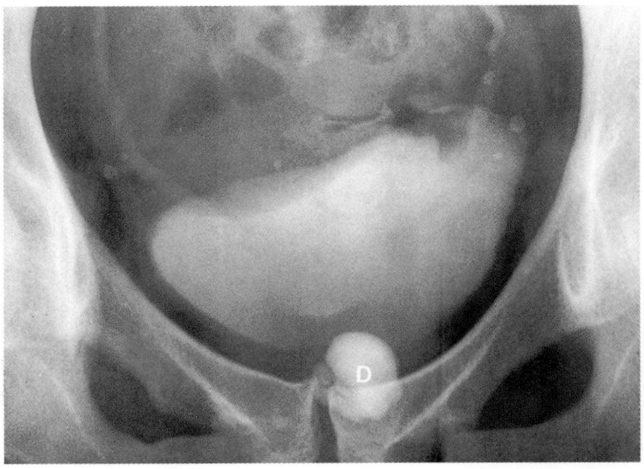

a

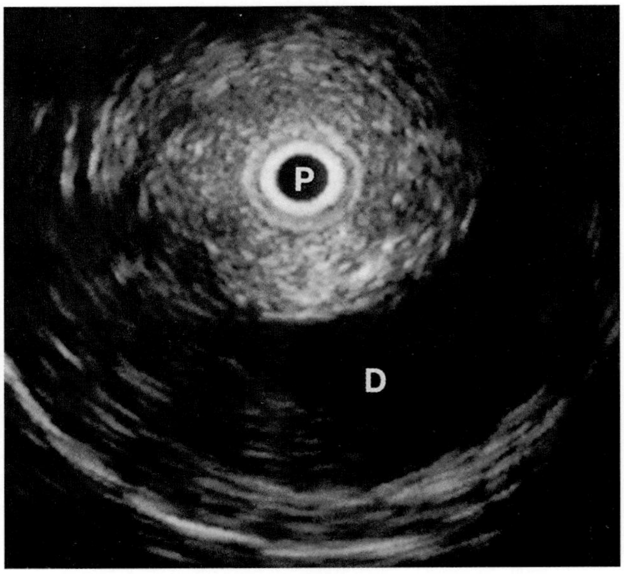

b

Figure 5.19 *Comparison of endoluminal ultrasound and voiding cystourethrogram of urethral diverticulum. (a) Urethral diverticulum (D) on voiding cystourethrogram. (b) Intraoperative endoluminal ultrasound clearly showing the diverticulum (D) with internal debris. P, probe.*

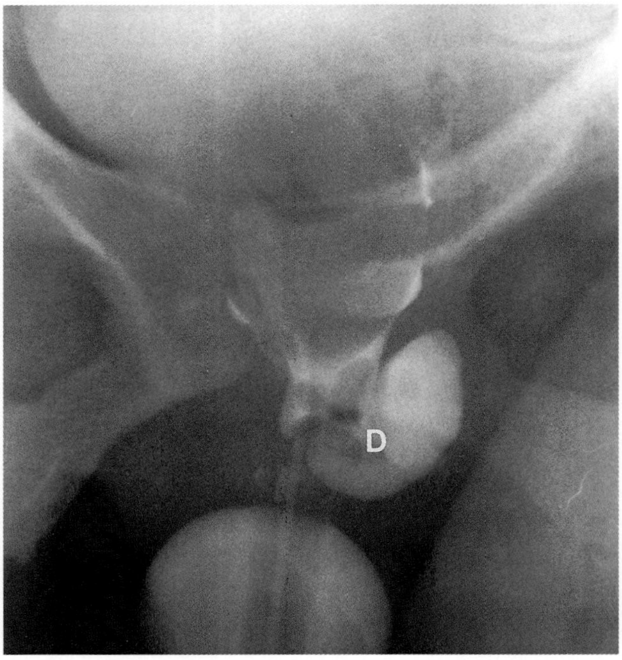

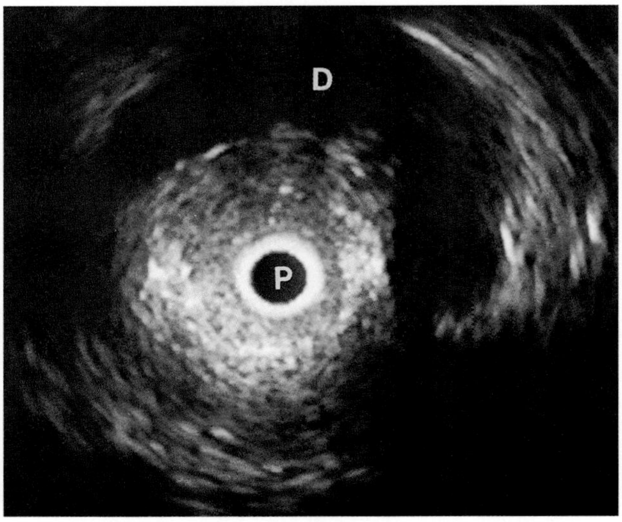

a *b*

Figure 5.20 *(a) A large urethral diverticulum (D) seen on voiding cystourethrogram. (b) Endoluminal ultrasound imaging of the diverticulum (D). Note the horseshoe configuration of the diverticulum that wraps around the urethra from 3 o'clock to 9 o'clock. P, probe.*

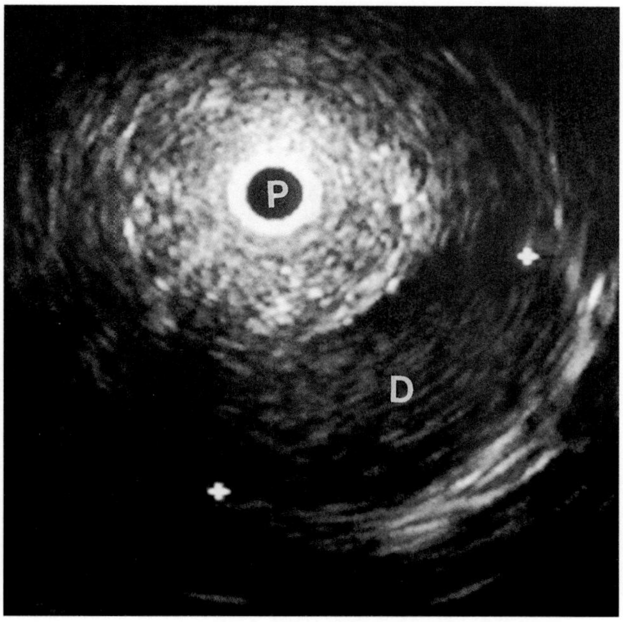

Figure 5.21 *Endoluminal ultrasound imaging of a urethral diverticulum (D) with sludge corresponding with an infective diverticulum. P, probe.*

(Fig. 5.21). Even the point of connection of diverticula with the urethral lumen could be visualized with endoluminal ultrasound in some patients.

One patient presenting with a symptomatic anterior vaginal mass, diagnosed clinically as a urethral diverticulum, was found to have a solid lesion using endoluminal ultrasound. This imaging modality enhanced the resection of this lesion, ensuring extirpation while protecting contiguous structures. Histologic examination revealed a leiomyoma of the proximal urethra and bladder neck. None of the women developed postoperative stress, urinary incontinence or urethrovaginal fistulae. None of the patients had clinical symptoms of urethral diverticulum postoperatively.

The one male in this study was a paraplegic after traumatic spinal cord injury. His incontinence, caused by neurogenic vesical dysfunction, had been managed with an external condom catheter urine-collecting device. Experiencing difficulty with maintaining catheter application, he had increasingly applied pressure to the condom-retaining band wrapping the penis. This resulted in aneurysmal dilation immediately proximal to the condom strap, unnoticed because of his neurologic impairment and decreased sensation. Subsequently, a diverticulum formed, which eventually eroded a fistula to the scrotal skin. Utilizing endoluminal ultrasound, it was possible not only to quantify the diameter of the urethra and the urethral diverticulum, but also to identify the location and opening of the fistula tract. The high resolution of the ultrasound image greatly facilitated the planning and execution of this complex urethral reconstruction.

Endoluminal ultrasound is an atraumatic procedure; no complication was attributed to its use. In all cases, it was possible to obtain complete cross-sectional images from the various lumina entered, determining not only wall thickness but also sonographic textural patterns of normal and pathologic structures. As the ultrasound probe was passed through the urethra, it was possible to visualize a variety of anatomic structures. The delineation of areas of abnormality, including plaque, stricture, calculi, and solid or cystic tumors, was also possible.

Our experience indicates several advantages to using endoluminal ultrasound intraoperatively when treating urethral diverticula. The primary advantage is the diagnostic confirmation that a diverticulum is actually present, especially when the diverticulum is not easily palpable. Once the diagnosis is established, endoluminal ultrasound helps determine the surgical approach to the lesion by defining its size, shape and location. Planning its dissection is further enhanced by the ability of endoluminal ultrasound to define the extent of periurethral inflammation, wall thickness and the distance from the diverticular wall to the urethral lumen. With this information, troublesome areas can be anticipated and care taken to avoid dissection of noninvolved tissue. Urethral or bladder neck injury could be avoided. With enhanced imaging of the neck of the diverticulum during surgery, recurrence rates should be minimized. Confirmation of the complete excision of all diverticular components by endoluminal ultrasound should eliminate the potential for the persistence of subepithelial cystic remnants which may remain infected, inflamed and symptomatic. Calculi and malignancy have previously been reported to be associated with urethral diverticula.[54,55] Endoluminal ultrasound can effectively differentiate cystic and solid components within the diverticulum, helping to determine whether a diverticulum has a secondary pathologic process, such as calculus or tumor, which may modify the surgical approach.

The role of endoluminal ultrasound as a preoperative test for urethral diverticula is presently unexplored. Its sensitivity and specificity intraoperatively were 100% in this limited series. The two most common complications of the surgical repair of urethral diverticula are urinary incontinence and urethrovaginal fistula. In the 12 patients in this series, no short- or long-term complications occurred. No patient experienced recurrence of preoperative symptoms. We feel that the use of endoluminal ultrasound significantly contributed to therapeutic benefit by supplying information, which would otherwise be unavailable, which helped to modify the surgical technique.

The only limitation of intraoperative urethral endoluminal ultrasound is the difficulty in maintaining a precise 360° orientation since this may change with manipulation of the transducer-containing catheter. This shortcoming can be alleviated by using a reference probe in the vagina to continuously monitor its orientation. In conclusion, this technique proved valuable in assisting in the identification of anatomic landmarks such as the bladder neck, confirming the excision of all diverticular components, and ensuring there is no inadvertent disruption of the urethral and bladder neck structures.

URINARY INCONTINENCE

The assessment of female urinary incontinence by transvaginal sonography was first reported by Debus-Thiede et al in 1985.[56] They evaluated changes in the orientation of a urethral catheter depending on the hold and bear-down maneuvers in both normal women and patients with urinary incontinence, and measured the posterior vesicourethral angle and the postvoiding bladder residue. Since then, many investigators have used transvaginal, transperineal and transrectal ultrasound to evaluate the urethra and bladder neck in patients with stress incontinence.[57–61] Real-time ultrasonography has been combined with the urodynamic manometer to obtain accurate morphologic and dynamic images of the urethra and bladder base.[62]

More recently, Kirschner-Hermanns et al[63] used 20 MHz catheter-based endoluminal ultrasound to examine the urethra in 12 healthy women and 32 women with stress urinary incontinence. They found that endoluminal ultrasound provided high-resolution imaging of the urethra and surrounding tissues. The whole length of the urethra was visualized. The external sphincter was easily recognized as an oval-shaped, hypoechoic structure. The average area of the sphincter muscle was 1.03 cm^2 (SD 0.3) for normal subjects and 0.73 cm^2 (SD 0.4) for incontinent patients. The average sphincter circumference was 3.61 cm (SD 0.5) for normal subjects and 2.97 cm (SD 0.71) for incontinent patients. Examination of women with and without stress incontinence revealed a negative correlation between the external urethral sphincter (area and circumference) and the grade of stress incontinence ($P < 0.01$). Intraurethral ultrasound provided a simple way to image the urethra, the external sphincter and the periurethral tissue. Knowledge of the sphincter size might help in choosing adequate treatment of incontinence. With use of MRI, the sphincter can be identified but its size cannot be measured.[64,65] Endoluminal ultrasound allows evaluation of the urethral sphincter beyond the capability of conventional radiographic and cystoscopic modalities.

Periurethral injections of polytetrafluoroethylene paste (Teflon, Polytef) have been used since 1970 for the treatment of stress urinary incontinence.[66] The disadvantages are distant particle migration and granuloma formation.[67–69] Therefore, a strong impetus exists for the development of better substances for the purpose of periurethral bulking (Fig. 5.22).

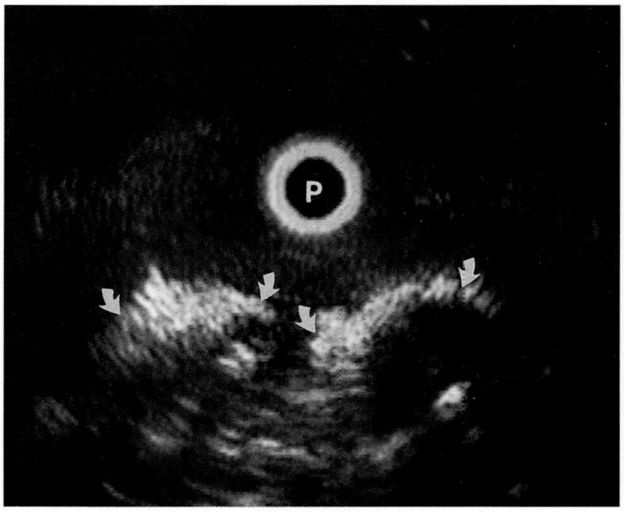

Figure 5.22 *Endoluminal ultrasound imaging showing the hyperechoic Teflon paste (arrows) located at the neck of the periurethral region. P, probe.*

Glutaraldehyde cross-linked bovine (GAX) collagen was approved by the Food and Drug Administration in 1993 for the treatment of stress urinary incontinence caused by intrinsic sphincteric deficiency.

Studies on periurethral injections of Contigen[R] have yielded promising results.[70,71] The major disadvantage of this material is reabsorption, requiring repeat injection in some patients in order to maintain therapeutic efficacy. Furthermore, there is presently no way of predicting which patients may develop reabsorption of significant magnitude to require reinjection. Review of the medical literature is inconclusive as to the optimal depth of collagen injection required to produce durable clinical efficacy. Endoluminal ultrasound shows promise in improving the accuracy and success of periurethral collagen injection.

Animal Study

Yucatan mini-pigs weighing 15 kg were preanesthetized with intramuscular atropine 0.04 mg/kg and ketamine 20 mg/kg. The collagen injections and ultrasound examinations were performed in the supine position under intravenous thiopental anesthesia.[72] The urethra and bladder were initially examined visually using a 21 Fr cystoscope with a 30° lens, and then ultrasonographically with a 20 MHz transducer mounted on a 6.2 Fr endoluminal ultrasound catheter passed through the cystoscope. Bladder volume and bladder and urethral wall thickness were quantified ultrasonically. Collagen was then injected under endoluminal ultrasound guidance using a 22 gauge needle mounted on a urethral catheter passed through the cystoscope. This project received prior institutional Animal Review Board approval.

The collagen was injected at three different depths (submucosal, intramuscular and periadventitial) in both bladder and urethral sites. One millilitre of collagen was injected at each site. In the bladder, 2 cm separated each injection site, while in the urethra, the collagen was injected at three different sites corresponding to the 3, 5 and 9 o'clock positions when viewed endoscopically. Endoluminal ultrasound examination was repeated after 3 h, at which time the hypoechoic collagen could be identified only in the submucosal and intramuscular depths, in both the bladder and urethral walls, but not at the periadventitial locations. Under anesthesia, both endoluminal ultrasound imaging and cystoscopy with biopsy of the injection sites was performed at 1 week and after 1, 2, and 3 months in order to determine the appearance of the injected collagen. Urine cultures were obtained at the time of each follow-up endoscopic and ultrasound evaluation.

Collagen was also injected into the subcutaneous and intramuscular tissue of the right lateral thigh of each animal. At each injection site, marked with tattoos, 1.0 ml of collagen was injected into both the superficial, subcutaneous and intramuscular tissue under linear array ultrasound guidance.

The animals were sacrificed after 3 months, at which time the bladder and urethra of each was examined with endoluminal ultrasound and removed. The injected area of the thigh was examined with linear-array ultrasound and the tissue then excised. The specimens were fixed in 3.8% formalin and embedded in paraffin. The tissue was then mounted for histopathological examination and stained with trichrome stain. The ultrasound images were then correlated with the histologic appearance under light microscopy.

Using endoluminal ultrasound, a discrete hypoechoic mass became apparent where the collagen was injected in the submucosal and intramuscular depths of the lower urinary tract. The injections into the urinary tract submucosa appeared more distinct than did the intramuscular injections, both acutely and over time. The collagen appeared as a discrete, hypoechoic area which persisted not only after 3 h, but also after 1 week. On further follow-up at 1, 2 and 3 months, the appearance of the collagen was less discrete. After injection beyond the bladder or urethral wall into periadventitial sites, the collagen dispersed immediately and could not be localized ultrasonographically; no localized collection could be identified.

Under direct cystoscopic vision, a bulge at the site of injection developed initially only with the submucosal and intramuscular sites, however, beyond 2 and 3 months visual localization of the collagen bulk was not possible.

Where the collagen was injected into the lateral thigh, linear array ultrasound demonstrated a discrete hypoechoic sphere, similar to the endoluminal ultrasound appearance, in both the subcutaneous and intramuscular layers. The ultrasound measurement of this sphere correlated closely with the 1 ml volume of the injected collagen (0.7–1.0 cm diameters). One month after injection, the collagen could still be clearly visualized ultrasonographically at both tissue depths.

Histologic analysis of the collagen implant one month after injection revealed a fine fibrous tissue capsule and peripheral fibroblast infiltration. The periphery of the implant adjacent to muscle demonstrated a more pronounced infiltration by fibroblasts. Following hematoxylin and eosin staining, the center of the implant was still intact and appeared with its typical granular structure staining pale pink. In the periphery, however, newly formed endogenous collagen which stained intensely pink was noted.

Biopsies at 2 and 3 months postinjection revealed approximately the same histologic findings as those removed 1 month after injection. The implants examined at 3 months, however, demonstrated increased infiltration by fibroblasts, which had reached the center of the injected collagen. The implants had the appearance of being partly compartmentalized by newly formed type 1 and 2 collagen fibers.

Minimal inflammation was noted near the site of collagen injection at all tissue depths and locations. Infiltration by histiofibroblasts and neovascularization appeared to begin in the periphery of the injected collagen and the extent appeared to be time-related, i.e. the longer the collagen had remained in place, the greater the number of histiofibroblasts and amount of neovascularity. The injection of collagen was well tolerated by the mini-pigs. Neither anaphylaxis nor urinary tract infection resulted from the injections.

A direct correlation between the ultrasonic localization and the histologic presence of the collagen implant has been established. The ultrasound data suggests that submucosal injection has the greatest ultrasonically visible longevity and the least histologic evidence of absorption, and thereby the greatest chance for durable clinical success. Periadventitial urethral injections are to be avoided because of the immediate dispersion and early resorption of the collagen, which would impair clinical efficacy.

The host-collagen interaction and its effect on implant longevity may differ from patient to patient.[73] Although granuloma formation did not occur, infiltration by histiofibroblasts and neovascularization into the injected collagen occurred in all cases, but to a variable degree. The injected collagen also demonstrated replacement with native collagen to a variable degree.

In animals, a direct correlation was established between the ultrasound localization and the histologic presence of the collagen implant. These ultrasound findings suggest that periurethral injections (beyond the bladder or urethral walls) are to be avoided due to the immediate dispersion and early resorption of the collagen. Submucosal injection appears to have the greatest ultrasonographically visible longevity and the least histologic evidence of absorption.

These results suggest that endoluminal ultrasound is a promising method for evaluating the injection of periurethral collagen. The location, depth and volume of each injection could be precisely defined. Clinical trials using endoluminal ultrasound to guide periurethral collagen injections and to monitor results in the treatment of incontinent patients are ongoing.

Clinical Study

We have used intraoperative endoluminal ultrasound during injection of collagen in over a dozen men and women with stress urinary incontinence. Collagen injection is performed using the transurethral technique in men using a 21 gauge injection needle inserted through a cystoscopy port. The needle is inserted submucosally and collagen is injected under visual guidance. In women, collagen injection may be done transurethrally or periurethrally. The preiurethral technique involves placing a shorter 21 gauge needle, much like a spinal needle, a few millimeters from the urethral meatus and inserting it parallel to the urethral lumen. The needle is inserted to the level of the proximal urethra near the bladder neck. A cystoscope is then positioned in the urethra to confirm the proximity of the needle in the submucosal layer of the urethral walls. The perceived advantage of the periurethral technique is that the needle does not perforate the mucosa. Therefore, there is less chance of collagen extravasion into the urethral lumen. However, there has been no study to demonstrate any clinical advantage of this periurethral technique. Most clinicians use a transurethral technique because it is easier to learn, and it is less time consuming to properly place the needle tip within the submucosal layer of the proximal urethra.

Endoluminal ultrasound has been used with both transurethral and periurethral injection techniques. With the transurethral technique the ultrasound catheter is inserted in one port of the cystoscope while the collagen injection needle is positioned in the second port. Care is required to avoid roughly pushing back and forth the injection needle, which could cause accidental puncture of the ultrasound catheter. With the periurethral injection technique, only the ultrasound catheter is inserted through the port of the cystoscope.

Prior to collagen injection it is possible to identify scarring of the bladder-urethral anastomosis in men who have undergone radical prostatectomy for

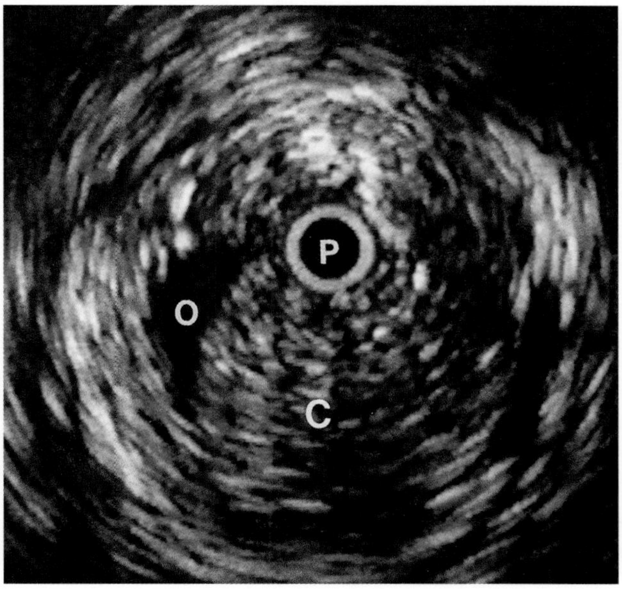

Figure 5.23 *Intraoperative transurethral ultrasound showing hypoechoic submucosal collagen (C) injected into the lateral wall of the urethra. Note that the bulging collagen has compressed and closed the urethral opening (O). P, probe.*

prostatic cancer. The area of the external sphincter appears fibrotic and fixed open, rather than having the normal muscular structure which is closed and sealed at rest. With high-resolution endoluminal ultrasound the metallic injection needle is easily visualized and the depth of the needle in the urethral walls is also clearly delineated. Collagen appears hypoechoic and localized in the submucosa after injection (Fig. 5.23). The calculated volume of injected collagen at each site correlates closely with the actual volume of collagen injected (Fig. 5.24). Improper needle location can be easily determined. If the tip of the injection needle is inserted too far and it enters the bladder, gross extravasation of the collagen can be seen. This alerts the surgeon to stop injection and reposition the needle to avoid wasting the collagen, which is quite expensive.

The most interesting application of endoluminal ultrasound with collagen injection is in its follow-up. Endoluminal ultrasound can visualize any residual collagen mass. The longer the time from injection, the less hypoechoic the collagen appears (Fig. 5.25). The boundaries around the injected collagen appear

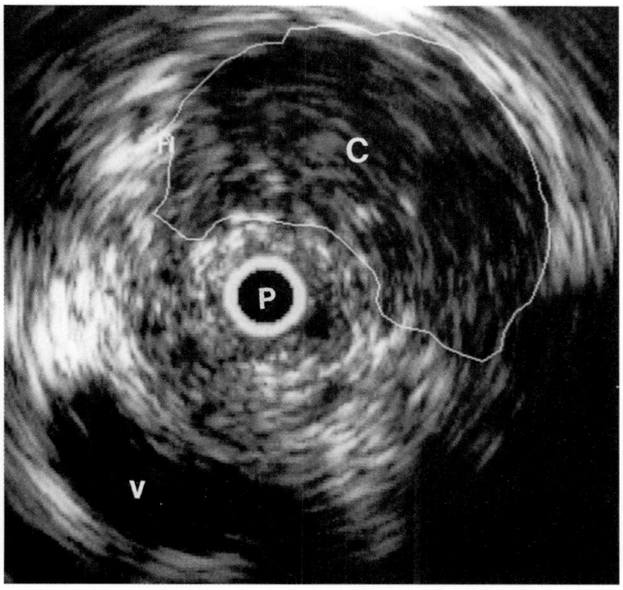

a

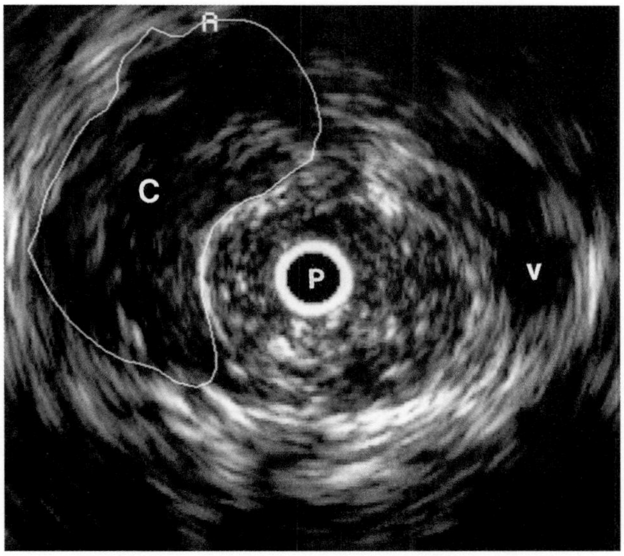

b

Figure 5.24 *Endoluminal ultrasound was used for the localization and deployment of the collagen injection. (a) Injected collagen (C) at 11 to 3 o'clock and (b) injected collagen (C) at 7 to 12 o'clock. The volume of injected collagen can also be calculated. P, probe; V, blood vessel.*

less discrete after several months compared to the time of the initial injection. There was a remarkable difference in the residual collagen mass among different patients (Fig. 5.26). Those with good clinical

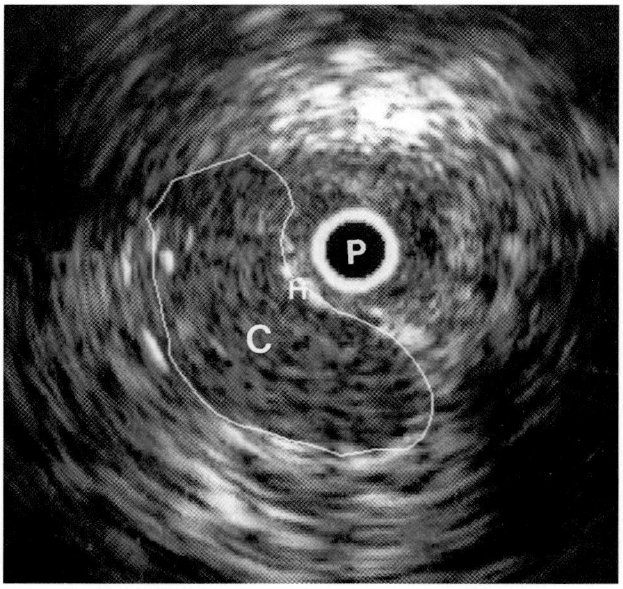

Figure 5.25 *The follow-up ultrasound examination demonstrates the residual collagen mass (C) with less hypoechoic and less discrete appearance. P, probe.*

improvement in their incontinence always have a significant amount of residual collagen remaining in the urethral walls. Patients with return of incontinence after previous injection generally have little or no collagen visible on endoluminal ultrasound.[38]

OTHER APPLICATIONS

In the urethra, it has been possible to visualize various anatomic structures and to delineate areas of abnormality including calcified plaque or fibrosis (Fig. 5.27). Urethral strictures appear as hyperechoic urethral walls associated with lumen narrowing. The length of the stricture and the depth of fibrosis can be identified with endoluminal ultrasound. In addition, as the ultrasound catheter passes through the prostatic portion of the urethra, this structure can be imaged, especially the periurethral region. It should be pointed out that the posterior and lateral aspects of the prostate are best delineated with transrectal ultrasound. However, initial results suggest

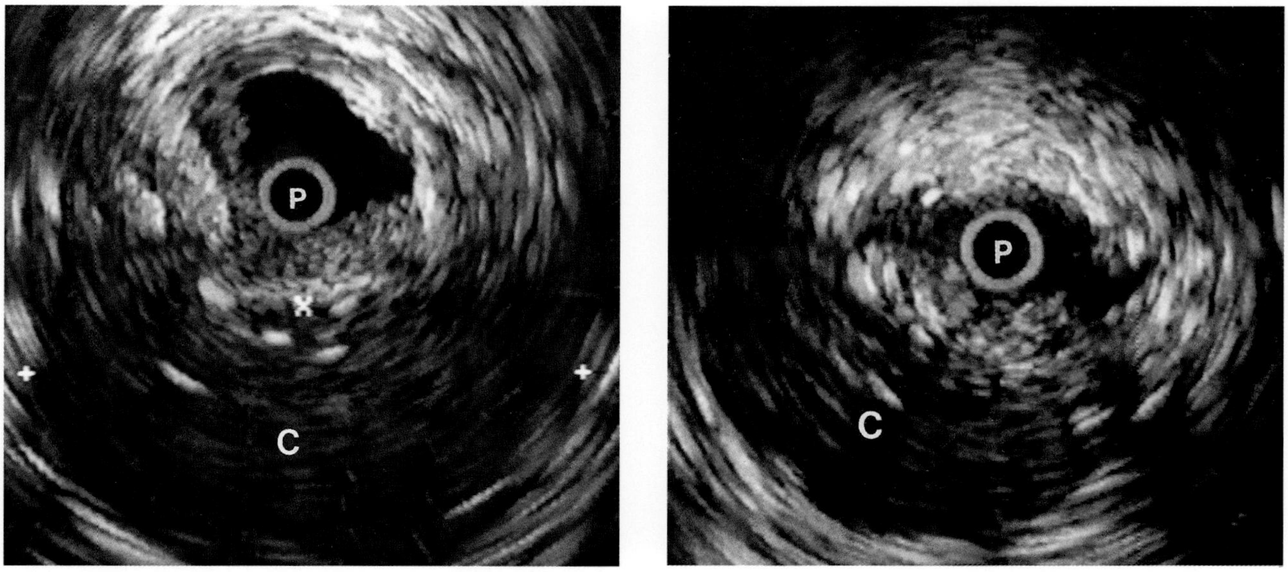

a *b*

Figure 5.26 *(a) Endoluminal ultrasound obtained just after injection of the collagen (C) showing a hypoechoic area measuring 2 × 1 cm. (b) After 6 months, follow-up examination demonstrated the collagen mass reduced to 1.2 × 0.7 cm. P, probe.*

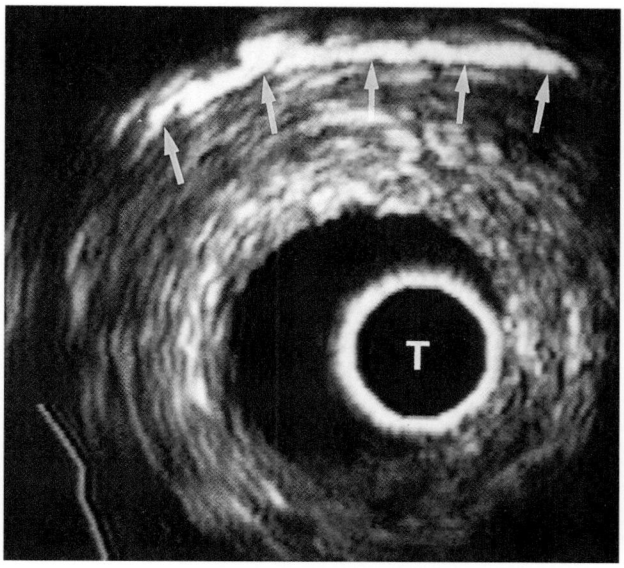

Figure 5.27 *The catheter-based transducer (T) located within the penile urethra demonstrates a hyperechoic linear area (arrows) consistent with a region of plaque.*

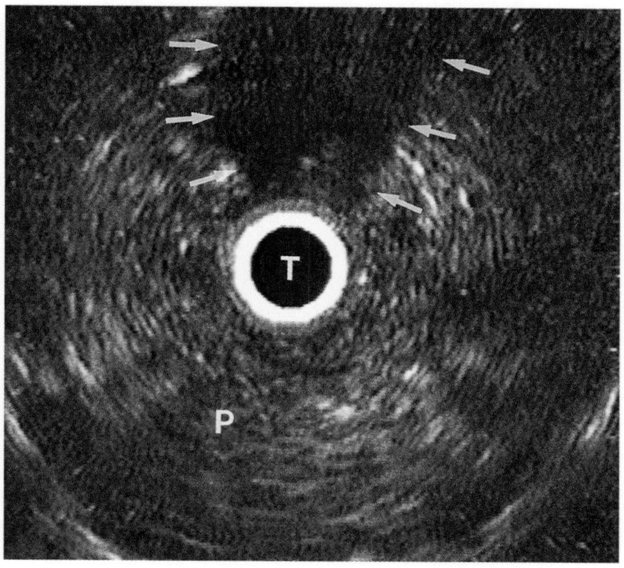

Figure 5.28 *During transurethral prostectomy the site of tissue removal has been delineated (arrows). P, prostate; T, transducer.*

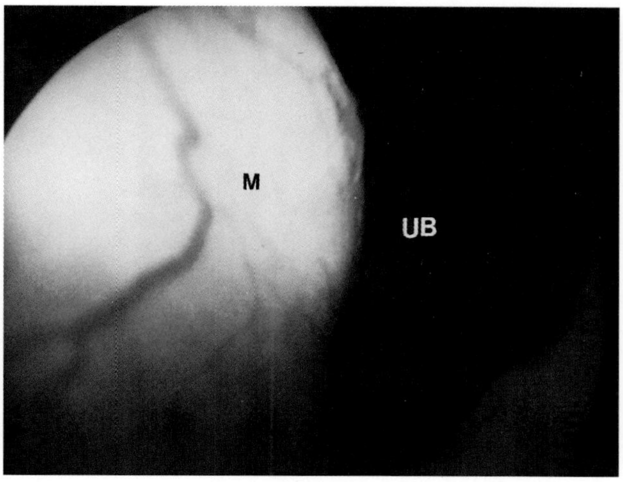

a

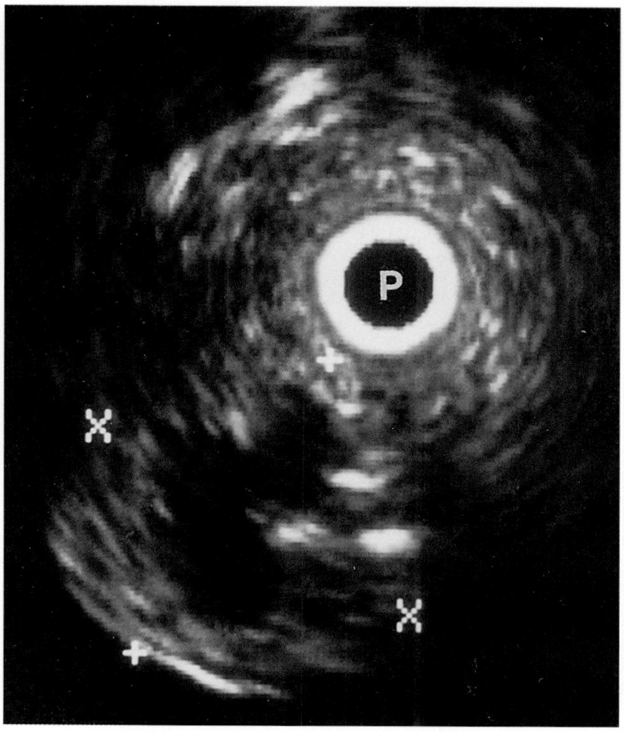

b

Figure 5.29 *(a) Cystoscopic view shown a bulging area (M) from the neck of the bladder (UB). (b) Transurethral ultrasound demonstrated a polyp-like mass (× and +) projecting into the bladder from the proximity of the urethra consistent with a urethral polyp. P, probe.*

that the more central portion is easier to evaluate with an endourethral approach. These catheters have also been used before, during and after transurethral prostatectomy, allowing the urologist to monitor the extent of tissue removal (Fig. 5.28).

Polyps of the urethra are uncommon. They can present with irritative and obstructive symptoms and can occur in any segment of the urethra.[74] We have observed an interesting polyp of the bladder neck during a work-up for hematuria. The polyp was easily seen with endoluminal ultrasound (Fig. 5.29). We have also observed a granulomatous reaction of the bladder neck secondary to surgical foreign body reaction.

LIMITATIONS

There are presently several limitations of urethral endoluminal ultrasound for lower urinary tract examination. Precise bladder and urethral orientation can be difficult. It is impossible to diagnose whether a solid lesion is benign or malignant. Penetration is too shallow for most lesions within the prostate. The cost of endoluminal catheters and transducers is another shortcoming of this exciting new technology.

FUTURE DEVELOPMENTS

Presently, urethral endoluminal ultrasound is a valuable adjunct in the evaluation of a variety of urethral abnormalities. This new ultrasound application permits visualization of the precise size, location, orientation and characteristics of urethral diverticula, fistulae and surrounding tissues. Endoluminal ultrasound is also helpful for the evaluation of urethral endoluminal stents and periurethral bulking agent injections. Through enhanced imaging, surgical success is facilitated.

Efforts to improve urinary continence are in progress using injectable substances to provide coadaptation of urethral and bladder neck urothelial surfaces. The depth at the injection site is difficult to define using the current method of direct-vision urethroscopy for such maneuvers. Endoluminal ultrasound should enable a more accurate periurethral injection of substances such as collagen, increasing the efficacy of treatment for stress urinary incontinence. It should be possible to inject periurethral collagen using only endoluminal ultrasound guidance. With improving depth of visualization, adequate examination of the prostate for benign and neoplastic diseases should become possible. Endoluminal ultrasound may also be important for the staging of transitional carcinoma of the bladder and urethra, allowing for assessment of depth of penetration. It should become a useful test for urethral stricture where determination of length and depth of scar and inflammatory tissue is an important predictor for treatment planning and outcome. Endoluminal ultrasound may also become a valuable test in the evaluation of stress urinary incontinence because of its ability to visualize the urinary sphincter.

REFERENCES

1. Dake MD, Intravascular ultrasound, *Current Opin Radiol* 1991; **3**:181–7.
2. Goldberg BB, Liu JB, Merton DA et al. Endoluminal US: experiments with nonvascular uses in animals, *Radiology* 1990; **175**:39–43.
3. Goldberg BB, Bagley D, Liu JB, Merton DA, Alexander A, Kurtz AB, Endoluminal sonography of the urinary tract: preliminary observations, *AJR* 1991; **156**:99–103.
4. Goldberg BB, Liu JB, Kuhlman K, Merton DA, Kurtz AB. Endoluminal gynecologic ultrasound: preliminary results, *J Ultrasound Med* 1991; **10**:583–90.
5. Liu JB, Miller LS, Goldberg BB et al, Transnasal US of the esophagus: preliminary morphologic and function studies, *Radiology* 1992; **184**:721–7.
6. Miller LS, Liu JB, Klenn PJ et al, Endoluminal ultrasonography of the distal esophagus in systemic sclerosis, *Gastroenterology* 1993; **105**:31–9.
7. Goldberg BB, Steiner RM, Liu et al, Ultrasound-assisted bronchoscopy with use of miniature transducer-containing catheters, *Radiology* 1994; **190**:233–7.
8. Alexander AA, Miller LS, Liu JB, Feld RI, Goldberg BB, High resolution endoluminal sonography of the anal sphincter complex, *J Ultrasound Med* 1994; **13**:281–4.
9. Bagley DH, Liu JB, Grasso M, Goldberg BB, Endoluminal sonography in evaluation of the obstructed ureteropelvic junction, *J Endourol* 1994; **8**:287–92.
10. Grasso M, Liu JB, Goldberg BB, Bagley DH, Submucosal calculi: endoluminal sonographic diagnosis and treatment options, *J Urol* 1995; **153**:1384–9.
11. Braechman J, Keuppens F, Denis L, Transurethral echography, *Prog Clin Biol Res* 1988; **263**:231–5.
12. Tanagho EA, Anatomy of the lower urinary tract. In: Walsh PC, Retik AB, Stamey TA, eds, *Campbell's Urology*, 6th edn: (WB Saunders: Philadelphia PA, 1992).

13. Holm HH, Northeved A, A transurethral ultrasound scanner, *J Urol* 1974; **111**:238–48.
14. Rutila H, Resnick MI, Ultrasonography of the urinary bladder, *World J Urol* 1992; **10**:135–41.
15. Resnick MI, Kursh ED, Transurethral ultrasonography of the urinary bladder, *World J Urol* 1988; **6**:22–6.
16. Devonec M, Chapelon JY, Codas J, Dubernard JM, Revillard JP, Cathignol D: Evaluation of bladder cancer with a miniature high frequency transurethral ultrasonography probe, *Br J Urol* 1987; **59**:550–3.
17. Roth RA, Aretz HT, Transurethral ultrasound-guided laser-induced prostatectomy (TULIP procedure): a canine prostate feasibility study, *J Urol* 1991; **146**:1128–35.
18. Goldberg BB, Liu JB, Endoluminal urologic ultrasound, *Scand J Urol Nephrol Suppl* 1991; **137**:147–54.
19. Alexander AA, Liu JB, McCue P, Gomella LG, Ross RP, Lattime EC, Intravesical growth of murine bladder tumors assessed by transrectal ultrasound, *J Urol* 1993; **150**:525–8.
20. Chin J, Kadhim S, Garcia B, Kim YS, Karlik S, Magnetic resonance imaging for detecting and treatment monitoring of orthotopic murine bladder tumor implants, *J Urol* 1991; **145**:1297–301.
21. Hricak H, Urologic cancer: methods of early detection and future developments, *Cancer* 1987; **6(3Suppl)**:677–85.
22. Itzchak Y, Singer D, Fischelovithc Y, Ultrasonographic assessment of bladder tumors: I. tumor detection, *J Urol* 1981; **126**:31–3.
23. Malone PR, Weston-Underwood J, Aron PM, Wilkinson KW, Joseph AE, Riddle PR, The use of transabdominal ultrasound in the detection of early bladder tumors, *Br J Urol* 1986; **58**:520–2.
24. Brun B, Gammelgaard J, Christofferson J, Transabdominal dynamic ultrasonography in detection of bladder, *J Urol* 1984; **132**:19–20.
25. Devonec M, Chapelon JY, Codas H, Dubernard JM, Revillard JP, Cathignol D, Evaluation of bladder cancer with a miniature high frequency transurethral ultrasonography probe, *Br J Urol* 1987; **59**:550–3.
26. Grups JW, Gruss A, Frohmuller HGW, Evaluation of the T stage of carcinoma of the bladder by transurethral ultrasonography, *Urol Int* 1989; **44**:132–4.
27. Salo JO, Intravesical ultrasound for staging bladder tumours, *Scand J Urol Nephrol* 1987; **21**:203–7.
28. Schulze S, Holm-Nielsen A, Mogensen P, Transurethral ultrasound scanning in the evaluation of invasive bladder cancer, *Scand J Urol Nephrol* 1991; **25**:215–17.
29. Braeckman J, Denis L, The practice and pitfalls of ultrasonography in the lower urinary tract, *Eur Urol* 1983; **9**:193–201.
30. Lopatkin NA, Darenkov AF, Iguashin NS, Ultrasonic diagnosis of vesical neoplasms, *Urol Nephrol* 1983; **4**:3–9.
31. Nakamura S, Niijima R, Staging of bladder cancer by ultrasonography: a new technique by transvesical scanning, *J Urol* 1980; **124**:341–4.
32. Paoletti PP, Tenti S, Fiorelli C, Francalanci R, Paoletti MC, L'echografia endocavitaria transrethrale, *Urologia* 1982; **49**:648–54.
33. Schuller J, Walther V, Schmiedt E, Staehler G, Bauer HW, Schilling A, Intravesical ultrasound tomography in staging bladder carcinoma, *J Urol* 1982; **128**:264–6.
34. Kaisary AV, Intravesical BCG therapy in the management of multiple superficial bladder carcinoma, *Br J Urol* 1987; **59**:554–8.
35. Jaeger N, Radeke HW, Adolphs HD, Penkert A, Bertermann H, Vahlensieck W, Value of intravesical sonography in tumor classification of bladder carcinoma, *Eur Urol* 1986; **12**:76–84.
36. Chancellor MB, Rivas DA, Ackman D et al, Multicenter trials of Urolume™ Endourethral Wallstent® prosthesis for the urinary sphincter in spinal cord injured men, *J Urol* 1994; **152**:924–30.
37. Chancellor MB, Karasick S, Erhard MJ et al, Intraurethral wire mesh prosthesis placement in the external urinary sphincter of spinal cord injured men, *Radiology* 1993; **187**:551–5.
38. Liu JB, Alexander AA, Chancellor MB, Merton DA, Rivas DA, Goldberg BB, Endoluminal urethral ultrasound: clinical applications, *Radiology* 1994; **193**(P): 168.
39. Anderson MJF, The incidence of diverticula in the female urethra, *J Urol* 1967; **98**:96–8.
40. Benjamin J, Elliot L, Cooper JF, Bjornson L, Urethral diverticulum in adult female. Clinical aspects, operative procedures, and pathology, *Urology* 1974; **3**:1–7.
41. Drutz HP, Urethral diverticula, *Obstet Gynecol Clin North Am* 1989; **16**:923–9.
42. Lee RA, Diverticulum of the urethra: clinical presentation, diagnosis, and management, *Clin Obstet Gynecol* 1984; **27**:490–8.
43. Abet L, Natho W, Schulze B, Richter J, Hegenscheid F, Urethrography versus vaginal ultrasonography in urethral diverticula, *Gynakol Rundschau* 1990; **30**(Suppl 1):238–41.
44. Summitt RL, Stovall TG, Urethral diverticula: evaluation by urethral pressure profilometry, cystourethroscopy, and the voiding cystourethrogram, *Obstet Gynecol* 1992; **80**:695–9.
45. Lee TG, Keller FS, Urethral diverticulum: diagnosis by ultrasound, *AJR* 1977; **128**:690–1.
46. Wexler JS, McGovern TP, Ultrasonography of female urethral diverticula, *AJR* 1980; **134**:737–40.
47. Pliskow N, Silver TM, Ultrasonic diagnosis of urethral diverticulum, *Urology* 1980; **15**:625–6.
48. Baert L, Willemen P, Oyen R, Endovaginal sonography: new diagnostic approach for urethral diverticula, *J Urol* 1992; **147**:464–6.
49. Pavlica P, Viglietta G, Losinno F, Veneziano S, Dalla RS, Diverticula of the female urethra. A radiological and ultrasound study, *Radiol Med* 1988; **75**:521–7.
50. Keefe B, Warshauer DM, Tucker MS, Mittelstaedt CA, Diverticula of the female urethra: diagnosis by endovaginal and transperineal sonography, *AJR* 1991; **156**:1195–7.
51. Martenssonn O, Duchek M, Translabial ultrasonography with pulsed colour-Doppler in the diagnosis of female urethral diverticula, *Scand J Urol Nephrol* 1994; **28**:101–4.
52. Kim B, Hricak H, Tanagho EA. Diagnosis of urethral diverticula in women: value of MR imaging, *AJR* 1993; **161**:809–15.
53. Chancellor MB, Liu JB, Rivas DA, Intraoperative endoluminal ultrasound evaluation of urethral diverticulum, *J Urol* 1995; **153**:72–5.
54. Hinman F Jr, Cohlan WR, Gartner's duct carcinoma in a urethral diverticulum, *J Urol* 1960; **83**:414–15.
55. Frydenberg M, Lover CJ. Calculus in urethral diverticulum formed upon a nylon suture, *Br J Urol* 1988; **62**:614.
56. Debus-Thiede G, Wagner U, Schurmann R, Christ F, Erste erfahrungen mit der transvaginalen sonographie von urethra and blase in rahmen der inkontinenz diagnostik, *Geburtshilfe Frauenheilkd* 1985; **45**:891–4.

57. Richmond DH, Sutherst J, Transrectal ultrasound scanning in urinary incontinence: the effect of the probe on urodynamic parameters, *Br J Urol* 1989; **64**:582–5.
58. Kohorn EI, Scioscia AL, Jeanty P, Hobbins J, Ultrasound cystourethrography by perineal scanning for the assessment of female stress urinary incontinence, *Obstet Gynecol* 1986; **68**:269–70.
59. Quinn MJ, Beynon J, Mortenson NJM, Smith PJB, Transvaginal endosonography: a new method to study the anatomy of the lower urinary tract in urinary stress incontinence, *Br J Urol* 1988; **62**:414–18.
60. Beco JL, Sulu MS, Schaaps JJ, Transvaginal sonography of micturition and urinary incontinence. In: Fornage BD (ed.), *Endosonography* (Kluwer Academic Publishers, 1989) 121–8.
61. Bernaschek HK, Perinealsonography in the assessment of urinary incontinence in the female, *Geburtsh u Frauenheilk* 1989; **49**:498–501.
62. Beco J, Sulu M, Schaaps JP, Lambotte R. Une nouvelle approche morphodynamique des troubles de la continence chez la female: L echoghraphie urodynamique par voie vaginale, *J Gynecol Obstet Biol Reprod* 1987; **16**:987–98.
63. Kirschner-Hermanns R, Klein HM, Muller U, Schafer W, Jakse G, Intra-urethral ultrasound in women with stress incontinence, *Br J Urol* 1994; **74**:315–18.
64. Klutke C, Golomb J, Raz S et al, The anatomy of stress incontinence: magnetic imaging of the female bladder neck and urethra, *J Urol* 1990; **143**:563–6.
65. Hricak H, Secaf E, Buckley DW et al, Female urethra: MR imaging, *Radiology* 1991; **178**:527–37.
66. Politano VA, Small MP, Harper J, Lynne CM, Periurethral Teflon injection for urinary incontinence, *J Urol* 1974; **111**:180–3.
67. Ferro MA, Smith JHF, Smith PJB, Periurethral granuloma: unusual complication of Teflon periurethral injection, *Urology* 1988; **31**:422–3.
68. Malizia AA, Reiman HM, Myers RP, Migration and granulomatous reaction after periurethral injection of polytef (Teflon), *JAMA* 1984; **251**:3277–81.
69. Claes H, Stoorbants D, van Meerbenk J, Verbeken E, Knockaert D, Baert L, Pulmonary migration following periurethral polytetrafluorethylene injection for urinary incontinence, *J Urol* 1989; **142**:821–2.
70. Appell RA, Injectables for urethral incompetence, *World J Urology* 1990; **8**:208–11.
71. Shortliffe LMD, Freiha FS, Kessler R, Stamey TA, Constantinou CE, Treatment of urinary incontinence by the periurethral implantation of cross-linked collagen, *J Urol* 1989; **141**:538–41.
72. Rivas DA, Chancellor MB, Liu JB, Hanau C, Bagely DH, Goldberg B, Endoluminal ultrasound and histological evaluation of periurethral collagen injection, *J Endourology* 1996; **10**:61–6.
73. DeLustro F, Smith ST, Sundsmo J, Salem G, Kincaid A, Ellingsworth L, Reaction to injectable collagen: results in animal models and clinical use, *Plast Reconstr Surg* 1987; **21**:581–94.
74. Caro PA, Rosenberg HK, Snyder HM III, Congenital urethral polyp, *AJR* 1986; **147**:1041–2.

Chapter 6 Upper gastrointestinal tract

Ji-Bin Liu, Thomas D Schiano and Larry S Miller

INTRODUCTION

Placement of an endoluminal ultrasound probe into the gastrointestinal (GI) tract was first performed in 1956 by Wild and Reid,[1] who used an ultrasound transducer in the rectum to examine malignant tumors. Since that time, there have been significant technical improvement as well as clinical advances in endoluminal ultrasound. In the early 1980s several separate groups of investigators developed the concept of combining a flexible endoscope with an ultrasound transducer to image the GI tract with the use of 7.5–12.5-MHz transducers. Using these transducers, it was possible to image both the mural structures of the GI tract and structures adjacent to the GI tract wall.[2–4]

Endoluminal ultrasound was developed to overcome the limitations of standard transabdominal ultrasound. The use of transabdominal ultrasound is restricted because its lower frequency leads to limited resolution, due to interposed structures which limit imaging (i.e. ribs, lungs, fat and bowel gas), and because there is general inability to image mural lesions of the upper GI tract. Endoscopic ultrasound overcomes these limitations by the use of higher-frequency transducers which allow for increased resolution. In addition, by placing the probe close to the organ being imaged, there is elimination of artifact due to bony structures, obesity and bowel gas.

Currently, clinical imaging of the GI tract is usually accomplished with dedicated endoscopic ultrasound scopes. Using these scopes, imaging is done by one of three techniques. First, the scope can be placed directly in contact with the mucosa. This technique is commonly used in the esophagus and duodenum. Second, a balloon around the ultrasound transducer can be inflated with water to promote acoustic coupling. This technique is used in the esophagus, stomach and duodenum. Finally, viscera can be filled with de-aerated water and imaging accomplished through the water. This technique is commonly used in the stomach.

There are two types of dedicated echoendoscopes in clinical use today. The side-viewing Olympus echoendoscope with a 360° sector scan is widely used and has a rigid tip which contains the ultrasound transducer with side-viewing optics. The ultrasound sector scan is perpendicular to the shaft axis of the instrument. The endoscopic controls are those of a typical fiberoptic or video-endoscope, and the ultrasound frequency can be switched from 7.5 to 12 MHz. Although experience with the Pentax FG32 UA echoendoscope is somewhat more limited than with the Olympus scopes, it is being used more frequently. This echoendoscope uses a curvilinear array and provides a sector scan which is oriented along the axis of the scope. These echoendoscopes also have color and spectral Doppler capabilities, and ultrasound-guided biopsies can be done through the biopsy channel.[5]

ANATOMY OF UPPER GI TRACT AND ADJACENT STRUCTURES

ESOPHAGUS AND STOMACH

The esophagus is a muscular tubular structure about 25 cm long that joins the pharynx to the stomach. The esophagus comprises the cervical, thoracic and abdominal portions, with the majority of the esophagus lying within the thorax. The esophagus enters the abdomen through an opening in the right crus of the diaphragm. Clinically, the esophagus is divided into three portions: upper esophageal sphincter, body esophagus, and lower esophageal sphincter (Fig. 6.1). The average distance of the cardia from the upper incisor teeth is approximately 40 cm, but in some tall individuals this distance may be as much as 42 or 43 cm.

Histologically, the esophagus, like other parts of the GI tract, is composed of a mucosa, a submucosa, a muscularis and an adventitia. The mucosa is made up of epithelium, lamina propria and muscularis mucosae. The submucosa is quite dense and contains both elastic and collagen fibers. The

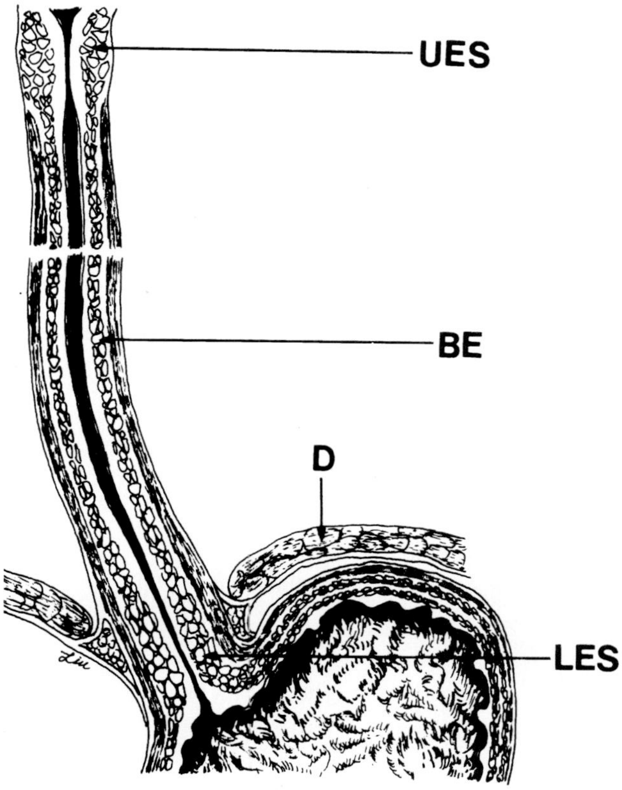

Figure 6.1 *Diagrammatic representation of the esophageal anatomy in frontal section. UES, upper esophageal sphincter; BE, body esophagus; D, diaphragm; LES, lower esophageal sphincter.*

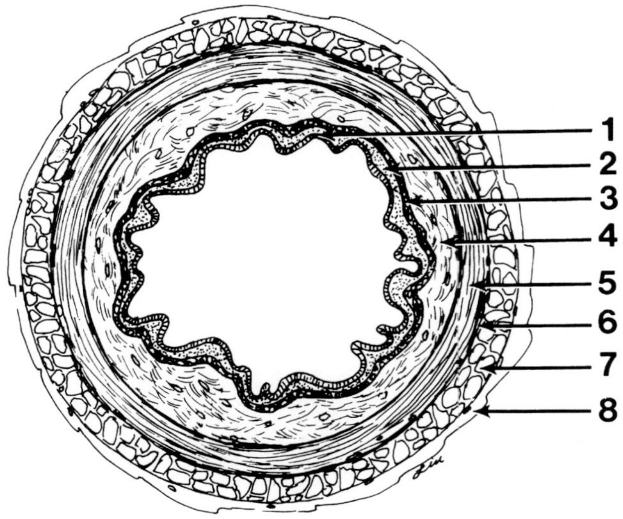

Figure 6.2 *A schematic cross-sectional view of histologic structures of the esophagus. 1, epithelium; 2, lamina propria; 3, muscularis mucosae; 4, submucosa; 5, inner circular smooth muscle; 6, intermuscular connective tissue; 7, longitudinal smooth muscle; 8, adventitia.*

muscular coat consists of an inner circular layer and an outer longitudinal layer. A thin layer of connective tissue called the intermuscular connective tissue is spread between the two muscular layers. The adventitia consists of loose connective tissue, connecting the esophagus to its surrounding structure (Fig. 6.2).

The stomach is a dilated portion of the alimentary canal and is situated in the upper part of the abdomen, extending from the left hypochondriac region into the epigastric and umbilical areas. It is roughly J-shaped and has two openings, the cardiac and pyloric orifices, and two curvatures known as the greater and lesser curvatures. The stomach is usually divided into the following parts: (1) the fundus, which is dome-shaped and projects upward and to the left of the cardiac orifice and is often full of gas; (2) the body of the stomach, which extends from the level of the cardiac orifice to the level of the incisura angularis; and (3) the pylorus, which is the most tubular part of the stomach and the thick muscular wall of which forms the pyloric sphincter (Fig. 6.3). With the use of a high-frequency catheter-based ultrasound probe (20 MHz), detailed histologic structures of the esophagus and stomach have been demonstrated. We will discuss this separately.

Using dedicated endoscopic ultrasound scopes (7.5–12 MHz), the wall of the upper GI tract usually appears as a five layered structure. Each of the layers corresponds to a specific histologic layer. Correlation of these various layers is as follows: the first hyperechoic layer corresponds to the acoustic interface between the water balloon and the mucosa; the second hypoechoic layer to the deep mucosa and possibly the muscularis mucosa; the third hyperechoic layer to the submucosa; the fourth hypoechoic layer to the muscularis propria; and the fifth hyperechoic layer to the serosa or adventitia (Fig. 6.4).[6]

EXTRAMURAL AND RETROPERITONEAL STRUCTURES

In addition to imaging mural structures, endoscopic ultrasound is capable of imaging extramural and retroperitoneal structures. The following is a brief

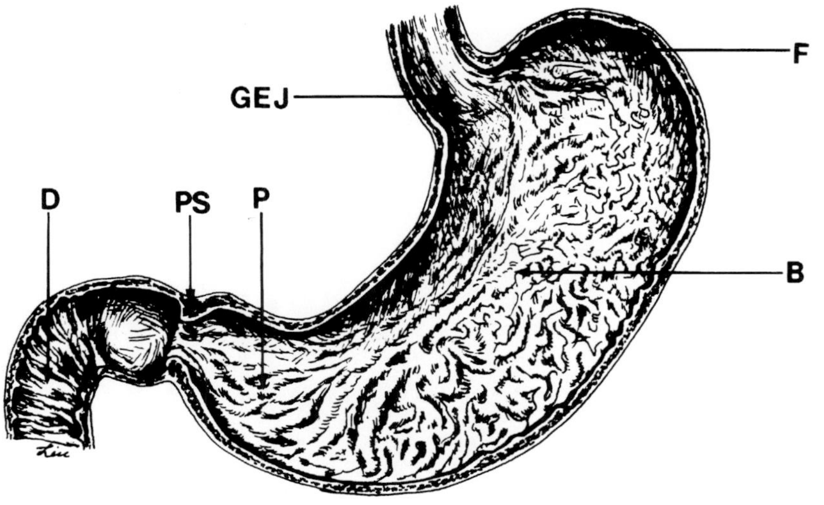

Figure 6.3 *A schematic illustration of the gastric anatomy. GEJ, Gastroesophageal junction; F, fundus of the stomach; B, body of the stomach; P, pylorus; PS, pyloric sphincter; D, duodenum.*

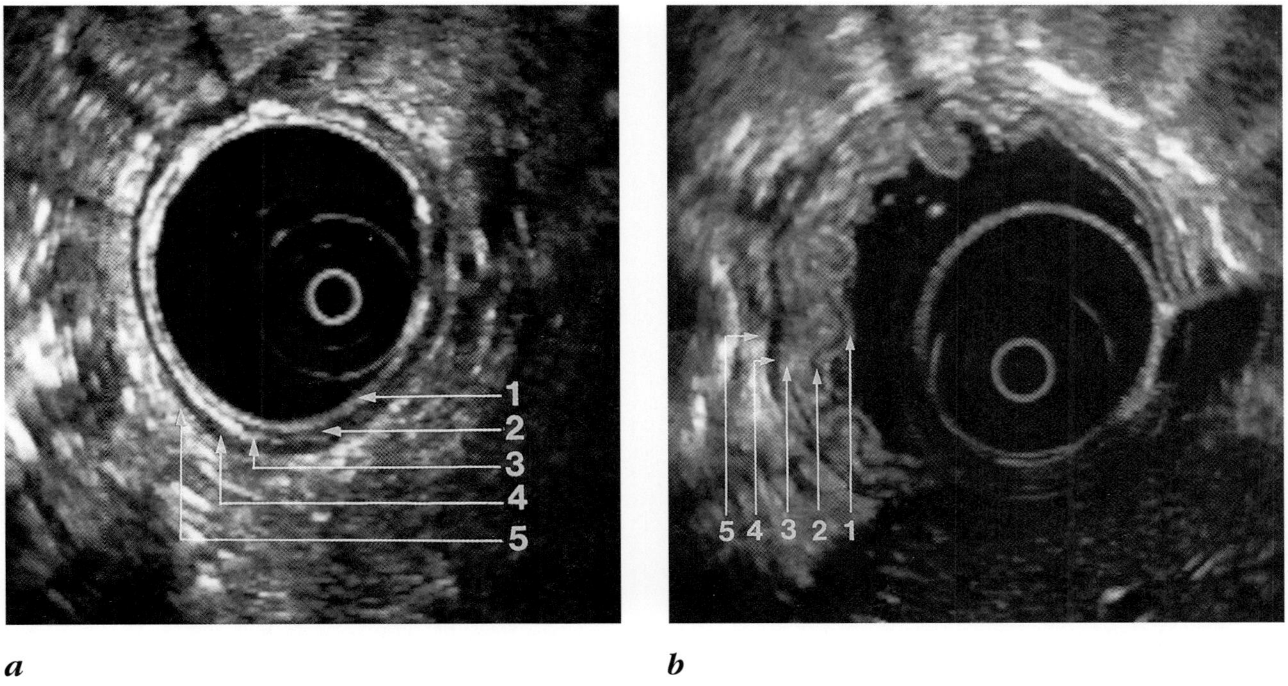

Figure 6.4 *Endoscopic ultrasound images obtained from the distal esophagus (a) and the body of the stomach (b) demonstrate cross-sectional structures of the esophageal and gastric wall. They are the first hyperechoic mucosa (1), the second hypoechoic deep mucosa and possibly the muscularis mucosa (2), the third hyperechoic submucosa (3), the fourth hypoechoic muscularis propria (4), and the fifth hyperechoic adventitia (5).*

review of the extramural anatomy which can be imaged by endoscopic ultrasound.

The pancreas is divided into three portions: the head, which lies in the concavity of the duodenum, the neck, which overlies the portal vein, and the body, which tapers to form the tail toward the spleen. The uncinate process is the portion of the head that curves back toward the spleen under the mesenteric vessels. The pancreatic ductal system is formed by fusion of the duct of Santorini in the dorsal pancreatic anlage with Wirsung's duct in the ventral anlage. The minor papilla drains Santorini's duct, while the major papilla represents the common termination of Wirsung's duct and the bile duct.[7]

The gallbladder lies on the inferior surface of the liver in a fossa marking the division of the liver into its anatomic right and left lobes. In the liver hilum, the bile ducts are generally ventral to the portal vein and hepatic artery. The common hepatic duct lies along the anterolateral aspect of the portal vein. The common bile duct, formed by the union of the cystic and common hepatic ducts, is a direct continuation of the common hepatic duct. It passes behind the first portion of the duodenum and through the pancreatic head to enter the descending portion of the duodenum (Fig. 6.5).[8]

The falciform ligament divides the liver into right and left lobes. Only the left lobe can be imaged with endoscopic ultrasound. The hepatic artery arises as one of the three major branches of the celiac axis (Fig. 6.6), ascending to the porta hepatis, branching off the right gastric and gastroduodenal arteries. The portal vein is formed by the confluence of the superior mesenteric vein (SMV) and the splenic vein behind the pancreas.

The duodenum is divided into four portions: the bulb, the second (directly posteriorly), the third (descending to form the C-loop) and the fourth (transverse from the C-loop to the ligament of Treitz) (Fig. 6.5). The fourth portion cannot be reached with the endoscopic ultrasound scope. To adequately image the pancreaticobiliary system, the tip of the echoendoscope is first placed into the third portion of the duodenum. Controlled withdrawal of the instrument allows imaging of the uncinate process, distal common bile duct, ampulla, ventral pancreas, superior mesenteric and portal veins and, occasionally, the right kidney. Continued withdrawal into the bulb affords imaging of the pancreatic head with its upper border delineated by the gastroduodenal artery. The gallbladder, portal vein, hepatic artery and inferior vena cava are also imaged from this position. Further imaging of the pancreatic body, gallbladder and splenic and portal veins is performed in the gastric antrum. The pancreatic tail, the spleen and its hilar vessels and, occasionally, the left kidney are imaged from the gastric fundus. Technical limitations include a small field of view and operator dependency in maneuvering the scope into the appropriate imaging position.[9–12]

The pancreatic body and tail are located adjacent to the posterior gastric wall with the echoendoscope within the stomach; the left hepatic lobe and portal

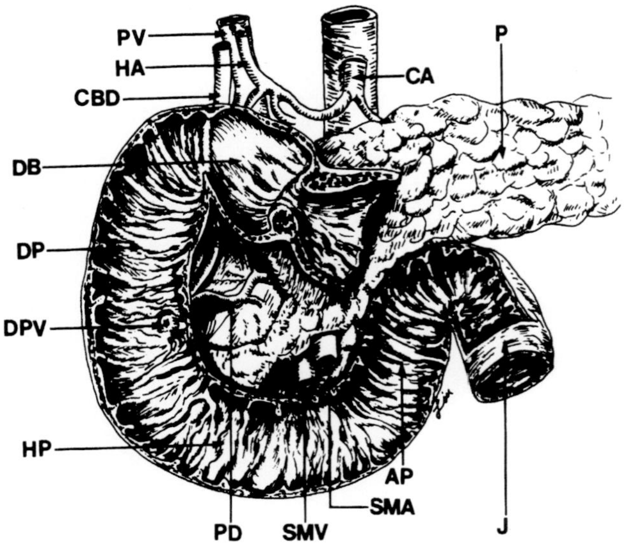

Figure 6.5 *Diagrammatic representation of the duodenum and adjacent structures in frontal view. PV, portal vein; HA, hepatic artery; CBD, common bile duct; CA, celiac artery; P, pancreas; DB, duodenal bulb; DP, descending part; DPV, duodenal papilla of Vater; HP, horizontal part; PD, pancreatic duct; SMV, superior mesenteric vein; SMA, superior mesenteric artery; AP, ascending part; J, jejunum.*

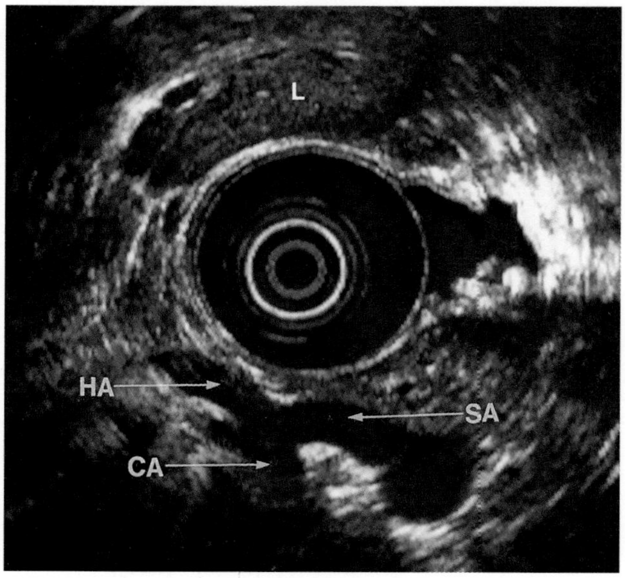

Figure 6.6 *Endoscopic ultrasound image demonstrates a celiac artery (CA) and its branches of the hepatic (HA) and splenic arteries (SA). L, left lobe of liver.*

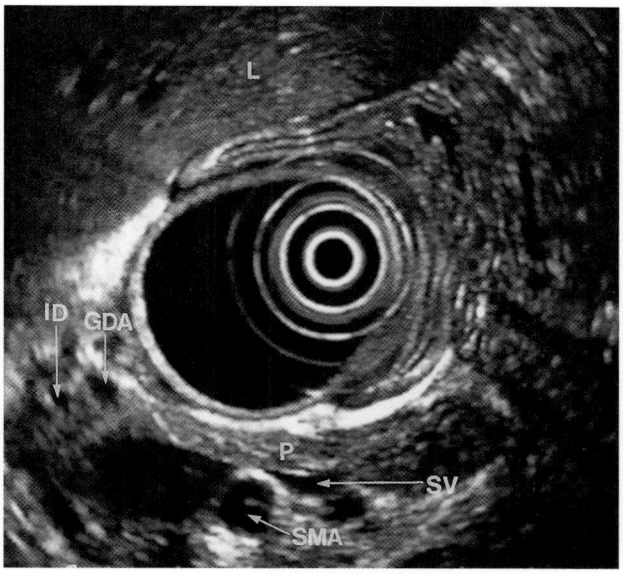

Figure 6.7 *Endoscopic ultrasound image shows normal pancreas (P) and surrounding structures, i.e. splenic vein (SV), superior mesenteric artery (SMA), intrapancreatic bile duct (ID), gastroduodenal artery (GDA) and the liver (L).*

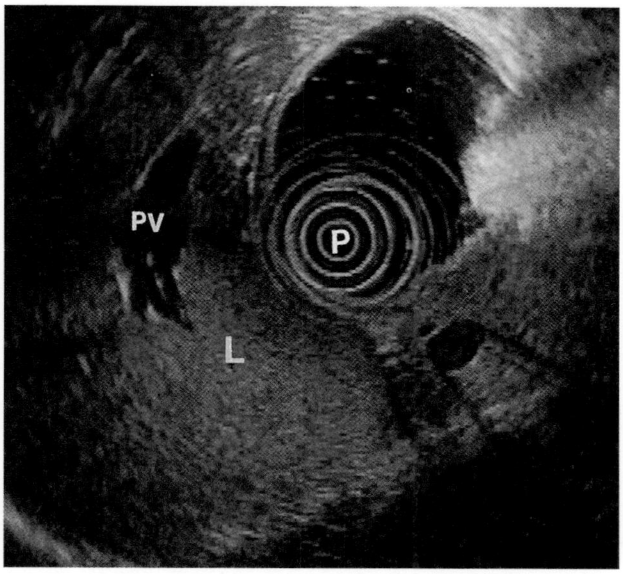

Figure 6.9 *Endoscopic ultrasound image shows the left lobe of the liver (L) with intrahepatic portal vein (PV). P, endoscopic probe.*

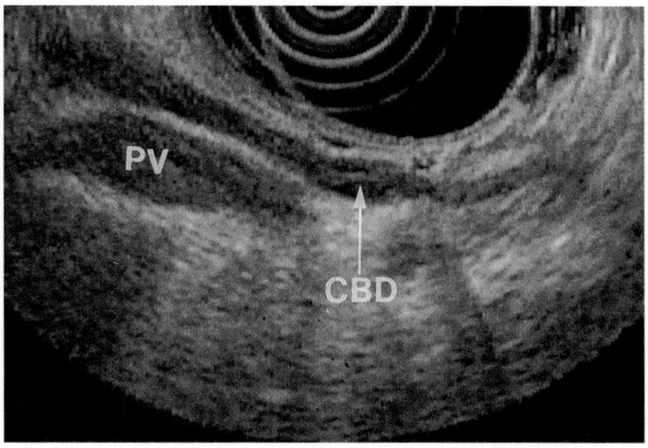

Figure 6.8 *Endoscopic ultrasound image shows a normal-sized distal common bile duct (CBD) and main portal vein (PV).*

vein are used as landmarks for imaging. The entire pancreas can be imaged in more than 95% of patients (Fig. 6.7). The normal main bile duct is visualized in 80–90% of cases, while a dilated common duct is almost always seen endosonographically (Fig. 6.8). The liver hilum with the hepatic branches is more difficult to delineate, with success only being achieved 50–60% of the time. Because only small parts of the left lobe and none of the right lobe of the liver can be visualized, systematic examination of the intrahepatic bile ducts is not possible (Fig. 6.9).[10–12]

While imaging the duodenum, the aorta should be placed at 5 o'clock and the vena cava at the 7 o'clock position, with the anechoic spine being visualized between these two great vessels. The superior mesenteric artery (SMA) can often be seen branching from the aorta in the direction of the transducer. The SMV or splenic vein is immediately ventral to the SMA. These mesenteric vessels are located to the left of the aorta. The gastroduodenal artery, which originates from the hepatic artery, can be imaged between the duodenum and ventral pancreas in close proximity to the common bile duct. The uncinate process is localized between the aorta and mesenteric vessels. The branch of the pancreatic duct that drains the uncinate process is found ventrally from the superior mesenteric vein or splenic vein. The main pancreatic duct is ventral to the aorta and vena cava. The trifurcation created by the portal and splenic veins and SMV can often be visualized. The common bile and common hepatic ducts are imaged using the portal vein as a guide. The bile duct is parallel to the portal vein and

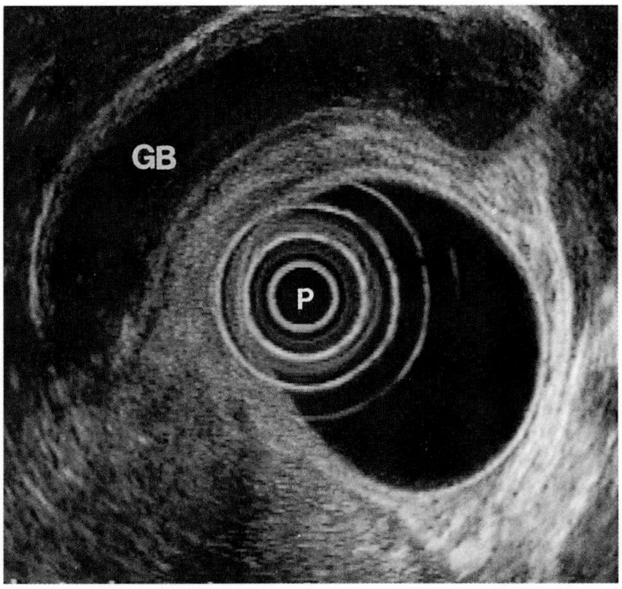

Figure 6.10 *Endoscopic ultrasound image obtained from within the second part of the duodenum shows a bile-filled gallbladder (GB). P, endoscopic probe.*

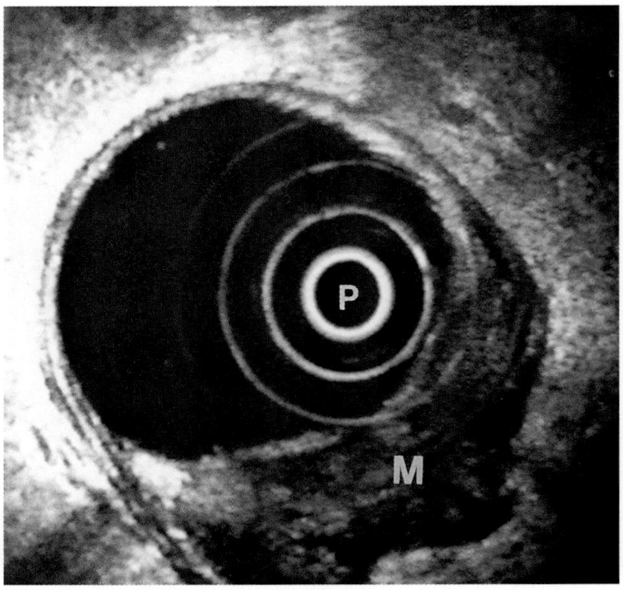

Figure 6.11 *Endoscopic ultrasound image shows a hypoechoic mass (M) at the level of the distal esophagus. P, endoscopic probe.*

adjacent to the duodenum. The cystic duct and gallbladder are variable in location, with the former often found close to the ampulla or adjacent to the hilum (Fig. 6.10). The papilla is visualized as a raised area in the duodenal wall containing the common bile and pancreatic ducts. The common channel connecting the two can often be delineated.[10–12]

By filling the gastric lumen with water, the spleen can also be used as a landmark. It is distinguished from the liver by the absence of the intrahepatic branches of the portal vein, and the spleen's proximity to the pancreatic tail and left kidney. The splenic vein and artery course together into the splenic hilum. The splenic vein is located on the immediately dorsal aspect of the pancreas, continuing along the pancreatic body and tail into the hilum. The main pancreatic duct is found ventral to the splenic vein.

APPLICATION OF DEDICATED ENDOSCOPIC ULTRASOUND PROBES

The main clinical indications for the use of endoscopic ultrasound in the upper GI tract are for the evaluation of neoplasms in the esophagus and stomach, to assess the depth of infiltration and the presence or absence of regional lymphadenopathy, and in the evaluation of submucosal lesions.

ESOPHAGEAL CARCINOMA

Endoscopic ultrasound is the most accurate diagnostic tool available for local tumor staging in esophageal carcinoma. With endoscopic ultrasound, esophageal carcinoma generally images as a hypoechoic or mixed echoic circumscribed mass or diffuse wall thickening (Figs 6.11 and 6.12). Endoscopic ultrasound has been found to be a useful imaging modality for the T classification of the TNM staging system. This classification is as follows: T1 = tumor involving the mucosa and submucosa but leaving the muscularis propria intact (Fig. 6.13); T2 = tumor infiltration into the muscularis propria but confined by this layer (Fig. 6.14); T3 = tumor invasion into the adventitia resulting in an irregular outer margin with tumorous pseudopodia (Fig. 6.15); and T4 = tumor invasion into other structures or adjacent organs such as the aorta, azygous vein, left atrium, or trachea.[13]

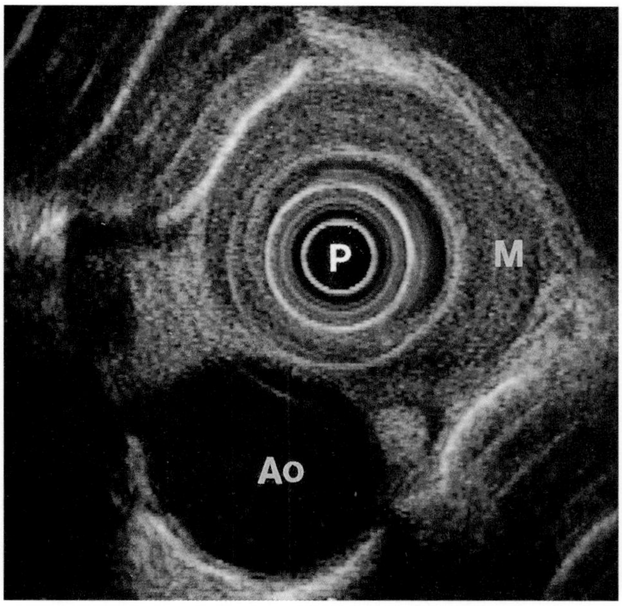

Figure 6.12 *Endoscopic ultrasound image demonstrates diffuse wall thickening (M) at the mid-portion of the esophagus. Endoscopic biopsy proved this to be an esophageal carcinoma. Ao, aorta; P, probe.*

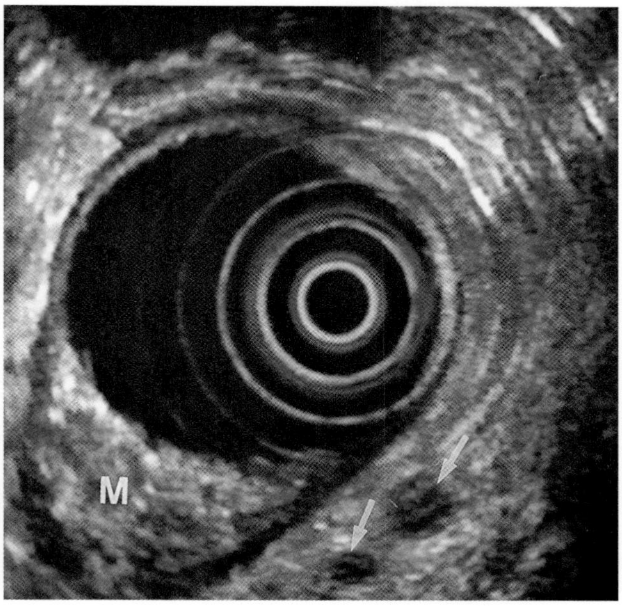

Figure 6.13 *Stage T1 esophageal carcinoma. A cross-sectional ultrasound image detects a mixed echogenic mass (M) within the esophageal submucosa without involvement of the muscularis propria. Two round-shaped lymph nodes (arrows) are also seen.*

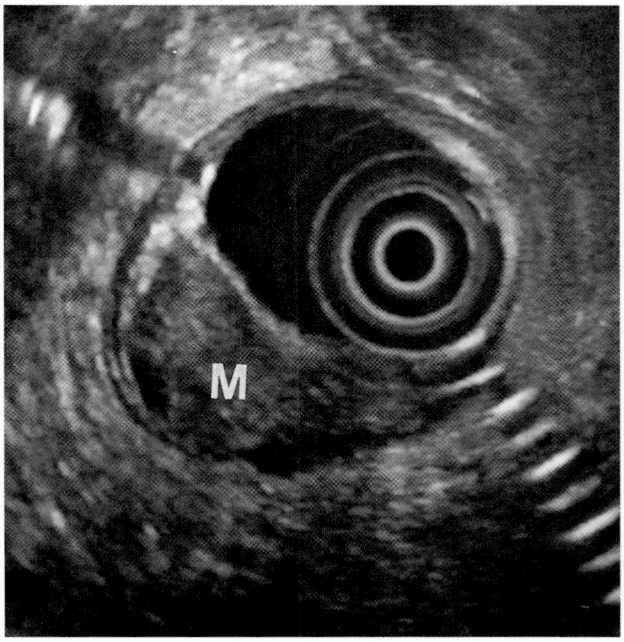

Figure 6.14 *Stage T2 esophageal carcinoma. A cross-sectional ultrasound image of the esophagus demonstrates a hypoechoic mass (M) infiltrating into the muscularis propria.*

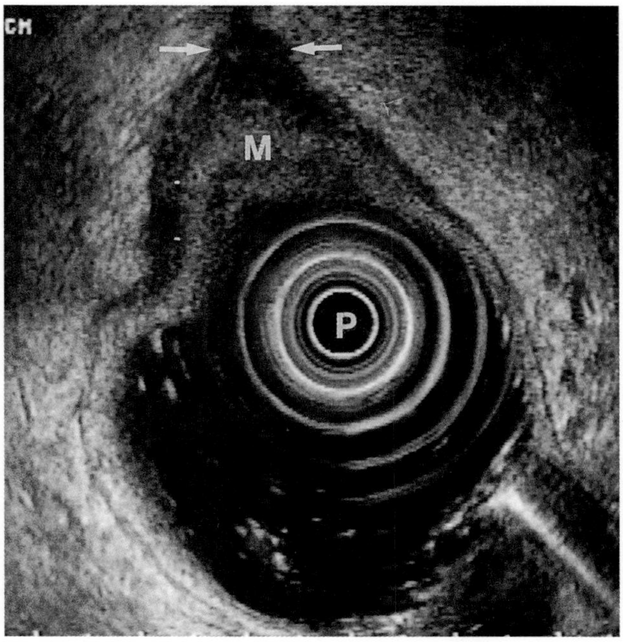

Figure 6.15 *Stage T3 esophageal carcinoma. An esophageal ultrasound image demonstrates a hypoechoic mass (M) invading beyond the adventitia (arrows). P, probe.*

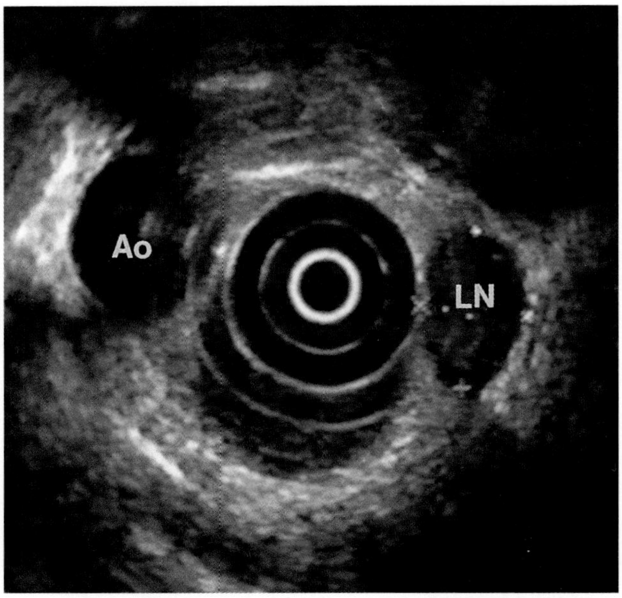

Figure 6.16 *In a patient with esophageal carcinoma, endoscopic ultrasound demonstrates an enlarged lymph node (LN) adjacent to the esophagus. Ao, aorta.*

There is no consensus opinion existing as to criteria for defining stage N0 or N1. Recently, Catalano et al[14] evaluated endosonographic features that were thought to characterize lymph node metastasis in 100 patients with esophageal carcinoma. Endosonographically imaged lymph nodes were evaluated according to size, shape, border demarcation and central echo pattern. The sensitivity and specificity of endosonography in detecting lymph node metastasis were 89.1% and 91.7%, respectively. When lymph nodes were imaged endosonographically, regardless of the specific features, the likelihood of N1 disease was 86%, whereas when no lymph nodes were imaged, the chance of N0 disease was 79%. Endosonographic features predictive of malignancy, in increasing order of importance, were echopoor (hypoechoic) structure, sharply demarcated borders, rounded contour, and size greater than 10 mm. Collectively, the endoscopic ultrasound features produced an additive effect with respect to accuracy in the prediction of malignant lymph node involvement. Malignancy could be predicted with 100% accuracy when all four features were present (Fig. 6.16). Distant metastases cannot be detected by endoscopic ultrasound, because of the limited depth of penetration.

A number of studies have shown that endoscopic ultrasound is highly accurate when compared to surgery in the T and N staging of esophageal carcinoma.[15–26] In addition, endoscopic ultrasound is accurate in predicting outcome in terms of curative resectability and palliative resectability or nonresectability.[16,20] When compared with CT, endoscopic ultrasound is far superior in correctly predicting the T and N stages.[18,19,21,24,27] Endoscopic ultrasound is also reliable in detecting anastomotic recurrence of carcinoma.[28]

Problems with endoscopic ultrasound in the evaluation of esophageal carcinoma include mis-staging due to microscopic infiltration or peritumorous inflammation. In addition, because of the size of the current dedicated scopes, it is often difficult to traverse a stricture area in the esophagus.

GASTRIC CARCINOMA

With endoscopic ultrasound, gastric tumors also appear as hypoechoic or mixed echoic lesions (Figs 6.17 and 6.18). The following is the endoscopic ultrasound staging classification according to the TNM system: T1 = thickening or tumor infiltration of the mucosal and submucosal layers, leaving the muscularis propria intact; T2 = infiltration of the muscularis propria or the subserosa (Fig. 6.17); T3 = tumor penetration through the serosa without invasion of adjacent structures (Fig. 6.18). T4 = tumor invasion of adjacent structures or vasculature. Discrete flat or slightly depressed early gastric cancers cannot be visualized by endoscopic ultrasound. In these cases, the absence of any transmural tumor growth or histologic proof of carcinoma can be taken as evidence for a T1 lesion. Since the subserosa cannot be differentiated from the serosa by endoscopic ultrasound except in patients with ascites, problems arise in differentiating between stages T2 and T3. Linitis plastica (leather-bottle stomach) is characterized by diffuse hypoechoic wall thickening (Fig. 6.19). In local tumor staging, a number of studies have shown endoscopic ultrasound to be accurate in predicting the T stage but somewhat less accurate in predicting the N stage.[29–42] Endoscopic ultrasound is far superior to CT in predicting the T and N stages of gastric carcinoma (Fig. 6.20).[33,34,38]

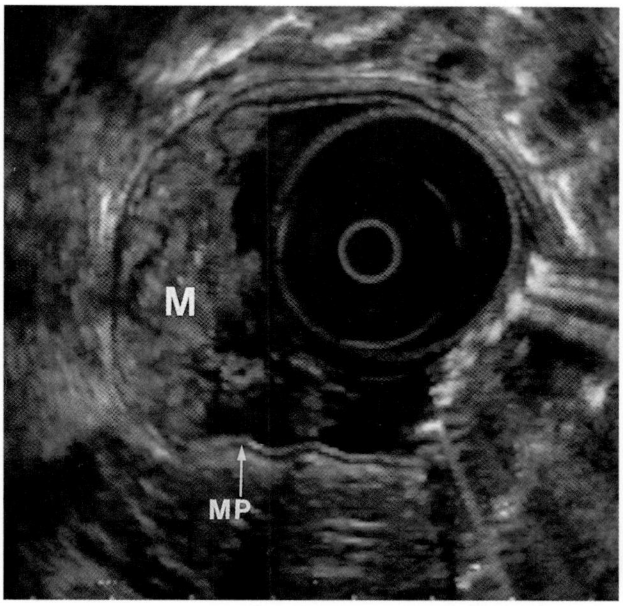

Figure 6.17 *Endoscopic ultrasound image of the stomach shows a heterogeneous echogenic mass (M) without involving the muscularis propria (MP). This was pathologically confirmed as stage T1 gastric carcinoma.*

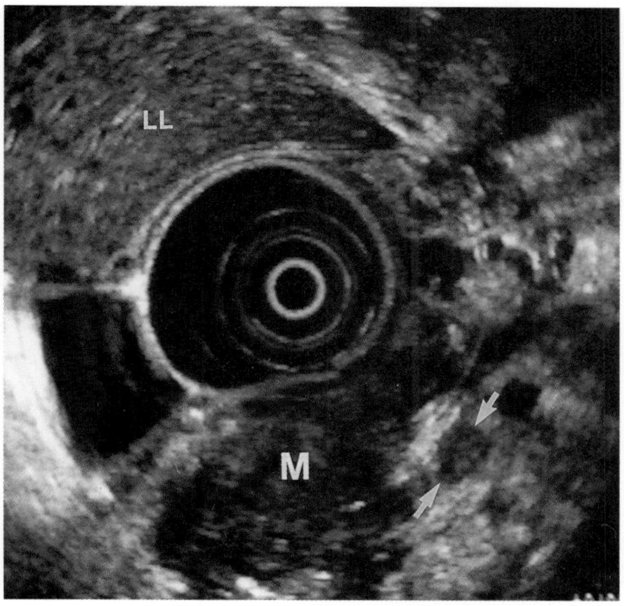

Figure 6.18 *Endoscopic ultrasound image shows a hypoechoic mass (M) with penetration through the serosa of the stomach. A round-shaped lymph node is also seen (arrows). LL, left lobe of the liver.*

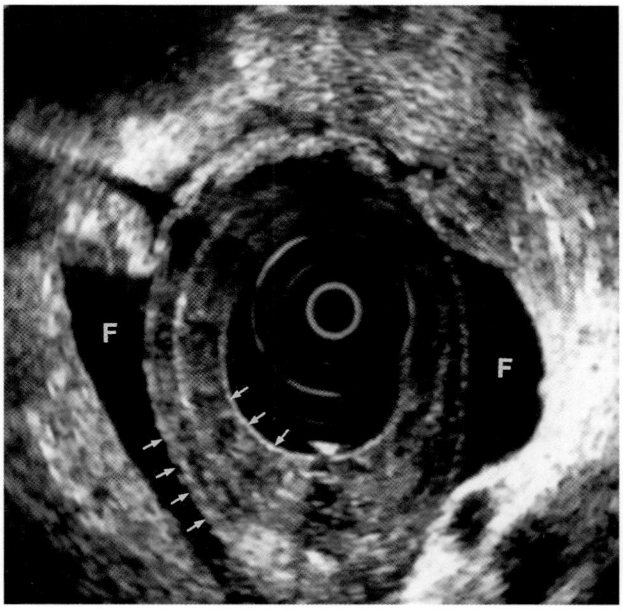

Figure 6.19 *Endoscopic ultrasound demonstrates a diffuse wall thickening (arrows) of the stomach surrounded by ascites (F). These findings corresponded to linitis plastica (leather-bottle stomach).*

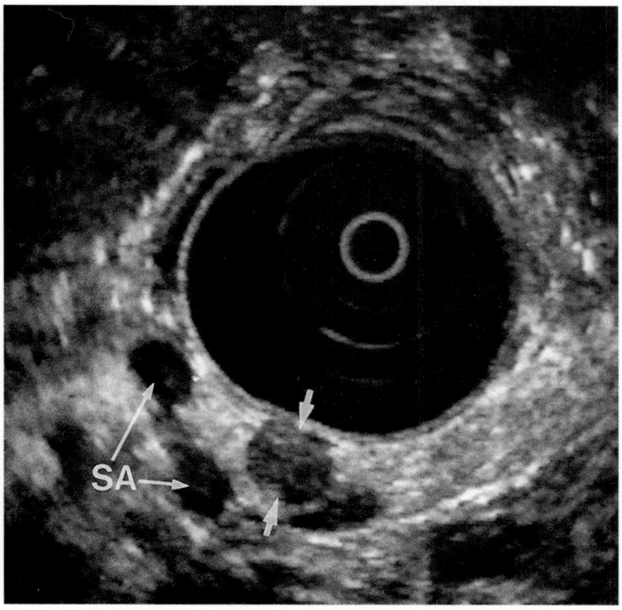

Figure 6.20 *In a patient with gastric carcinoma, endoscopic ultrasound detects an enlarged round-shaped lymph node (arrows) adjacent to the splenic artery (SA), which was not seen on CT scan.*

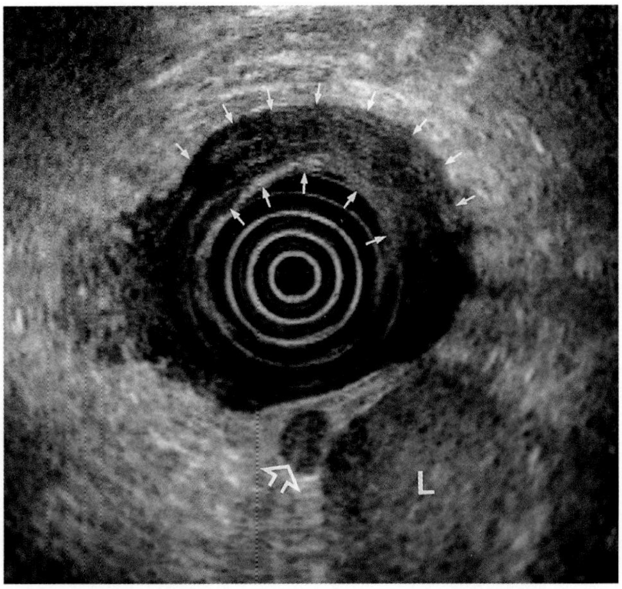

Figure 6.21 *In a patient with biopsy-proven gastric lymphoma, the hypoechoic tumor (arrows) is located circumferentially in the stomach and invades through all the wall layers into the surrounding tissue. Note a lymph node (open arrow) adjacent to the gastric wall. L, liver.*

GASTRIC LYMPHOMA

The typical appearance of gastric lymphoma with endoscopic ultrasound is that of diffuse or localized hypoechoic infiltration of the second and third layers (Fig. 6.21). However, transmural tumor growth or infiltration of other organs may also occur. Metastatic lymph nodes usually show an echo pattern similar to that of the primary tumor. As in gastric carcinoma, endoscopic ultrasound has been found to be accurate in delineating tumor extent and in detecting perigastric lymph node metastasis. However, because of lack of penetration, more distant metastases cannot be demonstrated.[43-50]

THICK GASTRIC FOLDS

Giant gastric folds develop in several benign and malignant diseases. In a study by Songur et al,[51] endoscopic ultrasound was used to evaluate patients with thickened gastric folds. The thickness of the gastric wall and each layer was measured and compared with the endosonographic findings of healthy subjects. Endoscopic ultrasound revealed that the second layer alone was thickened in Menetrier's disease (Fig. 6.22), and the third layer alone enlarged in anisakiasis. Most of the patients with scirrhous carcinoma showed an abnormally enlarged third and fourth layer. The second layer, together with the third layer, was thickened in healthy subjects with simple hyperregosity and in patients with gastric lymphoma. However, the fourth ultrasound layer corresponding to the muscularis propria was significantly thickened only in malignant conditions.

In another study, Mendis et al[52] examined the utility of endoscopic ultrasound in the diagnostic evaluation of large gastric folds. Twenty-five consecutive patients with endoscopically or radiographically diagnosed large gastric folds were studied. All patients underwent endoscopic ultrasound investigation to determine the anatomic wall layer of enlargement. Endoscopic ultrasound demonstrated enlargement of layer 2 only (deep mucosa) in 64%, primarily of layer 3 (submucosa) in 14% and of layer 4 (muscularis propria) in 21%. Malignancy did not develop in any of the patients with gastric wall thickening limited to layer 2 and negative biopsy results. Abnormalities involving the muscularis propria in the absence of ulceration strongly suggest malignancy and should be investigated further if endoscopic biopsy findings are negative.

SUBMUCOSAL LESIONS

Endoscopic ultrasound is used in the evaluation of submucosal tumors, to differentiate true submucosal tumors from extramural compression, to help differentiate benign from malignant lesions, and to rule out varices or other vascular structures prior to biopsy.

Submucosal lesions can be differentiated by endoscopic ultrasound via consideration of the following criteria: the echo layer from which it originates, the echo pattern, the tumor margins and whether or not the lesion arises from an extraluminal site. Submucosal lesions can arise from the muscularis mucosa, submucosa, or the muscularis propria. The echo pattern is critical in the differentiation of various submucosal lesions; the three echo patterns that are seen are hyperechoic (bright), hypoechoic (dark) and anechoic (echo-free).

The most frequently encountered submucosal lesion is the leiomyoma (Fig. 6.23). This lesion

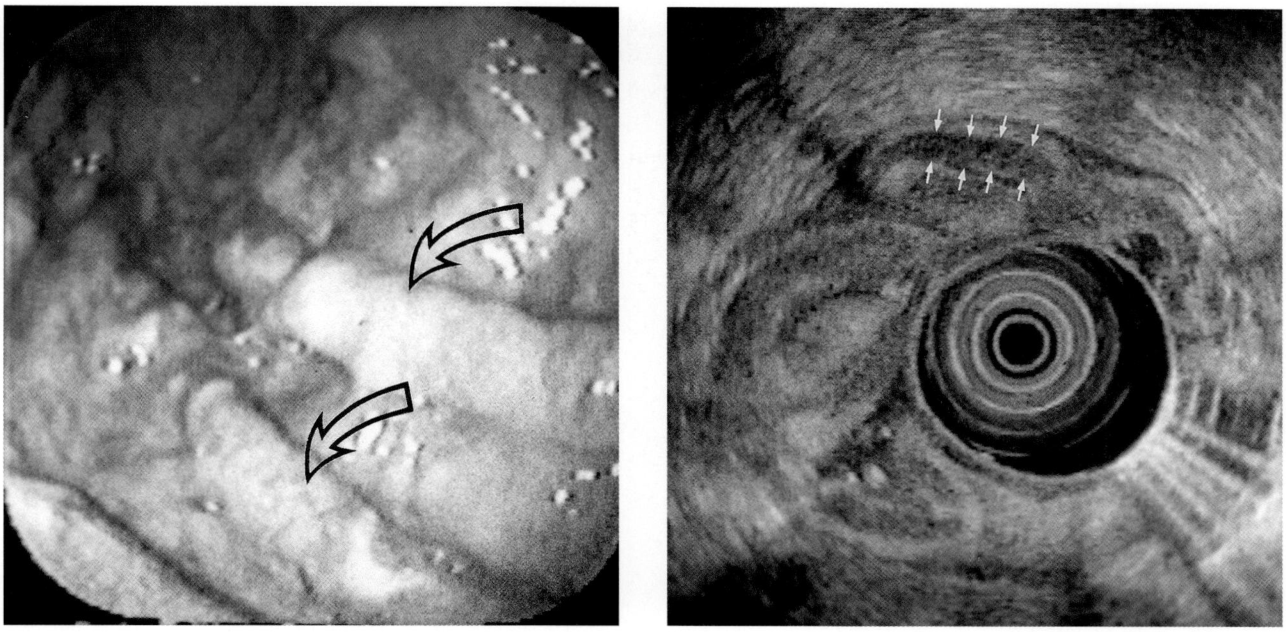

a *b*

Figure 6.22 *(a) This patient was found to have markedly enlarged gastric folds (arrows) on endoscopy. However the diagnosis could not be made by endoscopy alone since enlarged folds can be seen in a number of different disease processes. (b) Endoscopic ultrasound revealed hypoechoic marked thickening of the second layer (arrows) of the gastric wall consistent with a diagnosis of Menetrier's disease.*

arises in the fourth layer, consistent with the muscularis propria. It is typically hypoechoic and homogeneous with smooth margins. The second hypoechoic layer is occasionally reported as the origin of leiomyomas. Leiomyoblastomas and leiomyosarcomas can also arise from the fourth hypoechoic layer and also appear hypoechoic. Although these lesions cannot be differentiated from the more benign leiomyoma by endoscopic ultrasound, some characteristics, such as larger size and increased degenerative changes representing tumor necrosis and calcification, may denote a higher risk potential for malignancy. In addition, the tumor margin may be irregular, which is more commonly seen in malignant lesions as opposed to the smoother margin seen in leiomyomas.[53–61]

Lipomas arise from the submucosa and are hyperechoic and well demarcated (Fig. 6.24). Aberrant pancreatic tissue or pancreatic rests also arise within the submucosa and appear well demarcated. These

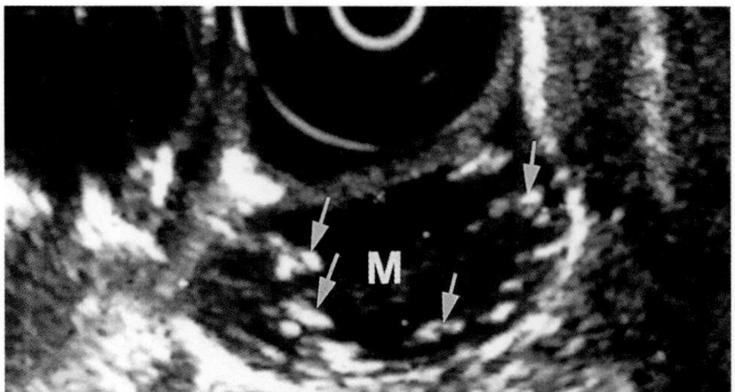

Figure 6.23 *Endoscopic ultrasound of the stomach demonstrates a hypoechoic mass (M) with smooth margins arising from the posterior wall of the stomach. Scattered bright reflectors (arrows) within the mass represent calcifications or fibrosis. Biopsy of this mass proved to be a leiomyoma.*

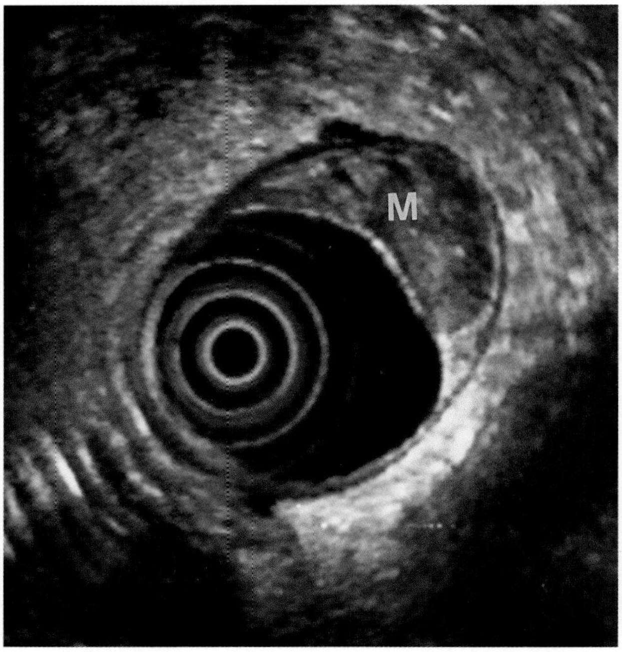

Figure 6.24 *A hyperechoic mass (M) arising from the submucosa of the esophagus is detected by endoscopic ultrasound. This lesion has uniform echotexture with smooth contours. Biopsy has proven it to be a lipoma.*

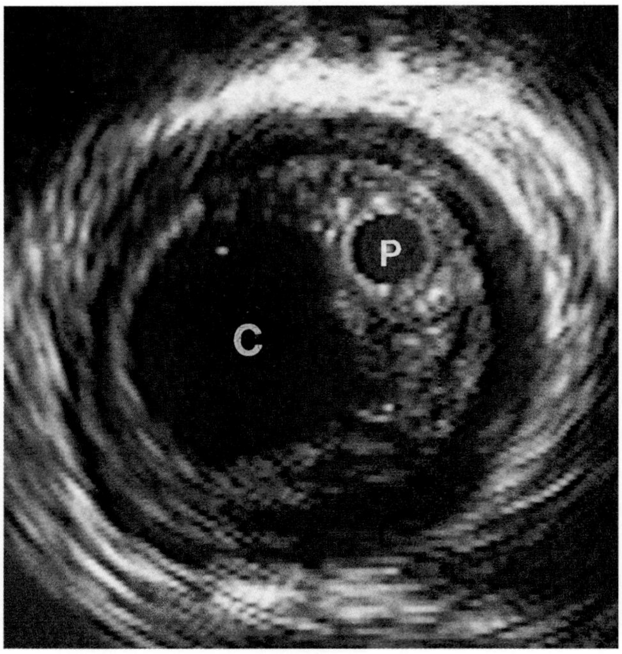

Figure 6.25 *A cross-sectional ultrasound image identified a cystic lesion (C) within the submucosa of the esophagus. P, probe.*

lesions are typically hypoechoic with smooth margins and fine scattered hypoechoic spots and, occasionally, duct-like structures. Cysts are typically anechoic, well-demarcated structures within the submucosa (Fig. 6.25).

Extramural compression may be due to normal viscera, tumor infiltrated organs, normal vascular structures or cystic structures outside the wall of the GI tract. These extramural compressions can usually be differentiated from true submucosal lesions via endoscopic ultrasound.[53,55,61–64] The shortcoming of endoscopic ultrasound is that it cannot distinguish between benign and malignant lesions with certainty and a biopsy is almost always needed.

PANCREATIC CARCINOMA

The entire pancreas can be imaged using the lower-frequency dedicated ultrasound scopes. From the posterior wall of the stomach, the body and the tail of the pancreas as well as the pancreatic duct can be well imaged. From the first portion of the duodenum and the duodenal bulb, the head of the pancreas and the uncinate process can be imaged. Adenocarcinoma in the pancreas appears as a hypoechoic tumor infiltrating into the pancreatic parenchyma. Often, pancreatic carcinoma will cause obstruction of the pancreatic and/or common bile duct. When obstruction occurs, dilated pancreatic and common bile ducts can be well visualized as hypoechoic fluid-filled tubular structures (Fig. 6.26). Pancreatic carcinoma can also be seen infiltrating into the common bile duct and surrounding structures. The celiac axis can also be imaged to evaluate for metastatic lymph nodes from the pancreatic carcinoma.

CATHETER-BASED ULTRASOUND PROBES

As opposed to the dedicated endoscopic ultrasound scopes, ultrasound probes are catheters that contain high-frequency ultrasound transducers. These

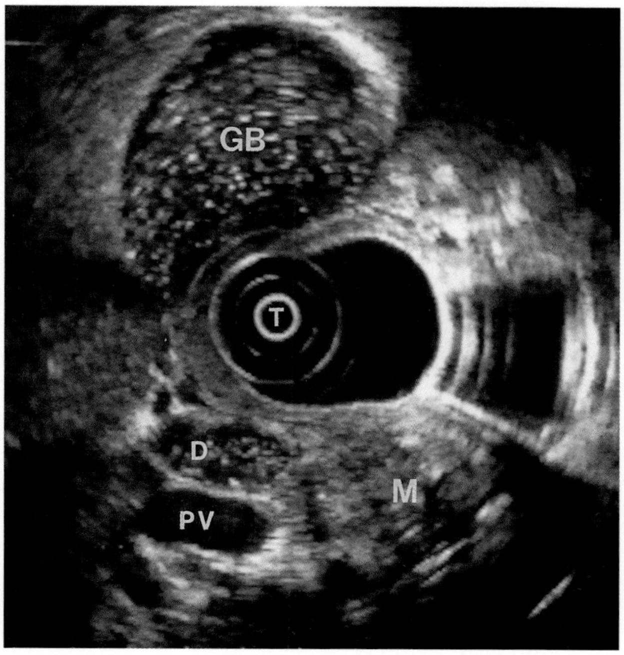

Figure 6.26 *This picture shows a hypoechoic mass (M) within the head of the pancreas with a remarkably dilated common bile duct (D) and gallbladder (GB) filled with sludge. The sludge appears as hyperechoic speckled images. A portal vein (PV) can also be seen just inferior to the dilated common bile duct (D). T, transducer.*

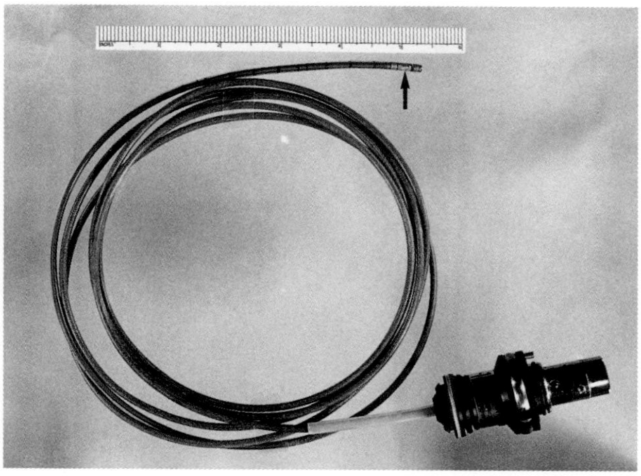

Figure 6.27 *The Olympus 7.5-MHz ultrasound probe has a length of 250 cm and a diameter of 3.4 mm. The transducer (arrow) produces a 360° cross-sectional image.*

catheters are thin (1–3 mm in diameter) and can be passed through the biopsy channel of an endoscope or through a nasogastric tube. The advantages of these catheter-based ultrasound probes are that they are able to pass tight strictures, can be placed endoscopically while imaging sonographically, and are often of higher frequency, which allows for better resolution. Disadvantages are that they have a limited life expectancy, have poor depth penetration and lack a balloon, and therefore frequently lose acoustic coupling.

There are several endoluminal catheter-based ultrasound probes that have been used to image the GI tract. For example, the Sonoprobe SP101 from Fuginon has a length of 150–180 cm and a diameter of 2.6 mm. Its principle of ultrasound scanning is via linear compound scanning (B-mode). Its ultrasound frequency is 15–20 MHz with a linear ultrasound view. The Olympus UM1W ultrasound probe has a length of 250 cm and a diameter of 3.4 mm. Its principle of scanning is radiomechanical and produces 360° cross-sectional imaging; the ultrasound frequency is 7.5 MHz (Fig. 6.27). The EndoSound™ catheter (Microvasive/Boston Scientific Corporation, Natick, MA) has a length of 95–126 cm and a diameter of 4.8, 6.2 or 9 Fr (Fig. 6.28). Its single-element transducer is mounted on the end of a wire core which is connected to a motor on the ultrasound instrument (HP100, or IVUS, Diasonics). The motor is rotated to produce a 360° transaxial real-time image. Sterile water (0.5–1.0 ml) is introduced between the probe core and the catheter to eliminate air, which can interfere with the transmission of the ultrasound beam. The transducer sends and receives the ultrasound signal at a 10° angle from the perpendicular to the long axis of the catheter. The operating frequency of 20 MHz results in an axial resolution of 0.1 mm and a penetration of about 2 cm. Real-time images can be recorded on videotape for off-line evaluation.[65]

This higher frequency increases the axial resolution of the image so that mural GI structures can be seen in much greater detail. Although the axial resolution of these transducers is greater, the penetration of the ultrasound waves is limited by the higher frequency.

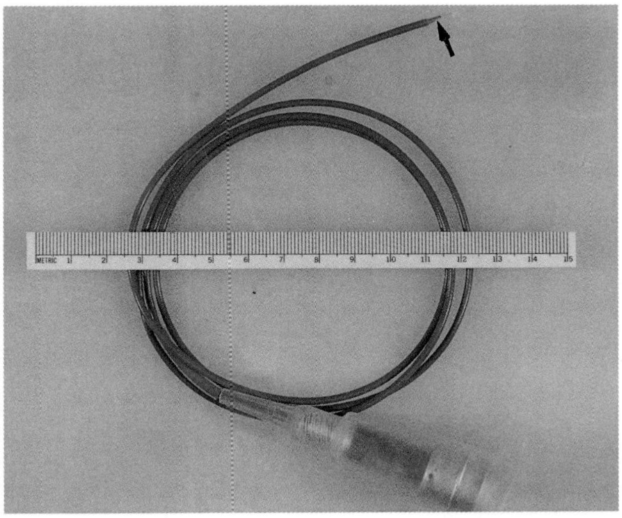

Figure 6.28 *The EndoSound™ 20-MHz ultrasound transducer (arrow) is mounted on the distal end of a wire core and is housed within a 6.2 Fr catheter.*

Therefore, structures surrounding the GI tract are often not imaged, so there is limited ability of these transducers to stage large or advanced tumors. Another advantage is that these transducers are not surrounded by a water-filled balloon, as are the transducers embedded in dedicated endoscopes. Because of the smaller size and the lack of compression, there is much less distortion of small mural structures such as esophageal varices. A disadvantage is that there may be loss of acoustic coupling in organs filled with air, such as the stomach and the small intestine.

IN VITRO STUDIES

The initial studies performed using 20-MHz catheter-based ultrasound transducers were animal studies using sheep esophagus. Freshly resected specimens were placed in a water bath, and the transducer-containing catheter was inserted into the lumen of the esophagus. To eliminate near-field transducer artifact, 15 ml of saline was injected into the lumen of the esophagus. After ultrasound imaging, the specimens were fixed in 10% formalin and embedded in paraffin; histologic cross-sections were prepared that corresponded to the ultrasound imaging planes. The recorded ultrasound images demonstrated seven layers of the esophageal wall.[65] Correlation of the histologic findings with these ultrasound images showed that the innermost (hyperechoic) layer represented the squamous epithelium and superficial mucosa; the second (hypoechoic) layer, the deep mucosa and muscularis mucosa; the third (hyperechoic) layer, the submucosa; the fourth (hypoechoic) layer, the circular smooth muscle; the thin fifth (hyperechoic) layer, the intermuscular connective tissue; the sixth (hypoechoic) layer, the longitudinal smooth muscle; and the seventh (hyperechoic) layer, the adventitia (Fig. 6.29). Using the lower-frequency 7.5- or 12-MHz echoendoscope, the esophageal wall appears as only five sonographic layers with different echogenicities.[66] This difference is probably due to compression of the esophagus wall by the water-filled balloon and poor resolution.[67]

The human esophagus was first evaluated using autopsy specimens.[68] These were infused with various volumes of water and placed in a water bath. The catheter containing the ultrasound transducer was introduced into the esophagus, and an image of the entire esophagus was then obtained. Silk sutures were placed on the esophageal adventitial surface at various imaging locations. The esophagus was then fixed in 4% buffered formalin, and sections for histologic evaluation were taken at the suture levels. Histologic examination was performed on standard paraffin-embedded specimens, which were stained with hematoxylin-eosin and Masson's trichome; the results were correlated with the cross-sectional endoluminal ultrasound image at corresponding levels. Analysis of these images revealed seven reproducible and distinct alternating hyperechoic and hypoechoic layers in the esophageal wall. The difference between the non-fluid-filled and the fluid-filled esophagus was that the first layer in the non-fluid-filled esophagus appeared as a mixed echoic layer corresponding to the squamous epithelium, lamina propria and muscularis mucosa. This is thought to be due partly to the first three histologic layers (squamous epithelium, lamina propria and muscularis mucosa) being folded and contracted around the transducer (Fig. 6.30).[65]

IN VIVO STUDIES

Because the miniature ultrasound transducers demonstrated a very high resolution in both the in

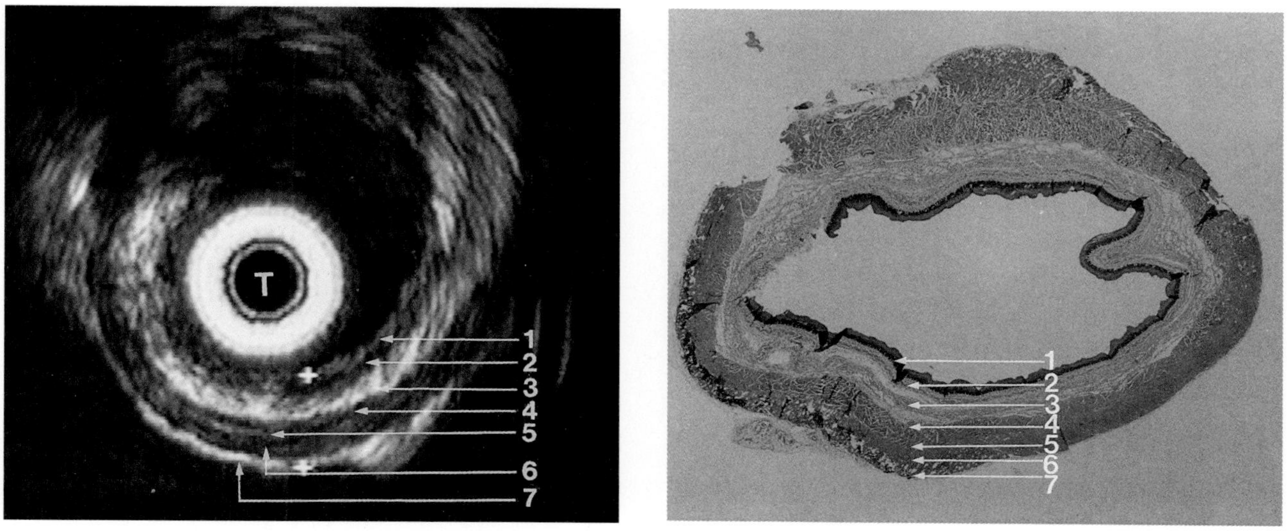

a *b*

Figure 6.29 *(a) The 20-MHz ultrasound transducer (T) located within the saline-distended sheep esophagus delineates seven layers of the esophageal wall. (b) Close correlation between the cross-sectional histologic slice and the ultrasound image in (a) can be seen. 1, squamous epithelium and superficial mucosa; 2, deep mucosa and muscularis mucosa; 3, submucosa; 4, circular smooth muscle; 5, intermuscular connective tissue; 6, longitudinal smooth muscle; 7, adventitia. (Reproduced with permission from Liu et al.[65])*

vitro animal esophagus and in human esophageal autopsy specimens, similar transducers were used in normal human volunteers to see if the findings could be reproduced in vivo. In a human study, a 16 Fr nasogastric tube was introduced transnasally through the esophagus into the stomach, and then an ultrasound catheter was inserted through it into the stomach (Fig. 6.31). By manipulating the nasogastric tube and the ultrasound catheter, it was possible to image the entire esophagus and most of the stomach and duodenum.[65]

In normal volunteers, all of the layers seen in autopsy esophageal specimens were also seen in the in vivo human esophagus. With the esophagus at rest, six layers were seen as in the non-fluid-filled autopsy esophageal specimens. During the swallowing of a 5–10-ml water bolus, seven layers were seen, similar to the fluid-filled autopsy esophageal specimen. In the area of the lower esophageal sphincter (LES), the muscle layers were significantly thicker than the regions above the LES (Fig. 6.32). By using a digital computer analysis system (MicroSonic™, Indianapolis), repetitive measurements could be made of the circular smooth muscle, longitudinal smooth muscle and total muscle thickness in each individual subject (Fig. 6.33). Each muscle layer was significantly thicker at the LES when compared to the same structure 5–10 cm above the LES (Table 6.1). In addition, it was also found that the circular smooth muscle was significantly thicker than the longitudinal smooth muscle, both at the level of the LES and 5–10 cm above it.[65] The area of the LES was consistently round, and the diaphragm was seen in that area as a hypoechoic band just outside the wall of the esophagus (Fig. 6.34). However, in its middle and upper portions, the esophagus was asymmetric. This configuration appeared to be due to compression from various periesophageal structures. The esophageal submucosa was consistently brighter (hyperechoic) in the area just below the upper esophageal sphincter than at the LES. This may be due to the increased number of glands found in the submucosa in that area (Fig. 6.35).

The upper esophageal sphincter forms a slit-like tonically contracted segment in the upper esophagus. With swallowing, this segment can be seen to immediately relax, allowing the bolus through, and then to immediately contract once again. Average pressures measured in the anterior and posterior upper esophageal sphincter far exceed pressures

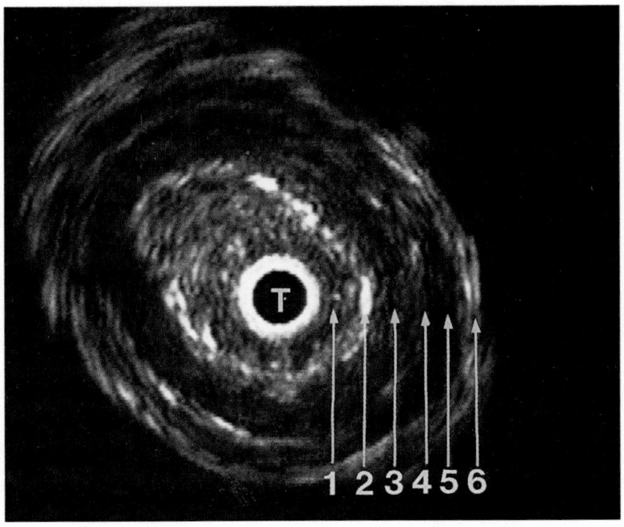

a

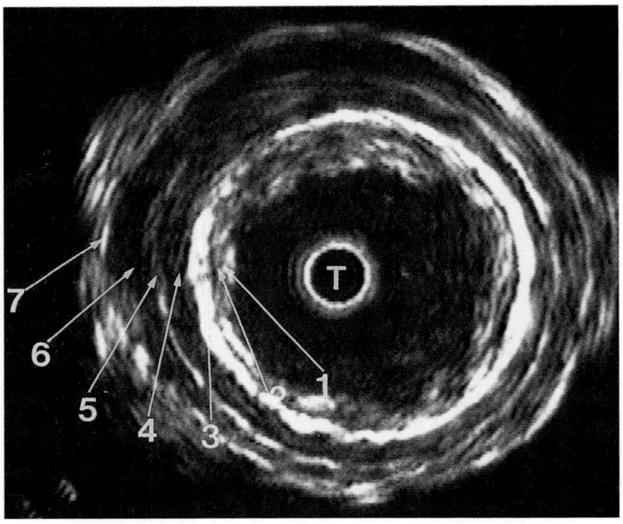

b

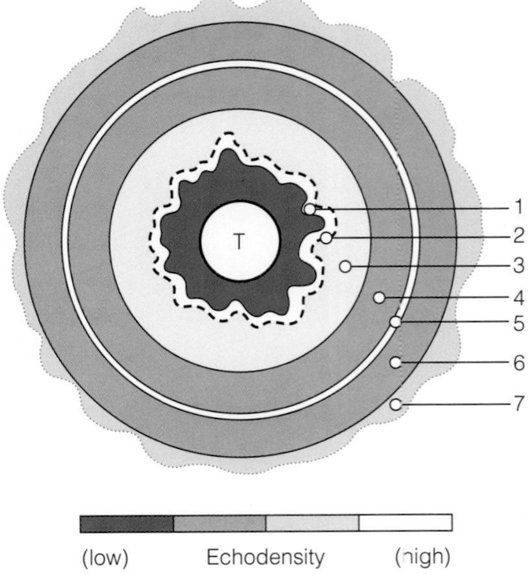

c

Figure 6.30 *(a) The 20-MHz ultrasound transducer (T) located within the non-fluid-filled human specimen esophagus delineates six layers of the esophageal wall. 1, mucosa; 2, submucosa; 3, circular smooth muscle; 4, intermuscular connective tissue; 5, longitudinal smooth muscle; 6, adventitia. (b) With same specimen filled with a fluid, seven layers of the esophageal wall are identified. (c) Schematic drawing demonstrates the esophageal wall structures in cross-section. In (b) and (c), 1, squamous epithelium and superficial mucosa; 2, deep mucosa and muscularis mucosa; 3, submucosa; 4, circular smooth muscle; 5, intermuscular connective tissue; 6, longitudinal smooth muscle; 7, adventitia.*

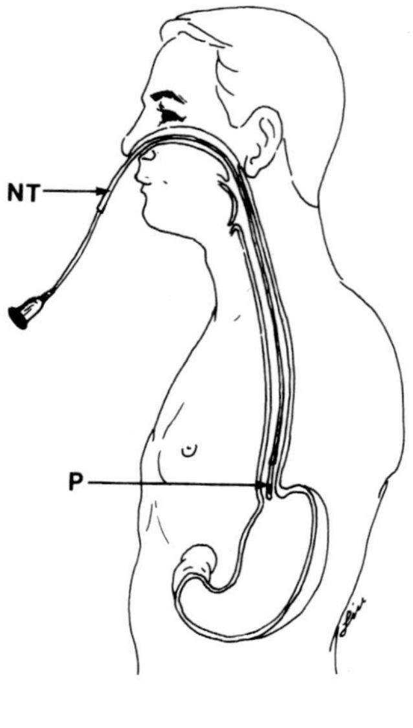

Figure 6.31 *Schematic representation shows the catheter-based ultrasound probe (P) passed transnasally through the nasogastric tube (NT) into the esophagus and stomach. (Reproduced with permission from Liu et al.[65])*

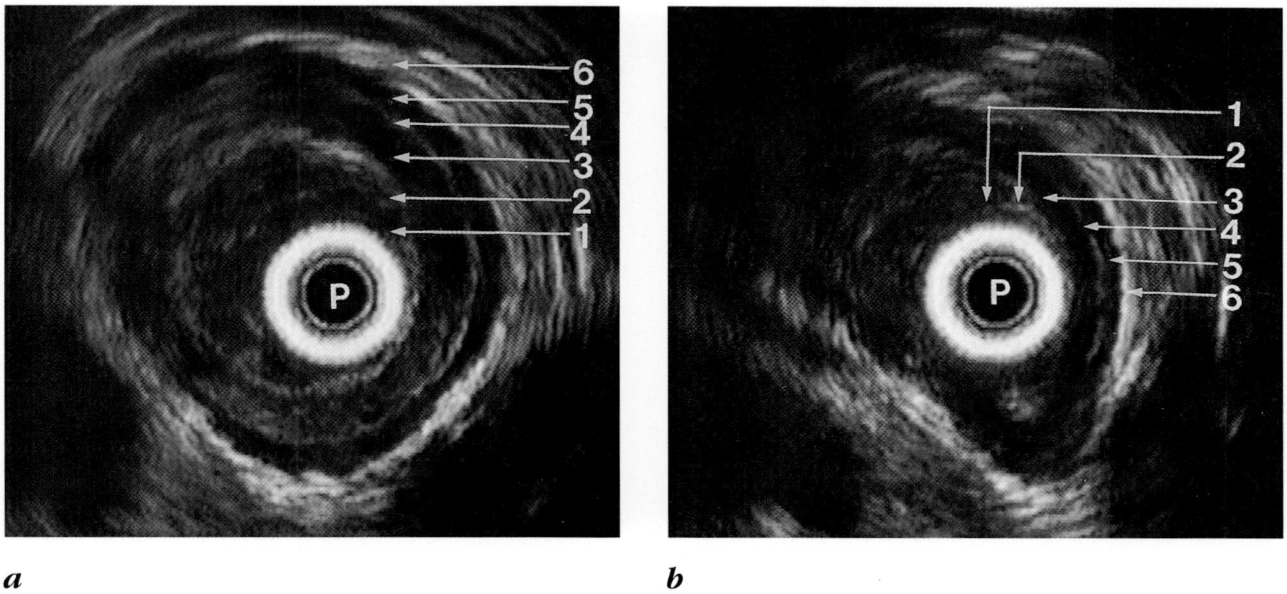

Figure 6.32 *Endoluminal ultrasound transducer (P) positioned within the LES region (a) and 8 cm above the LES (b) in a healthy subject delineates the various normal layers of the esophageal wall. Note that the thicknesses of the muscular layers in the LES region are different from the thicknesses of those in the body of the esophagus. 1, mucosa; 2, submucosa; 3, circular smooth muscle; 4, intermuscular connective tissue; 5, longitudinal smooth muscle; 6, adventitia.*

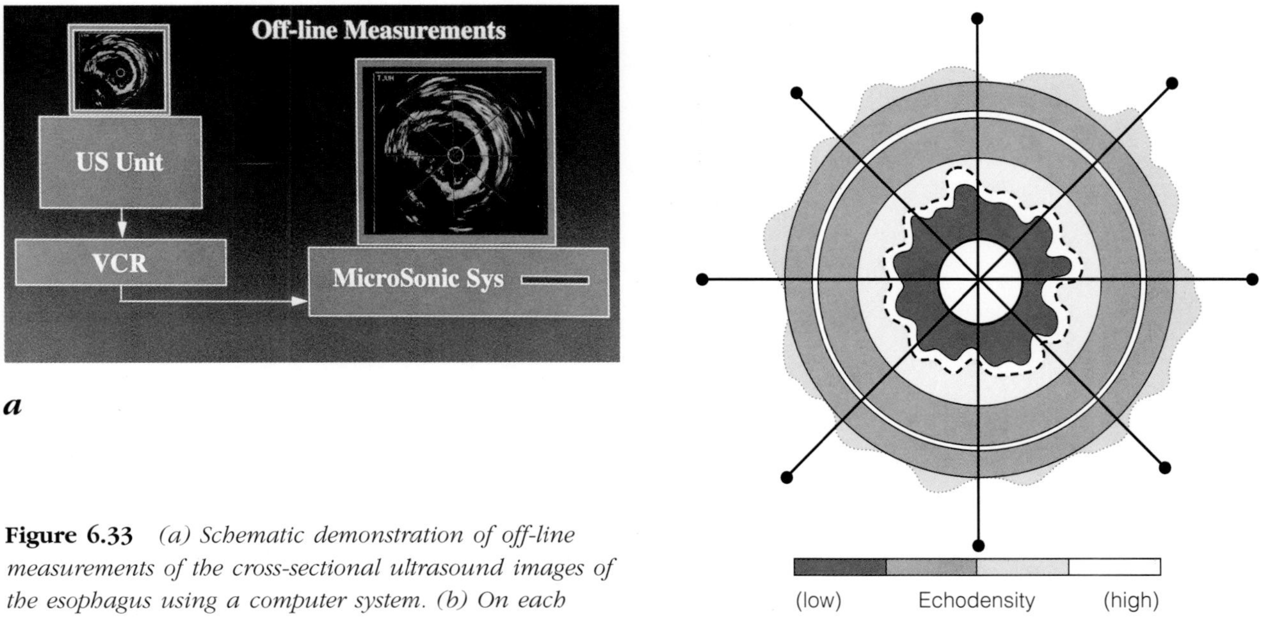

Figure 6.33 *(a) Schematic demonstration of off-line measurements of the cross-sectional ultrasound images of the esophagus using a computer system. (b) On each image, the thickness of each muscle can be measured at eight radial octants.*

Table 6.1 Mean muscle thickness at the lower esophageal sphincter and 5-10 cm above the lower esophageal sphincter (N = 17).

Region	*Circular smooth muscle (cm)*	*Longitudinal smooth muscle (cm)*	*Total width of muscle (cm)*
LES	0.134 ± 0.034	0.079 ± 0.013	0.236 ± 0.046
5–10 cm above LES	0.072 ± 0.026	0.051 ± 0.011	0.130 ± 0.039

Reproduced with permission from Liu et al.[65]

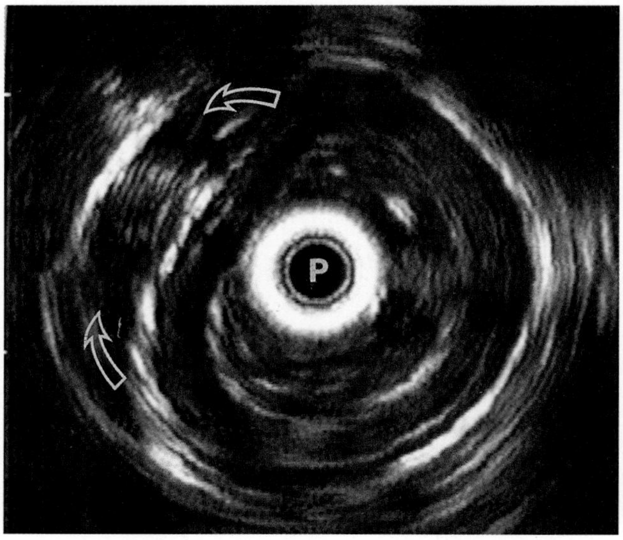

Figure 6.34 *Endoluminal cross-sectional ultrasound image obtained at the gastroesophageal junction shows a hypoechoic region (arrows) adjacent to the esophageal wall, representing the diaphragm. P, probe. (Reproduced with permission from Liu et al.[65])*

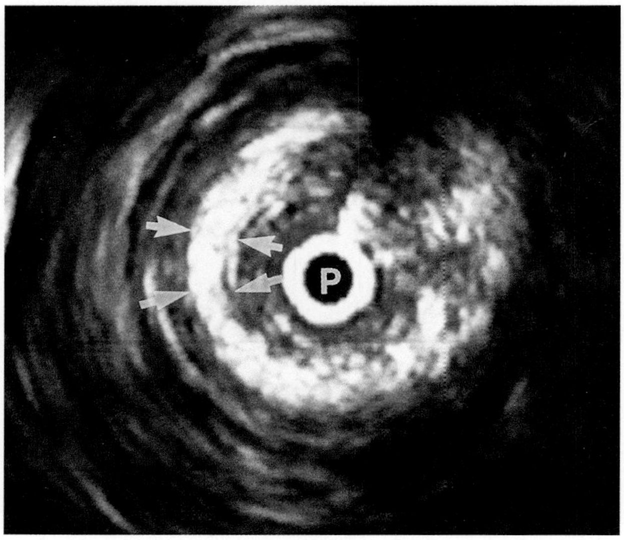

Figure 6.35 *Endoluminal ultrasound image obtained from the area just below the upper esophageal sphincter shows a hypoechoic submucosal appearance (arrows) compared with the submucosa in areas below this level. This may be due to the abundance of submucosa glands in this area.*

measured laterally. This is consistent with the anatomic organization of the upper esophageal sphincter as seen on high-resolution endoluminal sonography (Fig. 6.36). Although the penetration of the transducer was only about 2 cm, it was possible to image some periesophageal structures such as lymph nodes and blood vessels (Fig. 6.37).[65]

Sequential ultrasound imaging has been obtained both at the level of the LES and in the body of the esophagus during swallowing of 5–10 ml boluses of water in normal subjects. Initially, when the lumen of the esophagus was distended, there was an associated decrease in esophageal wall thickness. This was most marked in the two muscular layers. Following the distention, the two smooth muscle layers contracted and the lumen narrowed, resulting in an increased wall thickness. The circular smooth muscle layer also increased in echogenicity during this

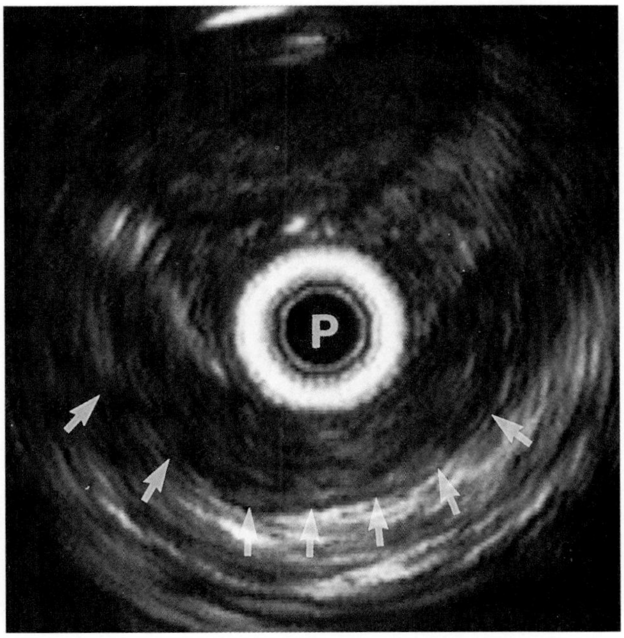

Figure 6.36 *Ultrasound transducer (P) is positioned in the center of the slit-like upper esophageal sphincter. Arrows outline the muscle forming the upper esophageal sphincter. Note the asymmetry of the muscle.*

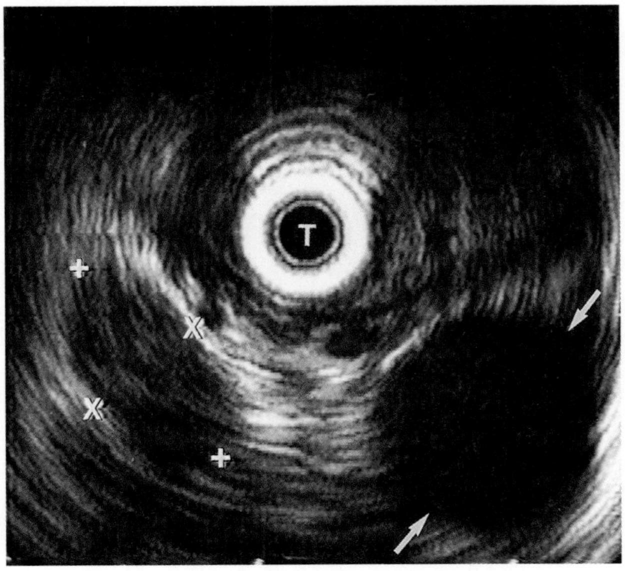

Figure 6.37 *Endoluminal ultrasound transducer (T) located within the distal esophageal lumen shows a hypoechoic structure (cursors), which is a lymph node. The predominantly anechoic area (arrows) is an artery and pulsation can be seen during real-time imaging. (Reproduced with permission from Liu et al.[65])*

phase. Subsequently, the esophagus returned to the resting position (Fig. 6.38).[65]

The stomach and duodenum can also be imaged using a 20-MHz catheter-based ultrasound transducer. In the stomach five layers are visualized, similar to that seen with lower frequency endoscopic ultrasound (Fig. 6.39). The stomach is imaged by having the subject drink 400–600 ml of water, and the transducer is then placed within the water to promote acoustic coupling. By manipulating the transducer and repositioning the subject, most of the stomach can be imaged. The pyloric area of the stomach can be entered and imaged with the ultrasound catheter, with the pyloric sphincter appearing as a markedly thickened muscle layer (Fig. 6.40). In addition, the ultrasound catheter can often be inserted into the proximal duodenum (Fig. 6.41). In the duodenum and pylorus, peristaltic contraction can be seen in real-time imaging.

CLINICAL STUDIES

Once the normal sonographic anatomy of the upper GI tract was defined in vivo using the 20-MHz ultrasound transducer, it was possible to look for abnormalities in patients with various disorders in the upper GI tract.

Achalasia

Achalasia is a motility disorder of the esophagus defined as loss of peristalsis in the body of the esophagus and failure of the LES to relax completely on deglutition. As a consequence, the esophagus may become dilated and filled with food debris and fluid. It is a common cause of dysphagia, nocturnal regurgitation and noncardiac chest pain. More importantly, patients with achalasia are at markedly increased risk of developing esophageal cancer.[69] Characteristic features of achalasia are demonstrated on manometric evaluation (incomplete relaxation of the LES on deglutition and loss of peristalsis) and barium radiography (a dilated esophagus with a symmetrically tapered 'bird-beak' appearance at the LES).

Although endoscopic ultrasound has been used previously to image the area of the LES in patients with achalasia, a number of technical problems have been encountered, resulting in rather inconsistent findings. Four prior studies have used endoscopic ultrasound to examine the esophagus and gastroesophageal (GE) junction in patients with achalasia.

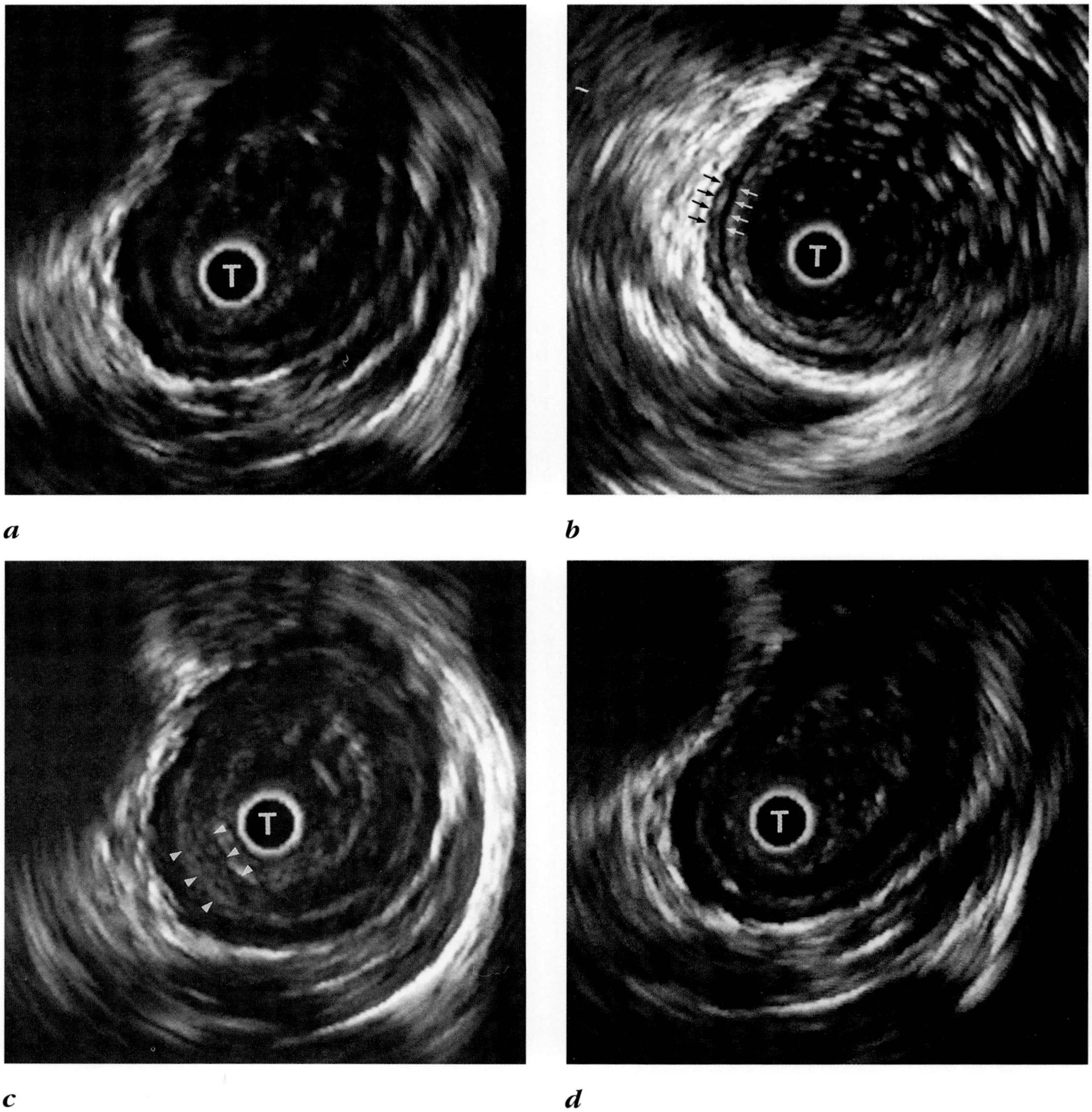

Figure 6.38 *Sequential ultrasound images obtained at the level of the LES demonstrate the swallowing process in a normal subject. (a) Cross-sectional image of the esophagus in its resting state. (b) Image obtained after lumen of the esophagus was distended by the swallowing of 10 ml of water. Note that the two muscle layers have become thinner (arrows) and that all seven layers of the esophageal wall can be identified. (c) Image of peristaltic contraction of the muscular layers associated with increased wall thickness. During peristaltic contraction, the circular muscle layer increases in echogenicity (arrowheads) while the longitudinal muscle layer shows no change. (d) Image of the esophagus following return to its resting state. T, transducer.*

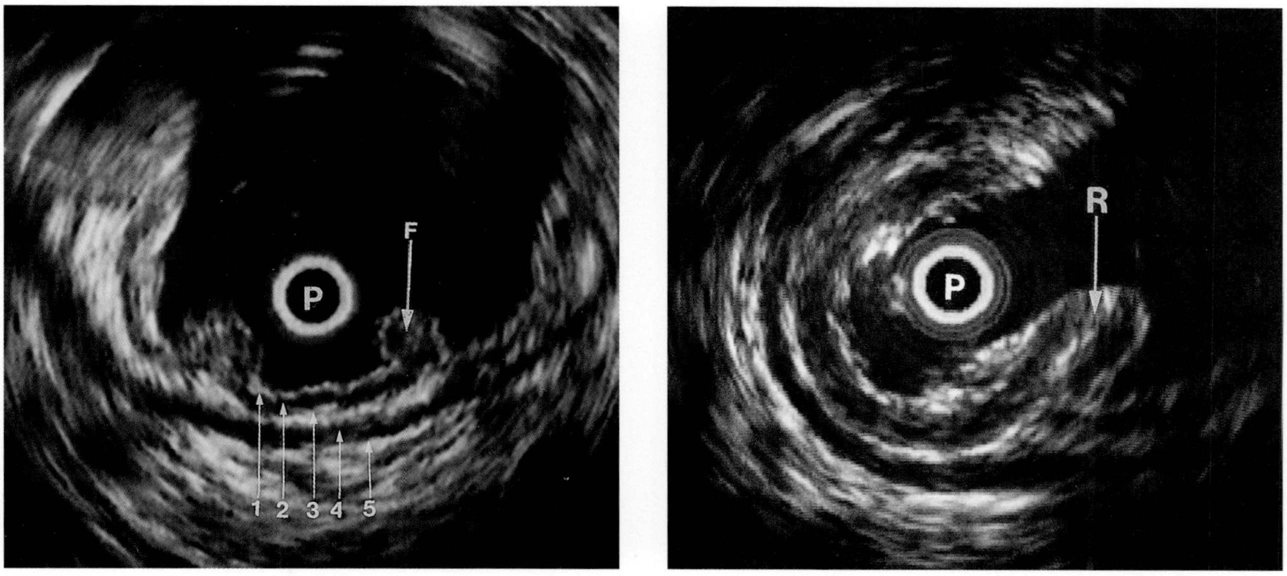

a *b*

Figure 6.39 *(a) Endoluminal ultrasound image obtained from the body of the stomach demonstrates the normal five layers of the gastric wall, which are: 1, the hyperechoic mucosa; 2, hypoechoic deep mucosa and muscularis mucosa; 3, hyperechoic submucosa; 4, hypoechoic muscularis propria; 5, hyperechoic serosa. P, probe; F, fold. (b) This ultrasound image shows the fundus of the stomach in a normal subject. The rugal fold (R) is clearly visualized. P, probe.*

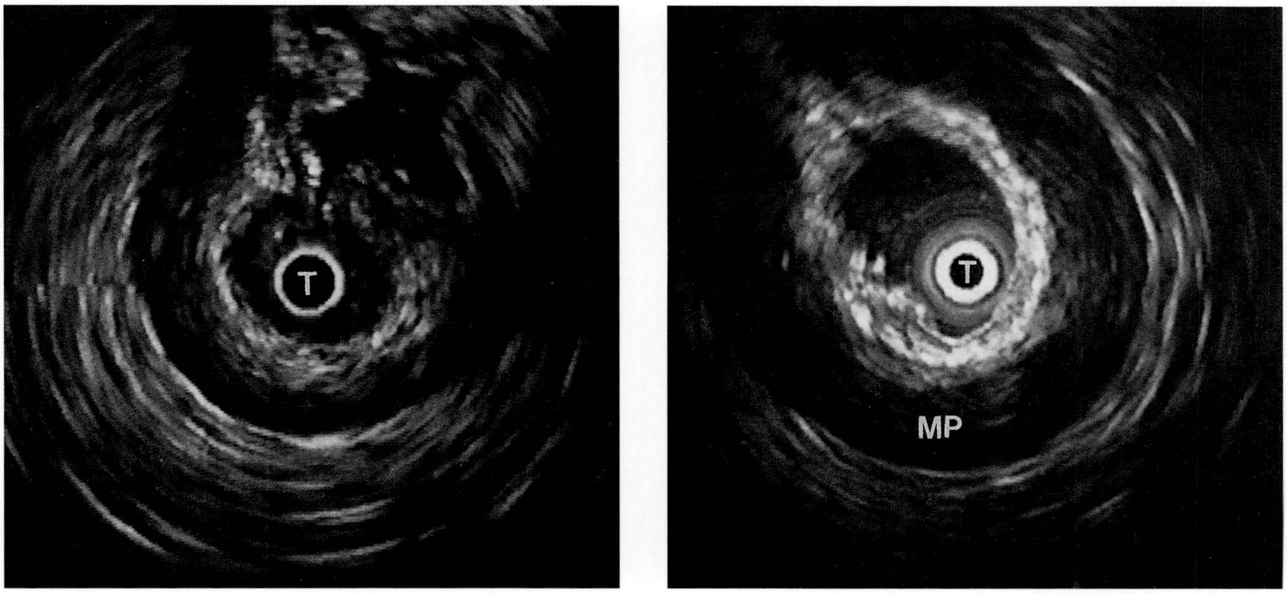

a *b*

Figure 6.40 *The 20-MHz catheter-based ultrasound images obtained from within the pylorus of the stomach (a) and at the level of the pyloric sphincter (b) show five layers of the gastric wall. Note that the muscularis propria (MP) is much thicker in the pylorus area and pyloric sphincter region compared with the muscularis propria in the body of the stomach. T, transducer.*

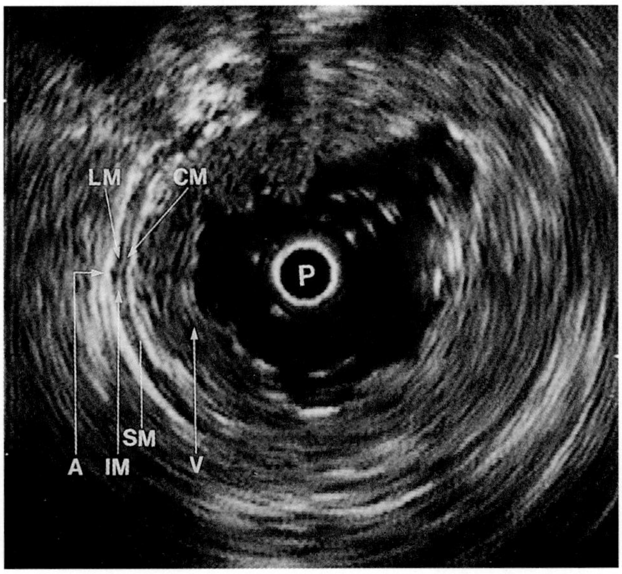

Figure 6.41 *A cross-sectional image obtained from fluid-filled duodenal lumen delineates six layers of the duodenal wall, which are villi (V), submucosa (SM), circular muscle (CM), intermuscular connective tissue (IM), longitudinal muscle (LM), and adventitia (A). P, probe.*

In the first study, Deviere et al[70] examined six patients with known achalasia using the Olympus GFUM 20 7.5-MHz ultrasound endoscope. They demonstrated enlargement of the echolayers corresponding to the muscularis propria in five patients, ranging from 0.8-1.6 cm thick. This was greater than the mean thickness (3 mm) of the esophageal wall demonstrated in 280 other patients without known esophageal pathology. However, because of the relatively low resolution of the transducer and the compressive effect of the balloon around it, the investigators were unable to distinguish between or measure the width of the individual circular smooth muscle and longitudinal smooth muscle components. They were also unable to visualize the intermuscular connective tissue component between these two muscle layers. The same investigators subsequently reported that they had examined several more achalasia patients, thus bringing the total to 14, in whom 9 had enlargement of their muscularis propria.

Ponsot et al[71] found that 5 of 17 patients (31%) with achalasia had a 1–3-mm enlargement of the muscularis propria. There was no correlation between either the duration of dysphagia or the manometric findings and the enlargement of the muscularis propria. They concluded that the enlargement of the muscularis propria detected by endoscopic ultrasound was only slight and not a consistent feature in achalasia. In another study, Ziegler et al[72] evaluated 16 patients suspected of having achalasia using a prototype linear-array ultrasonic probe (Siemens, West Germany), which had a 7.5-MHz transducer fixed to the tip of a Pentax FG28 gastroscope. Fifteen of these patients had normal endoscopic ultrasound appearance of the wall of the GE junction without hypertrophy of the smooth muscle layer. In the remaining case, endoscopic ultrasound detected an intramural tumor.

Trowers et al[73] used the high-frequency Fuginon Sonoprobe to evaluate the muscle thickness in patients with achalasia. The probe was 150–180 cm in length with a diameter of 2.6 mm, and a linear compound B-mode scanner was used with an ultrasound frequency of 20 MHz. It was used to evaluate the histologic layers of the esophagus in six achalasia patients and six normal controls. As a group, the achalasia patients showed an increased thickness of the muscularis propria. The investigators reported that achalasia patients had muscle thicknesses significantly greater than two standard deviations above normal and that the greatest thickness was in the inner circular muscle layer.

We have used the EndoSound 20-MHz transducer to evaluate the width of various muscle layers at the GE junction in normal volunteers and patients with achalasia.[65,74] The resolution achieved with this 20-MHz ultrasound transducer is superior to that obtained with the other transducers, because the ultrasound transducer makes contact with the mucus and water layer on the mucosal surface at the LES. Therefore, acoustic coupling is accomplished without a water-filled balloon around the transducer which can compress the wall of the esophagus and distort the native anatomy of the esophagus. Because the esophagus above the LES is usually markedly dilated, acoustic coupling can be accomplished only in the area of the LES. To perform this high-resolution endoluminal sound (HRES) above the LES, water must be placed into the esophageal lumen. With the relatively high resolution of these endoluminal transducers, each component muscle layer at the LES could be imaged and measured quite accurately.

Table 6.2 Muscle thickness measurements at the LES in achalasia patients (N = 8).

	Maximum (cm)	*Minimum (cm)*	*Mean ± SD (cm)*
CSM	0.600	0.187	0.339 ± 0.161
LSM	0.145	0.092	0.119 ± 0.020
TM	0.783	0.333	0.496 ± 0.180

CSM, circular smooth muscle; LSM, longitudinal smooth muscle; TM, total muscle.
Reproduced with permission from Liu et al.[65]

In order to resolve the issue of whether or not the muscularis propria layers at the LES were thickened, the muscle width was measured in a baseline resting state at the LES. This was accomplished by leaving the transducer at the level of the LES for a considerable length of time and making sure that the patient did not swallow during this period. Tangential artifacts were excluded by moving the transducer within the LES to a position where the thicknesses of the muscularis propria layers were symmetrically equal circumferentially around the transducer.

This in vivo study demonstrated that the mean width of the muscle layers was increased in achalasia patients when compared to normal controls (Table 6.2) (Fig. 6.42). Although there was a statistically significant increase in thickness at the LES, there was also an overlap in the muscle width thicknesses between achalasia patients and controls. Therefore, a thickened muscularis propria cannot be used to clinically diagnose achalasia. Upon retrospective review of clinical, manometric and radiographic data, achalasia patients with marked thickening of the muscularis propria could not be differentiated from achalasia patients without this muscular thickening. In addition, the response to the swallowing of a 10-ml water bolus in the control group was compared with the swallowing response in the achalasia patients. Distention of the lumen at the LES in the achalasia patients was only 5–30% of that in the control group. The water did not completely pass through the LES into the stomach; a portion was retained in the dilated esophagus proximal to the LES (Fig. 6.43). Air above this fluid level resulted in gas artifact. Furthermore, the typical peristaltic contraction seen in control subjects was absent in the dilated segment of the esophagus in achalasia patients.[65]

Esophageal imaging with lower-frequency transducers that have less resolution does not allow for precise measurements of the width of the muscularis propria layer. In addition, component muscle layers cannot be differentiated and measured individually. The larger size of the lower-frequency transducers and the fact that they are surrounded by a water-filled balloon can cause compression artifact, thus distorting the width of the muscularis propria at the LES. These limitations may explain the previous conflicting results observed in achalasia patients. The fact that a 20-MHz catheter is so small, is not surrounded by a balloon and has much better resolution allows for more precise measurement of the layers of the muscularis propria at the LES in achalasia.

Schiano et al[75] have employed HRES to determine how much wall damage occurs at the GE junction after both pneumatic dilation and injection of botulinum toxin in the treatment of achalasia. The HRES transducer was passed through the biopsy channel of a standard 34 Fr endoscope to the level of the GE junction. The layers of the esophageal wall were imaged before, immediately after, and 24 h after pneumatic dilation or intrasphincteric injection of botulinum toxin. Measurement of the thicknesses of the mucosa/submucosa and the circular smooth muscle (CSM) and longitudinal smooth muscle (LSM) layers at the level of the diaphragm were made before and after treatment.

In this study, HRES revealed similar pretreatment mucosa/submucosa diameter thicknesses for botulinum toxin injection and pneumatic dilation patients, respectively. These were similar to those seen in normal controls. There was a significant increase in the mucosa/submucosa diameter thickness of the esophageal wall immediately after pneumatic dilation and no significant difference in the mucosa/submucosa after botulinum toxin injection. The increase in mucosa/submucosa diameter thickness was diffuse after pneumatic dilation, consistent with edema and/or hematoma formation (Fig. 6.44). The twofold increase in the mucosa/submucosa diameter and cross-sectional surface area in pneumatic dilation patients normalized within 24 h, indicating a transient traumatic insult. In addition, there was no statistically significant change in the thickness or character of the muscle layers immediately after either botulinum toxin injection or pneumatic dilation, or at 24 h posttreatment. In comparing the subjective symptomatic response to the objective HRES measurements, no correlation was found between the improvement in symptoms and

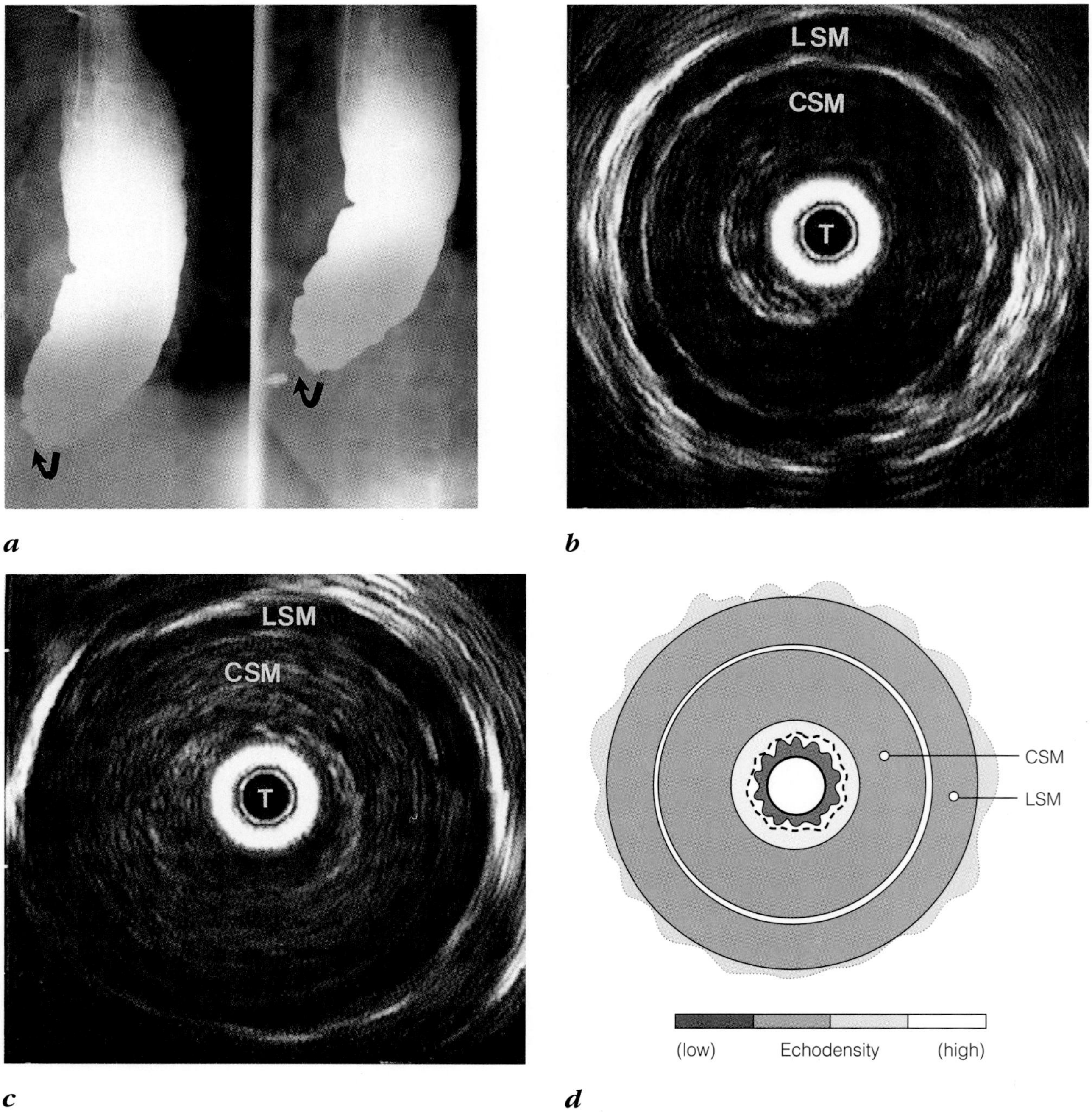

Figure 6.42 *(a) In a patient with advanced achalasia, barium study shows dilated, aperistaltic esophagus with a narrowing at the gastroesophageal junction (curved arrows). (b) Transnasal esophageal ultrasound demonstrates increased thickness of the two muscular layers in the LES region. Note that the circular smooth muscle (CSM) is much thicker than the longitudinal smooth muscle (LSM). (c) In another achalasia patient, endoluminal ultrasound demonstrates increased thickness of the two muscular layers with consistent CSM contraction even in the resting stage. (d) Schematic illustration of ultrasound appearance in achalasia. T, transducer. (6.42b reproduced with permission from Liu et al.[65])*

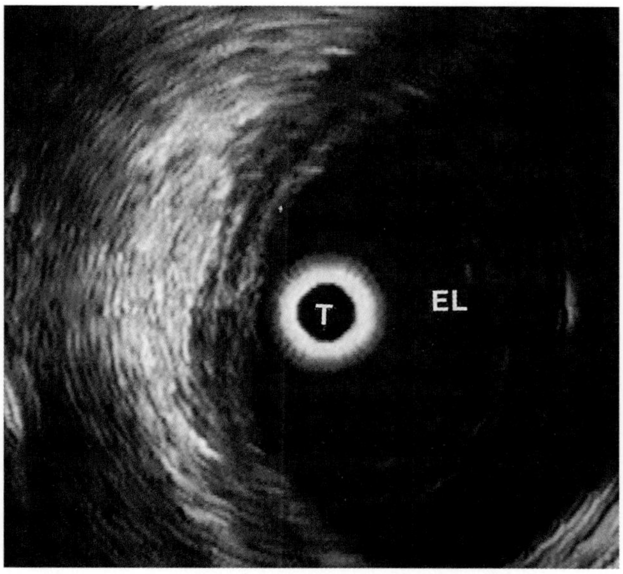

Figure 6.43 *Endoluminal ultrasound transducer (T) located within the esophageal lumen demonstrates a dilated esophagus (EL) filled with fluid proximal to the LES in a patient with achalasia.*

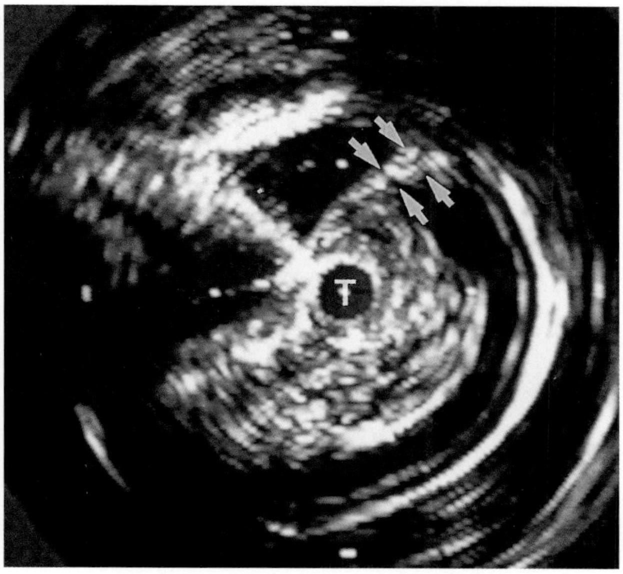

Figure 6.45 *Endoluminal ultrasound image obtained at the level of the LES demonstrates a hyperechoic disruption of the muscle layers (arrows) corresponding to scar after Heller cardiomyotomy. T, transducer.*

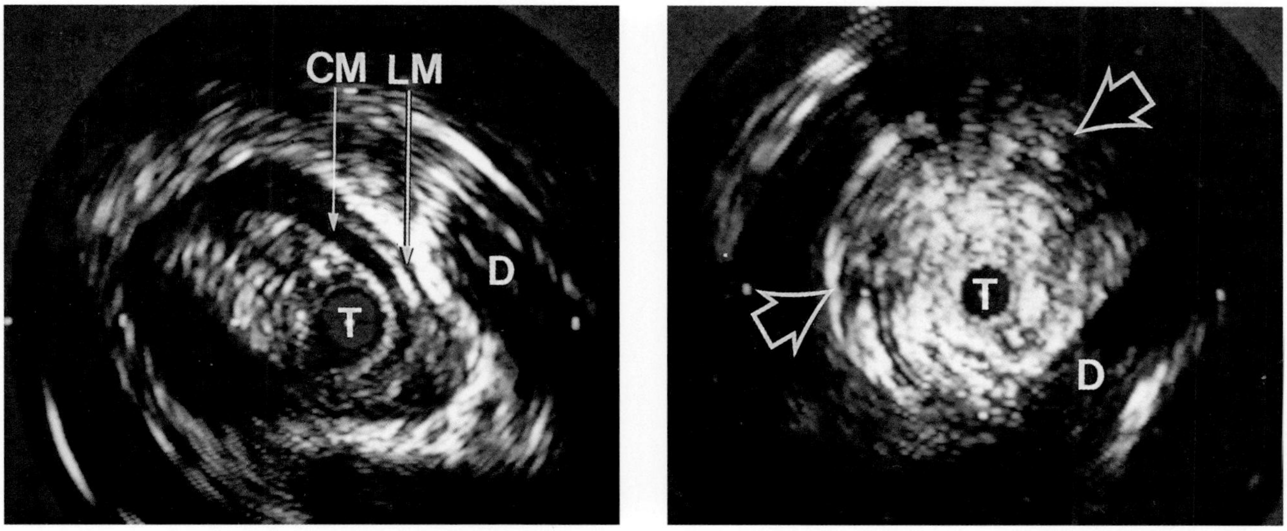

a ***b***

Figure 6.44 *Before pneumatic dilation. (a) The transducer (T) is at the level of the diaphragm (D) and the LES made up of the circular smooth muscle (CM) and longitudinal smooth muscle (LM). Note that the mucosa/submucosa is bordered by the inner aspect of the CM. (b) After pneumatic dilation, the transducer remains at the same level in the LES but the mucosa/submucosa has expanded (arrows) in cross-sectional area. This is consistent with edema, inflammation and hemorrhage.*

the change in the submucosal thickness of the esophageal wall post-pneumatic dilation.

Muscle fibrosis and other postoperative changes can be seen in achalasia patients after Heller cardiomyotomy (Fig. 6.45). The mucosa/submucosa appears normal, but the muscle layers are disrupted by hyperechogenicity, consistent with scar tissue formation from the myotomy.

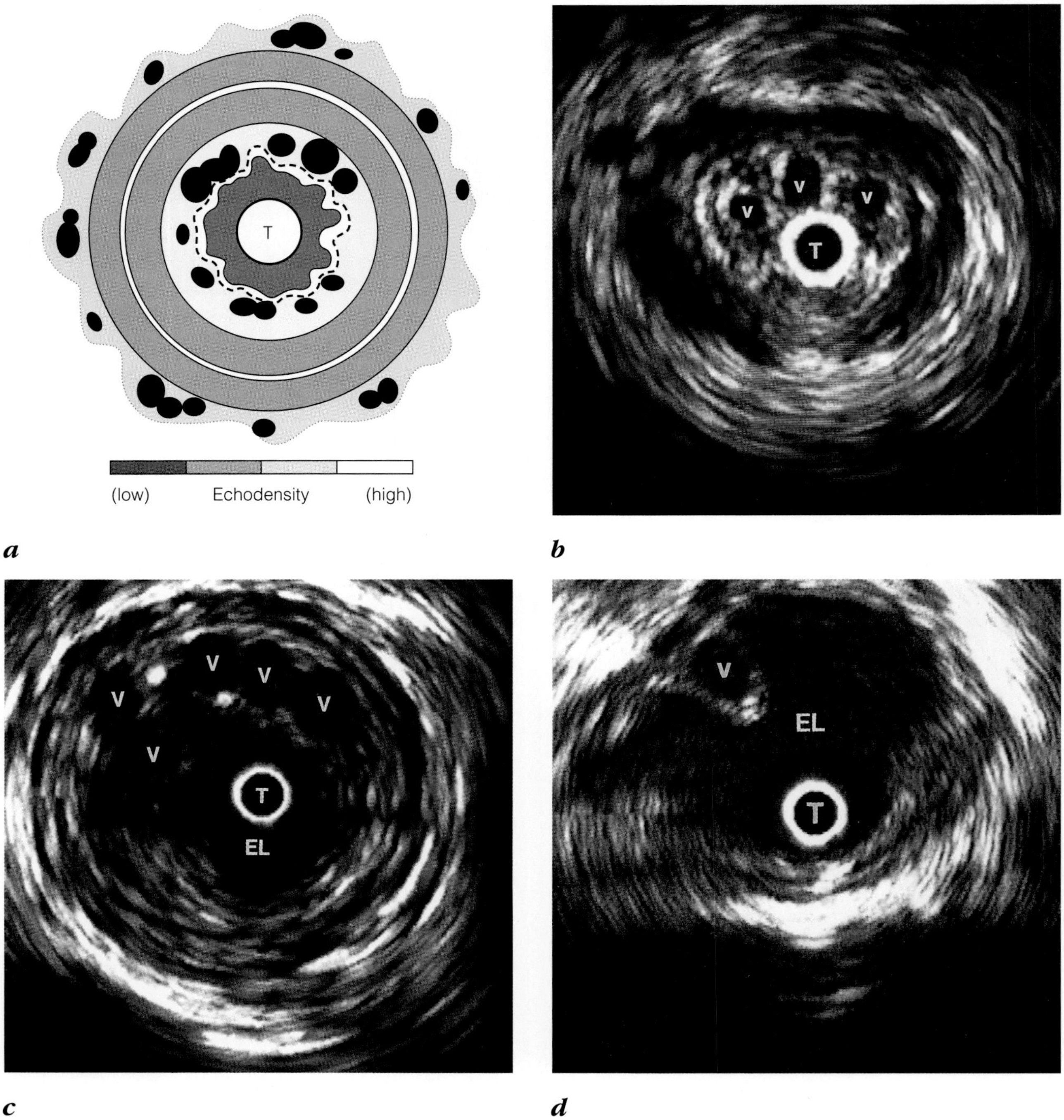

Figure 6.46 *(a) Schematic representation of endoluminal ultrasound image of esophageal varices. In a patient with portal hypertension, transnasal ultrasound image demonstrates esophageal varices appearing as anechoic areas within the submucosa as demonstrated in upper (b), middle (c), lower (d) portions of the esophagus. T, transducer; V, varices; EL, esophageal lumen.*

Esophageal and Gastric Varices

Esophageal and gastric varices result from transmission of portal venous pressure through the coronary (left gastric) vein into the periesophageal and perigastric venous plexus. Blood can then travel retrogradely through the azygos system to the superior vena cava and, finally, into the right atrium, decompressing the portal system. There are several methods with which to evaluate esophagogastric varices; barium swallow radiography has been the traditional method. Dilated submucosal veins appear as serpiginous filling defects in the distal esophagus and cardia of the stomach. However, despite careful attention to detail and use of various modifications in the technique, the diagnostic accuracy of barium swallow examination for varices has remained low.[76–78] Percutaneous transhepatic portography provides the best anatomic definition of varices and collateral circulation, but it is a highly invasive and a technically complex procedure that has a high complication rate. Although some reports reveal a close correlation between findings at endoscopy and those at radiography, the outcomes of most comparative studies indicate that results at endoscopy are superior to results at radiography for recognition of varices unless the varices are large.[79,80] However, even endoscopy has a high interobserver variability.

Endoscopic ultrasound has been used to evaluate esophagogastric varices and periesophageal collateral veins.[81,82] Prior studies using a lower-frequency transducer by Caletti et al[83] found that esophageal varices were seen by endoscopic ultrasound in only half of patients in which varices were demonstrated by endoscopy. In Caletti's study,[83] endoscopic ultrasound demonstrated varices in only 14% of the patients with endoscopic (EGD) grade 1 esophageal varices, 78% of patients with grade 2 varices, and 50% of patients with grade 3 varices. In addition, periesophageal varices were demonstrated by endoscopic ultrasound in 57% of grade 1 varices, 89% of grade 2 varices, and all patients with grade 3 varices. Endoscopic ultrasound was felt to be inferior to EGD in detecting and grading esophageal varices ($P < 0.0005$), but superior in the detection of varices in the gastric fundus ($P < 0.0005$).

To overcome the limitations of the current endoscopic ultrasound technology, we have used a miniature 20-MHz catheter-based transducer to image and quantify esophageal and gastric varices. Esophageal and gastric varices as well as periesophageal and perigastric varices can be clearly imaged with this technique (Figs. 6.46–6.50). On cross-sectional ultrasound images, varices appear as multiple serpiginous anechoic structures. In some cases, perforating vessels were seen communicating between the periesophageal and submucosal varices. Because of the higher resolution and lack of compression of the varices by the catheter-based transducer, submucosal varices in the esophagus are well delineated, and their size can be precisely measured. Interobserver variation between two investigators for measurements of the largest esophageal varix in each patients had r values of 0.99 for diameter, 0.99 for cross-sectional surface area, and 0.98 for circumference. It was found that, compared to HRES, video-endoscopy had a sensitivity of 48% and a specificity of 50% for the detection of gastric varices, and a sensitivity of 94% and a specificity of 17% for the detection of esophageal varices. The inability to define the presence or absence of gastric varices is probably due to the endoscopist's inability to discriminate between varices and normal gastric folds.[84]

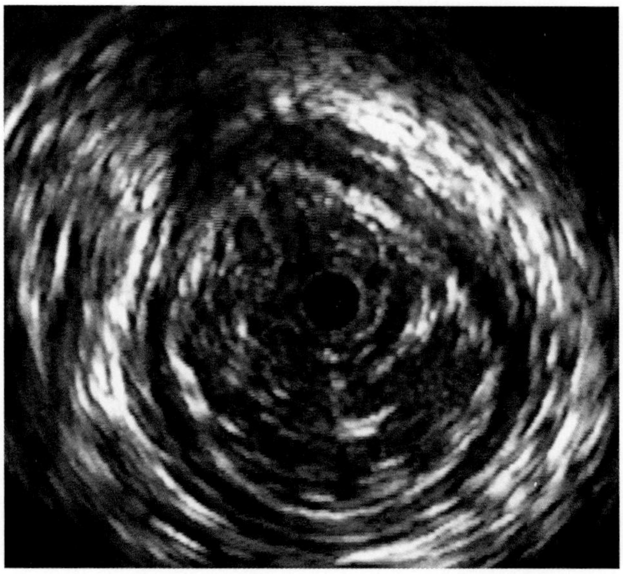

Figure 6.47 *In this case, esophageal varices appear as mixed-echoic areas within the submucosa, representing red cell reflections in the slow-motion flow of the varices.*

There are three reasons why HRES appears to be better than conventional endoscopic ultrasound in quantifying the size of esophageal varices: the higher-frequency (20 MHz) ultrasound imaging

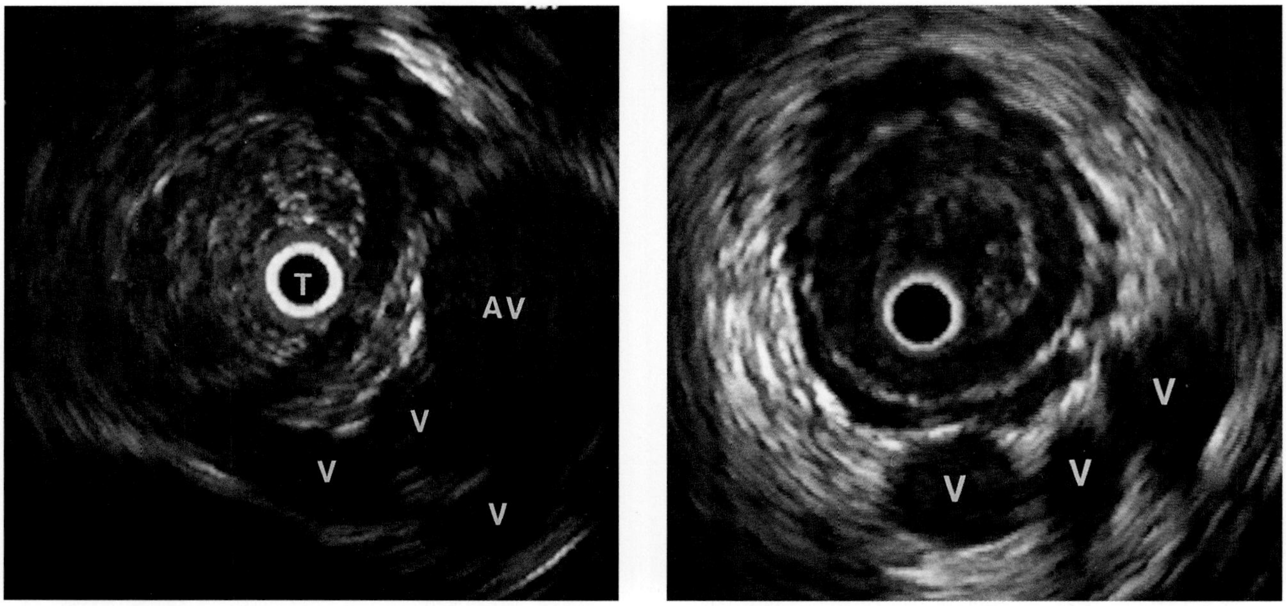

a *b*

Figure 6.48 *In a patient with portal hypertension, endoluminal ultrasound image demonstrates the dilated azygos vein (AV) (a) and periesophageal varices (V) (b) outside the wall of the esophagus. T, transducer.*

allows for improved resolution of submucosal structures, there is no water-filled balloon around the transducer to distort the anatomy of the esophagus and varix, and the catheter-based transducer itself is so small that it does not distort the size or shape of the varix.

Miller et al[85] used HRES to compare the size of esophageal varices at and 5 cm above the esophageal high-pressure zone. HRES was performed in 36 patients with esophageal varices using a 20-MHz, 6.2 Fr transducer passed through an endoscope and used to image esophageal varices as it was slowly withdrawn through the high-pressure zone (the level at which the diaphragm was imaged) and into the body of the esophagus. The mean, total and percentage of cross-sectional surface area occupied by varices was calculated and then compared at and 5 cm above the esophageal high pressure zone (Fig. 6.51).

Six patients (17%) were found to have no varices imaged at the high-pressure zone, but did have varices imaged in the distal esophagus. The mean cross-sectional surface area per varix at the high-pressure zone (0.036 ± 0.006 cm^2) was significantly less than that 5 cm above it (0.142 ± 0.018 cm^2) ($P \leq 0.0001$). The average total cross-sectional surface area occupied by varices at the high-pressure zone (0.137 ± 0.034 cm^2) was significantly less than the average 5 cm above it (0.672 ± 0.080 cm^2) ($P \leq 0.0001$). The mean percentage esophageal wall cross-sectional surface area occupied by varices at the high pressure zone (16%) was significantly less than that 5 cm above it (49%) ($P \leq 0.0001$). These findings suggest that it might be possible to use HRES to observe modifications of variceal size with pharmacologic intervention directed at the esophageal high-pressure zone.

Several clinical and endoscopic parameters have been associated with the identification of patients at risk for variceal bleeding. It has been suggested that the risk of variceal bleeding increases with variceal size, and that the actual rupture of a varix depends on its wall tension. Theoretically, the Laplace equation ($T = p_t \times r/w$) can be used to determine the wall tension of a varix in the esophagus based on the measurement of three separate variables (p_t, r, w): T = wall tension, p_t = transmural pressure between

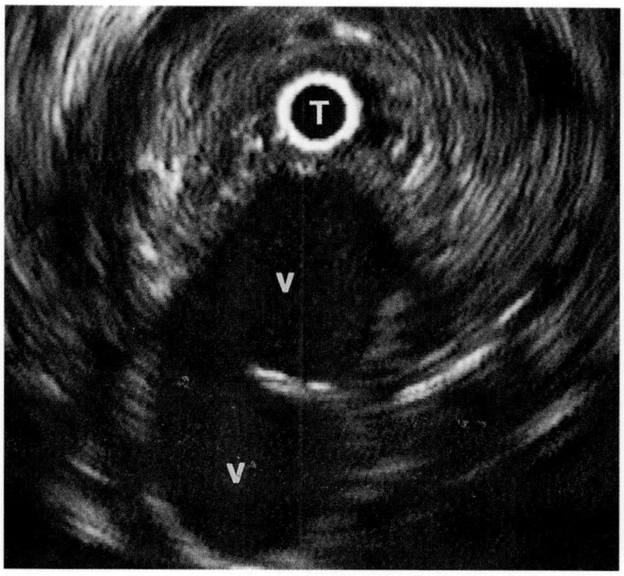

a

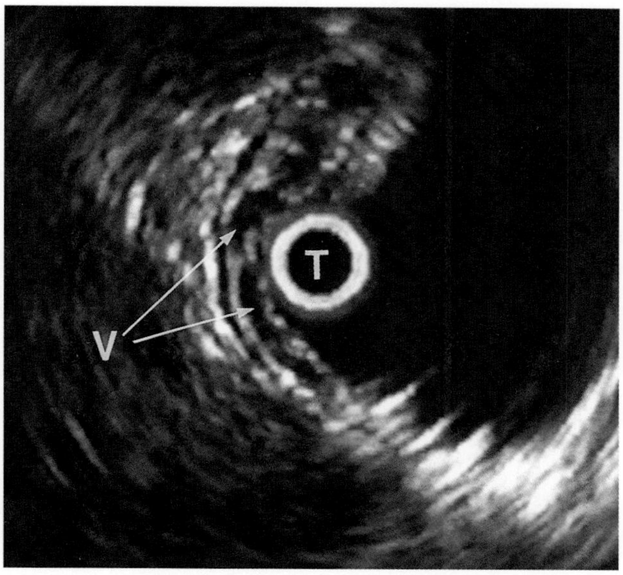

b

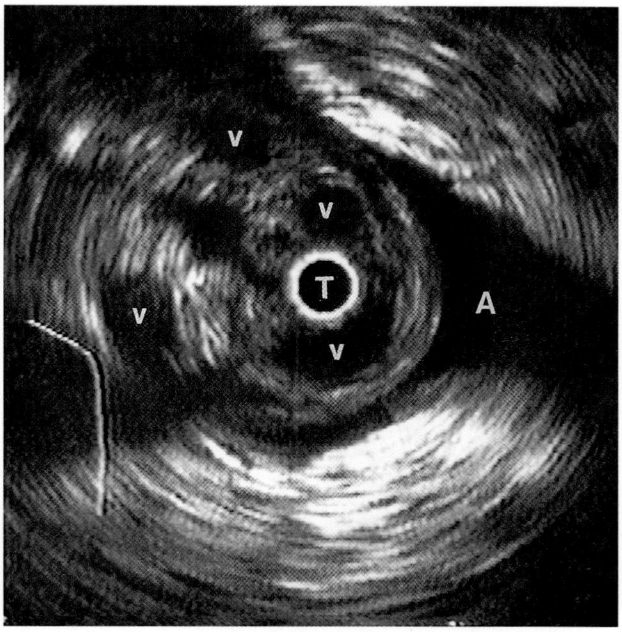

c

Figure 6.49 *Endoluminal ultrasound images obtained in patients with portal hypertension demonstrate multiple anechoic varices (V) within the submucosa of the stomach. Some small varices, such as in (b), may not be detected by endoscopy. Ascites (A) can also be seen through the gastric wall in (c). T, transducer.*

the varix and the esophageal lumen, r = radius of the varix, and w = wall thickness of the varix. To date, only p_t has been measured in vivo, and no method has been found to accurately measure or calculate r or w.

Miller et al[86] sought to evaluate esophageal variceal radius and wall thickness in an attempt to derive and correlate the two previously undetermined variables of the Laplace equation. Water was placed into the esophageal lumen through the biopsy channel of an endoscope to distend the esophagus. Using HRES, all measurements were made at a cross-section of the varix where the varix appeared circular, in order to avoid tangential imaging (Fig. 6.52). Multiple varices

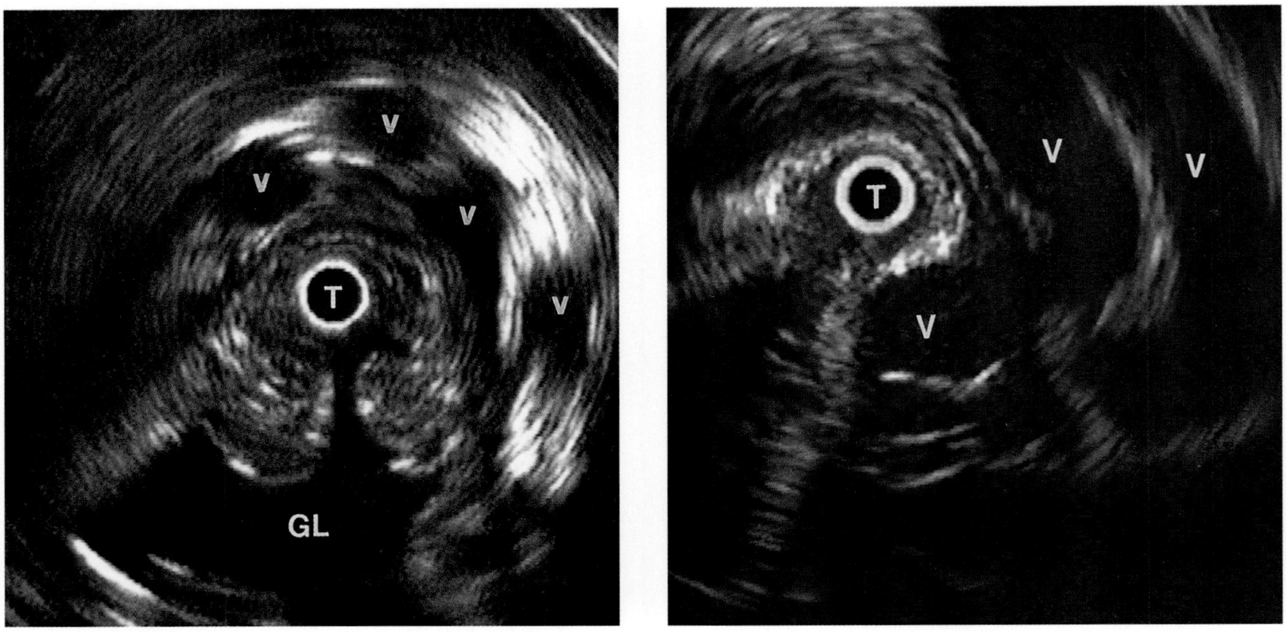

a *b*

Figure 6.50 *Perigastric varices (V) can be visualized as anechoic round or tubular areas just outside of the wall of the stomach. T, transducer; V, varices; GL, gastric lumen. (Reproduced with permission from Liu et al.*[65]*)*

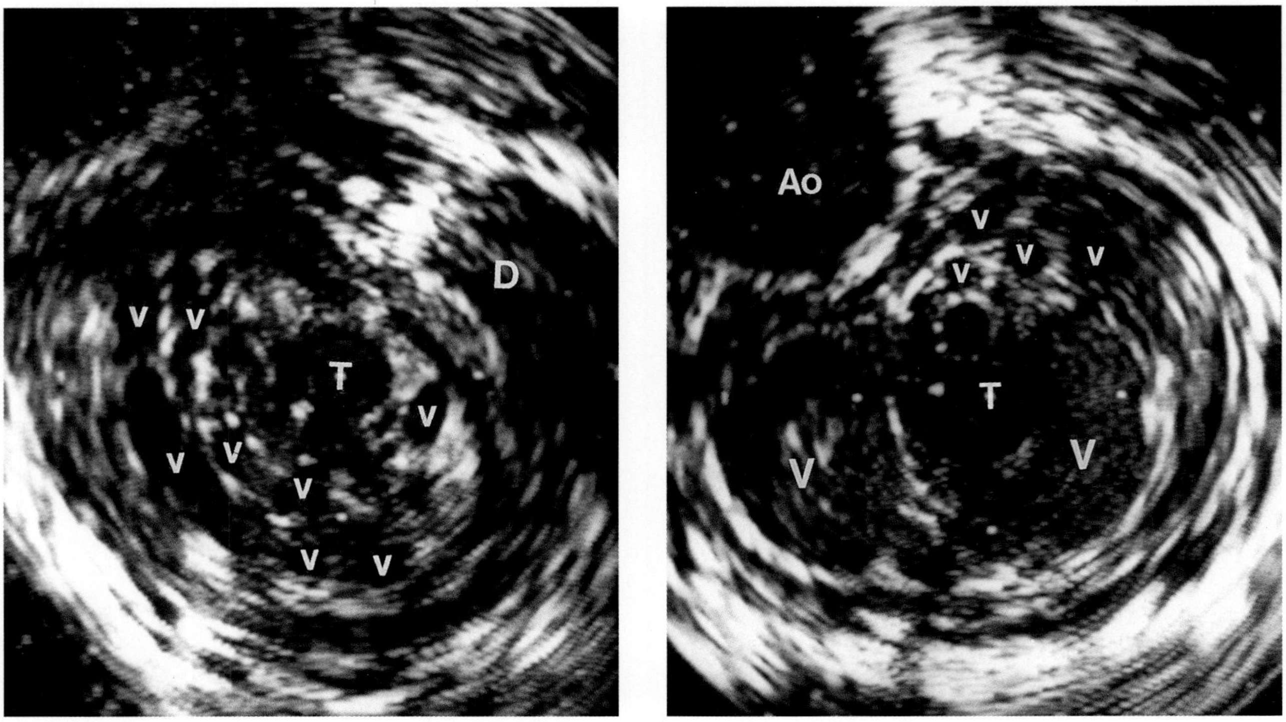

a *b*

Figure 6.51 *Endoluminal ultrasound images obtained from patient with portal hypertension. (a) Varices (V) at the high-pressure zone in the distal esophagus appear small. This is due to the intrinsic anatomy of the varices at this level as well as to compression due to the lower esophageal sphincter and diaphragm (D). (b) Varices (V) above the high-pressure zone appear much larger. T, transducer; Ao, aorta.*

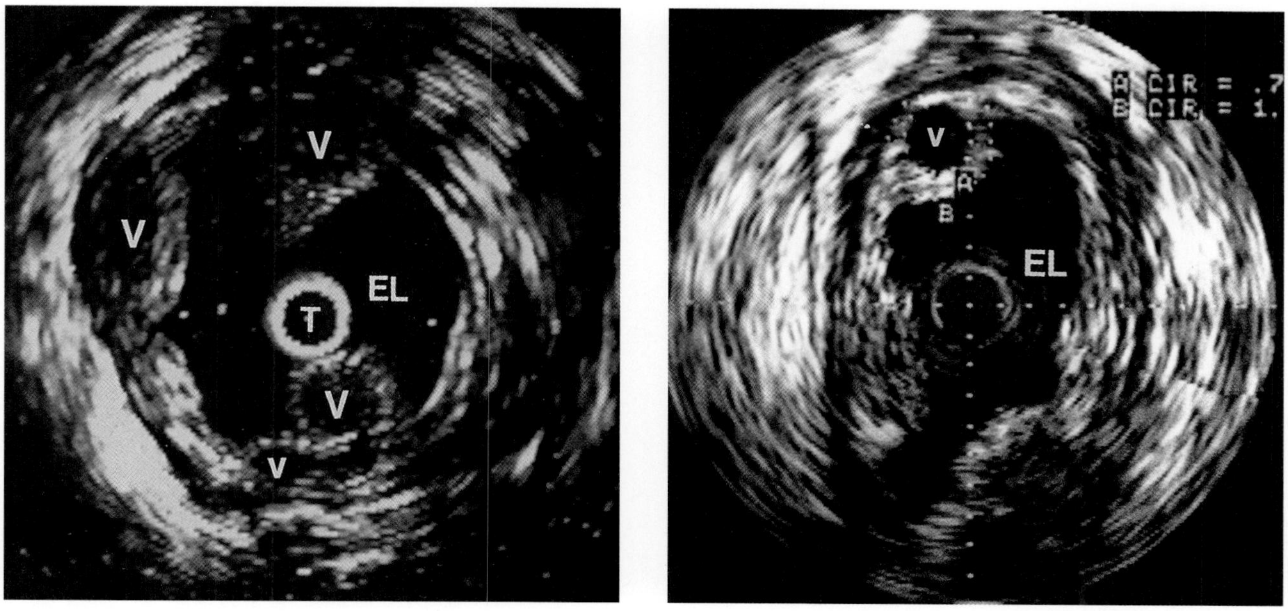

a *b*

Figure 6.52 *(a) The hypoechoic variceal lumen (V) can be clearly seen surrounded by the hyperechoic wall of the varix. (b) The esophageal lumen (EL) is distended with water in order to image the hyperechoic walls of the varices (V). The inner and outer variceal circumferences can be measured and the wall thickness of the varix can be calculated. In this case the inner circumference is 0.74 cm and the outer circumference is 1.13 cm. T, transducer.*

were imaged at different levels of the esophagus in each of 36 patients. Measurement of the outer (C_o) and inner (C_i) circumference of the varices was made. The outer circumference was measured at the border between the hypoechoic fluid-filled esophageal lumen and the hyperechoic mucosa where the varix protruded into the esophageal lumen. In the intramural portion of the varix, the outer circumference was measured at the border between the hyperechoic submucosa and hypoechoic muscularis propria. The inner circumference was measured at the border of the hypoechoic blood-filled variceal lumen and hyperechoic inner wall of the varix (Fig. 6.52). The radius of each varix was calculated using the formula $r = C_o/2\pi$. The variceal wall thickness (w) was then calculated using the formula $w = (C_o - C_i)/2\pi$.

All normal controls were identified by HRES as not having varices. Varices in the patients with portal hypertension appear as hypoechoic fluid-filled, round structures within the hyperechoic submucosa. The varices protrude into the hypoechoic fluid-filled esophageal lumen.

This study demonstrated that variceal size (radius) and variceal wall thickness can be measured directly using HRES. Furthermore, there was no direct correlation found between variceal size and variceal wall thickness. This lack of correlation implies that variceal wall tension cannot be accurately estimated by endoscopic observation of variceal size alone or even by size measurements combined with intravariceal pressure measurements. These findings have important clinical implications. The direct measurement of variceal wall tension may allow for the prediction of impending variceal bleeding, thus allowing for non-emergent intervention. Endoscopic sclerotherapy or band ligation can be undertaken, beta-blockers and/or nitrates can be started, or their pre-existing doses can be increased.

HRES was used by Miller et al[87] to image and measure esophageal varices in controls and patients with portal hypertension and compared with endoscopic findings. Nine control patients and 68 patients with known cirrhosis or non-cirrhotic portal hypertension underwent videotaped HRES and videotaped esophagoscopy (EGD). Two blinded

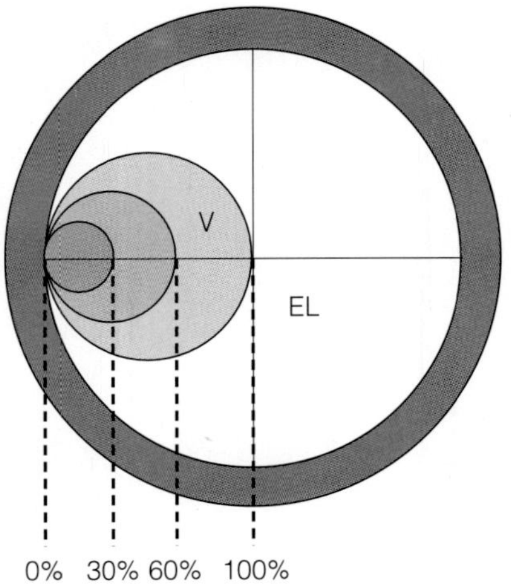

Figure 6.53 *A schematic illustration of the percentage of variceal size for endoscopic grading. Grade I, 0%; grade II, varices present but flatter with air insufflation (not shown); Grade III, 1-30%; grade IV: 31–60%; grade, V: 61–100%. EL, esophageal lumen; V, varix.*

investigators reviewed the videotapes to determine the presence and size of the largest esophageal varix in each patient. The largest varix by HRES was measured with the esophagus at rest at a point where the varix appeared most circular. The largest varix seen on EGD was graded on a five-point scale: grade I = no varices; grade II = varices present but flatten with air insufflation; grade III = varices 0–30% of the radius of the esophageal lumen; grade IV varices = 31–60% of the radius of the lumen; and grade V varices = 61–100% of the radius of the lumen (Fig. 6.53). All nine of the control patients were correctly identified by both EGD and HRES as grade I (no varices). Eight of the ten patients with no varices seen on EGD had varices identified by HRES. The interobserver correlation for HRES was $r = 0.88$ and for EGD was $r = 0.79$. The correlation between EGD and HRES was $r = 0.50$. HRES was found to be a more accurate, sensitive and reproducible imaging modality than esophagoscopy for the detection and sizing of esophageal varices. There was poor correlation between sonographic measurement and endoscopic grading of esophageal varices. Assessment of esophageal variceal presence and the measurement of variceal size by HRES is an accurate and reproducible method of determining the size of esophageal varices.

Thus, HRES may be more capable than EGD of detecting esophageal varices at an earlier stage of development. This information might allow for the earlier initiation of prophylactic beta-blocker therapy and for a more accurate assessment of objective response to other treatments undertaken to decrease variceal size (e.g. transjugular intrahepatic portosystemic shunt (TIPS)).

There are many potential clinical applications using HRES in the setting of portal hypertension. We have used this technology to determine the size of esophageal varices pre- and post-TIPS and to compare the results with those of endoscopy (Fig. 6.54). Although there were changes seen with both endoscopy and HRES, a statistically significant change was seen only with HRES. We have also used HRES to follow patients during sclerotherapy to determine the patency of the varices (Fig. 6.55) and to image the stomach for the presence or absence of gastric varices when endoscopy is equivocal. Hematocystic spots, which are red blister-like lesions seen endoscopically on varices, predict which patients will bleed from esophageal varices. These lesions can be seen sonographically as an aneurysmal dilation of the varix (Fig. 6.56). HRES is also sensitive for imaging portal gastropathy, in which very small varices in the submucosa of the stomach cannot be visualized at endoscopy (Fig. 6.57).

We have experienced no complications due to placement of the nasogastric tube or ultrasound catheter. However, we believe that caution is advised in blindly placing nasogastric tubes in patients with varices so as not to disrupt the varices and cause bleeding during the procedure.

In conclusion, the unique capabilities of transnasal endoluminal ultrasound make this new imaging modality an important supplement to endoscopic visualization of esophagogastric varices. This technique may become the new standard of reference for quantitative studies of varices in the upper GI tract.

Scleroderma

Scleroderma is a generalized connective tissue disorder characterized by fibrosis and microvascular obliteration in the skin, GI tract, lung, heart, and kidneys. The esophagus is the most frequent GI tract organ affected in scleroderma, with involvement usually accompanied by significant clinical symptomatology

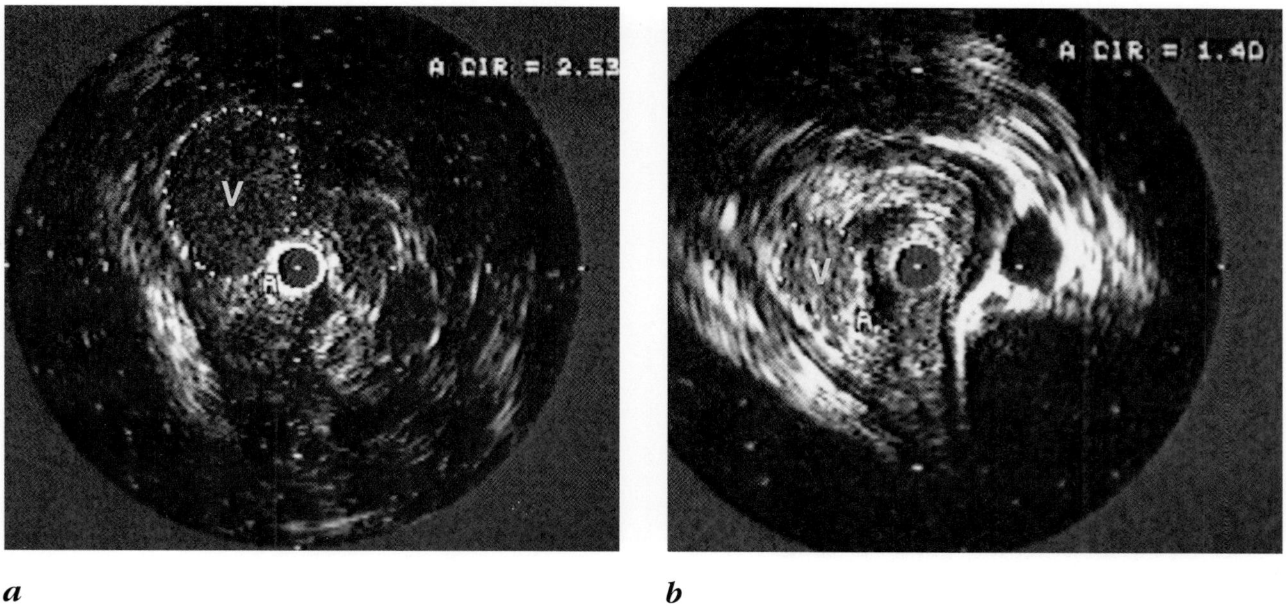

Figure 6.54 *(a) This endoluminal ultrasound image obtained before the TIPS demonstrated a largest varix (V) with circumference measurement of 2.53 cm. (b) In the same patient, the measurement of the largest varix (V) of 1.40 cm was obtained after TIPS.*

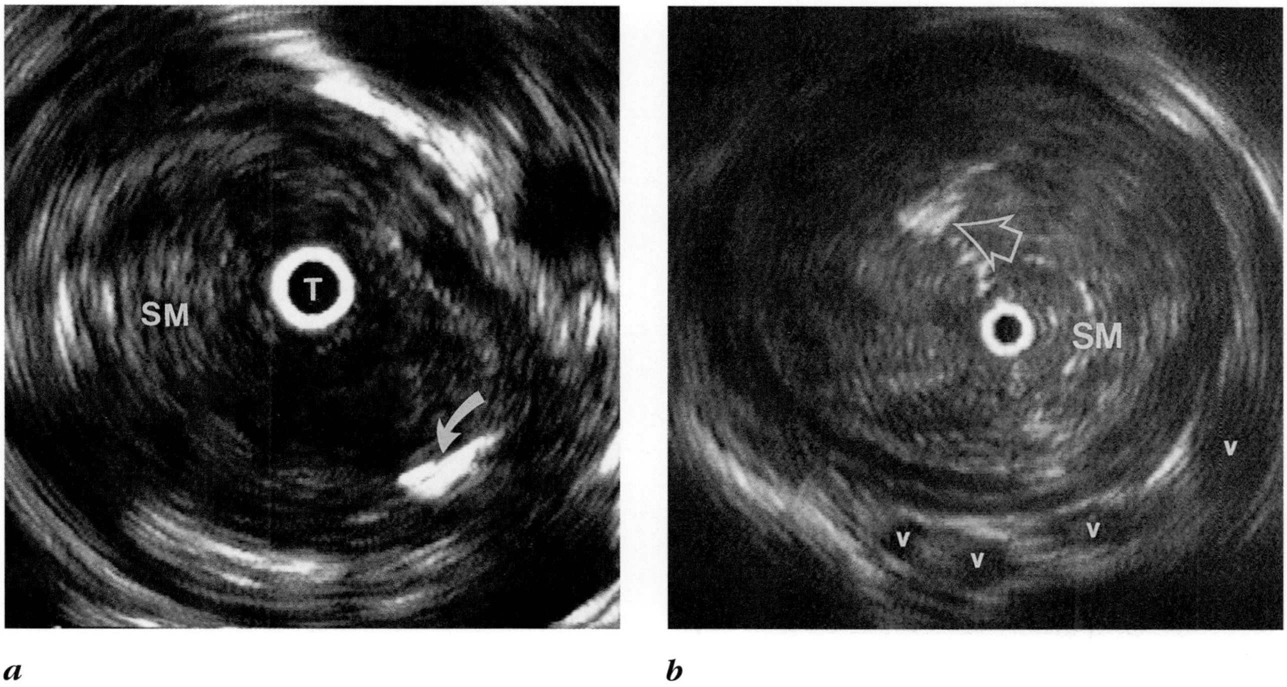

Figure 6.55 *(a,b) These endoluminal ultrasound images were obtained in patients who had undergone previous sclerotherapy. Bright reflective echoes (arrows) within the thickened submucosa (SM) are seen at the site of injection. Periesophageal varices (V) can still be seen adjacent to the wall of the esophagus. T, transducer.*

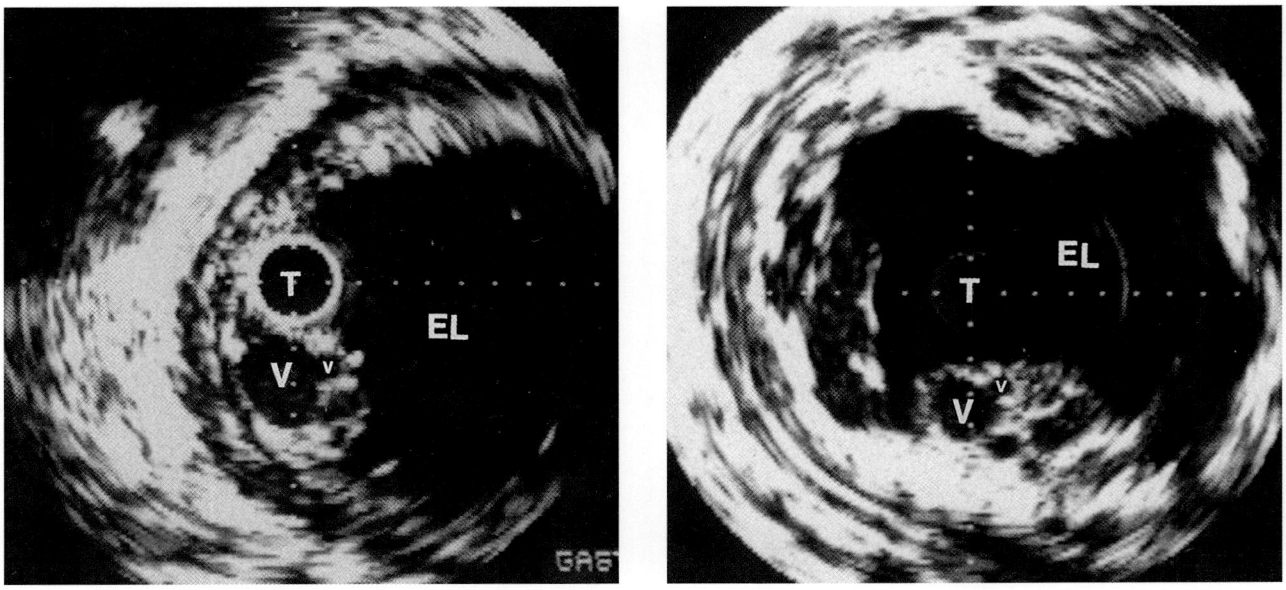

a *b*

Figure 6.56 *(a, b) Hematocystic spots, which are red blister-like lesions seen endoscopically on varices, have been demonstrated sonographically as an aneurysmal dilation of the varix. T, transducer; V, varix; EL, esophageal lumen.*

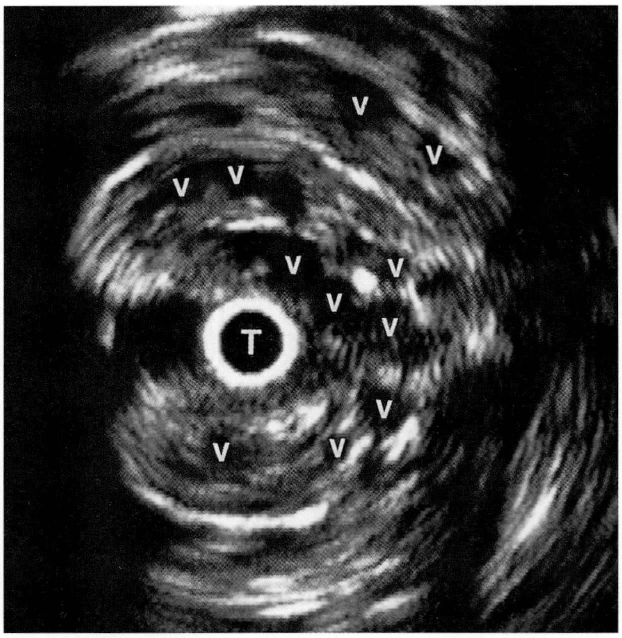

Figure 6.57 *Endoluminal ultrasound image demonstrates very small varices (V) in the submucosa of the stomach in patient with portal gastropathy. Endoscopically this appears as a red, inflamed cobblestone mucosa but small vessels cannot be seen endoscopically. (Reproduced with permission from Liu et al.[84])*

and subsequent morbidity. In another HRES study, Miller et al[88] correlated esophageal autopsy specimens histologically and sonographically from patients with scleroderma and with those of non-scleroderma patients. The esophagi of normal controls and scleroderma patients were then evaluated in vivo using HRES to determine whether or not there were HRES abnormalities consistent with the HRES images of the autopsy specimens. The degree of ultrasound abnormality seen in the scleroderma patients was then quantified and compared to esophageal manometric findings.

A hyperechoic abnormality was seen in the normally hypoechoic muscularis propria in specimens obtained from patients with scleroderma that was not detected in specimens from patients who died of non-esophageal-related diseases (Fig. 6.58). This hyperechoic abnormality correlated with the presence of fibrosis in histologic sections from these autopsy specimens (Fig. 6.59). Similar hyperechoic abnormalities (fibrosis) were seen in most patients with scleroderma, whereas no hyperechoic abnormalities were seen in the normal volunteers (Fig. 6.60). These hyperechoic abnormalities were graded using the following ultrasound grading system: grade 1 = normal appearing, no fibrosis (hyperechoic abnormalities) of the muscularis propria; grade

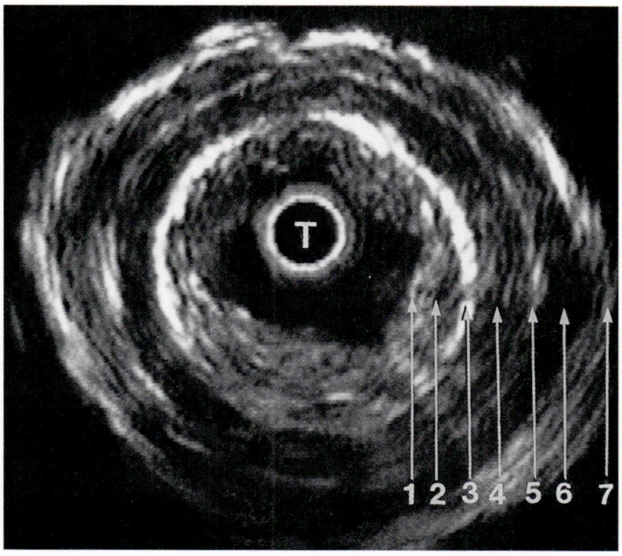

a

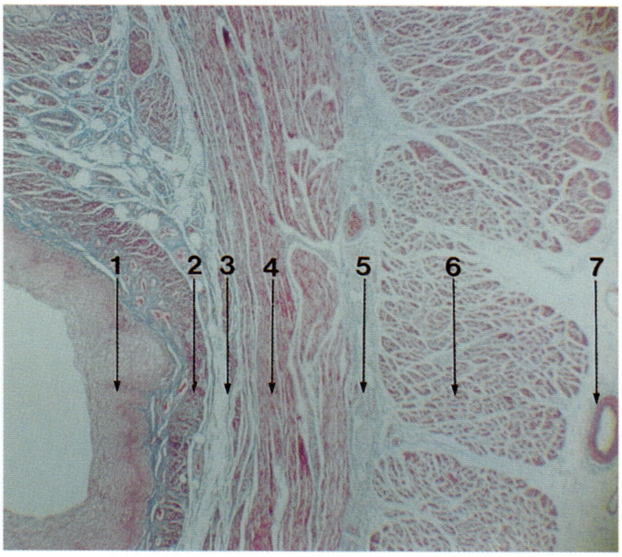

b

Figure 6.58 *(a) Cross-sectional ultrasound image from the postmortem esophagus in a patient who died of non-GI-related disease shows the seven layers of the esophageal wall. (b) Histologic section, stained with Masson's trichome stain, from the postmortem esophagus of the same patient and area seen in (a). 1, squamous epithelium and superficial mucosa; 2, deep mucosa and muscularis mucosa; 3, submucosa; 4, circular smooth muscle; 5, intermuscular connective tissue; 6, longitudinal smooth muscle; 7, adventitia. T, transducer.*

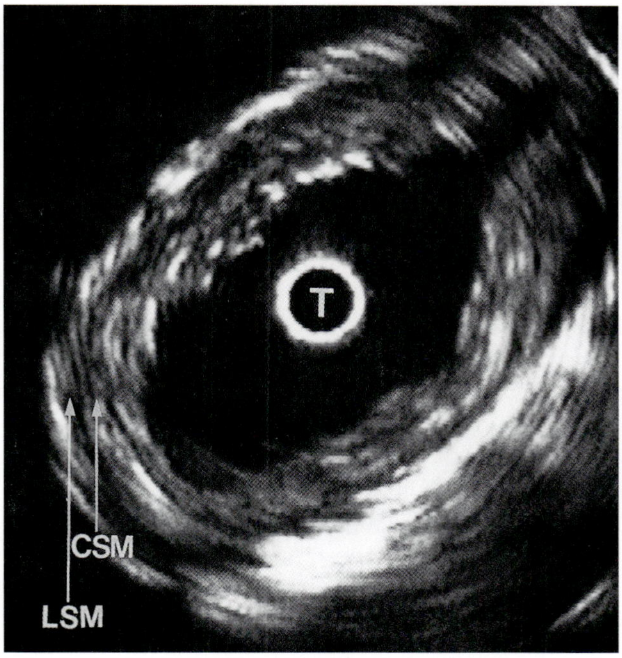

a

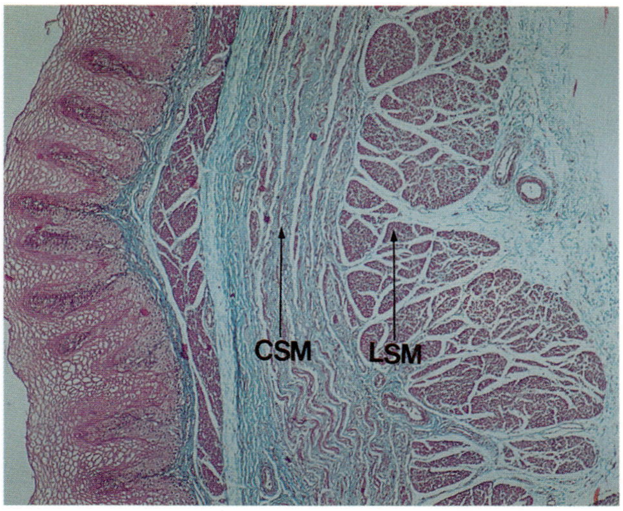

b

Figure 6.59 *(a) A cross-sectional ultrasound image of the esophagus in a patient with scleroderma demonstrates a hyperechoic abnormality (fibrosis) completely obliterating the circular smooth muscle (CSM) and partially obliterating the longitudinal smooth muscle (LSM). T, transducer. (b) This esophageal histologic section with Masson's stain was taken from the same level as in (a). There is marked fibrosis (blue) obliterating the circular smooth muscle (CSM). However, the longitudinal smooth muscle (LSM) remains relatively well-preserved.*

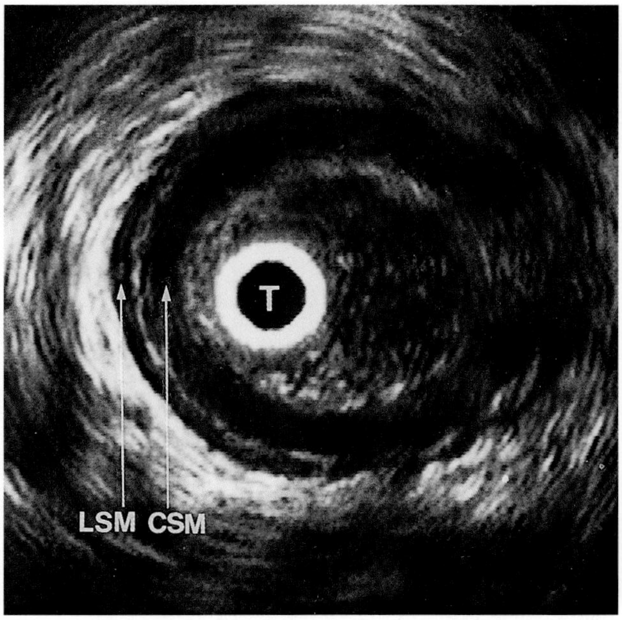

a

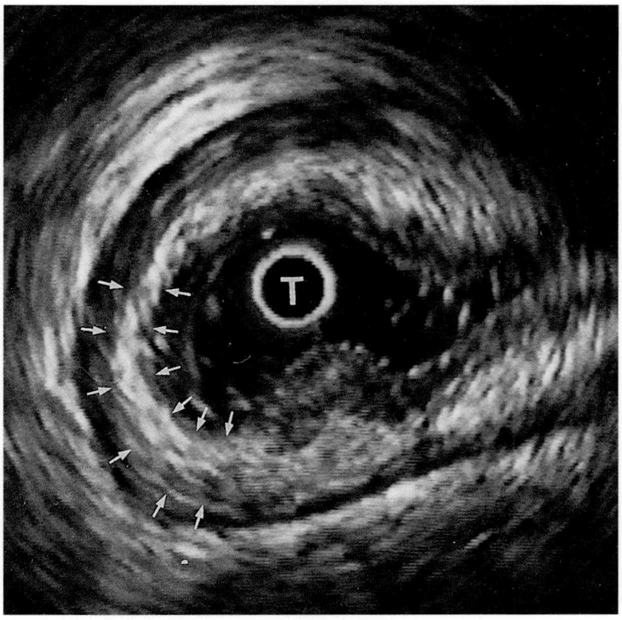

b

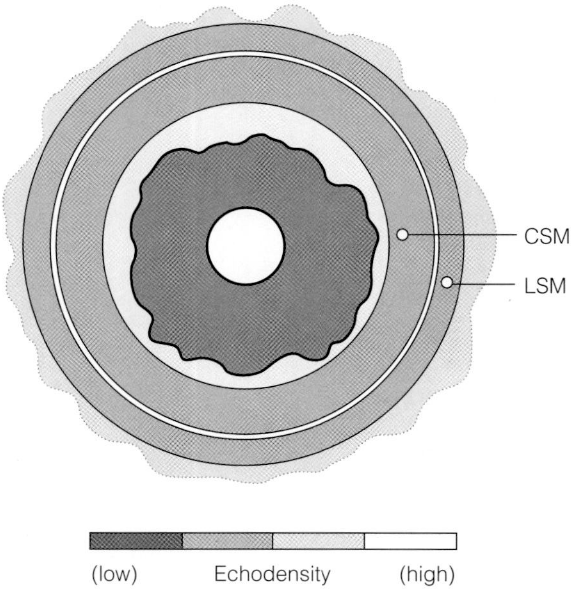

c

Figure 6.60 *(a) Endoluminal ultrasound image from the distal esophagus of a normal volunteer. CSM, circular smooth muscle; LSM, longitudinal smooth muscle; T, transducer. (b) Endoluminal ultrasound image obtained in the distal esophagus in a scleroderma patient shows diffusely increased echogenicity of the esophageal wall (arrows). The normal appearance of the various wall structures is no longer evident. T, transducer. (c) Schematic representation of sonographic appearance of the sclerodermatous esophagus. CSM, circular smooth muscle; LSM, longitudinal smooth muscle; T, transducer.*

2 = fibrosis into but not completely obliterating the inner circular smooth muscle; grade 3 = fibrosis obliterating the circular smooth muscle but not encroaching into the outer longitudinal smooth muscle; grade 4 = fibrosis obliterating the circular smooth muscle and extending into the longitudinal smooth muscle but not completely obliterating the longitudinal smooth muscle; grade 5 = complete replacement of the entire muscularis propria with fibrosis (Fig. 6.61).[88]

A significant correlation between the grade of manometric abnormality and degree of hyperechoic

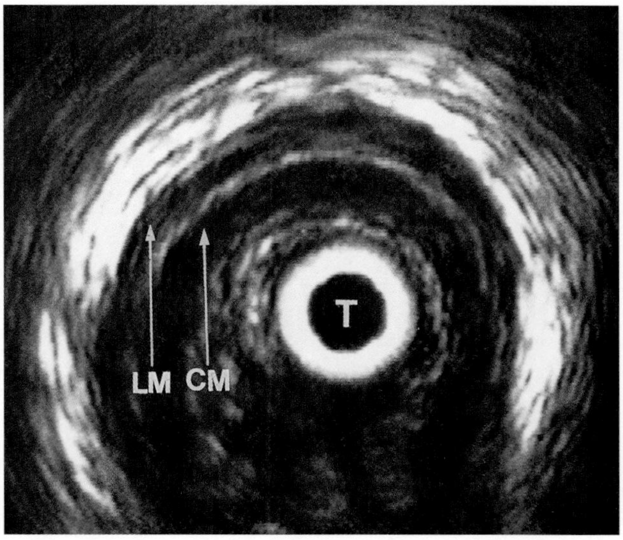

a

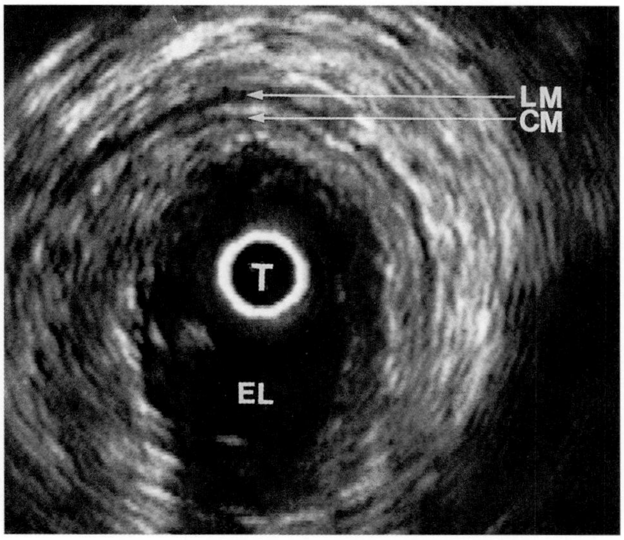

b

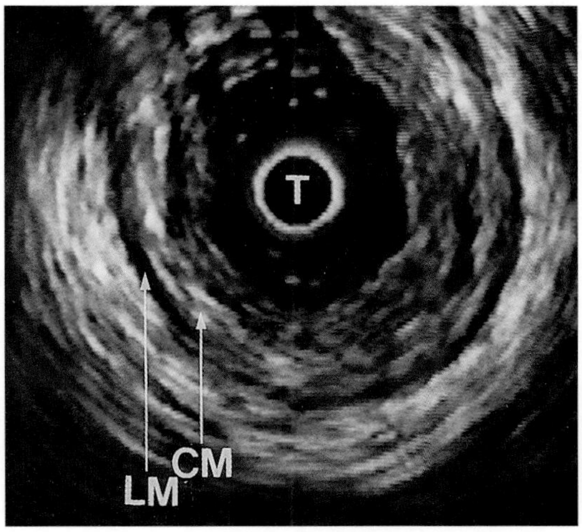

c

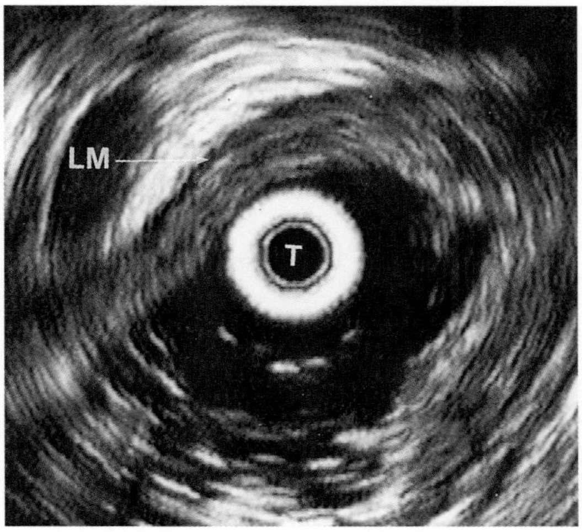

d

Figure 6.61 *HRES grading of the esophagus with sclerodermatous involvement. (a) Grade 1: there is no hyperechoic abnormality (fibrosis) in either layer of the muscularis propria. (b) Grade 2: hyperechoic abnormality in the muscularis propria involving but not completely obliterating the inner circular smooth muscle (CM). Longitudinal smooth muscle (LM) appears normal. (c) Grade 3: hyperechoic abnormality in the muscularis propria obliterating the CM but not involving the outer LM. (d) Grade 4: hyperechoic abnormality in the muscularis propria obliterating the CM and involving the LM but not completely obliterating the LM. (e) Grade 5: complete replacement of the entire muscularis propria with hyperechoic abnormality (arrows). T, transducer.*

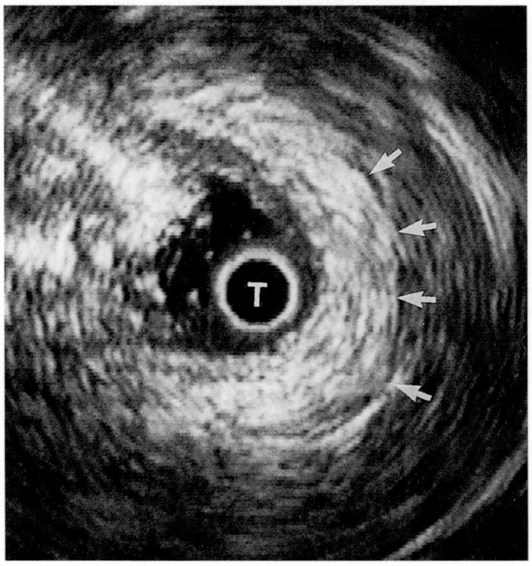

e

abnormality was found ($r = 0.89$). It was hypothesized that the hyperechoic abnormality represents fibrosis in the muscularis propria and that the degree of fibrosis can be accurately quantitated by evaluating the grade of hyperechoic abnormality in the muscularis propria according to the grading system described above. The distal esophageal lumen was slightly dilated at rest in 85% of patients with scleroderma (Fig. 6.62).[88] In contrast to the muscular contraction seen in the normal subjects, these patients showed weak or absent muscular contraction in response to a swallowed water bolus. In addition, one-third of the patients with scleroderma were found to have prominent periesophageal lymph nodes (Fig. 6.63). Comparison of CT with HRES in the detection of lymph nodes in the periesophageal area demonstrated that HRES was more sensitive. Because HRES reflects the degree of histologic fibrosis in the distal esophagus, it is anticipated that this technology may be used clinically in longitudinal studies to follow the progression of fibrosis in the esophagus. Furthermore, it may be useful in the evaluation of various therapeutic drug regimens that may modify the progression of fibrosis in the distal esophagus in scleroderma.

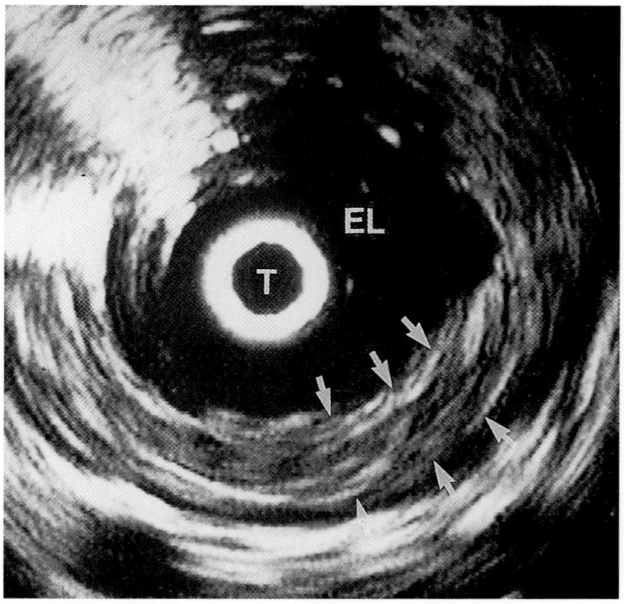

Figure 6.62 *Catheter-based ultrasound transducer (T) located in the distal esophagus in a patient with scleroderma shows diffusely increased echogenicity of the esophageal wall (arrows). Note that the esophageal lumen (EL) remains slightly dilated in the resting stage.*

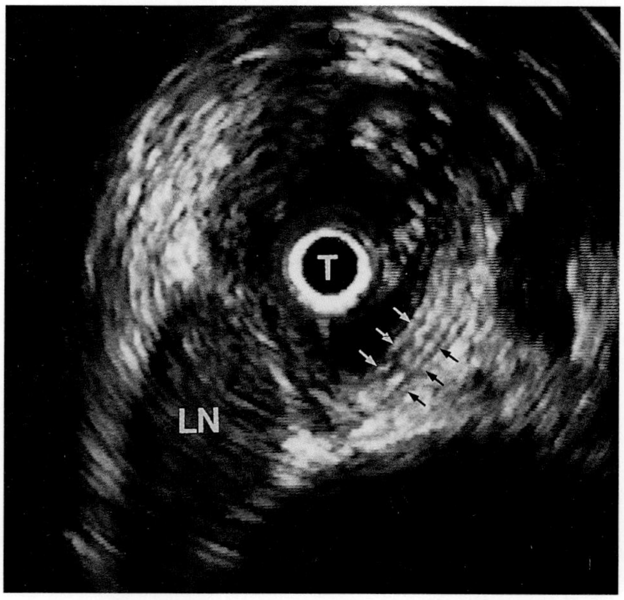

a

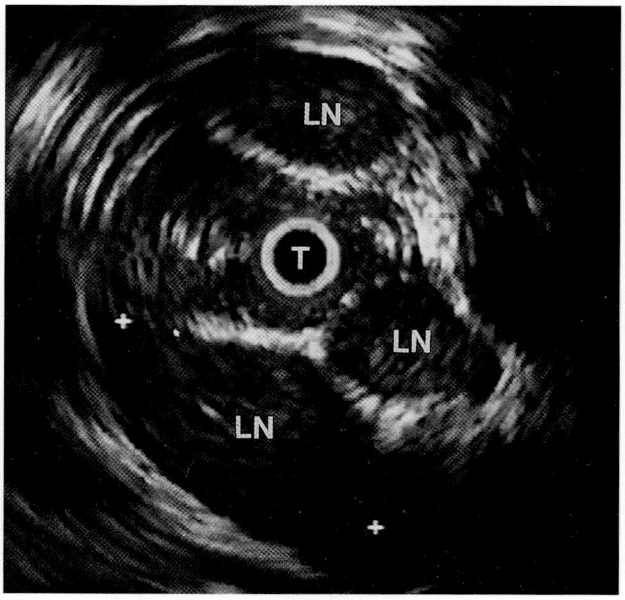

b

Figure 6.63 *(a,b) Cross-sectional ultrasound images obtained from patients with scleroderma detected enlarged lymph nodes (LN) adjacent to the esophageal wall. Sonographic fibrosis within the muscularis propria (arrows) can be seen. T, transducer.*

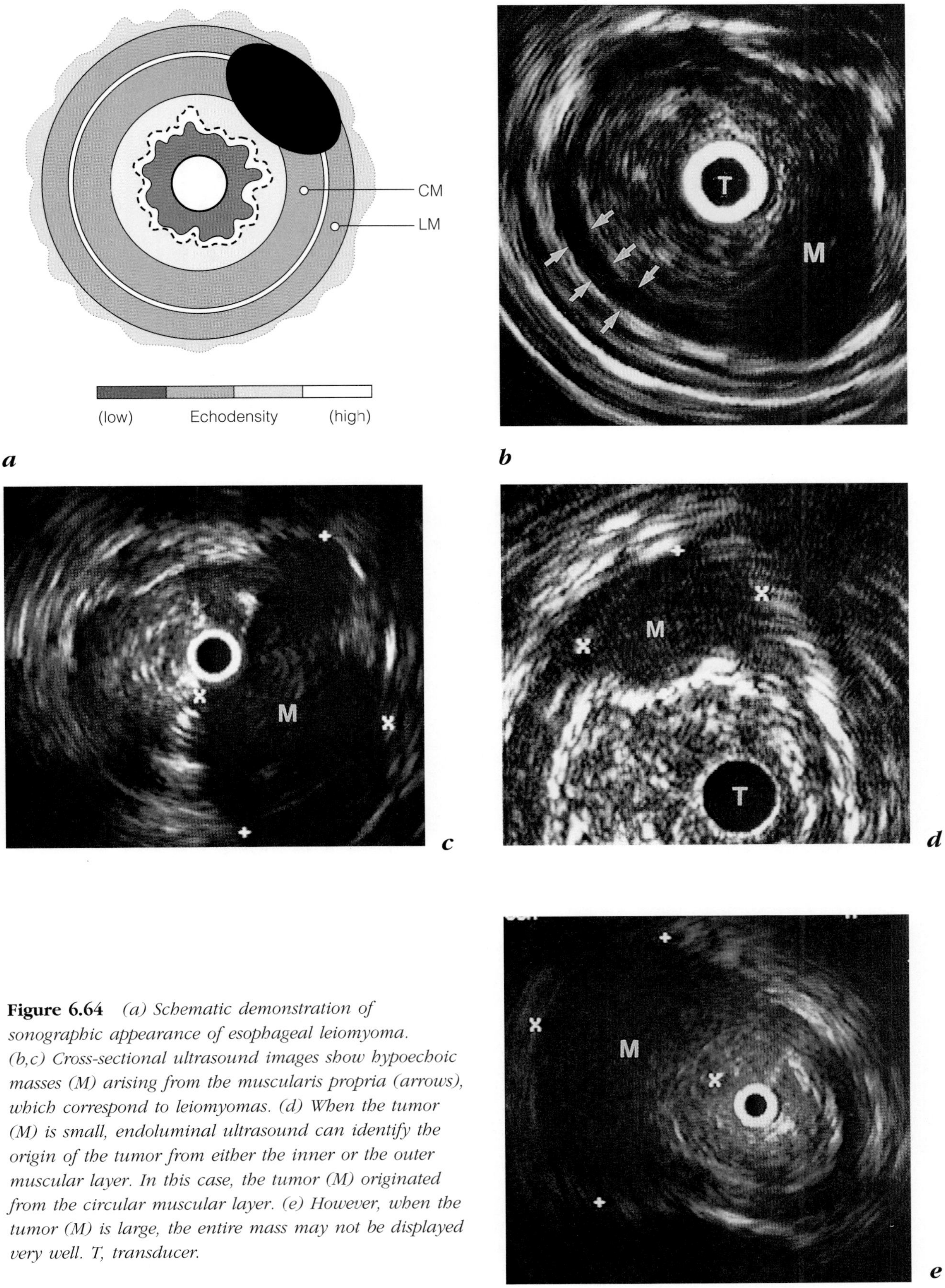

Figure 6.64 *(a) Schematic demonstration of sonographic appearance of esophageal leiomyoma. (b,c) Cross-sectional ultrasound images show hypoechoic masses (M) arising from the muscularis propria (arrows), which correspond to leiomyomas. (d) When the tumor (M) is small, endoluminal ultrasound can identify the origin of the tumor from either the inner or the outer muscular layer. In this case, the tumor (M) originated from the circular muscular layer. (e) However, when the tumor (M) is large, the entire mass may not be displayed very well. T, transducer.*

Neoplasms and Submucosal Lesions

Because of the high resolution of endoluminal ultrasound, imaging of the GI tract for submucosal lesions is exquisitely sensitive. As with lower frequency endoscopic ultrasound transducers, various submucosal lesions have characteristic echodensities and echotextures and arise from specific areas of the GI tract wall. The major advantage of HRES technology is that very small lesions can be imaged with high resolution and without compression artifact resulting from a water-filled balloon or a large-size transducer. However, a major disadvantage in imaging periesophageal structures with HRES is that if the abnormality is larger than 2 cm in the axial plain perpendicular to the transducer, the distal borders of the lesion will not be imaged. This is due to the limited penetration of the ultrasound beam.[89]

As with the lower-frequency endoscopic ultrasound scopes the principles of differentiating submucosal lesions by HRES depend on: the echo-layer from which it originates, the echo pattern, the tumor margins, and whether or not the lesion originates from an extraluminal site. Leiomyomas appear as hypoechoic masses arising from the muscularis propria. When the tumor is small, HRES can identify the origin of the tumor from either the circular smooth muscle or the longitudinal smooth muscle (Fig. 6.64). Lipomas, which arise from the submucosa, are hyperechoic and well demarcated (Fig. 6.65).

A number of patients with acute esophagitis documented by EGD and endoscopic biopsy have been imaged with HRES. Imaging of patients with acute esophagitis revealed specific abnormalities, including diffuse thickening in the submucosa, often 3-4 times the normal thickness, associated with small dilated vessels imaged within this region (Figs 6.66 and 6.67). This thickening is probably due to edema, inflammation and necrotic debris.

Barrett's esophagus is a metaplastic change in the mucosa lining the esophagus. The mucosa changes from its normal squamous appearance to a columnar-type mucosa. This change is brought about by chronic reflux esophagitis and has an overall prevalence of approximately 10% in patients with reflux

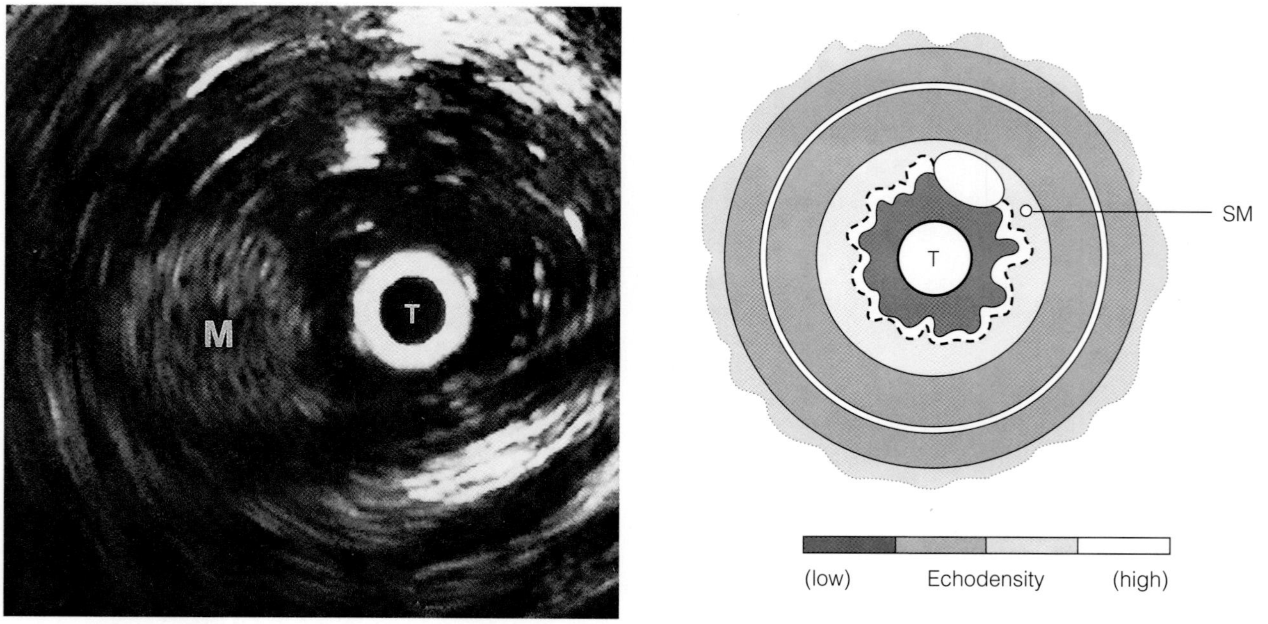

a *b*

Figure 6.65 *(a) Endoluminal ultrasound image demonstrates a hyperechoic mass (M) arising from the layer of the submucosa. Transendoscopic biopsy proved this to be a lipoma. (b) Schematic demonstration of sonographic appearance of the esophageal lipoma. SM, submucosa; T, transducer.*

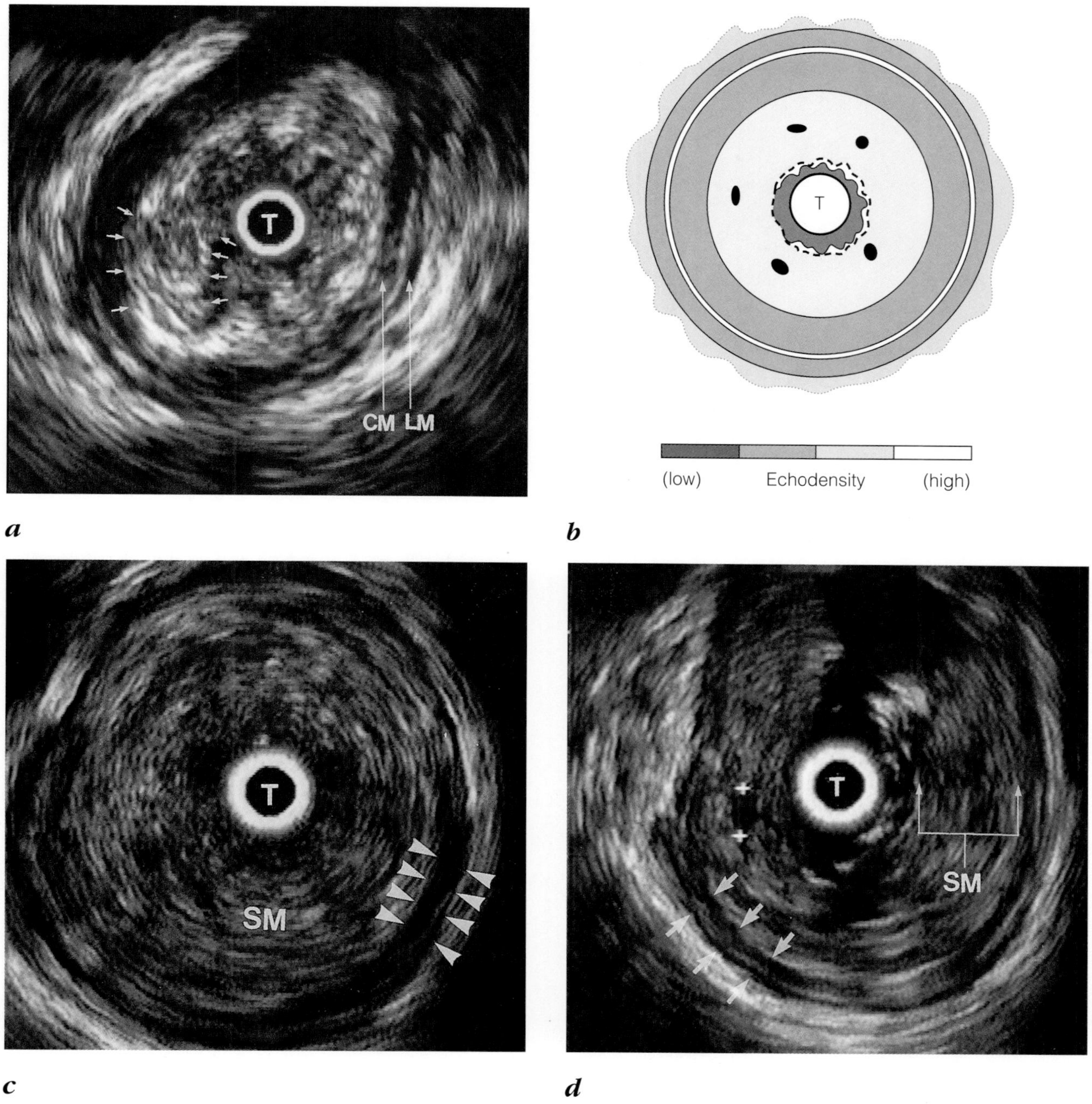

Figure 6.66 *Endoluminal ultrasound demonstrates diffusive submucosal thickening (arrows) and normal muscularis propria, which correspond to esophagitis (a). Schematic representation of sonographic appearance of the esophagitis (b). CM, circular smooth muscle; LM, longitudinal smooth muscle. Cross-sectional esophageal ultrasound image demonstrates loss of the mucosa and thickening of the submucosa (SM) in the lower portion of the esophagus at the resting state (c) and during the water swallowing (d). Dilated vessels (cursors) can be seen within the submucosa. Note that the two muscular layers (arrowheads) are not involved in the disease process. These findings are consistent with severe reflux esophagitis, which correlated with the endoscopic diagnosis of ulcerative esophagitis. T, transducer. (Reproduced with permission from Liu et al.[65])*

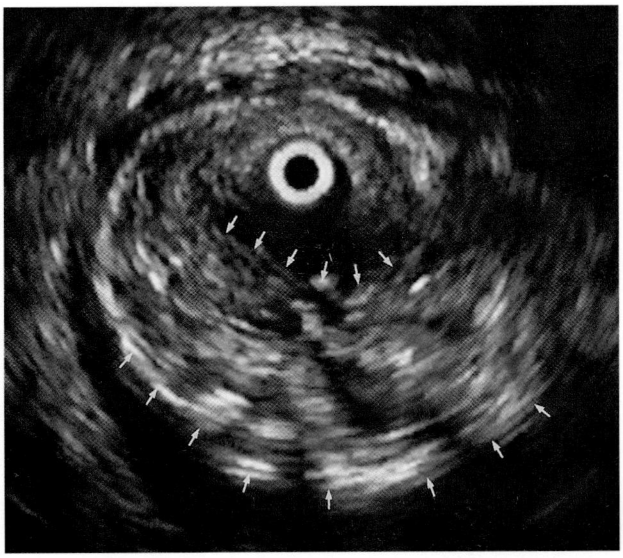

Figure 6.67 *In this case, endoluminal ultrasound image shows a focal thickening (arrows) of submucosa at the lower segment of the esophagus, which corresponds with focal esophagitis.*

Figure 6.68 *HRES images (a,b) obtained from the two different cases showing diffusive thickening (arrows) of the mucosa at distal esophagus with normal appearance of the submucosa (SM) and muscularis propria (MP). The sonographic findings are consistent with the endoscopic and pathologic diagnosis of Barrett's esophagus. (c) Schematic representation of sonographic appearance of Barrett's esophagus. M, mucosa; SM, submucosa; T, transducer.*

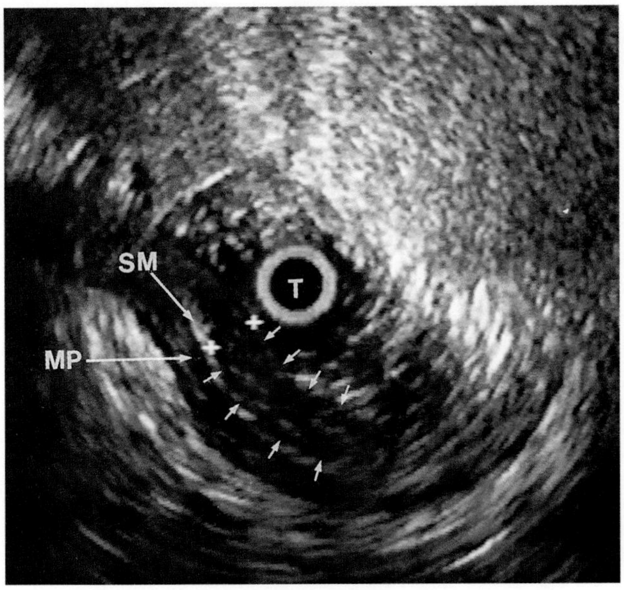

b

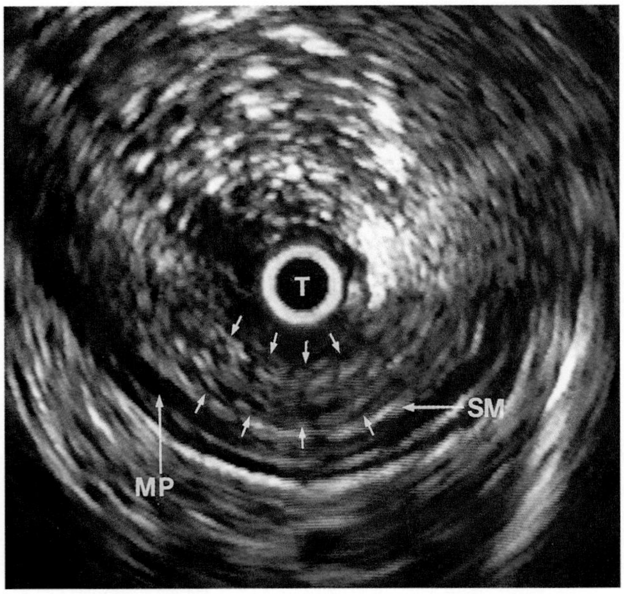

a

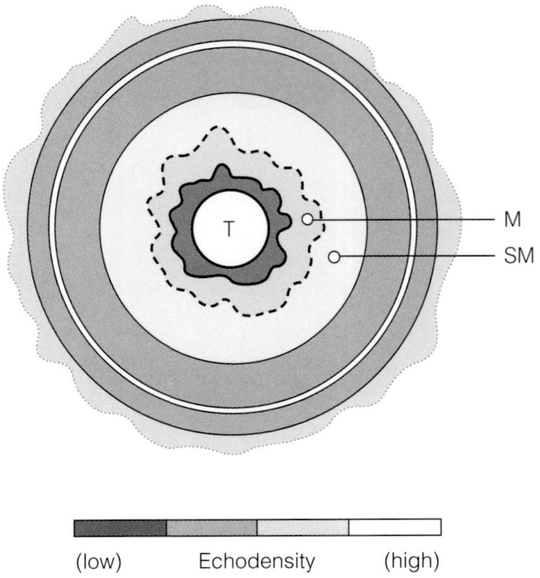

c

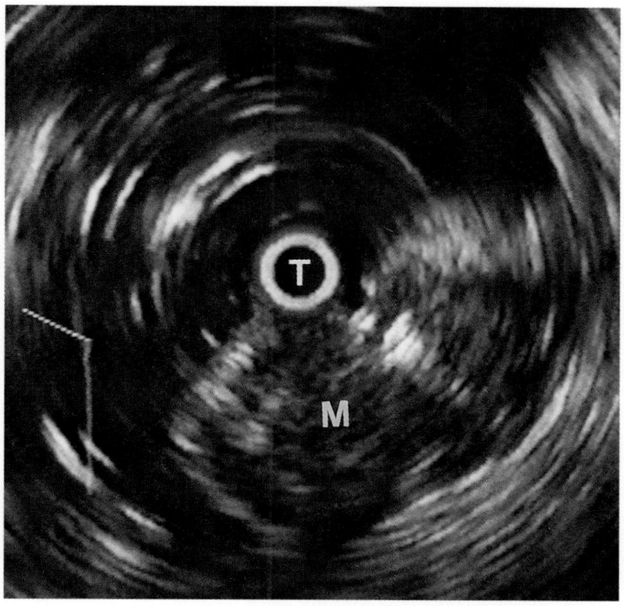

Figure 6.69 *Endoluminal ultrasound image obtained from the body of the stomach shows a hypoechoic solid mass (M). Transendoscopic biopsy proved this to be a gastric carcinoma. T, transducer.*

disease. When the metaplasic mucosa is specialized intestinal metaplasia, Barrett's becomes a premalignant condition with an increased risk for adenocarcinoma. With HRES the hyperechoic layer of the mucosa appears thicker than the normal squamous mucosa. The submucosa remains preserved as a hyperechoic layer below the mucosa (Fig. 6.68).

HRES is useful in detecting hypoechoic or hyperechoic esophageal and gastric malignancies. Small masses can be detected and staged with great accuracy because the high resolution of the transducer provides accurate delineation of the area of interest (Fig. 6.69). However, the low penetration (2 cm) limits the direct application of these ultrasound transducers in large malignancies because extension far beyond the wall of the esophagus, as well as lymph nodes, will be out of range of the penetration of the ultrasound beam. A major advantage of the 6.2 Fr ultrasound catheters is that they can traverse almost any stricture caused by either esophageal carcinoma or radiation fibrosis and, therefore, can image the area of narrowing as well as the area beyond the stenosis.[89]

Preliminary results from McLoughin et al indicate that HRES can be used to stage esophageal malignancy. Primary esophageal carcinoma was staged correctly in six of seven (85.6%) cases by HRES but in only three of seven (42.9%) patients by CT scanning. However, lymph node assessment correlated poorly with pathologic findings for both HRES and CT.[90]

The TNM system has been utilized for staging esophageal carcinoma as follows: T1 invades lamina propria or submucosa; T2 invades muscularis propria; T3 invades adventitia; T4 invades adjacent structures. Regional lymph node involvement is staged as follows: N0, no lymph node involvement; N1, regional lymph nodes involved (Fig. 6.70). HRES is particularly good for staging early malignancies of the esophagus (T1, T2 and T3) (Fig. 6.71). While the dedicated ultrasound scopes may cause compression of the mucosa/submucosa due to the water filled balloon, HRES catheters cause no compression artifact. The high frequency allows for excellent resolution of mucosa/submucosa structures. However, the lack of penetration of the HRES probes does not allow for staging higher grades (T4) of esophageal carcinoma.

Evaluation of Swallowing Function

Liu et al[65] had previously utilized HRES in human subjects to examine wall motion of the esophagus during deglutition. Taniguchi et al[91] used HRES to evaluate swallowing in the sheep esophagus. Using a 20-MHz M-mode suction ultrasound probe, they observed thickening of the circular smooth muscle but none of the longitudinal smooth muscle during occlusive contractions.

Miller et al[92] have developed a method to quantitate the changes in esophageal wall motion by measuring the width of the muscularis propria during swallowing in the esophageal body, correlating these changes in muscle width and lumen circumference with changes in intraluminal pressure and defining various HRES phases of the swallowing sequence based on manometrically defined pressure changes in the esophageal lumen.

In order to obtain a simultaneous sonographic image and manometric tracing, a modified ultrasound/manometric catheter (a 3 Fr angiographic catheter attached to a 4.8 Fr EndoSound catheter with cyanoacrylate glue) was used (Fig. 6.72).[91] This

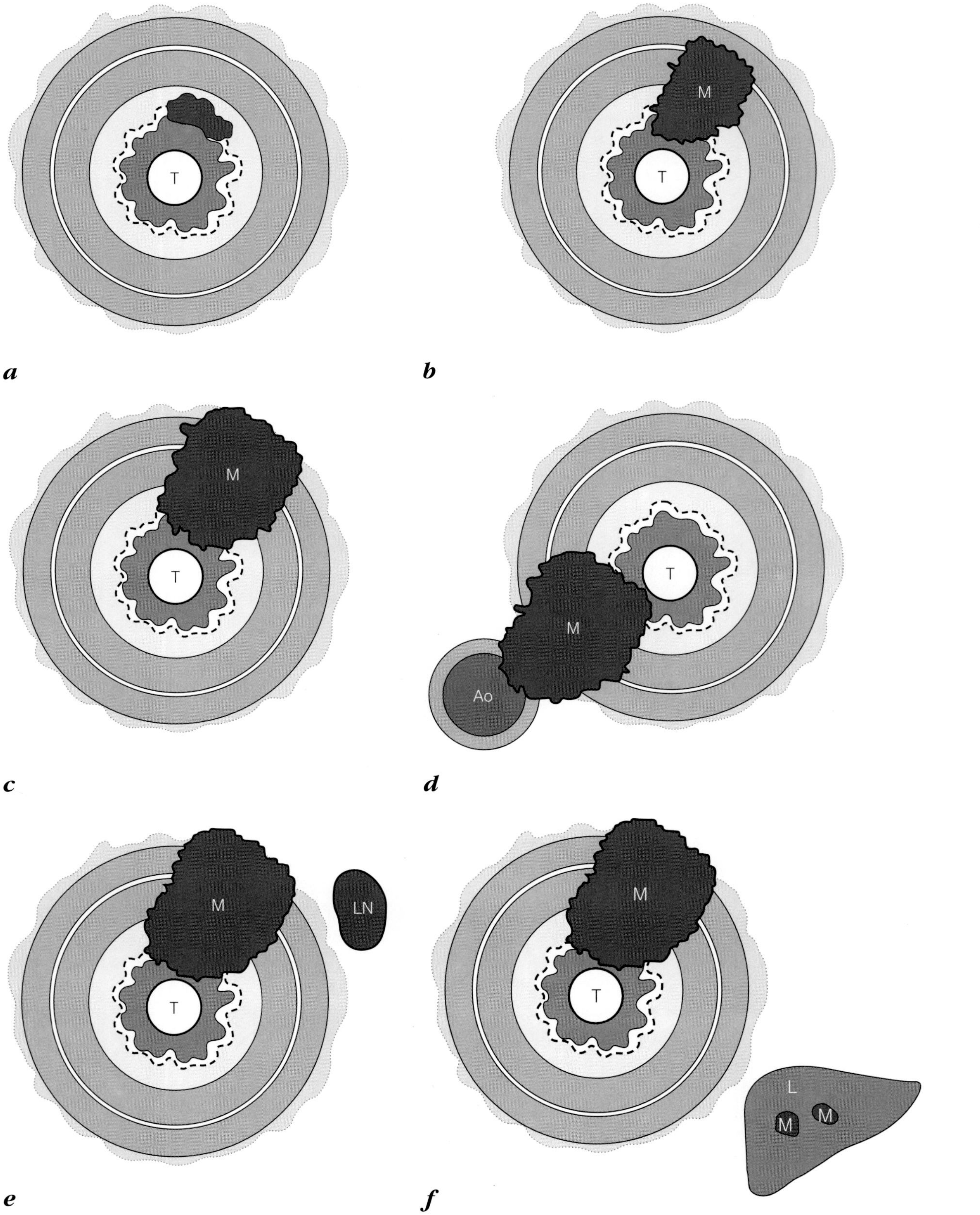

Figure 6.70 *Schematic representation of the TNM system for staging of the esophageal tumor. (a) T1 tumor; (b) T2 tumor; (c) T3 tumor; (d) T4 tumor; (e) T3N1 tumor, (f) T3 M1. T, transducer; M, mass, LN, lymph node; A, aorta, L, liver.*

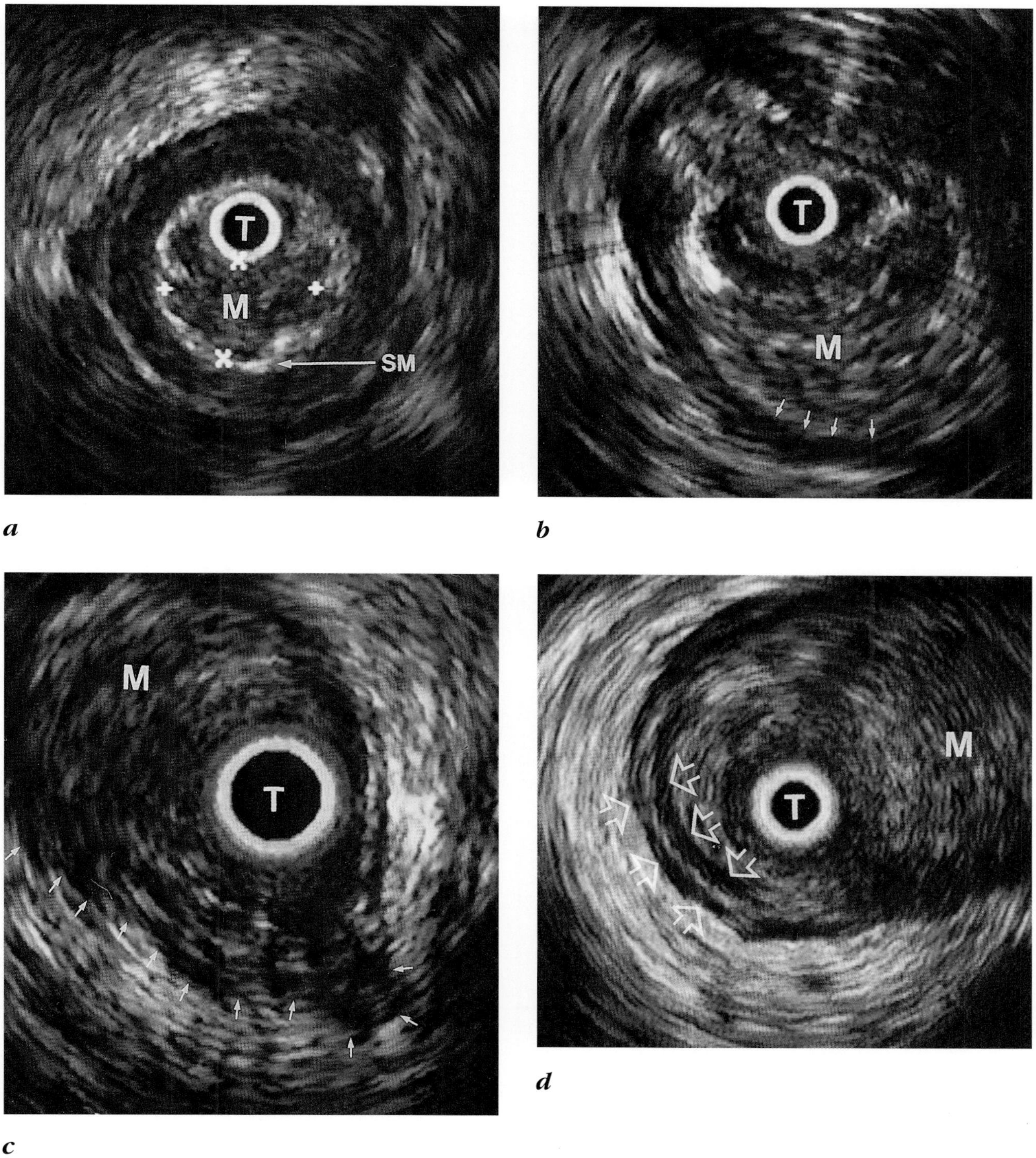

Figure 6.71 *(a) Stage T1 esophageal carcinoma: tumor (M) confined within the mucosa and submucosa (SM). (b) Stage T2 esophageal carcinoma: tumor (M) invaded into the muscular propria (arrows). (c) Stage T3 esophageal carcinoma: tumor (M) infiltrated beyond the adventitia (arrows). (d) Stage T4 esophageal carcinoma: tumor (M) invaded beyond the wall of the esophagus into the mediastinum. The normal appearance of the muscular layers (arrows) is preserved in the noninvolved portion of the esophagus. However, the outer margin (1 to 3 o'clock) of the tumor cannot be imaged by this high-frequency transducer because of the limited penetration of the ultrasound beam. Pathologic findings confirmed this to be a stage T4 esophageal carcinoma. T, transducer.*

assembly allowed sonographic images to be acquired while a manometric tracing was obtained (Fig. 6.73).

Since the HRES transducer and manometry catheter are glued together, they moved as one in the esophagus. Therefore, the resulting ultrasound image evaluated the same area as the pressure transducer.

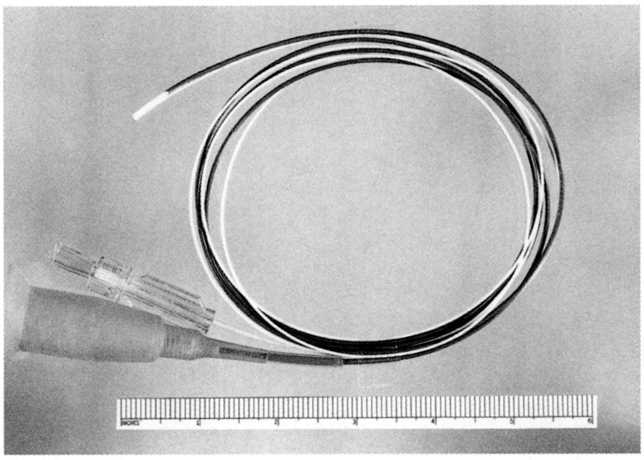

Figure 6.72 *A modified simultaneous ultrasound/manometric catheter assembly.*

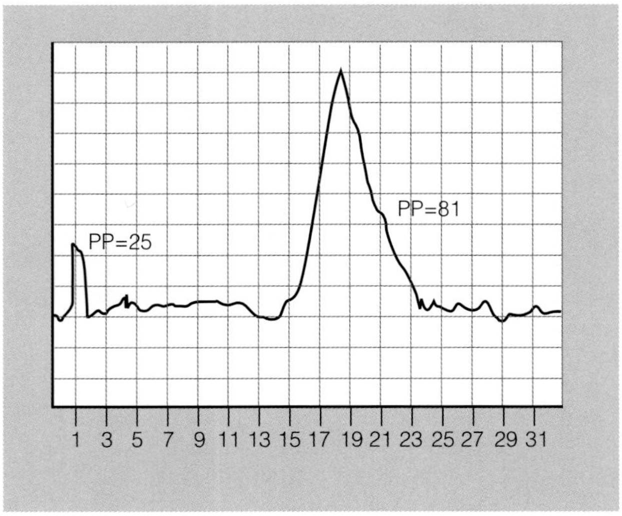

Figure 6.73 *A typical manometric tracing of esophageal swallowing. The reference mark is the square wave marked with peak pressure (PP) equal to 25. The baseline is divided into 500 ms intervals. (Reproduced with permission from Miller et al.[92])*

Although there was shortening of the esophagus in response to swallowing, this did not present a technical problem.

With the use of this technique, Miller et al[92] demonstrated four phases of the peristaltic sequence: phase I, a resting phase; phase II, a passive distention phase; phase III, a contraction phase; and phase IV, a relaxation phase (Fig. 6.74). During phases I and II there was no change in the esophageal pressure. In addition, there was no change in lumen circumference or muscle thickness. However, the passage of a gelatin bolus forced the esophageal lumen to open and the muscle to thin during phase II. Phase III began with the upstroke of the pressure recording and continued until peak pressure was attained. It was during phase III that there was a rapid decrease in the esophageal lumen circumference. A progressive increase in the muscle width of all of the muscular layers was observed as the lumen pressure increased progressively. Phase IV began as the pressure started to decline from maximal pressure and concluded when the pressure reached baseline resting pressure. During phase IV a marked decrease in muscle width was observed in all the layers of the muscularis propria. A return of the esophageal shape to its resting configuration was also demonstrated.

Increasing muscle width was the sonographic correlate of increasing lumen pressure as measured by manometry. The inner circular smooth muscle is thought to be the main contributor to the amount of intraluminal pressure generated during a contraction. Decreasing muscle width was the sonographic correlate of decreasing luminal pressure (Figs 6.75 and 6.76) (Table 6.3).

Table 6.3 Sonographic muscle width during phases of peristaltic sequence.

	Phase of peristaltic sequence		
	Phase 1 (mean, CM)	*Phase 2 (mean minimum thickness) (cm)*	*Phase 3 (mean maximum thickness) (cm)*
CSM	0.067 ± 0.009	0.050 ± 0.009	0.165 ± 0.027
LSM	0.068 ± 0.007	0.049 ± 0.010	0.123 ± 0.045
TMT	0.123 ± 0.014	0.091 ± 0.011	0.279 ± 0.028

CSM, circular smooth muscle; LSM, longitudinal smooth muscle; TMT, total muscle thickness.

Reproduced with permission from Miller et al.[92]

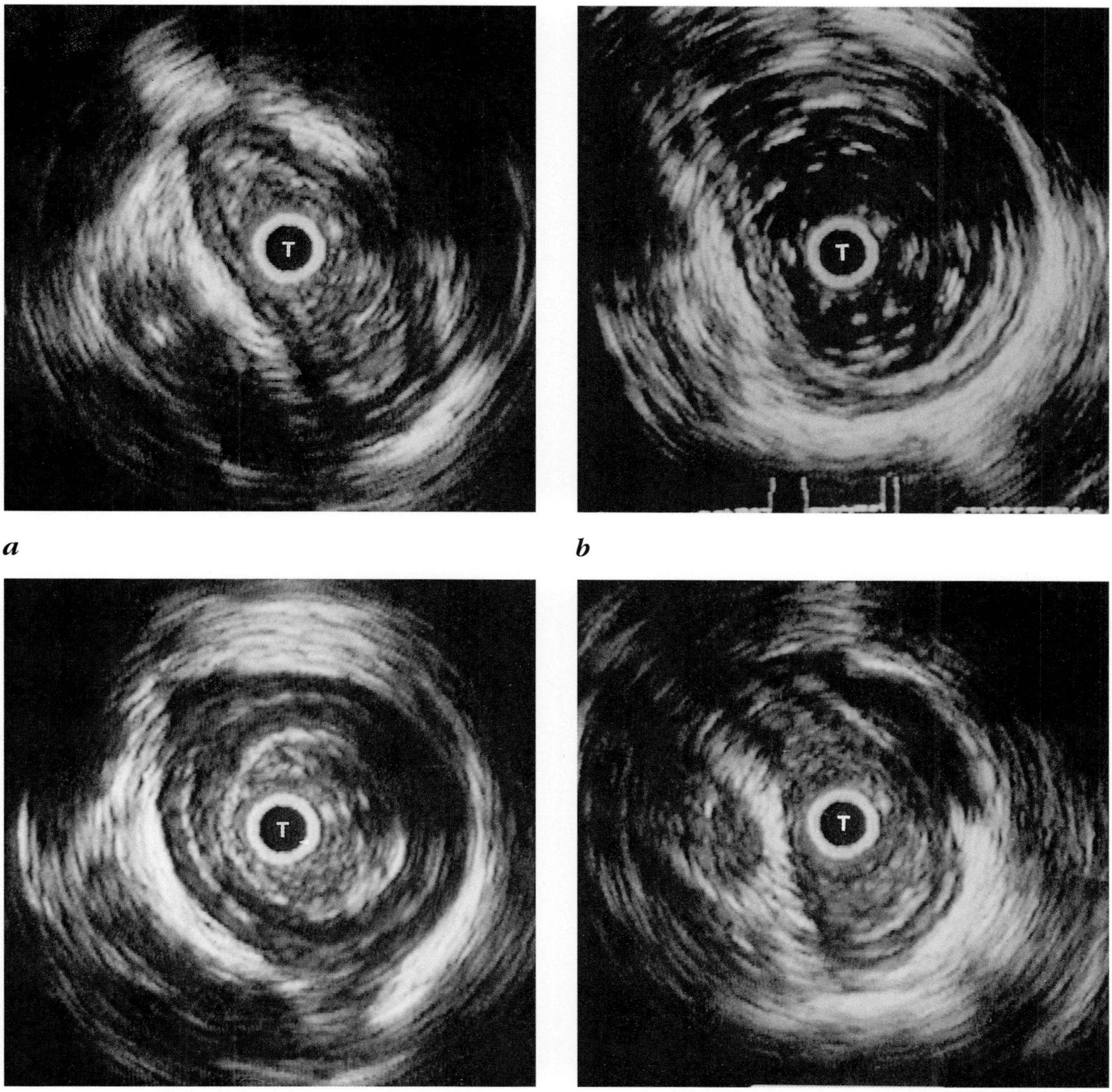

a *b* *c* *d*

Figure 6.74 *Sonographic image of the esophageal peristalsis sequence during resting phase I (a), passive distention phase II (b), contraction phase III (c), and relaxation phase IV (d). T, transducer. (Reproduced with permission from Miller et al.[92])*

The study demonstrated a number of previously unrecorded phenomena in the human esophagus: the rate of esophageal muscular wall thickening and thinning during the peristaltic sequence, the rate of luminal opening and closing measured sonographically during esophageal peristalsis, the maximum and minimum muscle thickness and lumen circumference during the peristaltic sequence, and the manometric

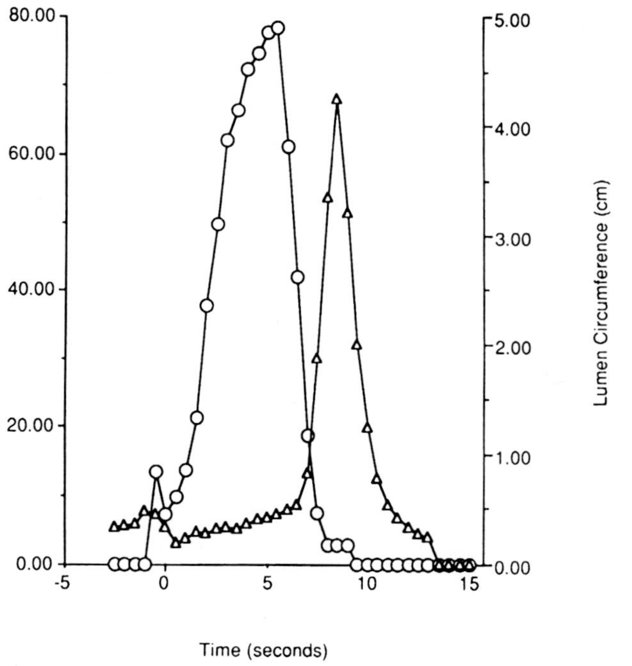

Figure 6.75 *This graph shows the mean esophageal lumen circumference (○) vs. the mean esophageal pressure (△). (Reproduced with permission from Miller et al.[92])*

correlation. With this technique, it may be possible to study esophageal motor disorders in the skeletal and smooth muscle segments of the esophagus and the LES before, during and after swallowing in patients with various motility disorders.

NEW APPLICATIONS AND FUTURE DEVELOPMENT

THREE-DIMENSIONAL ENDOLUMINAL SONOGRAPHY

In a preliminary study Kalimanis et al[93] evaluated the ability of three-dimensional endoscopic ultrasound to elucidate normal esophageal anatomy and pathologic conditions as compared with information obtained by two-dimensional endoscopic ultrasound. Using an Olympus EU-M20 echogastroscope, the scope was withdrawn through the esophagus in a straight, slow and stabilized manner. Using a frame grabber, approximately 80 individual images were digitized and stored on an optical disk. The stored two-dimensional images were than reconstructed with software

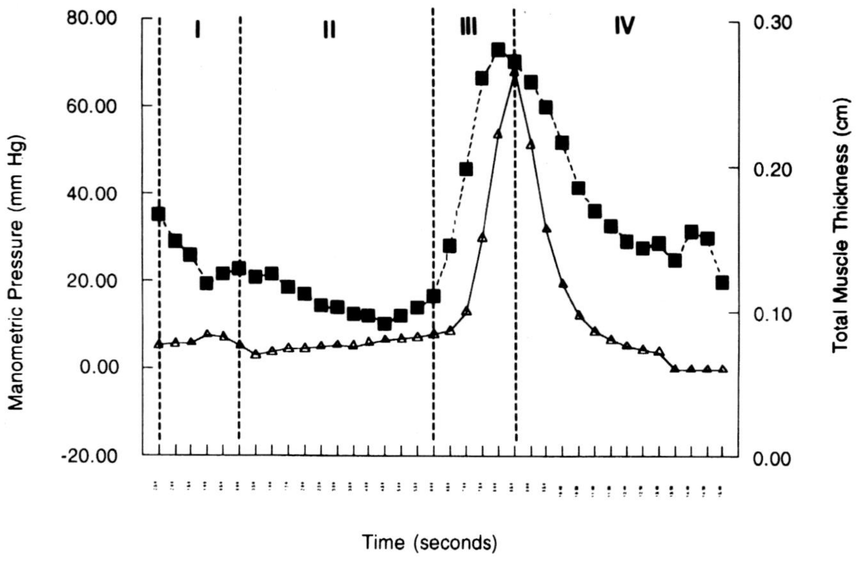

Figure 6.76 *This graph shows the mean total muscle thickness (■) versus the mean esophageal pressure (△). The four phases of the peristaltic sequence (I–IV) are shown. (Reproduced with permission from Miller et al.[92])*

that executed interpolation, boundary formation and surface rendering.

The authors of this study felt that three-dimensional reconstruction provides information that is an adjunct to conventional two-dimensional images. Three-dimensional reconstruction offers a format in which a series of two-dimensional images can be assessed and related to each other more readily. The observer may rapidly gain an overview of the local anatomy and its relationship to the target lesions. The three-dimensional format also offers the advantage of displaying the profile of lesions in the optimal viewing plane, which can be determined by real-time rotation of the three-dimensional model.

ULTRASOUND-GUIDED FINE NEEDLE BIOPSY

A number of recent studies have demonstrated the safety and efficacy of the use of endosonographically directed fine needle aspiration biopsies. Wiersema et al[94] demonstrated the utility of this method using either the Olympus EUM20 echoendoscope or the Pentax FG-32UA linear electronic array ultrasound endoscope. Fifty-six consecutive patients with extrinsic or submucosal masses, gastric ulcers or surgical anastomoses suspected of malignancy but with previously negative findings on conventional forceps biopsy or brush cytology underwent endoscopic ultrasound investigation followed by fine needle aspiration for cytology. Real-time ultrasound guidance for biopsy was not used in this study. Endoscopic ultrasound was first performed to characterize the exact size, location, vascularity and echotexture of the lesion. This was followed by routine endoscopy with fine needle aspiration. Diagnostic cytology results were obtained in 37 of 50 (74%) patients. In all patients endosonography was useful for identifying the extent of the lesion and detailing regional anatomy to permit an assessment of the safest and most appropriate site for needle biopsy. The highest yield was found in evaluating tumors extrinsic to the GI tract that were impinging on the lumen (14 of 15, or 93%). In 14 patients who underwent subsequent surgical therapy, the accuracy of fine needle aspiration cytology was 86% (12 of 14). No complications occurred.

Several case reports were described at approximately the same time as the above study by Wiersema[94–96] in which real-time endoscopic ultrasound-guided fine needle aspiration was done using a Pentax probe in conjunction with similar-caliber needles.

By the end of 1994, two back-to-back studies[97,98] were published which evaluated the use of real-time endoscopic ultrasound-guided fine needle aspiration. Chang et al[97] performed endoscopic ultrasound-guided fine needle aspiration in 38 consecutive patients with extraluminal and/or submucosal lesions. One hundred and sixty-three passes were made, with an average of 3.5 passes per lesion and 4.3 passes per patient. Adequate specimens were obtained from 91% of targeted lesions. The overall diagnostic accuracy was 87%. In patients with malignant lesions the sensitivity was 91% and the specificity was 100%. An initial tissue diagnosis of malignancy was made in 66% of cancer patients without a previous diagnosis and the preoperative staging was changed in 44% of cancer patients. The additional information gained by this modality influenced the decision not to perform surgery in 26% of patients with primary malignancy. No complications occurred.

In a second study, Wiersema et al[98] prospectively evaluated the use of endosonography-guided real-time fine needle aspiration biopsy. Endosonography-guided real-time fine needle aspiration biopsy was diagnostic in 18 of 20 patients (accuracy 90%). Overall, in 9 of 10 lesions in which visualization by CT was not possible, CT-guided fine needle aspiration was unsuccessful or prior nonsurgical biopsy techniques were unsuccessful, real-time fine needle aspiration biopsy was diagnostic.

Vilmann et al[99] have also published their experience with fine needle aspiration of lesions during real time endoscopic ultrasound. In most cases, an assistant is responsible for introduction of the needle and aspiration of material. This is necessary because the endoscopist has to maintain the transducer in contact with the GI wall during the needle puncture. The biopsy procedure is repeated until sufficient material has been aspirated as judged by the macroscopic appearance. The predictive value of the positive cytological diagnosis is 100% (89–100%) and the predictive value of the negative cytological diagnosis is 83% (36–100%), with a 95% confidence interval. Again, no complications were related to the biopsy procedures.[98]

ULTRASOUND CONTRAST AGENT

For endoscopic ultrasound of the stomach, de-aerated water is a good acoustic coupling medium whereas water that is not de-aerated can cause interference due to air bubbles. However, water is not an

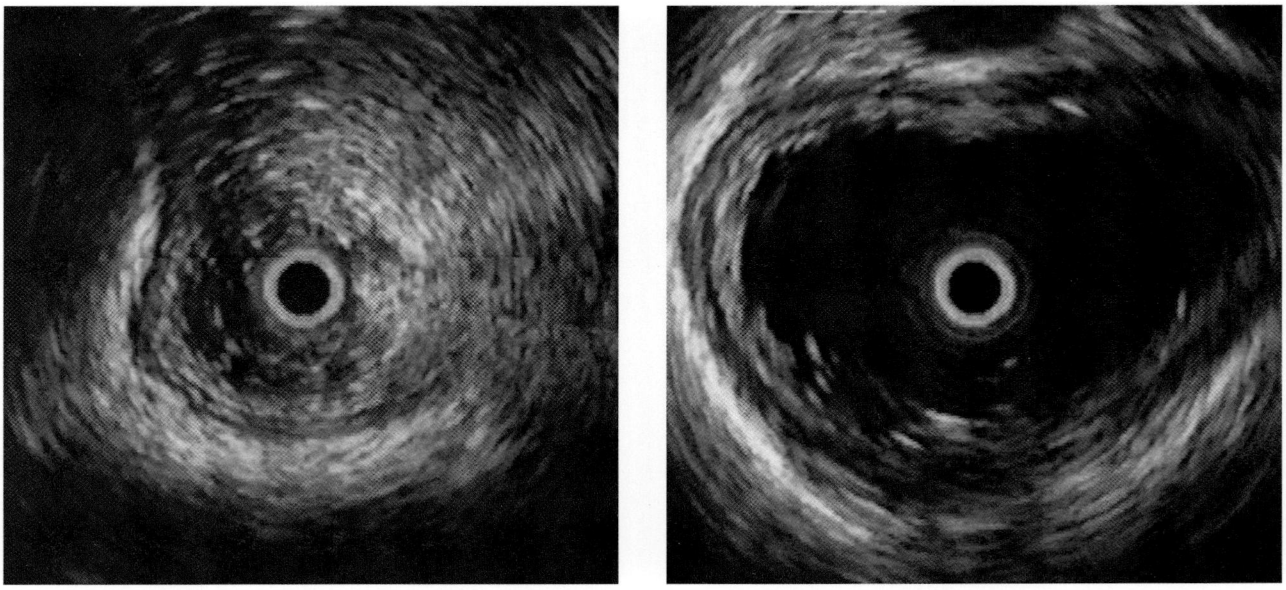

a *b*

Figure 6.77 *(a) Endoluminal ultrasound image of the esophagus during swallowing of a bolus of water. Air bubbles contained in the water cause the hyperechoic artifact seen between 12 and 5 o'clock. (b) Imaging of the esophagus in the same patient at the same level during swallowing of diluted Jello. Note that there is no longer artifact due to air bubbles. The mucosal and submucosal layers can be well imaged.*

optimum agent for the evaluation of swallowing function with endoluminal ultrasound techniques. We have tested various liquids and semisolids to improve endoluminal ultrasound imaging in the esophagus. We found that dilute Jello is a good acoustic coupling medium that can be used for swallowing studies, because it eliminates interference due to the formation of air bubble artifacts (Fig. 6.77). This technique has been used during simultaneous manometry and ultrasound to evaluate swallowing function. More studies are under way.

CONCLUSION

Over the last 10 years, endoscopic ultrasound has been found useful in the evaluation of upper GI malignancies in terms of diagnosis and staging and in the evaluation of submucosal lesions. A great deal of work has been done in these two areas and conventional endoscopic ultrasound has branched out to include malignancies of the biliary tract and pancreas. This chapter has reviewed the equipment and techniques of endoscopic ultrasound as well as numerous studies evaluating the clinical utility of conventional endoscopic ultrasound.

This chapter has also evaluated some of the newer uses of endoluminal ultrasound using special equipment and techniques. In particular, this chapter reviews the use of high-frequency probes in the evaluation of the normal esophagus, various esophageal motility disorders, swallowing function, and esophageal and gastric varices. This chapter also discusses the new modality of endoscopic ultrasound-directed biopsies and three-dimensional imaging.

Endoscopic ultrasound is a new imaging modality that has found a place in conventional gastroenterology. In addition, endoscopic ultrasound continues to evolve in equipment, technique and clinical utility.

REFERENCES

1. Wild JJ, Reid JM, Diagnostic use of ultrasound, *Br J Phys Med* 1956; **19**:248–57.
2. Fukuda M, Hirata K, Saito K et al, On the diagnostic use of echoendoscope in abdominal diseases. 1. Diagnostic experiences with a new type echoendoscope on gastric disease, *Proc Jpn Med Ultrasonography* 1980; **37**:409–15.
3. DiMagno EP, Reagan PT, Clain JE et al, Human endoscopic ultrasonography. *Gastroenterology* 1982; **83**:824–9.
4. Rifkin MD, Gordon SJ, Goldberg BB, Sonographic examination of the mediastinum and upper abdomen by fiberoptic gastroscope, *Radiology* 1984; **151**:175–80.
5. Rösch T, Classen M, *Gastroenterologic Endosonography* (Thieme Medical Publishers, Inc.: New York, 1992) 1–12.
6. Rösch T, Classen M, *Gastroenterologic Endosonography* (Thieme Medical Publishers, Inc.: New York, 1992) 36–44.
7. Rösch T, Classen M, Preoperative localization of endoscopic tumors of the pancreas, *Gastrointest Endosc Clin North Am* 1992; **2**:685–96.
8. Yasuda K, Mukai H, Fujimoto S, Nakajima M, Kawai K, The diagnosis of pancreatic cancer by endoscopic ultrasonography, *Gastrointest Endosc* 1988; **34**:1–8.
9. Vilmann P, Jacobson GK, Henriksen FW, Hancke S, Endoscopic ultrasonography with guided fine needle aspiration biopsy in pancreatic disease, *Gastrointest Endosc* 1992; **38**:172–4.
10. Lees WR, The pancreas: differential diagnosis and pancreatitis, *Gastrointest Endosc Clin North Am* 1992; **2**:657–71.
11. Tio TL, Endosonography in diagnosing and staging of pancreatic and ampullary cancer, *Gastrointest Endosc Clin North Am* 1992; **2**:673–84.
12. Dancygier H, Endosonographic evaluation of biliary tract disease, *Gastrointest Endosc Clin North Amer* 1992; **2**:697–713.
13. Rösch T, Classen M, *Gastroenterologic Endosonography* (Thieme Medical Publishers, Inc.: New York, 1992).
14. Catalano MF, Sivak MV Jr, Rice T, Gragg LA, VanDam J, Endosonographic features predictive of lymph node metastasis, *Gastrointest Endosc* 1994; **40**:442–6.
15. Tio TL, Coene PPLO, denHartog Jager FCA, Tytgat GNJ, Preoperative TNM classification of esophageal carcinoma by endosonography, *Hepato-Gastroenterology* 1990; **37**:376–81.
16. Dittler HJ, Bollschweiler E, Siewert JR, Was leistet die Endosonographie im praoperativen Staging des Osophaguskarzinoms? *Dtsch Med Wschr* 1991; **116**:561–6.
17. Vilgrain V, Mompoint D, Palazzo L et al, Staging of oesophageal carcinoma: comparison of results with endoscopic sonography and CT, *AJR* 1990; **155**:277–81.
18. Botet JF, Lightdale CJ, Zauber G, Gerdes H, Urmacher C, Brennan MF, Preoperative staging of esophageal cancer: comparison of endoscopic US and dynamic CT, *Radiology* 1991; **181**:419–25.
19. Grimm H, Maydeo A, Hamper K, Maas R, Noar M, Soehendra N, Results of endoscopic ultrasound and computed tomography in preoperative staging of esophageal cancer: a prospective controlled study, *Gastrointest Endosc* 1991; **37**:279 (Abstract).
20. Rosch T, Lorenz R, Zenker K et al, Local staging and assessment of resectability in carcinoma of the esophagus, stomach and duodenum by endoscopic ultrasonography, *Gastrointest Endosc* 1992; **38**:460–7.
21. Ziegler K, Sanft C, Zeitz M et al. Evaluation of endosonography in TN staging of esophageal cancer, *Gut* 1991; **32**:10–16.
22. Sugimachi K, Ohno S, Fujushima H, Kuwano H, Mori M, Misawa T, Endoscopic ultrasonographic detection of carcinomatous invasion and of lymph nodes in the thoracic esophagus, *Surgery* 1990; **107**:366–71.
23. Rice TW, Boyce GA, Sivak MV, Esophageal ultrasound and the preoperative staging of carcinoma of the esophagus, *J Thorac Cardiovasc Surg* 1991; **101**:536–44.
24. Heintz A, Hohne U, Schweden F, Junginger T, Endosonographie versus Computertomographie bei der praoperativen Stadienbeurteilung von Osophaguskarzinomen, *Z Gastroenterol* 1991; **29**:49–52.
25. Date H, Miyashita M, Sasajima K et al. Assessment of adventitial involvement of esophageal carcinoma by endoscopic ultrasonography, *Surg Endosc* 1990; **4**:195–7.
26. Takemoto T, Itoh T, Fukumoto Y, Aibe T, Okita K, Endoscopic ultrasonography in preoperative staging of esophageal cancer. In: Dancygier H, Classen M, eds, *5th International Symposium on Endoscopic Ultrasonography* (Demeter Verlag: Munich, 1989) (*Z Gastroenterol* suppl.) 34–8.
27. Tio TL, Cohen P, Coene PP, Udding J, denHartog Jager FCA, Tytgat GNJ, Endosonography and computed tomography of esophageal carcinoma, *Gastroenterology* 1989; **96**:1478–86.
28. Lightdale CJ, Botet JF, Kelsen DP, Turnbull AD, Brennan MF, Diagnosis of recurrent upper gastrointestinal cancer at the surgical anastomosis by endoscopic ultrasound, *Gastrointest Endosc* 1989; **35**:407–12.
29. Caletti GC, Brocchi E, Gibilaro M, Ferrari A, Carfagna L, Barbara L, Sensitivity, specificity and predictive value of endoscopic ultrasonography in the diagnosis and assessment of gastric cancer, *Gastrointest Endosc* 1990; **36**:194–5.
30. Ohashi S, Nakzawa S, Yoshino J, Endoscopic ultrasonography in the assessment of invasive gastric cancer, *Scand J Gastroenterol* 1989; **24**:1039–48.
31. Yasuda K, Nakajima M, Cho E, Kobayashi M, Kawai K, Benign versus malignant gastric ulcers: a role for endoscopic ultrasonography? In: Dancygier H, Classen M, eds, *5th International Symposium on Endoscopic Ultrasonography* (Demeter Verlag: Munich, 1989) (*Z Gastroenterol* suppl.) 50–6.
32. Murata Y, Suzuki S, Hashimoto H, Endoscopic ultrasonography of the upper gastrointestinal tract, *Surg Endosc* 1988; **2**:180–3.
33. Grimm H, Hamper K, Maydeo A, Maas R, Noar M. Soehendra N, Accuracy of endoscopic ultrasound and computed tomography in determining local/regional spread of gastric cancer; results of a prospective controlled study, *Gastrointest Endosc* 1991; **37**:279 (Abstract).
34. Akahoshi K, Misawa T, Fujishima H et al, Preoperative evaluation of gastric cancer by endoscopic ultrasound, *Gut* 1991; **32**:479–82.
35. Tio TL, Schouwink MH, Cikot RJ, Tytgat GN, Preoperative TNM classification of gastric carcinoma by endosonography in comparison with the pathological TNM system: a prospective study of 72 cases, *Hepatogastroenterol* 1989; **36**:51–6.

36. Sanft C, Ziegler K, Die bedutung der endosonographie fur das praoperative staging des magenkarzinoms, *Endoskopie Heute* 1989; **2**:30–3.
37. Aibe T, Fujimura H, Noguchi T et al, Endosonographic detection and staging of early gastric cancer. In: Dancygier H, Classen M, eds, *5th International Symposium on Endoscopic Ultrasonography* (Demeter Verlag: Munich, 1989) (*Z Gastroenterol* suppl.) 71–8.
38. Botet JF, Lightdale CJ, Zauber AG et al, Preoperative staging of gastric cancer: comparison of endoscopic US and dynamic CT, *Radiology* 1991; **181**:426–32.
39. Yoshimi M, Kusuyama A, Tashiro H et al, EUS approach to the regional lymph nodes in early gastric cancer. In: *Abstracts of the World Congresses of Gastroenterology*, Sydney 1990 (The Medicine Group (UK): Abingdon, 1990).
40. Saito N, Takeshita K, Habu H, Endo M, The use of endoscopic ultrasound in determining the depth of cancer invasion in patients with gastric cancer, *Surg Endosc* 1991; **5**:14–19.
41. Heintz A, Junginger T, Endosonographisches Staging von Karzinomen in Speiserohre und Magen, *Bildgenbung (Imaging)* 1991; **58**:4–8.
42. Bolondi L, Casanova P, Caletti GC, Grigioni W, Zani L, Barbara L, Primary gastric lymphoma versus gastric carcinoma: endoscopic US evaluation, *Radiology* 1987; **165**:821–6.
43. Caletti CG, Zani L, Bolondi L, Guizzardi G, Brocchi E, Barbarar L, Impact of endoscopic ultrasonography on diagnosis and treatment of primary gastric lymphoma, *Surgery* 1988; **103**:315–20.
44. Caletti GC, Brocchi E, Gibilaro M, Ferrari A, Carfagna L, Barbara L, Sensitivity, specificity and predictive value of endoscopic ultrasonography in the diagnosis of gastric lymphoma, *Gastrointest Endosc* 1990; **36**:195 (Abstract).
45. Fujishima H, Misawa T, Maruoka A, Chijiiwa Y, Masuda T, Nawata H, Primary gastric lymphoma in staging and follow-up by means of endoscopic ultrasonography. In: *Abstracts of the World Congresses of Gastroenterology*, Sydney (The Medicine Group (UK): Abingdon).
46. Tio TL, den Hartog Jager FCA, Tytgat GNJ, Endoscopic ultrasonography of non-Hodgkin lymphoma of the stomach, *Gastroenterology* 1986; **91**:401–8.
47. Tio TL, den Hartog Jager FCA, Tytgat GNJ, Endoscopic ultrasonography in the evaluation of non-Hodgkin lymphoma of the stomach: EUS versus computed tomography and endoscopy, *Gastroenterology* 1988; **94**:A461 (Abstract).
48. Wakabayashi N, Michinaka C, Kawamoto K, Ebisui S, Kodama T, Kashima K. Usefulness of endoscopic ultrasonography in the evaluation of gastric lymphoma, *Gastroenterology* 1991; **100**:A409 (Abstract).
49. Fujishima H, Misawa T, Maruoka A, Chijiiwa Y, Sakai K, Nawata H, Staging and follow-up of primary gastric lymphoma by endoscopic ultrasonography, *Am J Gastroenterol* 1991; **86**:719–24.
50. Schuder G, Feifel G, Koch B, Seitz G, Gross J, Endosonographisch gesteuerte therapie beim primaren non-Hodgkin lymphom des magens. Abstract presented during Ultraschall-Diagnostik 91, Lausanne October 17, 1991.
51. Songur Y, Okai T, Watanabe H, Motoo Y, Sawabu N, Endosonographic evaluation of giant gastric folds, *Gastrointest Endosc* 1995; **41**:468–74.
52. Mendis RE, Gerdes H, Lightdale CJ, Botet JF, Large gastric folds: a diagnostic approach using endoscopic ultrasonography, *Gastrointest Endosc* 1994; **40**:437–41.
53. Caletti GC, Zani L, Bolondi L, Brocchi E, Rollo V, Barbara L, Endoscopic ultrasonography in the diagnosis of gastric submucosal tumor, *Gastrointest Endosc* 1989; **35**:413–18.
54. Hashimoto H, Mistumaga A, Suzuki S, Kurokawa K, Obata H, Evaluation of endoscopic ultrasonography for gastric tumors and presentation of three-dimensional display of endoscopic ultrasonography, *Surg Endosc* 1989; **3**:173–81.
55. Kiyota K, Yasuda K, Fujimoto S, Najimoto S, Nakajima M, Kawai K, Endoscopic ultrasonography in the diagnosis of esophageal submucosal tumors. In: Dancygier H, Classen M, eds, *5th International Symposium on Endoscopic Ultrasonography* (Demeter Verlag: Munich, 1989) (*Z Gastroenterol* suppl.) 29–33.
56. Nakazawa S, Yoshino J, Nakamura T et al, Endoscopic ultrasonography of gastric myogenic tumor. A comparative study between histology and ultrasonography, *J Ultrasound Med* 1989; **8**:353–69.
57. Tio TL, Tytgat GNJ, denHartog Jager FCA, Endoscopic ultrasonography for the evaluation of smooth muscle tumors in the upper gastrointestinal tract: an experience with 42 cases, *Gastrointest Endosc* 1990; **36**:343–50.
58. Yamada Y, Kida M, Sakaguchi T, Matama S, Saigenji K, Differential diagnosis of submucosal tumors in the upper digestive tract using the endoscopic ultrasonography. In: *Abstracts of the World Congress of Gastroenterology*, Sydney,. 1990. (The Medicine Group (UK): Abingdon, 1990).
59. Yasuda K, Nakajima M, Yoshida S, Kiyota K, Kawai K, The diagnosis of submucosal tumors of the stomach by endoscopic ultrasonography, *Gastrointest Endosc* 1989; **35**:10–15.
60. Rösch T, Lorenz R, Dancygier H, VonWichert A, Classen M, Endosonographic ultrasonography of submucosal upper GI tract tumors, *Scand J Gastroenterol* 1992; **27**:1–8.
61. Murata Y, Yoshida M, Akimoto S, Ide H, Suzuki S, Hanyu F, Evaluation of endoscopic ultrasonography in the diagnosis of submucosal tumors of the esophagus, *Surg Endosc* 1988; **2**:51–8.
62. Heyder N, Obenauf G, Extragastric and submucosal lesions. In: Dancygier H, Classen M, eds, *5th International Symposium on Endoscopic Ultrasonography* (Demeter Verlag: Munich, 1989) (*Z Gastroenterol* suppl.) 79–82.
63. Takimoto Y, Inoue R, Hamashima H, Sakai M, Kita T, Value of endoscopic ultrasonography in diagnosis of submucosal tumor and extragastric lesion of the stomach, *Gastroenterology* 1989; **96**:502 (Abstract).
64. Amouyal P, Amouyal G, Palazzo L et al, L'echoendoscopie: une nouvelle technique d'exploration des tumeurs sous-epitheliales et des compressions extrinseques oeso-gastriques, *Gastroenterol Clin Biol* 1990; **14**:8–14.
65. Liu JB, Miller LS, Goldberg BB et al, Transnasal US of the esophagus: preliminary morphologic and function studies, *Radiology* 1992; **184**:721–7.
66. Kimmey MB, Martin RW, Haggitt RC, Wang KY, Franklin DW, Silverstein FE, Histologic correlates of gastrointestinal ultrasound images, *Gastroenterology* 1989; **96**:433–41.
67. Caletti G, Ferrari A, Brocchi E et al, Normal EUS anatomy: the gut wall. In: *Endoscopic Ultrasonography*, A Tutorial Course syllabus for a Symposium sponsored by the Cleveland Clinic Foundation, 21–22 March, 1992.
68. Miller L, Liu JB, Dhuria M, Goldberg B, Castell D, High frequency endoluminal sonography of the esophagus using a 20 MHz ultrasound transducer: correlation with cross-sectional histology in human anatomy specimen, *Gastroenterology* 1994; **102**:A486.

69. Sandler RS, Nyren O, Ekbom A, Eisen G, Yuen J, Josefsson S, The risk of esophageal cancer in patients with achalasia: a population-based study, *JAMA* 1995; **274**:1359–62.
70. Deviere J, Dunham F, Rickaert F, Bourgeois N, Cremer M, Endoscopic ultrasonography in achalasia, *Gastroenterology* 1989; **96**:1210–13.
71. Ponsot P, Chaussade S, Palazzo L et al, Endoscopic ultrasonography in achalasia, *Gastroenterology* 1990; **98**:253.
72. Ziegler K, Sanft C, Friedrich M, Gregor M, Riecken EO, Endosonographic appearance of the esophagus in achalasia, *Endoscopy* 1990; **22**:1–4.
73. Trowers EA, Kimmey MB, Yee HC, Martin RW, Taniguchi D, Silverstein FE, Assessment of esophageal muscle thickness in achalasia using a high frequency linear endoscopic ultrasound probe, *Gastrointest Endosc* 1992; **38**:244A.
74. Miller L, Liu J-B, Barbarevech CA et al, High-resolution endoluminal sonography in achalasia, *Gastrointest Endosc* 1995; **42**:545–9.
75. Schiano TD, Fisher RS, Parkman HP, Cohen S, Dabezies MA, Miller LS, Use of high-resolution endoscopic ultrasonography to assess esophageal wall damage after pneumatic dilatation and botulinum toxin injection to treat achalasia. *Gastrointest Endosc* 1996; **44**:151–7.
76. Brick IB, Palmer ED, Comparison of oesophagoscopic and roentgenologic diagnosis of esophageal varices in cirrhosis of the liver, *Am J Roentgenol Radium Ther Nucl Med* 1955; **73**:387–9.
77. Kirsh IE, Blackwell CC, Bennett HD, Roentgen diagnosis of oesophageal varices: comparison of roentgen and esophagoscopic findings in 502 cases, *Am J Roentgenol Radium Ther Nucl Med* 1955; **74**:477–85.
78. Evans KT, Oesophageal and gastric varices, *Br J Radiol* 1959; **32**:233–40.
79. Conn HO, Mitchell JR, Brodoff MG, A comparison of the radiologic and esophagoscopic diagnosis of esophageal varices, *N Engl J Med* 1961; **265**:160–4.
80. Waldram R, Nunnerley H, Davis M et al, Detection and grading of esophageal varices by fibre-optic endoscopy and barium swallow with and without buscopan, *Clin Radiol* 1977; **28**:137–41.
81. Caletti GC, Bolondi L, Zani L, Lab'o G, Technique of endoscopic ultrasonography investigation: esophagus, stomach, and duodenum, *Scand J Gastroenterol Suppl* 1986; **123**:1–5.
82. Caletti GC, Bolondi L, Zani L, Brocchi E, Guizzardi G, Lab'o G, Detection of portal hypertension and esophageal varices by means of endoscopic ultrasonography, *Scand J Gastroenterol Suppl* 1986; **123**:74–7.
83. Caletti G, Brocchi E, Baraldini M, Assessment of portal hypertension by endoscopic ultrasonography, *Gastrointest Endosc* **36**(suppl. 2):S21–7.
84. Liu J-B, Miller LS, Feld RI, Barbarevich CA, Needleman L, Goldberg BB, Gastric and esophageal varices: 20 MHz transnasal endoluminal US, *Radiology* 1993; **187**:363–6.
85. Miller LS, Schiano TD, McCray WH et al, In vivo comparison of esophageal varices at and above the diaphragmatic high pressure zone using high resolution endoluminal sonography. Submitted.
86. Miller LS, Schiano TD, McCray WH et al, Use of high resolution endoluminal sonography to measure the radius and wall thickness of esophageal varices. *Gastrointest Endosc* (accepted for publication).
87. Miller LS, Schiano TD, Liu JB et al, Comparison of high resolution endoluminal sonography to video-endoscopy in the detection and evaluation of esophageal varices. *Hepatology* (accepted for publication).
88. Miller LS, Liu JB, Klenn PJ et al, Endoluminal ultrasonography of the distal esophagus in systemic sclerosis, *Gastroenterology* 1993; **105**:31–9.
89. Liu JB, Miller LS, Goldberg BB, Endoluminal ultrasound in gastroenterology: application of new technology. In: Dubbins PA, Joseph AEA, eds, *Ultrasound in Gastroenterology* (Churchill Livingstone: New York, 1994).
90. McLoughlin RF, Cooperberg PL, Mathieson JR, Stordy SN, Halparin LS, High resolution endoluminal ultrasonography in the staging of esophageal carcinoma, *J Ultrasound Med* 1995; **14**:725–30.
91. Taniguchi DK, Martin RW, Trowers EA, Dennis MB, Odegaard S, Silverstein FE, Changes in esophageal wall layer during motility: measurements with a new miniature ultrasound device, *Gastrointest Endosc* 1993; **39**:146–52.
92. Miller LS, Liu JB, Colizzo FP et al, Correlation of high frequency esophageal ultrasonography and manometry in the study of esophageal motility, *Gastroenterology* 1995; **109**:833–7.
93. Kalimanis G, Garra BS, Tio TL et al, The feasibility of three-dimensional ultrasonography: a preliminary report, *Gastrointest Endosc* 1995; **41**:235–9.
94. Wiersema MJ, Wiersema LM, Khusro Q, Cramer HM, Tao LC, Combined endosonography and fine-needle aspiration cytology in the evaluation of gastrointestinal lesions, *Gastrointest Endosc* 1994; **40**:199–206.
95. Wiersema MJ, Kochman ML, Chak A, Cramer HM, Kessler KA, Real-time endoscopic ultrasound-guided fine-needle aspiration of a mediastinal lymph node, *Gastrointest Endosc* 1993; **39**:429–31.
96. Vilmann P, Jacobsen GK, Henriksen FW, Haneke S, Endoscopic ultrasonography with guided fine-needle aspiration biopsy in pancreatic disease, *Gastrointest Endosc* 1991; **38**:173–3.
97. Chang KJ, Katz KD, Durbin TE et al, Endoscopic ultrasound-guided fine needle aspiration, *Gastrointest Endosc* 1994; **40**:694–9.
98. Wiersema MJ, Kochman ML, Cramer HM, Hao LC, Wiersema LM, Endosonography-guided real-time fine-needle aspiration biopsy, *Gastrointest Endosc* 1994; **40**: 700–7.
99. Vilmann P, Hancke S, Henriksen FW, Jacobsen GK, Endoscopic ultrasonograph-guided fine-needle aspiration biopsy of lesions in the upper gastrointestinal tract, *Gastrointest Endosc* 1995; **41**:230–5.

Chapter 7 Lower gastrointestinal tract

Archie A Alexander, Larry S Miller, Thomas D Schiano and Ji-Bin Liu

INTRODUCTION

Since the introduction of endoluminal ultrasound for the evaluation of the lower gastrointestinal (GI) tract, it has assumed a greater role in the assessment of both inflammatory and neoplastic diseases of the colon, rectum and anal canal. The chief advantage of this technology comes from its use of sound energies for image production that, unlike other radiologic imaging technologies, avoids patient exposure to ionizing radiation and is relatively inexpensive. The ability to configure transducers with frequencies ranging from 7.0 to 20 MHz as either radial, linear or sector probes and incorporate them into endoscopes has enabled the sonographer to image multiple histologic layers within the wall of the lower GI tract.[1,2] More recently, endorectal probes have been made available for use in the anorectum, and miniature catheter-based ultrasound probes have been utilized to image the anorectal complex.[2]

In this chapter we will review the normal sonographic anatomy of the colon, rectum and anal canal. We will describe and evaluate the use of endosonography in various disorders of the lower GI tract, including benign and malignant neoplasms, inflammatory bowel disease, anal incontinence, anorectal abscesses, and fistulae. In addition, we will present techniques and applications of ultrasound-guided interventional procedures utilized in the diagnosis and treatment of colorectal disease. Finally, we will look at future applications of endosonography in the lower GI tract.

ENDOSONOGRAPHY OF THE COLON AND RECTUM

INSTRUMENTATION

The colon is usually imaged ultrasonographically during colonoscopy with a 7.5–12-MHz probe mounted on the end of an endosonoscope. The anorectum, on the other hand, may be imaged either with the endosonoscope or with endorectal probes specifically designed for this use.[1,3] These frequencies are usually obtained from mechanical or electronic transducers. Mechanical transducers produce ultrasound images by rotating elements in a radial fashion, generating a 90–360° image. Electronic transducers are motionless, relying on electrical impulses to create ultrasound images in a pie-shaped sector or rectangular (linear) configuration. Most of these transducers image in the transverse (axial) plane, except for the linear transducer, which produces a longitudinal image. With these transducer frequencies, sufficient depth of penetration and resolution should be available to image the multilayered rectal wall and any adjacent structures such as blood vessels, lymph nodes and visceral organs.

Higher-frequency transducers (12.5–20 MHz) are now available that acquire exquisitely detailed images of the colorectal wall layers over a short distance of 2–3 cm. Unfortunately, the reduction in optimum depth of penetration could pose a major limitation to sonographic detection of structures beyond this distance. Preliminary work has shown the feasibility of inserting miniature high-frequency ultrasound (20 MHz) catheters through the biopsy port of an endoscope to image the colon, and their ability to image the anorectum alone or in conjunction with the endoscope has been documented. With this approach, the endoscopist is able to visualize the superficial appearance of disease processes as well as their effects on the layers below the mucosal surface. Theoretically, the addition of this detailed information ought to improve the assessment and treatment of patients with colorectal disease.[2]

PREPARATION AND TECHNIQUES

For any endosonographic study of the lower GI tract, the transducer-containing portion of the probe is covered by a condom, which provides protection against fecal contamination. It also serves as a reservoir for water which, upon distention, provides a pathway for the conduction of sound waves from the transducer to the target. Additional important benefits obtained from the water-filled condom include a means to artificially adjust the focal depth of the transducer by altering the water volume, distend the bowel lumen, and displace gas and residual fecal debris away from the area of interest, reducing the potential for confusing pseudolesions. Distention of the condom is best achieved by injecting various amounts of degassed water from a catheter-tipped syringe through an extension tube attached to an injection port on the probe. All air bubbles must be purged from the fluid system, as air impedes the transmission of sound, degrading the image and reducing the resolution.

Performance of an adequate endosonographic study also relies on adequate preparation of the patient. It is critical to have performed a digital rectal examination prior to inserting any probe through the anorectum. If the lumen is too narrow to allow entry of a probe with a 2-cm diameter, a radial probe with a small shaft diameter may be considered.

If no contraindication exists, individuals undergoing colonic sonography should be prepared for colonoscopy. For ultrasonography of the anorectum, which is often done without the benefit of direct vision of the lesion, the patient may be given Fleet enemas to remove residual fecal debris from the rectosigmoid colon. This is usually done on the morning of the examination to reduce the potential for fecal debris pseudolesions.

Most patients are examined in the left lateral decubitus position with their knees toward their chest and their buttocks over the table edge. This position affords easy access to the patient, especially if ultrasound-guided interventional procedures are in order. In most cases imaging begins in the transverse (axial) plane but there are situations where a sagittal plane probe may be very helpful. Remember, that the examiner must be aware of image orientation throughout the entire scanning procedure.[3]

ANATOMY OF THE COLON AND RECTUM

COLON

The main portion of the colon lies within the abdomen as an inverted U-shaped structure that is anatomically divided from right to left into the cecum, and ascending, transverse and descending colon. The cecum is a blind-ending pouch-like structure which extends caudally below the ileocecal valve to occupy the right lower quadrant. The wormlike appendix projects from the inferior margin of the cecum to rest in the right lower quadrant in the majority of patients. The S-shaped sigmoid colon begins at the terminal aspect of the descending colon and enters the pelvis to become the rectum (Fig. 7.1). The ascending colon, descending colon and rectum below the third sacral vertebra are considered to be extraperitoneal structures.

The colon ascends through the right lateral and hypochondriac regions to the liver, bending sharply to the left at the hepatic flexure to become the transverse colon. The transverse colon is invested in

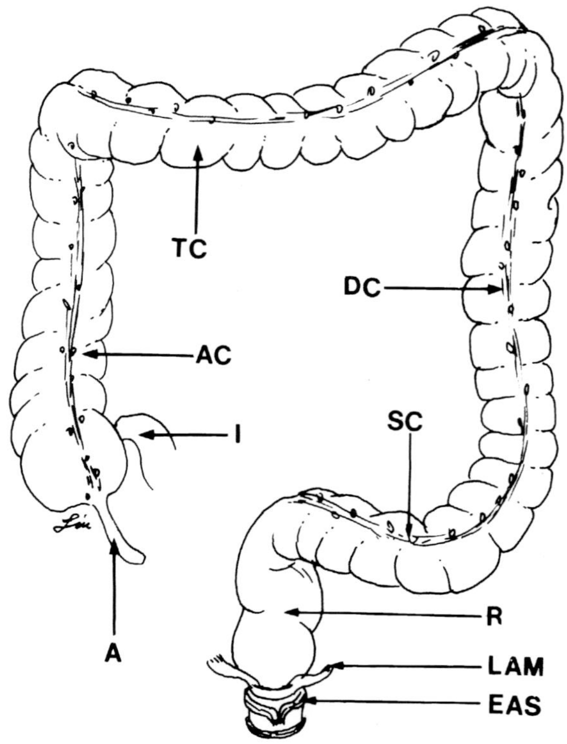

Figure 7.1 *Diagrammatic representation of the colon and anorectum in anterior view. A, appendix; I, ileum; AC, ascending colon; TC, transverse colon; DC, descending colon; SC, sigmoid colon; R, rectum; LAM, levator ani muscle; EAS, external anal sphincter.*

peritoneum and is suspended from the body wall by the transverse mesocolon. The transverse colon is the longest and most movable part of the colon, running leftward across the abdomen in the area of the umbilicus and left hypochondriac area below the spleen. At the spleen it bends to form the splenic flexure and then descends caudally through the left hypochondriac and lumbar region. It is covered anteriorly and laterally with peritoneum, which helps to fix it (Fig. 7.1).

The sigmoid colon is about 25–38 cm long and begins as a continuation of the descending colon in front of the left external iliac artery at the level of the pelvic brim (Fig. 7.1). Below, it becomes continuous with the rectum in front of the third sacral vertebra. The pelvic colon is attached to the posterior pelvic wall by the fan-shaped pelvic mesocolon. Anteriorly in the male is the urinary bladder; anteriorly in the female is the posterior surface of the uterus and the upper part of the vagina. Posteriorly is the rectum and the sacrum. The arterial supply to the pelvic colon is from the left colic branches of the inferior mesenteric artery. The veins correspond to the arteries and are tributaries of the portal system.

RECTUM

The rectum is about 13 cm long and begins in front of the third sacral vertebra as a continuation of the sigmoid colon. It ends 2.5 cm in front of the tip of the coccyx by piercing the pelvic diaphragm and becomes continuous with the anal canal. The lower part of the rectum lies immediately above the pelvic diaphragm and is dilated to form the rectal ampulla. The peritoneum covers the anterior and lateral surfaces of the first third of the rectum; only the anterior surface of the middle third and the lower third is not covered by peritoneum (Fig. 7.1).

The muscular coat of the rectum has outer longitudinal and inner circular smooth muscle layers. The three teniae coli of the sigmoid colon come together so that the longitudinal fibers form a broad band on the anterior and posterior surfaces of the rectum. Three folds, the transverse folds of the rectum, are formed by the mucous membrane and circular muscle layers. Two of these semicircular folds are on the left rectal wall and one is on the right rectal wall. The rectum is in contact with the sacrum and coccyx, the median sacral artery, and the periformis, coccygeus and levatores ani muscles. The sacral plexus and the sympathetic trunks are located posteriorly.

In the male the rectum is in contact anteriorly with the posterior surface of the bladder, the termination of the vas deferens, the seminal vesicles on each side, and the prostate. The upper two-thirds of the rectum is covered by peritoneum anteriorly and is related to the pelvic colon and coils of ileum that occupy the rectovesical pouch. In the female the upper two-thirds of the rectum is also covered by peritoneum and forms the pouch of Douglas. The lower third of the rectum, devoid of peritoneum, is related to the posterior surface of the vagina. The arterial supply to the rectum is from the superior, middle and inferior rectal arteries.

ENDOSONOGRAPHIC ANATOMY OF THE COLORECTUM

The exact anatomic correlation of the various layers of the wall of the colon and rectum with those imaged with ultrasound has at times been controversial.[4–14] Most investigators now agree that at least five layers of the wall can be detected with endosonography, depending on the level at which the colon or rectum is imaged and the frequency utilized.[4–14] Sonographically, each layer is represented by either a thin hypoechoic (dark or echo-poor) or hyperechoic (bright or echo-rich) band. The initial layer imaged is the echogenic wall of the water-filled condom as it interferes with the surface of the colonic mucosa. The next hyperechoic band represents the mucosa in both the colon and rectum, although some investigators believe that it may be a composite of both the mucosa and muscularis mucosa. The muscularis mucosa is not imaged as a discrete band, especially in the rectum, as its thickness is below the limit of resolution of the ultrasound frequencies utilized. The third sonographic layer is the hyperechoic submucosa which is the thickest layer in the wall. The fourth sonographic layer is the hypoechoic smooth muscle of the muscularis propria. The fifth and final layer is the hyperechoic colonic serosa.

The sonographic layers of the normal rectal wall are similar to those just described for the wall of the colon. The sonographer, however, should be aware of several important differences in the layers of rectal wall as compared to the more proximal colon. The peritoneal reflection occurs about the third sacral vertebral body and below this level the rectum is surrounded by hyperechoic perirectal fat, not serosa.[3] If a probe with 10-MHz or higher frequency transducer is employed, the hypoechoic muscularis propria of the rectal wall may appear as three distinct

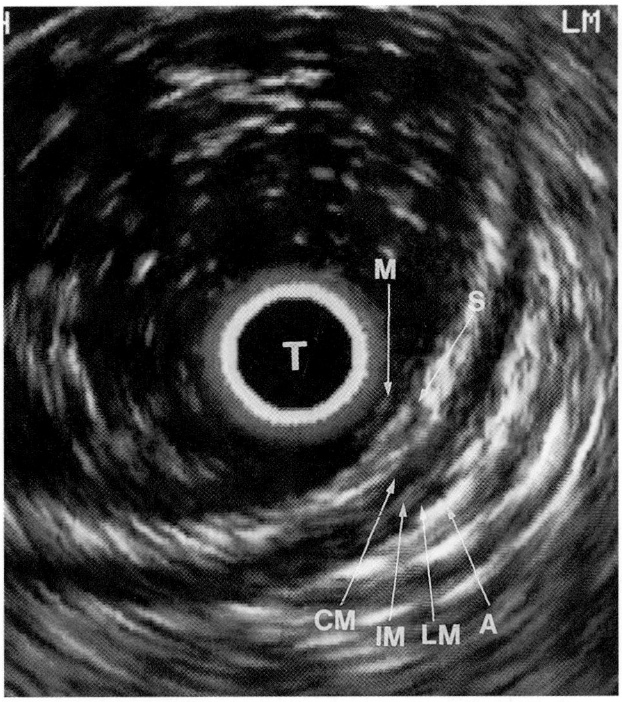

Figure 7.2 *A 20-MHz catheter-based ultrasound image obtained from within fluid-filled colon showing the six layers of the wall. From the colon lumen out, they are the hypoechoic mucosa (M), hyperechoic submucosa (S), hypoechoic circular smooth muscle (CM), hyperechoic intermuscular connective tissue (IM), hypoechoic longitudinal smooth muscle (LM), and hyperechoic adventitia (A). T, transducer.*

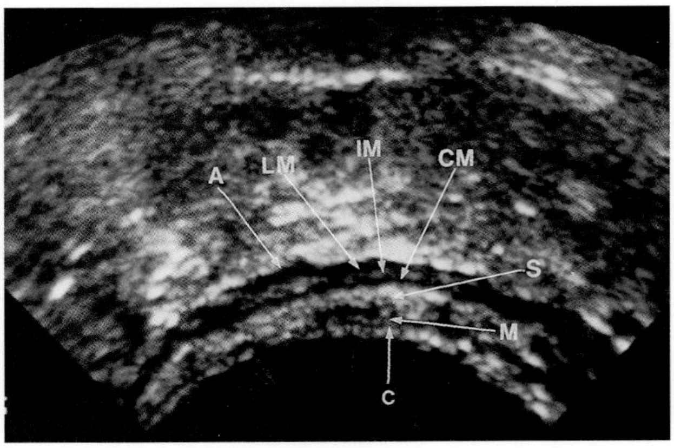

Figure 7.3 *A transrectal ultrasound image demonstrated the seven layers of the rectal wall. From the rectal lumen out, they are the hyperechoic condom interfacing with mucosa (C), hypoechoic mucosa (M), hyperechoic submucosa (S), hypoechoic circular smooth muscle (CM), hyperechoic intermuscular connective tissue (IM), hypoechoic longitudinal smooth muscle (LM), and hyperechoic adventitia (A).*

layers. The layer closest to the submucosa is the hypoechoic, inner circular muscle which lies adjacent to hyperechoic intermuscular connective tissue, and this is followed by the hypoechoic outer longitudinal muscle (Figures 7.2 and 7.3).[3]

With color flow and pulsed wave Doppler probes, the feeding perirectal and submucosal vessels can be demonstrated in the normal and abnormal rectal wall.[14,15] In the normal rectal wall, color signals have been detected arising from small extramural perirectal arteries just prior to their penetration through the muscularis propria. Within the wall proper color signals have also been detected within the submucosal layer which likely originate from the arterial segments of the submucosal vascular plexuses. The pulsed Doppler waveforms and pulsatility index (PI) measurements obtained from these vessels have high-impedance pattern (Fig. 7.4).[14,15]

As mentioned, the male rectum is related anteriorly to the bladder, the seminal vesicles and the prostate. The rectovesical septum, which is closely associated with the bladder, represents a potential cleavage plane between the rectum and the bladder. In the female the anterior relation of the rectum is the vagina. Tumors penetrating into the posterior wall of the vagina can be visualized transrectally. Blood vessels appear as hypoechoic or anechoic structures, which are easy to identify by Doppler imaging.

Anatomic structures such as lymph nodes adjacent to the colon and rectum may be seen. Generally, benign lymph nodes less than 2 mm are not detected with ultrasound but can be distinguished from vessels, which often have a traceable, serpiginous course.[16] Normal nodes will have an oval or kidney bean shape with an echogenic or bright center which represents the hilum. Male and female pelvic organs can be visualized with endosonography.[5–13,17–19]

The pelvic diaphragm, which consists of the levator ani and coccygeus muscles, form the pelvic floor. With an ultrasound probe in the anal canal, a

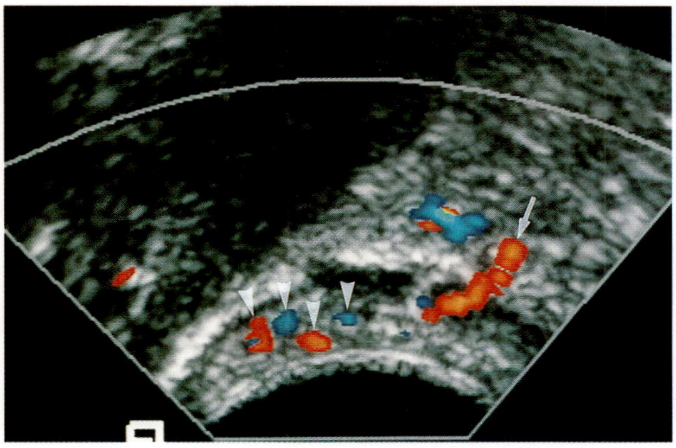

a

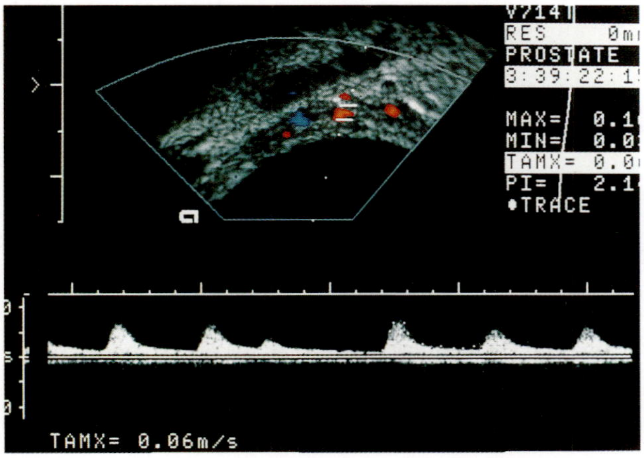

b

Figure 7.4 *(a) Transverse image of a normal rectal wall demonstrates a single peri-rectal artery (arrow) penetrating the hypoechoic layer of muscularis propria into the hyperechoic submucosa to form the submucosal arterial branches (arrowheads). (b) Both color flow and pulsed Doppler signals are recorded from one of the submucosal arterial branches in a normal rectal wall. A representative arterial waveform yields a high-resistance signal with a pulsatility index of 2.14. (Reprinted with permission from Alexander et al.[14])*

sonogram can demonstrate that the muscle sheet stretches between the pubis anteriorly and the coccyx posteriorly. The obturator internus muscle is seen as a hypoechoic band in front of the hyperechoic pubic ramus. The puborectalis muscle forms a sling at the junction of the rectum and the anal canal.

COLORECTAL DISORDERS

MALIGNANT COLORECTAL NEOPLASMS

The incidence of colorectal cancer is rising, and, with increased detection, colorectal cancer management has become a multidisciplinary effort.[20,21] Surgeons armed with new technologies, such as laser ablation techniques, have begun to offer patients with early local disease the option of local rather than more extensive radical resections. Likewise, management plans incorporating adjuvant treatment with high-dose preoperative radiation, with or without chemotherapy, have demonstrated reductions in tumor stage and improved local control.[21]

To select the appropriate therapy, both clinical and radiologic staging systems have been devised. Both the American Committee on Cancer (AJCC) and International Union Against Cancer (UICC) have proposed a staging system called the TNM classification. The TNM system is a popular staging system that incorporates information that influences local regional therapy.[20,21] 'T' is the depth of penetration of the tumor into the wall and extension beyond the wall into adjacent organs, 'N' is the presence or absence of metastatic lymph nodes, and 'M' is the extent of tumor spread to distant organs. Based on the TNM system, Hildebrandt et al[12,13] proposed an endosonographic staging: uT_1 confined to the mucosa and submucosa, uT_2 penetrating the muscularis propria but confined to the rectal wall, uT_3 penetrating into the perirectal fat, and uT_4 infiltrating into the surrounding organs (Fig. 7.5).

Although the colonoscopy for colon cancers and digital rectal examination for rectal cancers may provide some of this information, there are very important shortcomings. Therefore, surgical and medical oncologists have sought radiologic evaluation as a means of gathering more objective information.[20,21] In the preoperative staging of rectal cancer, endosonography has been shown to be more accurate for local staging (69–93%) (Table 7.1) than CT (33–70%). However, MRI (90–95%) may be as accurate or more accurate than endosonography.[22–49] Assessment of adjacent lymph nodes for metastatic disease is more problematic; accuracies achieved with endosonography (32–80%) (Table 7.2) and MRI (95%) are better than those with CT (25–73%).[22–49] For distant metastatic disease (M), both CT and MRI yield more information than endosonography.[22–49]

The typical colorectal cancer imaged with endosonography will appear as a hypoechoic mass,

Figure 7.5 *Diagram of ultrasonographic TNM staging system. (a) Stage* uT_1*: tumor confined to the mucosa and submucosa. 1, mucosa; 2, submucosa; 3, muscularis propria; 4, serosa. (b) Stage* uT_2*: extending into the muscularis propria but confined to the rectal wall. (c) Stage* uT_3*: penetrating into the serosa or perirectal fat. (d) Stage* uT_4*: infiltrating into the adjacent organs. V, vagina. (e) Stage* uT_2 *and* N_1*: rectal tumor with regional lymph node metastases. (f) Stage* uT_3 *and* M_1*: rectal tumor with distant metastases present. L, liver.*

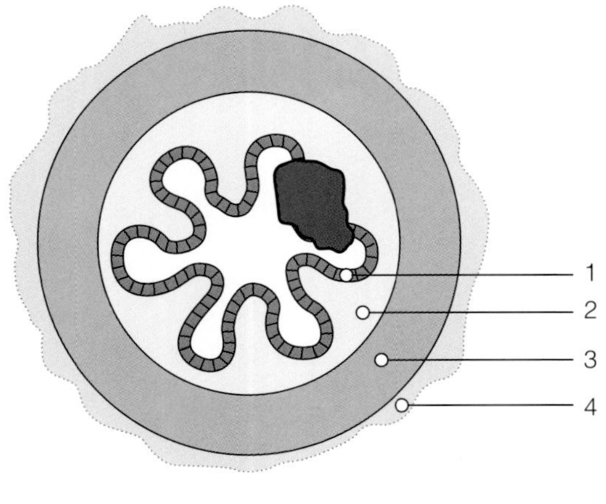

a

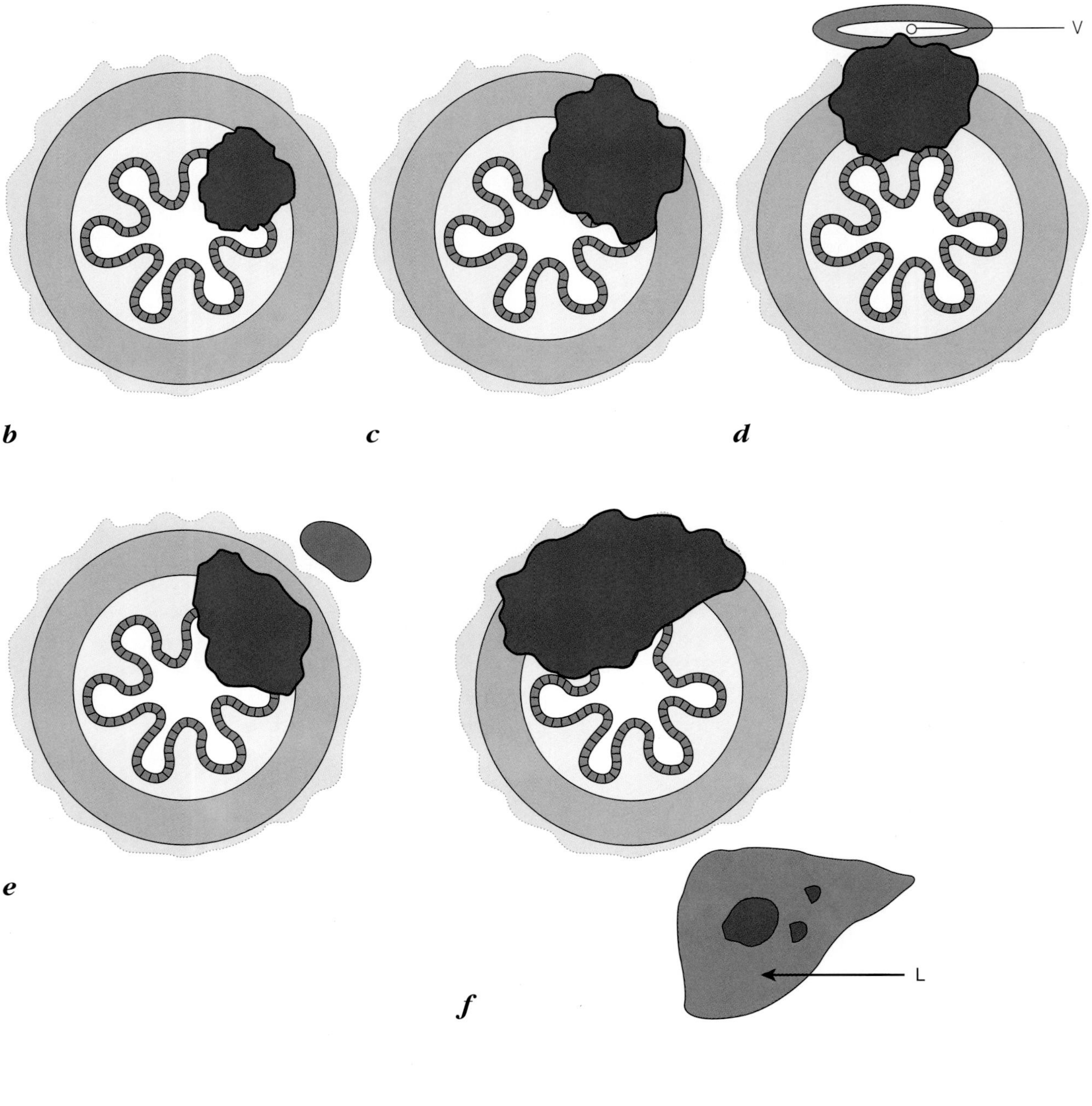

b ***c*** ***d***

e ***f***

Table 7.1 Accuracy and staging of endorectal sonography in detection of rectal tumors in series studies.

Study	*Year*	*No. of cases*	*Accuracy (%)*	*Understaging (%)*	*Overstaging (%)*
Rifkin et al[35]	1986	53	93	N/A	N/A
Wang et al[6]	1987	16	92.5	3.8	3.7
Heintz et al[7]	1989	66	87	6	7
Rotte et al[39]	1989	21	84	4	12
Zainea et al[52]	1989	27	90	4	6
Orrom et al[11]	1990	77	75	3	22
Roubein et al[48]	1990	9	69.3	0	30.7
Shimizu et al[49]	1990	53	84.9	N/A	N/A

N/A = not available.

Table 7.2 Accuracy of endorectal sonography in detection of neoplastic nodes compared to pathologic findings.

Study	*Year*	*No. of cases*	*Accuracy (%)*
Rifkin et al[35]	1986	55	81
Rotte et al[39]	1989	3	30
Zainea et al[52]	1989	6	67
Orrom et al[11]	1990	61	82
Roubein et al[48]	1990	9	69.3
Shimizu et al[49]	1990	6	67

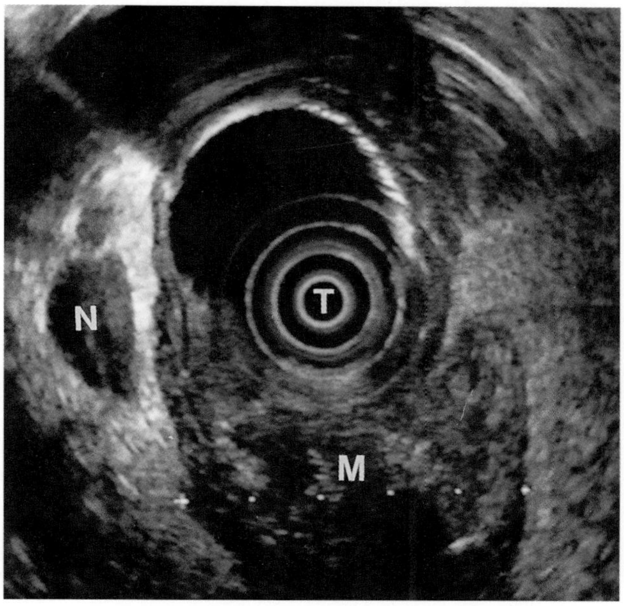

Figure 7.6 *An endosonographic image obtained from the distal colon demonstrated a hypoechoic mass (M) with a heterogeneous echotexture. An enlarged lymph node (N) adjacent to the tumor was also seen. T, transducer.*

although, on occasion, it may have a mixed echotexture with both bright and low-level internal echoes (Fig. 7.6). The mass may be lobulated or flat, mirroring the configuration of the tumor seen with endoscopy or palpated rectally.[1,3–13] The T stage or depth of penetration is based on the deepest layer involved by tumor.[12,13] More often than not, small mucosal lesions cannot be distinguished from adenomatous polyps, and mucosal lesions are lumped with submucosal lesions. Therefore, they are all staged as T_1 lesions (Fig. 7.7).[12,14,47] In the case of the villous adenoma, the sonographer may be unable to differentiate this lesion from a T_1 cancer.[46] Recognition of a moderately differentiated to well-differentiated T_1 rectal cancer less than 3 cm in diameter and lacking vascular or lymphatic invasion is of importance (Fig. 7.8). Patients having this lesion may be offered the option of local excision.[20] More advanced tumors extending into the muscularis propria are endosonographically staged as T_2 lesions (Fig. 7.9).[5–13] Sonographically, the hypoechoic muscularis propria may

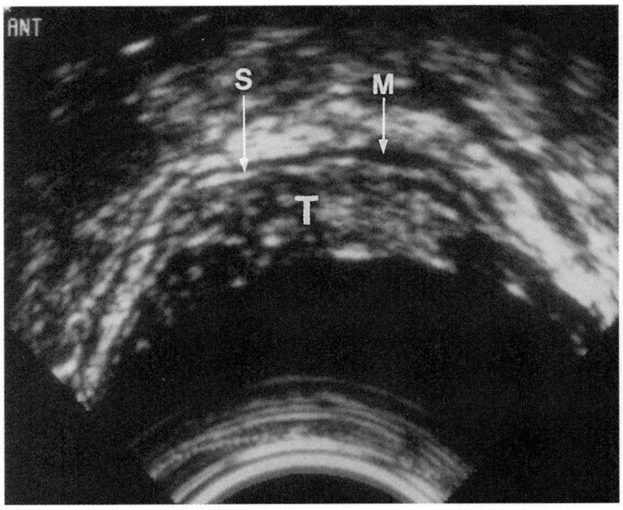

Figure 7.7 *Stage T_1 rectal carcinoma. Transrectal ultrasound image shows a hypoechoic mass (T) without penetration into the submucosa (S) and muscularis propria (M) corresponding to the stage T_1 rectal carcinoma.*

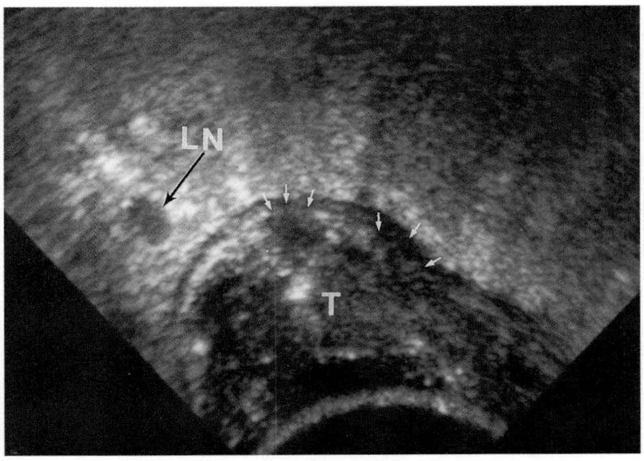

Figure 7.9 *Stage T_2 rectal carcinoma. Transrectal ultrasound image shows a hypoechoic mass (T) with irregularity of the hypoechoic muscularis propria (arrows). Note a lymph node adjacent to the tumor (LN).*

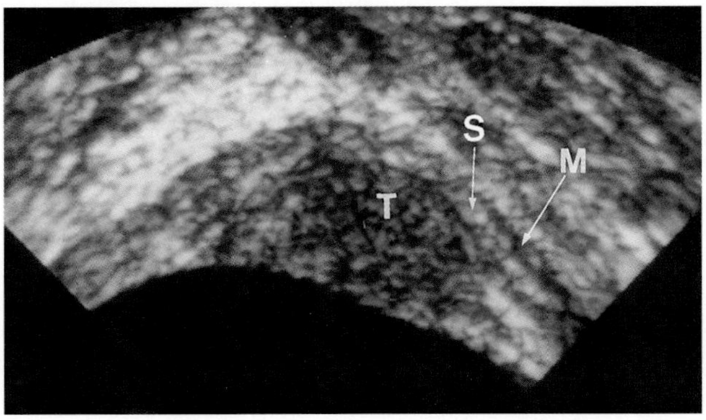

Figure 7.8 *Transrectal ultrasound image of a stage T_1 rectal carcinoma demonstrates a small hypoechoic mass (T) involving the submucosal layer (S) but not extending into the muscularis propria (M).*

be expanded or interrupted, but the adjacent outer white (hyperechoic or bright) line of colonic serosa or perirectal fat must be smooth and intact (Fig. 7.9).[47] Detection of T_3 disease relies on the sonographic recognition of a spiculated or irregular interface between the adjacent bright line of serosa or perirectal fat and the hypoechoic band of muscularis propria (Figs 7.10 and 7.11). If the tumor extends and involves adjacent blood vessels or visceral organs such as the uterus, ovaries, seminal vesicles, prostate gland, surrounding muscles or sacrum, it is staged as T_4 (Fig. 7.12).[3,5–10,13]

More recently, investigators utilizing endorectal Doppler probes have detected color flow and pulsed Doppler signals centrally and peripherally within the blood vessels feeding tumor masses.[14] Based on the pulsatility indices measured from arterial waveforms sampled from rectal cancer masses, the mean pulsatility indices ($PI = 1.36 \pm 0.021$) obtained from vessels feeding the central portion of the tumor were significantly lower than those ($PI = 2.10 \pm 0.87$) from the normal submucosal arterioles, but significantly higher than signals ($PI = 0.83 \pm 0.14$) acquired from more peripherally located vessels within the tumor (Fig. 7.13).[14] Similar observations were made in a series of rectal cancers studied by Jakob and co-workers. The mean pulsatility indices were slightly higher than those reported in the initial series.[15]

Immunohistochemical staining of the specimens obtained from the rectal carcinoma demonstrated that the tumor vessels possessing high-resistance flow were lined with smooth muscle coat and those with low-resistance arterial signals were lined with

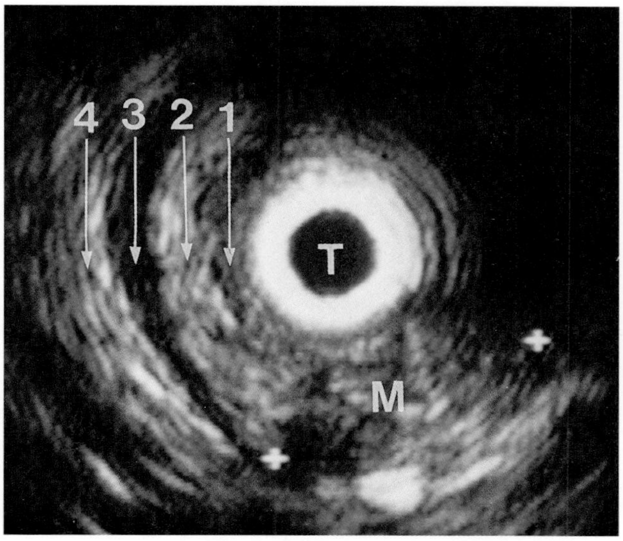

a

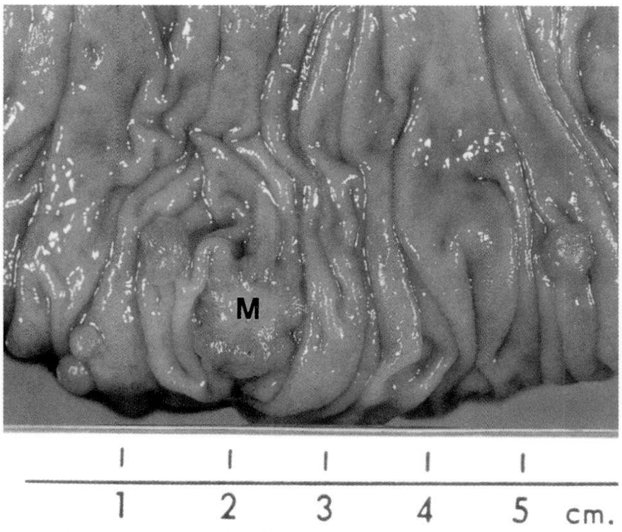

b

Figure 7.10 *(a) Catheter-based ultrasound transducer (T) positioned at distal colon images mixed echogenic mass (M) penetrating the rectal wall. (b) The gross specimen shows that the mass (M) has been excised and staged as T_3. 1, mucosa; 2, submucosa; 3, muscularis propria; 4, serosa.*

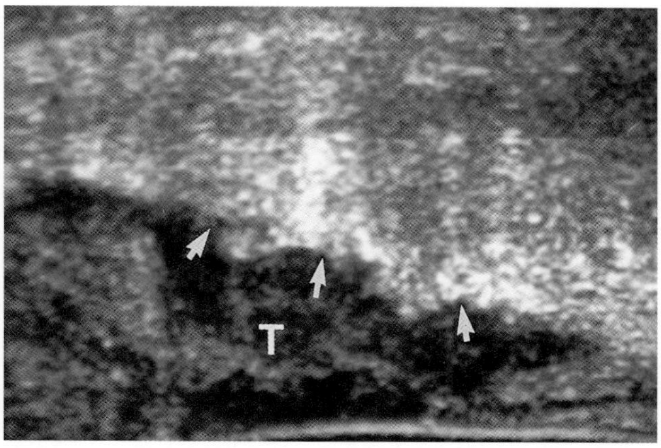

Figure 7.11 *Stage T_3 rectal carcinoma. Transrectal ultrasound image demonstrates a hypoechoic mass (T) extending beyond the muscularis propria into the perirectal fat which produces an irregular or spiculated interface (arrows).*

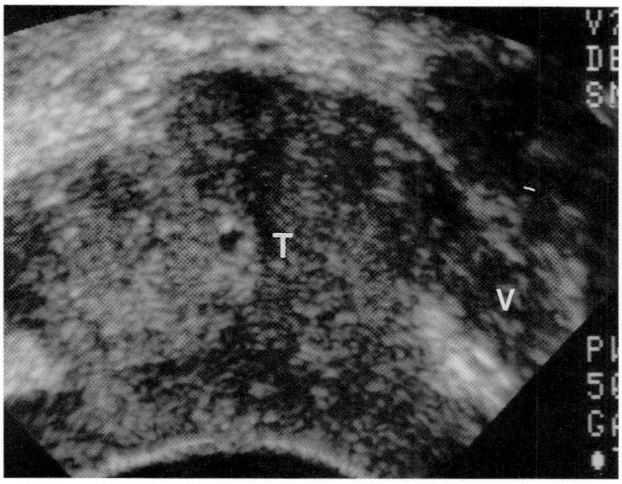

Figure 7.12 *Stage T_4 rectal carcinoma. Transrectal ultrasound image demonstrates a hypoechoic mass (T) involving adjacent vaginal wall (V).*

endothelium only (Fig. 7.14). The former may represent a native vessel that supplies the tumor, and the latter may be the product of tumor angiogenesis.[14] On the contrary, this increased flow was not detected in a small number of benign masses imaged by color flow and pulsed wave Doppler.[14] The significance, if any, of these differences between malignant and benign masses remains to be defined and is currently under investigation.

Caution is advised no matter what imaging technology is utilized for local staging, since over- and under-staging errors do occur. Over-staging errors

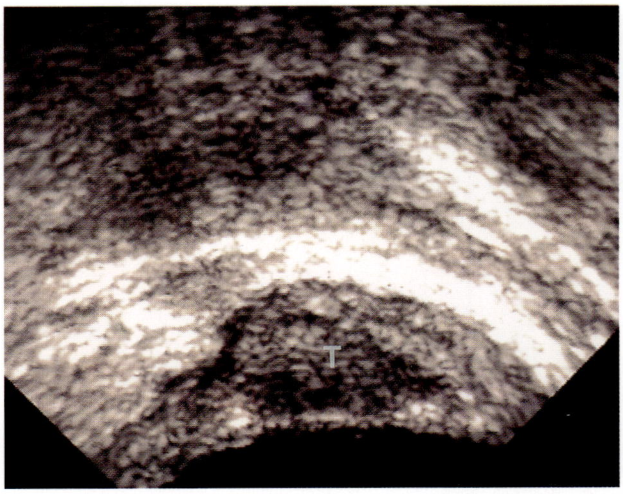

a

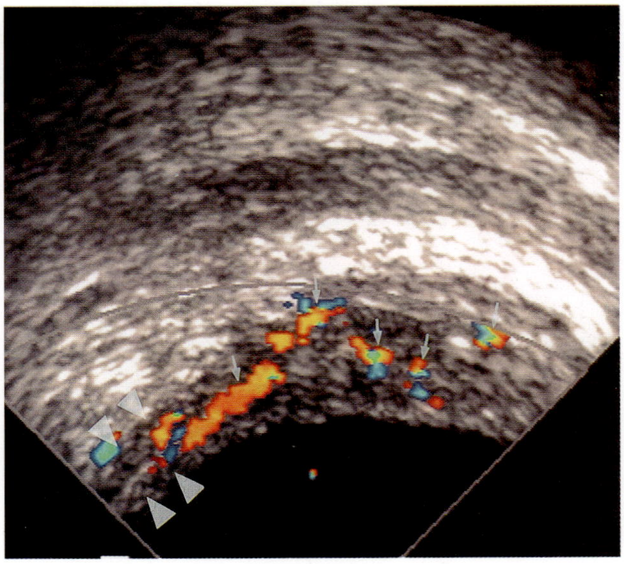

b

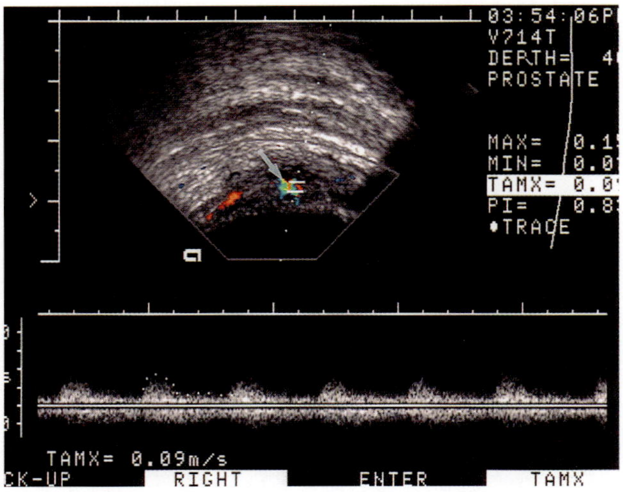

c

Figure 7.13 *(a) The gray-scale endorectal sonogram of a T_2 tumor (T) is imaged with color flow Doppler (b), which detects flow within the mass (arrows) and adjacent normal rectal wall (arrowheads). (c) Pulsed wave Doppler sample from a vessel (arrow) within the center of the mass has higher diastolic flow than the normal submucosal arteriole shown in Figure 7.4.*

may be the result of the inability of the sonologist to distinguish the sonographic changes due to peritumoral inflammation or post-biopsy edema and hemorrhage from frank tumor infiltration. The latter situation usually occurs after deep biopsies.[47] Understaging can occur when the sonologist fails to recognize early or minimal invasion into a deeper layer of the wall or when lesions cannot be completely evaluated due to the inability of the probe to pass beyond the entire lesion. Either of these situations can lead to under-staging, placing the patient at serious risk for undertreatment.[5–11,47]

Assessment of colorectal lymph nodes for metastatic invasion may present an even greater challenge to the sonographer than determination of the depth of invasion. If no lymph node metastasis is present, then it is assigned to N_0; if one to three lymph nodes are present, then the stage N_1 is assigned to the tumor; and if more than four lymph nodes are present, the tumor is staged as N_2. Criteria for evaluating lymph node metastasis vary, with the lymph node size, shape and echotexture being the most frequent sonographic indicators relied upon. Unfortunately, size may not be a reliable predictor, since it has been shown that lymph nodes as small as 5 mm are as likely to contain metastatic deposits as the 8-mm and larger lymph nodes often thought to contain tumor.[17–19,47] The central echogenicity of a

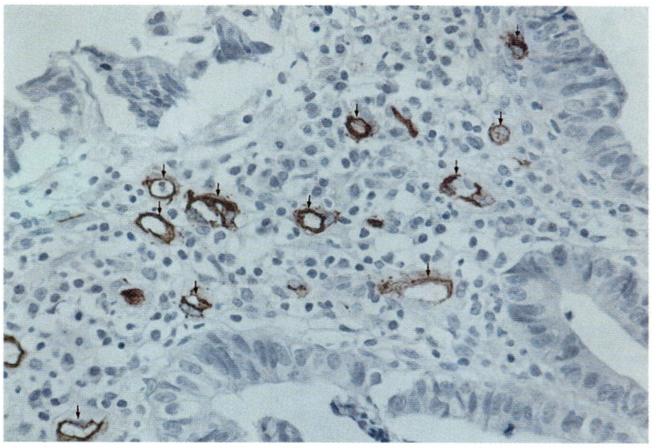

Figure 7.14 *Immunohistochemical staining with CD34 highlights endothelial lining of peripheral vessels (arrows) which lack a smooth muscle coat but are surrounded by stroma and tumor glands.*

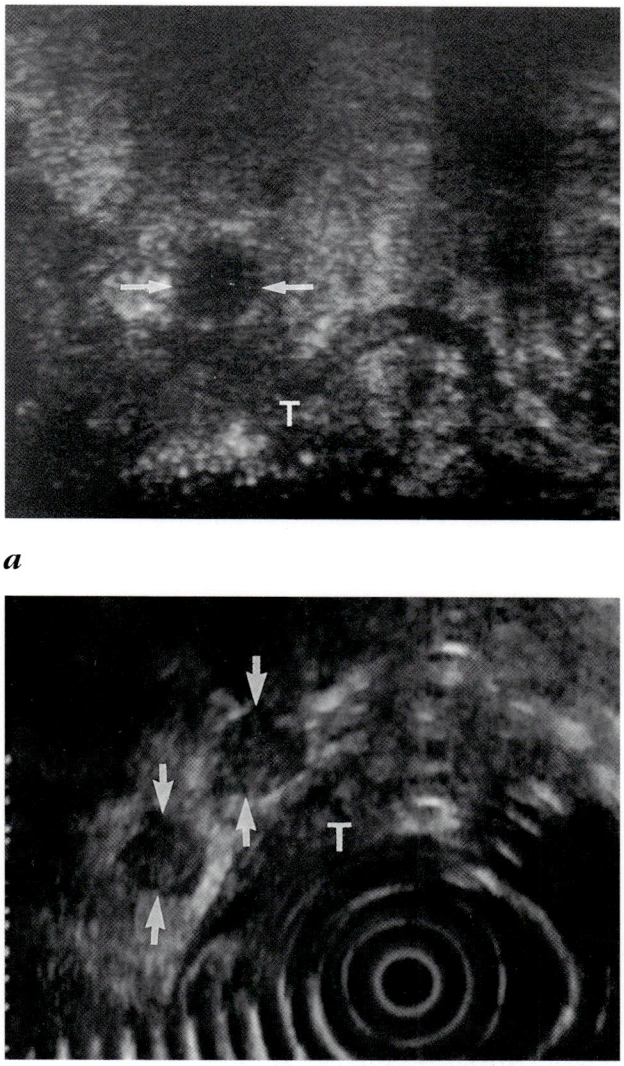

a

b

Figure 7.15 *(a) Transrectal ultrasound image of a round, central hypoechoic perirectal lymph node (arrows) adjacent to a rectal cancer infiltrating the rectal wall (T). (b) Occasionally, positive lymph nodes (arrows) will be rounded but their internal echogenicity is mixed (both hyper- and hypoechogenicity). These lymph nodes were pathologically confirmed and lie adjacent to an advanced rectal cancer (T).*

lymph node is another feature that should be carefully assessed with lymph nodes possessing a hypoechoic or echo-poor internal echotexture more likely to harbor metastatic disease than those maintaining their echogenic central hilum. Lymph node shape is also important, with a round shape being more characteristic of metastatic disease, as opposed to the oval or kidney-bean-shaped benign lymph nodes (Fig. 7.15).[1,3,17–19,47]

The need to perform endosonographic staging of irradiated rectal cancer has increased as high-dose radiation has been utilized to downstage advanced rectal cancers. The same principles described for the mural and nodal staging of non-irradiated colorectal cancers apply to tumors treated with high-dose preoperative radiation. Unfortunately, the endosonographic staging accuracies from the few series reported have not been as good as their pre-radiation counterparts.[50–52]

After high-dose preoperative radiation, the primary tumor frequently shrinks and its central echotexture becomes more echogenic as a result of increasing fibrosis.[53] The accompanying post-radiation edema and inflammation further confounds mural staging and has led some investigators to question whether or not mural staging of these tumors is possible (Fig. 7.16).[52] Lymph nodes also undergo sonographic changes following high-dose radiation. Lymph nodes may become centrally more echogenic and disappearance of benign-appearing nodes is known to occur.[50,51] Lymph nodes that remain round and hypoechoic should be considered to be positive for metastatic disease until proven otherwise.[51–53]

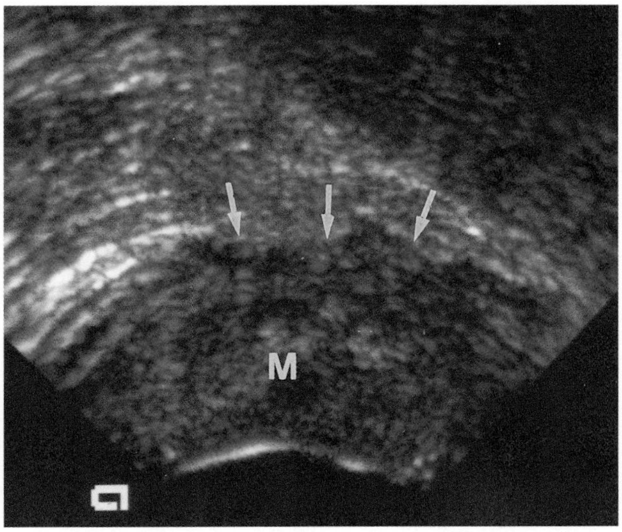

a

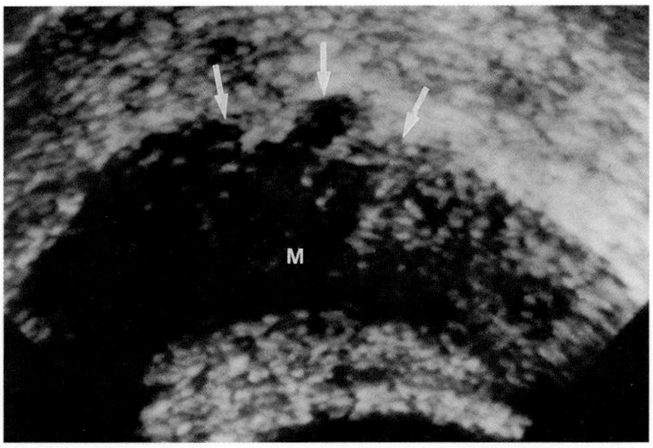

b

Figure 7.16 *(a) Transrectal ultrasound pre-radiation image demonstrates mixed echogenic mass (M) with spiculated muscle–fat interface (arrows) which was initially staged by ultrasound as a T_3 lesion. (b) After radiation, the mass (M) decreased in size and the border became less spiculated (arrows).*

BENIGN MUCOSAL AND SUBMUCOSAL TUMORS

The small benign adenoma and polyp may not be distinguished from the early mucosal carcinoma (Figs 7.17 and 7.18). Likewise, the large villous adenoma may contain clinically unrecognized cancer which is not detected by random superficial biopsies. The key point is recognizing that the lesion is not invading the hyperechoic submucosa, which is imaged as a continuous unbroken line.[47,54]

As in the upper GI tract, there are a number of benign tumors that involve the lower GI tract which arise from the layers beyond the mucosa. Lesions may originate from any of three mural layers (submucosa, muscularis mucosa and muscularis propria) and their sonographic appearance will reflect the histologic origin. These include leiomyomas, lipomas, carcinoid tumors, lymphangiomas and endometriomas.[1,55–57] Submucosal tumors are characterized by the echo layer from which they originate, sonographic appearance and tumor margins.

The most frequently encountered submucosal tumor is the leiomyoma, which arises from the hypoechoic muscularis propria, and is usually described as a smooth-margined, hypoechoic mass (Fig. 7.19).[1,55,56] Size may be the only feature that distinguishes this tumor from the larger leiomyoblastoma and leiomyosarcoma. Because of the large size, these latter tumors may also show degenerative changes of tumor necrosis and calcification, suggesting a higher potential for malignancy. Occasionally, the irregular margins of these tumors may be recognized as another feature of malignancy. Lipomas have been imaged as smooth-margined, hyperechoic submucosal masses (Fig. 7.20). Occasionally, anechoic cysts are encountered which appear as fluid-filled masses lacking internal echoes.

INFLAMMATORY BOWEL DISEASE

Ulcerative colitis has been classified by Shimizu et al,[58] using endosonography, into five different types. Classification criteria were based on thickening of the superficial versus deep layers and distensibility (Fig. 7.21). The role that endosonography plays in the diagnosis and management of the patient with ulcerative colitis remains unclear. One possible role would be surveillance of the patient with long-standing ulcerative colitis for the development of malignancy.

Crohn's colitis is a transmural inflammatory process which is often complicated by perirectal or perianal abscesses or fistulae. Endosonography has been shown to be an effective modality for imaging both fistulae and abscesses. Schratter-Sehn et al found 46 fistulae in 36 Crohn's patients and 4 individuals had abscesses.[59] Sonographically, abscesses may appear as complex masses (elements of both cystic and solid masses) with low level echoes internally which represent debris and white blood cells.[60] If gas is present

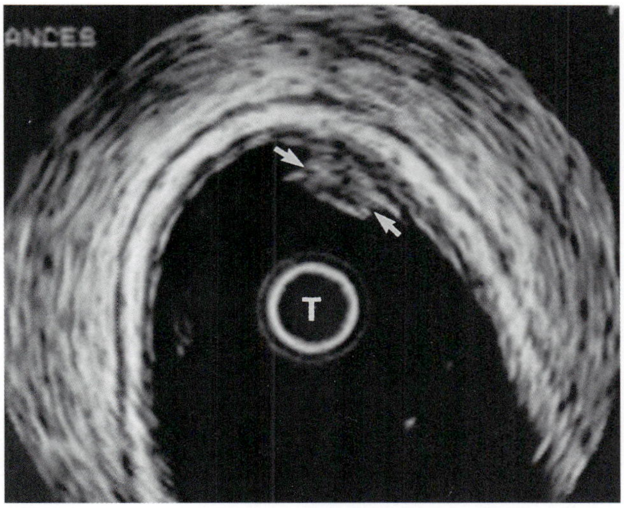

Figure 7.17 *High-frequency ultrasound image obtained from water-filled colon lumen demonstrated a small benign adenoma (arrows), which was proven by pathology. T, transducer.*

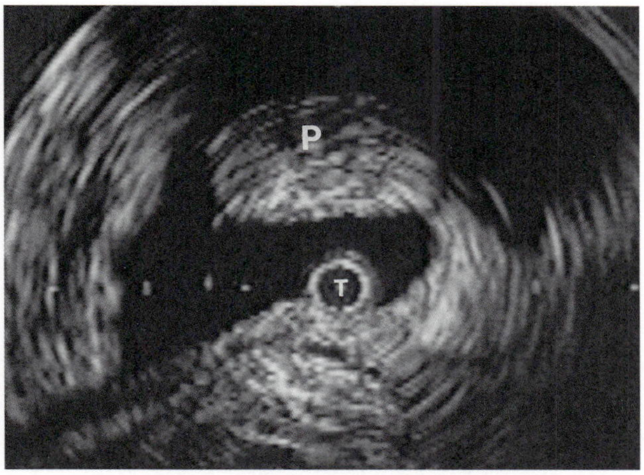

Figure 7.18 *A polyp-like mass (P) projecting into the lumen of the colon was clearly demonstrated by a catheter-based ultrasound transducer (T) with 20-MHz frequency. The mass was removed endoscopically and the specimen was confirmed pathologically to be a benign polyp.*

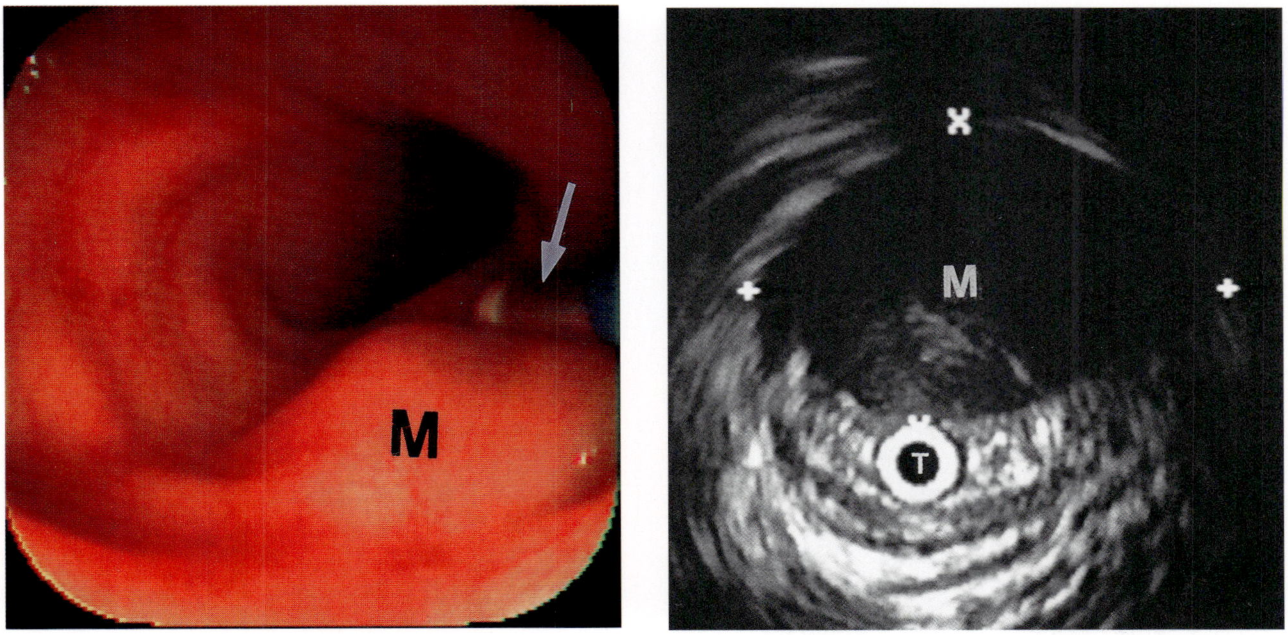

a *b*

Figure 7.19 *(a) An endoscopic view shown with a catheter-based ultrasound probe (arrow) scanning a mass (M) arising from the wall of the colon. (b) The corresponding cross-sectional endoluminal ultrasound image demonstrates a hypoechoic mass (M) with smooth margin arising from the muscularis propria. Also note that the sound transmission through the mass is attenuated at the posterior wall. Pathology has proven it to be a leiomyoma. T, transducer.*

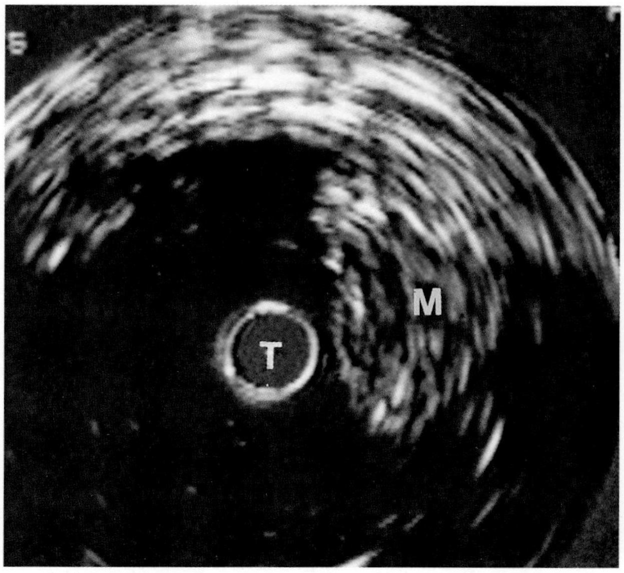

Figure 7.20 *An endoluminal ultrasound image of a hyperechoic mass (M) arising from the anterior wall of the descending colon was biopsied and proven to be a lipoma. T, transducer.*

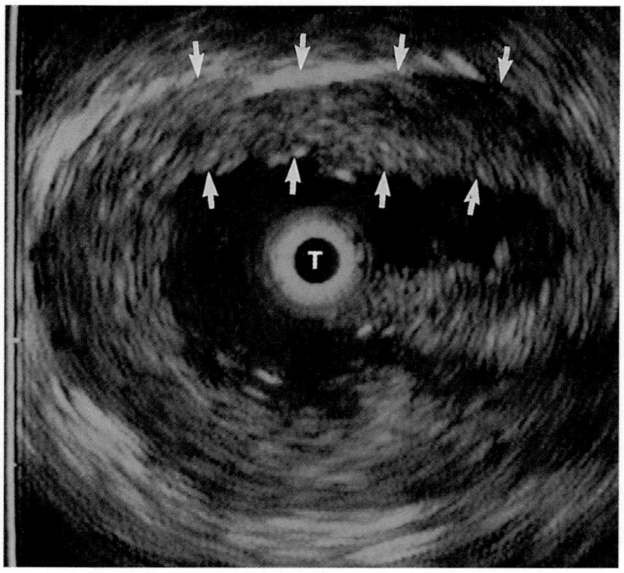

Figure 7.21 *Endoluminal catheter-based ultrasound image demonstrates thickening of the wall (arrows) in the descending colon in a known case of ulcerative colitis. The normal layers of the colon cannot be identified. T, transducer.*

there will be bright reflections and, if significant, even areas of acoustic shadowing. Less commonly, these masses may be echo-free.

Fistulae may be identified as small, hypoechoic structures and, when followed, may take a serpiginous-like course from an abscess cavity or bowel loop to exit via the skin or adjacent visceral structure. Sometimes the lumen of the fistula will appear hyperechoic as the result of air or gas trapped in the fistular tract. One difficulty that may limit endosonography is its inability to consistently identify the openings into the tracts. The precise role that endosonography will play in the evaluation of fistulae remains to be completely defined.[61,62]

DIVERTICULA

Diverticula are mucosal outpouches through a weakened muscularis propria. They may become obstructed and inflamed, leading to perforation or abscess formation. In asymptomatic patients, diverticula are rarely noticeable on the sonogram. However, when inflamed, diverticula are seen as outpouchings protruding beyond the lumen of the gut into or beyond the thickened colonic wall. They often contain shadowing echogenic material due to calcified fecaliths, fecal material or air. Catheter-based endoluminal ultrasound has been used to image diverticula through a working channel of the endoscope (Fig. 7.22).

TRANSRECTAL INTERVENTIONAL PROCEDURES

Endoscopic needle biopsies of mural masses within the colon and rectum have been performed with endosonographic assistance using the same technique described in the section on endosonography of the upper GI tract.[63,64] The main advantage of endosonographic guidance is derived from the increased control and, therefore, precision of the needle placement into the lesion. Endosonography-

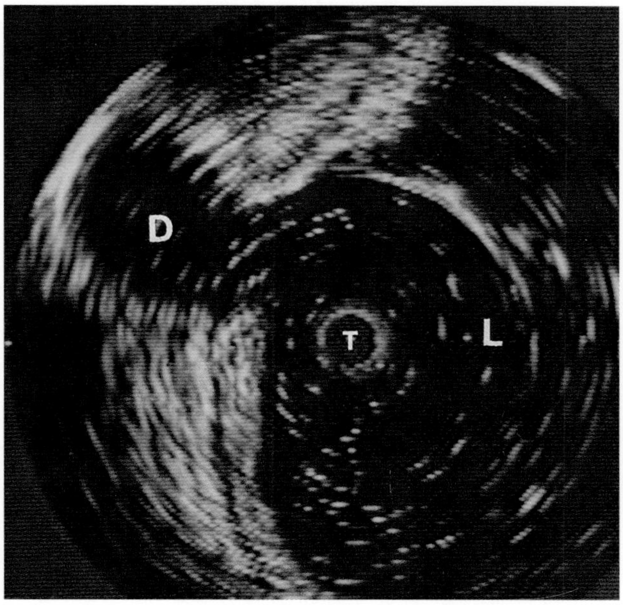

Figure 7.22 *Endoluminal ultrasound image clearly demonstrates a water-filled diverticulum (D) bulging out to the lumen (L) of the colon. T, transducer.*

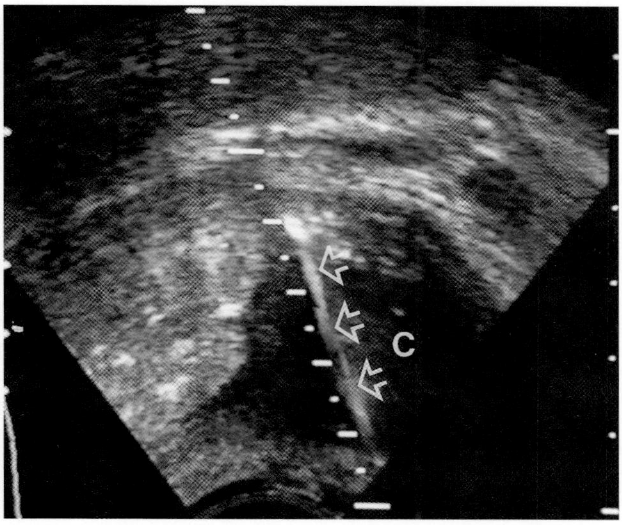

Figure 7.23 *Complex perirectal collection (C) in a febrile patient is imaged with transrectal ultrasound and the dash line of the ultrasound guide is superimposed for guidance. A needle (arrows) has been inserted across the rectum into the collection for aspiration.*

guided needle sampling of perirectal lymph nodes has provided cytological material to confirm the presence of metastatic disease.[47]

More recently, endosonography has been utilized to access deep pelvic collections unapproachable by the more conventional percutaneous routes.[65] To ensure the success of ultrasound-guided transrectal biopsies and drainages, some patient preparation is in order. Patients should be on the appropriate antimicrobial coverage, since needles and/or catheters must traverse the rectal wall. Patients are preferably positioned in the left lateral decubitus position, although the dorsilithotomy position may be used when necessary. A cleansing enema is suggested to remove as much of the rectal contents as possible. Sedation may or may not be necessary for fine needle aspiration; however, sedation is necessary in cases requiring placement of a drainage catheter. If sedation is given, then cardiac monitoring and anesthesia support should be available. The patient should be sterilely prepared and draped.[65]

Sizes of the fine needle may vary from 22 gauge for nodal aspiration to 18 gauge in cases of perirectal abscess aspiration. Abscess drainage catheters should be of the self-retaining variety, and the size chosen will vary according to the viscosity of the collection to be drained. In most cases, catheter sizes selected range from 8 to 10 Fr.[65]

The first step of catheter placement under endosonographic guidance requires localization of the perirectal collection by cross-sectional radiologic imaging. Once the collection is localized and the patient has been adequately prepared, a needle is guided into it (Fig. 7.23). After access, a suitable guidewire (0.38 or 0.35 inch) is passed through the needle under ultrasound guidance. Then the endosonographic probe is removed over the wire and the tract is sequentially dilated to allow placement of the catheter under fluoroscopic guidance. Location of the catheter tip within the collection is confirmed by contrast injection under fluoroscopic monitoring. As much of the contents of the abscess as possible is drained during the initial procedure. Afterwards, the catheter may be left for gravity drainage. Once placed, catheters are well tolerated in both pediatric and adult patients. They have not caused difficulties with defecation, and the use of self-retaining catheters has markedly reduced the incidence of spontaneous expulsions. Bacterial superinfection has not been a problem but continued antimicrobial coverage is necessary after catheter placement. The duration of catheter placement is governed by persistence of drainage, with removal following cessation of drainage.[65]

ENDOSONOGRAPHY OF THE ANAL CANAL

Endosonography of the anal canal and its surrounding structures has provided the colorectal surgeon with valuable anatomic information in patients with anorectal complaints.[66–72] Not only has endosonography demonstrated discontinuities of the muscles that comprise the anal sphincter complex, but it has also been able to image adjacent perianal and rectal abscesses as well as fistulae. Neoplasms arising within the anal canal and anorectal junction have also been evaluated with endosonography to define the size and level of mural invasion.[47]

The technical requirements for achieving an adequate endosonographic study of the anal canal are slightly more specialized than those of the routine endosonographic examination of the colon or rectum.[47,68–72] Radial or sector endosonography probes are usually chosen, with frequencies ranging from 10 to 12.5 MHz to provide the high resolution required to image the mucosa, submucosa and muscles of the anal sphincter complex.[2,47,68–72] Endosonographic probes may be equipped with a special cone to cover the ultrasound transducer.[47,69] Specially designed endoluminal ultrasound catheters, which are usually 9 or 6 Fr in size and 12.5 or 20 MHz in frequency, may also be used.[2] As previously mentioned, the shallow depth of penetration of the beam may limit the ability of the examiner to image the external sphincter and any structures adjacent to it.[2]

As in the endosonographic studies of the rectum or colon, patients are usually placed in the left lateral decubitus position or, when necessary, the dorsilithotomy position. Most patients are imaged by placing the endosonographic probe within the anal canal, but in the female patient very high quality images of the canal can be obtained by using a transvaginal approach as an acoustic window.[73,74] Although a cleansing enema may not be needed to study the canal proper, it may be advisable to administer one to patients with incontinence, since stool within the proximal rectal vault may be passed during the examination.[2,47,68–72]

ANATOMY OF THE ANAL CANAL

The anal canal is about 4 cm long and passes downward and backward from the rectal ampulla to the anus. Its internal walls are kept in opposition by the levatores ani muscles and the internal and external sphincters that form the anal sphincter complex.[2] In the perineum, the anal canal is related posteriorly to the anococcygeal body, a mass of fibrous tissue lying between the anal canal and the coccyx. Laterally it is related to the fat-filled ischiorectal fossae. In the male, it is related anteriorly to the perineal body, the urogenital diaphragm, the membranous part of the urethra and the bulb of the penis. In the female, it is related anteriorly to the perineal body, the urogenital diaphragm and the lower part of the vagina.

The mucosa of the upper half of the anal canal is lined by columnar epithelium and is thrown into vertical folds called anal columns, which join together at the lower ends by small semilunar folds called anal valves. The mucosa of the lower half of the anal canal is lined by stratified squamous epithelium, which gradually merges at the anus with the perianal epidermis.

The puborectalis fibers of the two sides form a sling, which is attached in front to the pubic bones and causes the rectum to join the anal canal at an acute angle. The muscular coats that form the anal sphincter complex of the anal canal are strongly developed. The downward continuation of circular smooth muscle from the muscularis propria of the rectum becomes thickened at the upper end of the anal canal and forms the involuntary internal sphincter. The internal sphincter is enclosed by a sheath of striped muscle that forms the voluntary external sphincter, which blends with the puborectalis part of the levatores ani muscles.

The external sphincter is a downward extension of striated muscle from the puborectalis muscle and extends more caudally than the muscle fibers of the internal sphincter.[66] Anatomically, three concentric bands of this sphincter surround the internal sphincter and are placed into the superficial and deep compartments. The subcutaneous and superficial

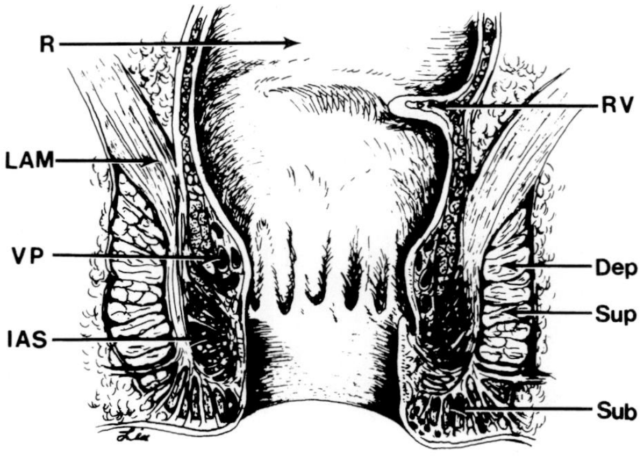

Figure 7.24 *A frontal sectional view of the anal canal and lower segmental rectum. R, rectum; LAM, levator ani muscle; VP, venous plexus; IAS, internal anal sphincter; RV, rectal valve; Dep, deep external sphincter muscle; Sup, superficial external sphincter muscle; Sub, subcutaneous external sphincter muscle.*

bands are within the superficial compartment, and the subcutaneous band of muscle is nearest the internal sphincter. The deep band is the outermost layer of striated muscle and may be subdivided into the deep circular fibers associated with the puborectalis muscle and the adjacent levator ani muscles.[2,66] The subcutaneous part encircles the lower end of the anal canal and has no bony attachments; the superficial part is attached to the coccyx behind and the perineal body in front; and the deep parts encircle the upper end of the canal and have no bony attachments (Fig. 7.24). The primary function of the anal sphincter complex is maintenance of fecal continence.[67]

ENDOSONOGRAPHIC ANATOMY OF THE ANAL CANAL

The anal sphincter complex muscles are imaged with endosonography as series of concentric bands. Most investigators are able to identify the first hypoechoic band or circular smooth muscle of the internal anal sphincter. This muscle may become thicker and more echogenic with age.[72] Changes associated with aging may be the result of fibrofatty infiltration and a concomitant degeneration of smooth muscle cells.[72] Utilizing the more conventional endosonographic probes fitted with a specialized cone, the thickness of the internal sphincter has been measured. The thickness varies depending on the series being reported. Burnett and Bartram reported ranges for the thickness of the normal internal sphincter based on age: 2.4–2.7 mm for patients less than 55 years old and 2.8–3.4 mm for patients more than 55 years of age.[72] They were also concerned about abnormally thick internal sphincter muscles in young adults, with internal sphincters measuring 4 mm or more. Others have reported the mean thickness of the internal sphincter muscle as 1.96 ± 0.61 mm or 6.5 mm (5.8–7.2 mm), and another series measured it as 2–3 mm.[66,69–71]

Transanal endosonography was routinely used to evaluate the anatomic structures of the anal canal until Sultan et al proposed transvaginal sonography as an alternative.[73] Both methods enable the sonologist to image the anal sphincter complex. Both allow the sonologist to determine whether or not the sphincter muscles are intact, but it is with a transvaginal approach that the anal canal is imaged in its natural, undisturbed state. With this technique, the sonographic anatomy of the anal canal includes the lumen of the canal, hypoechoic mucosa, echogenic submucosa, hypoechoic internal anal sphincter and part of the external anal sphincter (Fig. 7.25). The hypoechoic bands of the subcutaneous, superficial and deep muscle of the external sphincter cannot be consistently imaged. At the anorectal junction the puborectalis sling can be identified as a U-shaped hypoechoic structure (Fig. 7.26). In our study, the mean thickness of the internal anal sphincter measured with a MicroSonic computer system was 3.1 ± 0.57 mm (range, 1.9–3.9 mm). For individuals less than 55 years of age, the mean of 3.0 ± 0.56 mm was not significantly different from the mean of 3.23 ± 0.58 mm obtained from women greater than 55 years of age ($P = 0.31$).[74]

Alexander et al imaged the various components of the anal canal using a 9 Fr catheter containing a 12.5-MHz transducer. The anal mucosa and submucosa were described as hypoechoic and hyperechoic, respectively. The mean thickness of the internal sphincter was measured as slightly greater (3.5 ± 0.5 mm (range 2.6–4.3 mm)) and the muscle was uniformly hypoechoic (Fig. 7.27).[2]

Visualization of the entire external sphincter can be difficult. The sonographic description of this muscle varies but most investigators describe it as mixed with

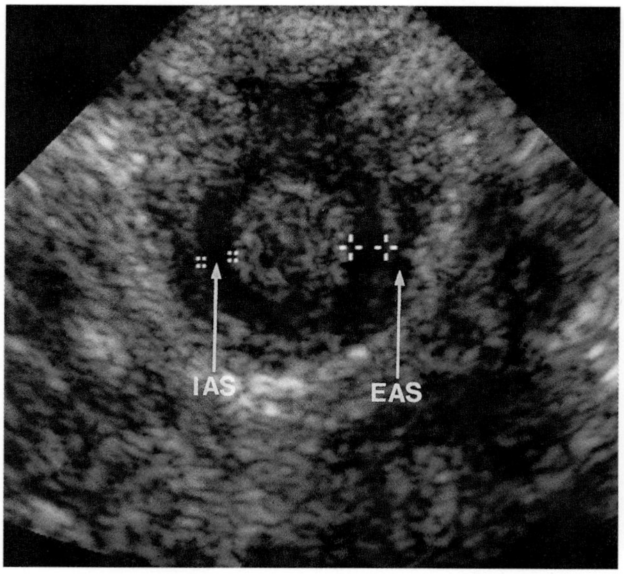

Figure 7.25 *A sonographic image of the normal anal canal using the transvaginal approach shows the intact hypoechoic internal anal sphincter (IAS) and part of the external anal sphincter (EAS).*

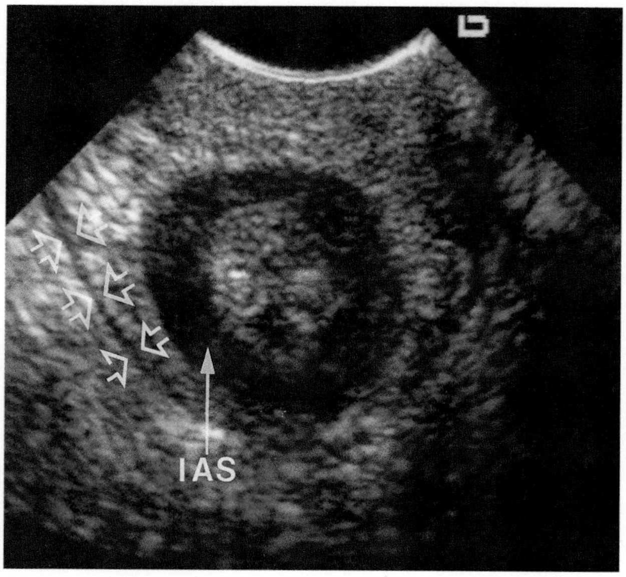

Figure 7.26 *This transvaginal ultrasound image shows a U-shaped hypoechoic puborectalis sling (open arrow) at the anorectal junction. IAS, internal anal sphincter. (Reprinted with permission from Alexander et al.[74])*

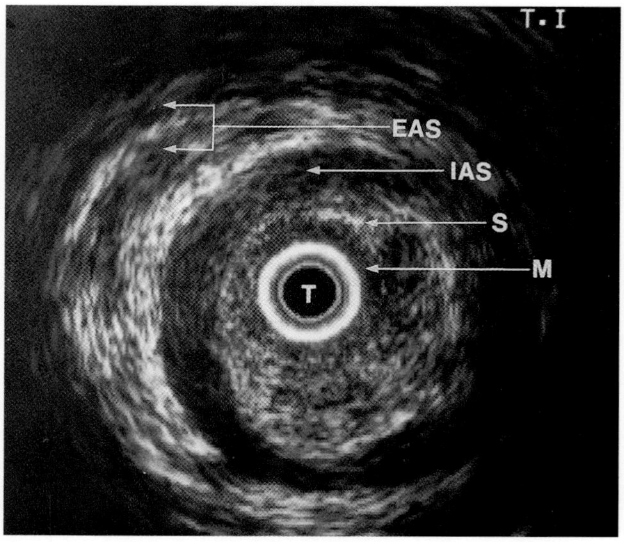

a

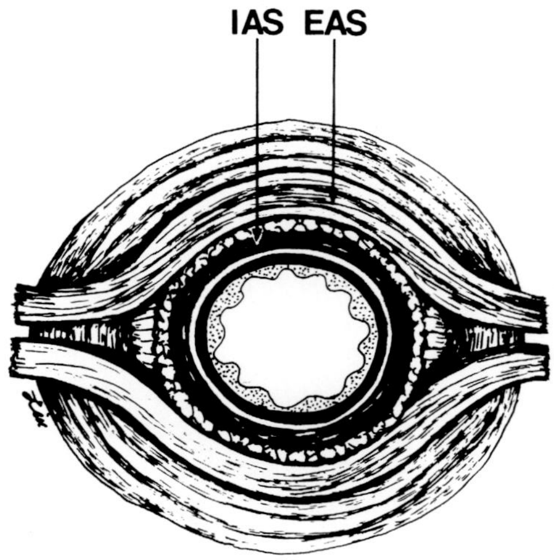

b

Figure 7.27 *(a) Transanal ultrasound image with the use of a catheter-based 20-MHz transducer (T) demonstrates hypoechoic mucosa (M), hyperechoic submucosa (S), internal anal sphincter (IAS), and a portion of external anal sphincter (EAS). (b) Diagrammatic representation of the internal anal sphincter (IAS) and external anal sphincter (EAS).*

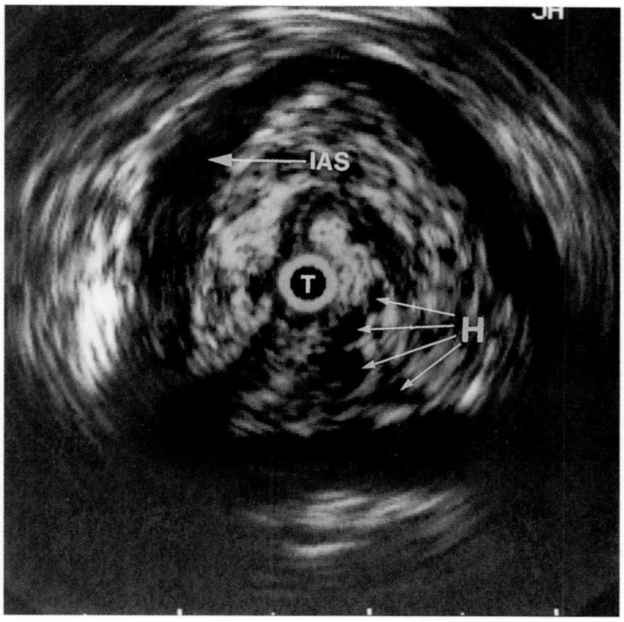

Figure 7.28 *This transanorectal image demonstrates hemorrhoids (H) within the mucosal–submucosal complex of the anal canal. IAS, internal anal sphincter; T, transducer.*

both bright and dark echoes. The median measurement reported is 6 mm with a range of 5–8 mm.[66–72] With high-resolution endoluminal catheters, multiple alternating hypoechoic and hyperechoic bands have been imaged. However, only a portion of the external sphincter muscle can be imaged and its mean was measured as 2.3 mm (range 1.6–3.2 mm).[2]

With use of the 20 MHz catheter-based transducer, hemorrhoids may be imaged within the mucosal-submucosal complex of the anal canal (Fig. 7.28). It may also be possible to monitor therapy of hemorrhoids by imaging before and after treatment with various therapeutic modalities, including rubber band ligation, infrared light coagulation, injection of sclerosant and bipolar electrocautery.

ANAL CANAL DISORDERS

ANAL INCONTINENCE

Endosonography has been frequently requested to give anatomic information about the anal canal in individuals complaining of fecal incontinence.[75–78] Although both sexes may be afflicted, it is frequently a problem reported in multiparous women.[79–81] Incontinence may arise after a traumatic mechanical or neurologic injury to the anal sphincter during childbirth, hemorrhoid repair or any traumatic insult to the anal canal.[80,81] In general, the work-up of this problem requires manometry and pudendal nerve motor latency studies to identify the location of the injury.[82–84] Both resting and squeeze pressures are obtained. Abnormally low resting pressures (<45 cmH_2O) are indicative of a defective internal sphincter. Abnormal squeeze pressures (<76 cmH_2O or twice the resting pressure) are indicative of an abnormal external sphincter.[82–84] Unfortunately, pressure measurements may vary for technical reasons and a superimposed neural injury may complicate the anatomic injury.[83] Therefore, pudendal nerve conduction studies are necessary to identify neural injuries leading to impairment or loss of external sphincter muscle function.[82–84]

Endosonography has been a very useful addition for the evaluation of fecal incontinence, because an actual disruption of the muscle can be identified. Because the injury may affect either the external sphincter, internal sphincter or both, it is very important to image both muscles.[75–84] Failure to image all injuries may result in a less than optimal surgical repair.[77] In women with incontinence after childbearing, the site of injury is usually along the line of tear from a third- or fourth-degree laceration.[79–81] An isolated injury to the external sphincter may result from a frank tear or midline episiotomy incision.[76]

The 20-MHz catheter-based transducers have been used transanally to detect anatomic abnormalities of the anal canal in patients with fecal incontinence. The site of injury will be recognized as a hyperechoic gap or disruption in the continuity of the affected sphincteral muscles (Figs 7.29 and 7.30). This hyperechoic appearance is due to fibrous scar tissue. Clinically, the information that the injury traverses the length of the canal is useful for the surgeon when performing the sphincter repair. It is also important to measure the thickness of the various muscle components, since an increase in internal sphincter muscle thickness has been associated with cases of idiopathic fecal incontinence.[72]

Transvaginal sonography of the anal canal is a satisfactory alternative to transanal sonography in the evaluation of female patients with fecal incontinence. Without disturbance of the natural state of the anal canal and compression of the sphincter muscles, transvaginal ultrasound often provides a better

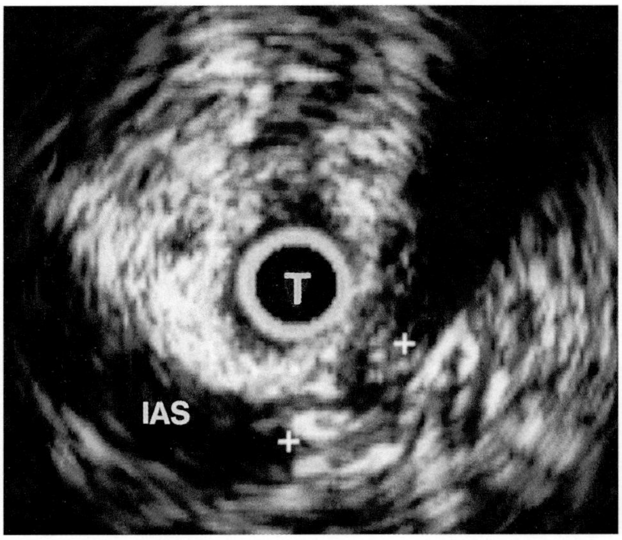

Figure 7.29 *In a patient with a history of anal canal injury, transanal ultrasound image using a catheter-based 20-MHz probe delineates a hyperechoic defect (+) within the internal anal sphincter (IAS). T, transducer.*

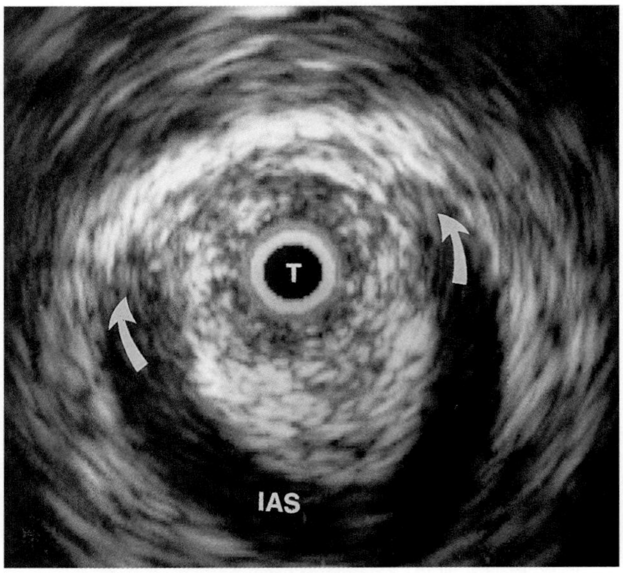

Figure 7.30 *This transanal ultrasound image obtained from a patient with history of the perianal abscess shows that one-third of the internal anal sphincter (IAS) is replaced by the hyperechoic fibrotic tissue (curved arrows). T, transducer.*

demonstration of the normal anatomy and abnormalities of the anal canal as well as adjacent structures (Fig. 7.31). Accurate sonographic demonstration of anatomic defects will allow the surgeon to appropriately select patients with fecal incontinence for surgery who may be cured or experience a marked improvement in their symptoms.[73,74]

ANORECTAL ABSCESSES AND FISTULAE

The anal glands are frequently the source of infections leading to formation of abscesses and fistulae in the perianal region. Anorectal abscesses and fistulae may also be associated with a disease entity such as Crohn's disease.[60–62,85,86] Depending on the source and its location, the infectious process may track proximally to form deep pelvic abscesses or distally to form ischiorectal fossa abscesses.[60] Although abscesses and fistulae may occasionally be palpated or imaged with alternative radiologic studies, endosonography may be able to localize the intersphincteric gland of origin, identify an occult opening of a fistulous tract and provide guidance for intervention.[60–62,85,86]

Before the insertion of a probe, the patient is positioned in the left lateral decubitus position and an inspection of the perianal region is performed to identify any suspected openings of fistular tracts onto the skin surface. A digital examination of the anorectum is then performed to detect defects in the muscles of the anal sphincter complex and to palpate for any adjacent but unsuspected abscesses. Afterwards, the endosonographic probe may be inserted. Depending on the probe used, the scanning technique will vary. If one scans with a conventional endosonographic probe, a plastic cone will cover the transducer, which is then placed into the anal canal. Another option would be for 9 Fr endoluminal ultrasound catheters to be inserted directly into the canal.[2] It is very important that a high-frequency transducer be utilized to obtain high-resolution images of the adjacent structures.[2,60–62,85,86] In addition, the transvaginal approach is another alternative to imaging the anorectal abscesses and fistulae. By injecting sterile water through a catheter located within the fistula,

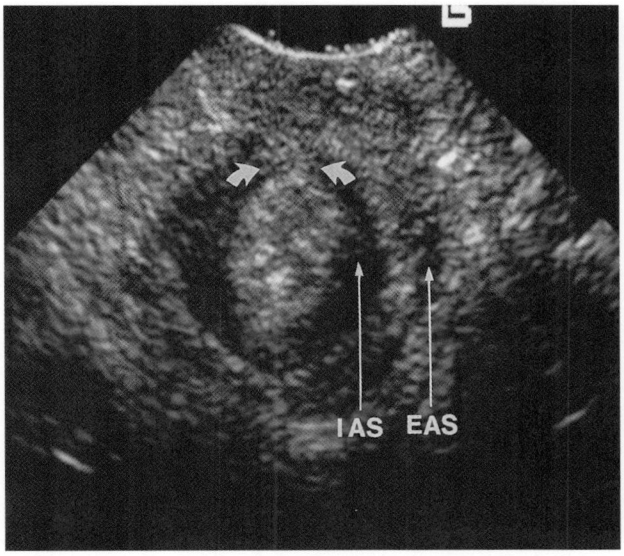

a

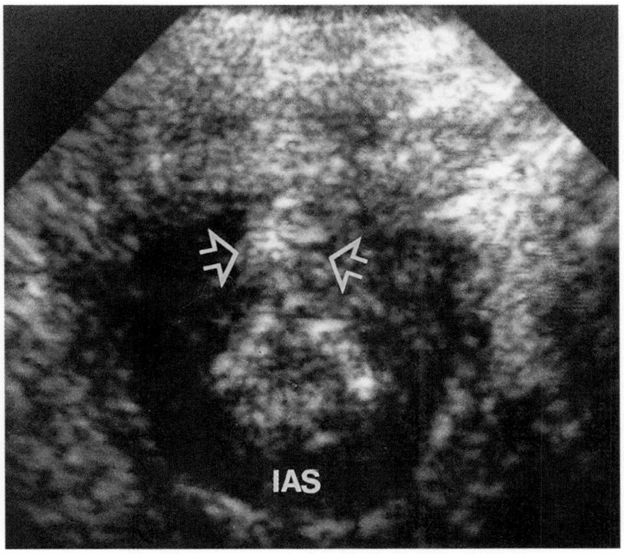

c

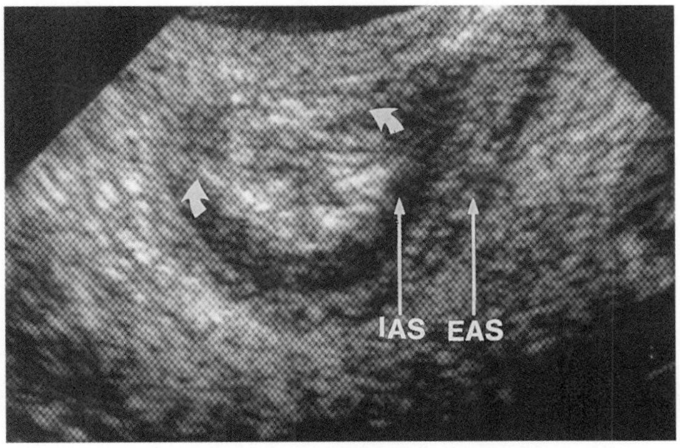

b

Figure 7.31 *(a–c) These transvaginal images obtained from different multiparous patients who suffered from failed repair of fourth degree lacerations reveal hyperechoic defects (arrows) which extend across both the internal (IAS) and external anal sphincters (EAS). (Reprinted with permission from Alexander et al.[74])*

the presence of the fistular connections to either the anorectum or vagina can be demonstrated and confirmed.

An abscess located adjacent to the anorectum will be identified sonographically as a mass which is either anechoic (without internal echoes) or hypoechoic (with internal echoes secondary to cellular debris) (Fig. 7.32). Fistular tracts may be identified as small, hypoechoic, round to oval structures that lie in an intersphincteric location when they are of cryptoglandular origin. Occasionally, internally they will be hyperechoic (increased or bright echoes) instead of hypoechoic as a result of gas or air within an abcess or a fistular tract (Fig. 7.33). The opening within the mucosa of the canal may present as a gap or disruption of the integrity of the mucosa (Figs 7.34 and 7.35). These tracts may be difficult to define and some have advocated injecting dilute hydrogen peroxide into the canal to fill the occult tract with hyperechoic gas. In cases of Crohn's disease, the thickness of the entire canal may be increased because of the transmural nature of the disease process.[60–62,85,86]

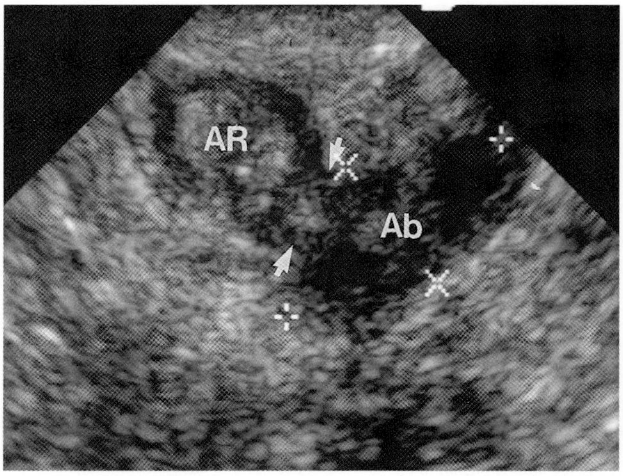

Figure 7.32 *In a women complaining of fecal incontinence, transvaginal ultrasound image demonstrates a fistula tract (arrows) at the anorectal junction (AR) draining an adjacent abscess (Ab). (Reprinted with permission from Alexander et al.[74])*

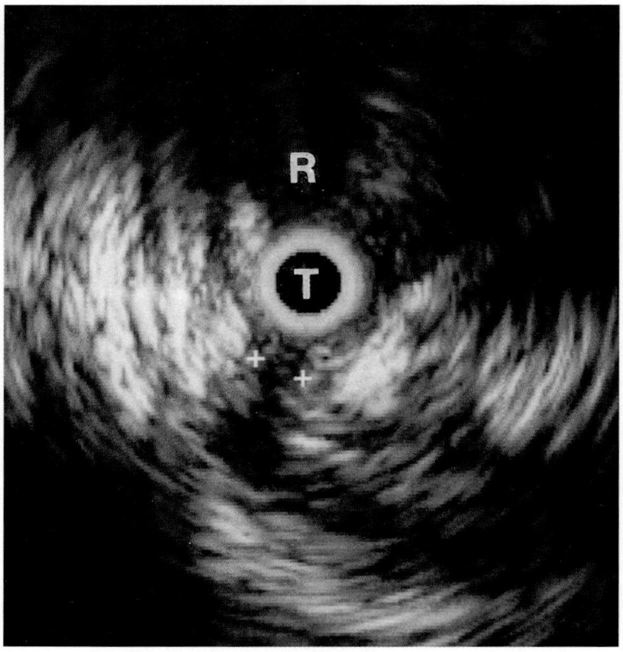

Figure 7.34 *Transanorectal ultrasound image demonstrates a fistular tract and its opening (+) into the lumen of the rectum (R).*

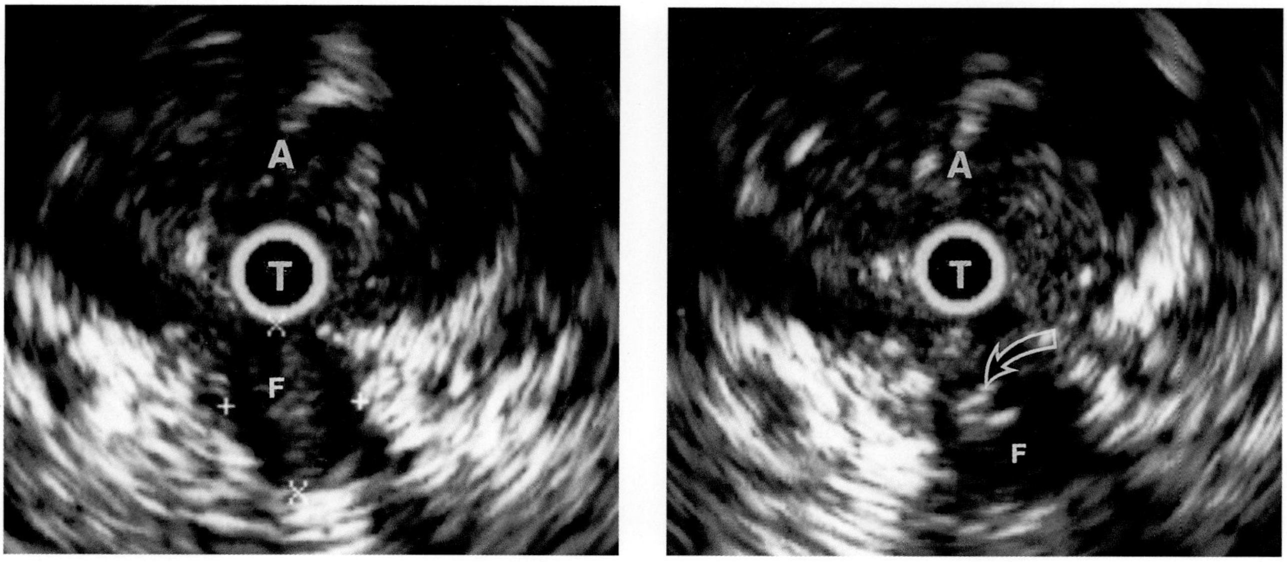

a ***b***

Figure 7.33 *(a) Endoluminal ultrasound image demonstrates a fistular tract (F) adjacent to the internal anal sphincter. The entire fistular tract can be imaged by real-time scanning within the anorectal canal (A). (b) Endoluminal ultrasound image shows hyperechoic gas reflection (open arrow) within the fistular tract (F). T, transducer.*

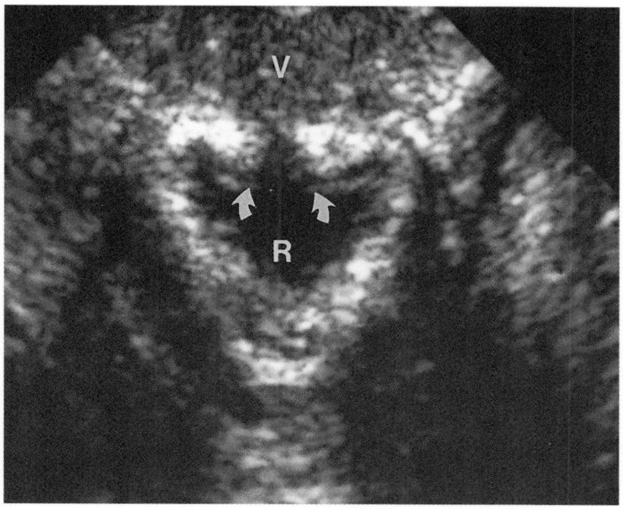

Figure 7.35 *A transvaginal ultrasound image at the anorectal junction obtained after a transanal injection of sterile water shows water flowing from the anorectal lumen (R) through the opening of the fistular tract (arrows) into the vagina (V). (Reprinted with permission from Alexander et al.[74])*

ANORECTAL MALIGNANCY

Endosonography may be requested to evaluate a mass palpated within the anal canal. The most commonly encountered primary cancers of the anal canal are squamous cell cancers. Epidermoid carcinomas may be staged by the TNM system and then treated with combined chemotherapy and radiation therapy.[87–89] Endosonography may provide helpful information such as tumor size, location, depth of mural penetration and extent beyond the canal into adjacent structures, which assists with staging (Fig. 7.36). After treatment, endosonography may have a role in the monitoring of the patient for local recurrence, since early tumor growth may be difficult to palpate within the scar tissue. In the latter situation, repeat studies to document an increase in the size of a lesion suspicious for recurrent disease or ultrasound-guided biopsy are usually necessary to distinguish recurrent tumor from scar.[87–89]

Ultrasonographically, a tumor will present as a hypoechoic mass which can be measured with a fair degree of accuracy. Depth of tumor invasion should

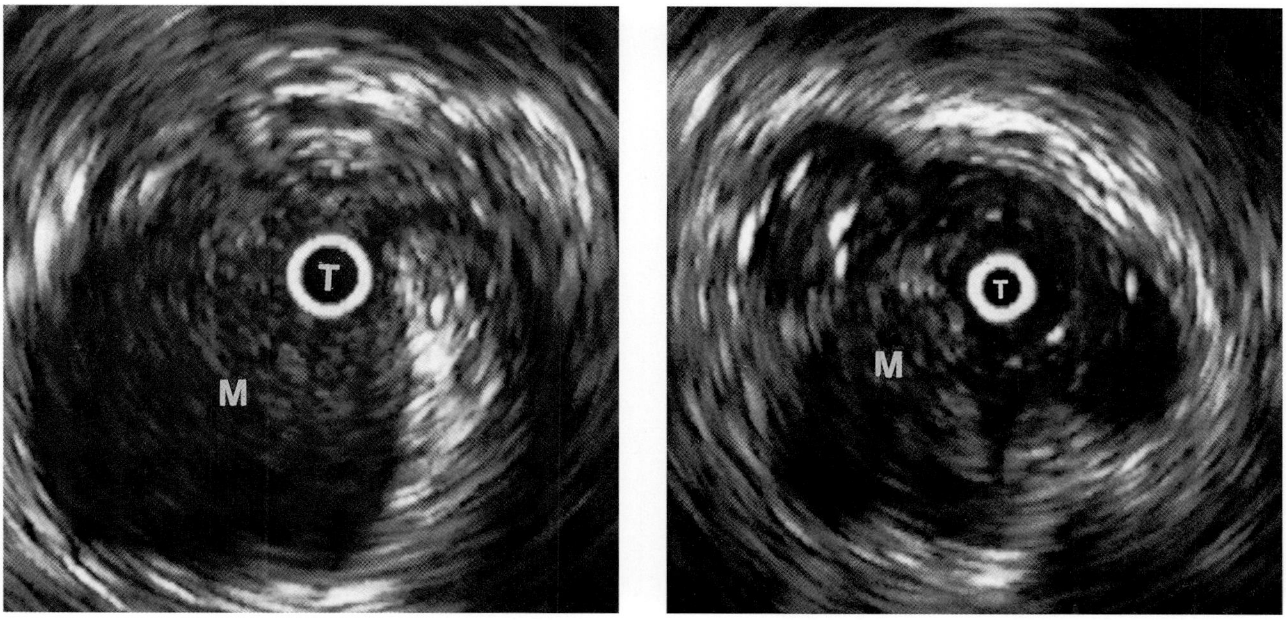

Figure 7.36 *(a) A catheter-based ultrasound transducer (T) located within the anorectal canal demonstrates a hypoechoic mass (M) at the level of the anorectal junction. (b) With water filling the lumen of the canal, the tumor location and its depth of mural penetration are better delineated. Surgical pathology showed an epidermoid carcinoma.*

be noted to determine whether the lesion is confined to the submucosa or invades the adjacent muscle or perirectal fat. Involvement of adjacent organs should be documented. In the same manner as staging of rectal cancers with endosonography, lesions may be staged as uT_1 if they are confined to the submucosa or uT_2 if they extend into the muscle. Lesions invading the adjacent fat are staged as uT_3, and are uT_4 if extension into the surrounding visceral structures has occurred.[87–89]

FUTURE POTENTIAL

Three-dimensional ultrasonography has been utilized in the study of the heart and, recently, this technology has been incorporated into endosonographic probes to evaluate the prostate.[90–93] In the upper GI tract, Kallimans et al have imaged the esophagus with an Olympus EU-M20 echogastroscope.[94] Images of the esophagus were obtained by pulling the scope through the esophagus and recording the images on 3/4-inch video tape. Approximately 80 images at 1–3-second intervals were taken with a frame grabber and digitized for storage on an optical disk. Computer translation of two-dimensional images into three dimensions was accomplished utilizing software that executed interpolation, boundary formation and surface renderings.[94] The main advantages offered to the observer were a quick overview of the anatomy and its relationship to the target lesion.[90–94] Although this technology has been applied to the upper GI tract, it could have applications in the evaluation and staging of colorectal lesions.

Miller et al[95] have developed a method to use simultaneous high-frequency ultrasound and real-time manometry to evaluate the physiologic processes involved in the peristaltic contraction of the esophagus. This same methodology could be used in the anal canal to better define normal anal physiology and to evaluate various disease processes in the anal canal.

CONCLUSION

Endosonographic technology has progressively improved over time and now provides diagnostic information not available from the clinical examination alone. Compared to CT and MRI, it is less costly and, unlike contrast radiography and CT, it does not utilize ionizing radiation. With endosonography, local staging of patients with cancers of the lower GI tract has been improved, possibly increasing local control and reducing local recurrence rates. With better staging, local rather than more radical surgical excisions may be performed with the hope of reducing patient morbidity.

Using a transrectal approach under sonographic guidance, drainage catheters can be placed into the abdomen and pelvis and aspiration and biopsies performed. Prior to endosonography, surgical intervention would have been required. These high-frequency probes can be placed through a sigmoidoscope or directly into the anal canal to obtain high-resolution images of the mural structures and abnormalities of the colon and anal-rectal area. Endosonographic evaluation can often identify a surgically correctable cause of fecal incontinence so that surgery may be performed successfully.

In conclusion, progressive improvements of ultrasound technology, especially endoluminal ultrasound, have greatly aided diagnostic evaluation of the lower GI tract. As an easily performed, relatively inexpensive noninvasive technique, endosonography has improved the assessment of the colorectum and anal canal and has shown promise in providing more useful information to the clinician in the diagnosis and management of malignant and nonmalignant diseases in the lower GI tract.

REFERENCES

1. Rosch T, Classon M, *Gastroenterologic Endosonography* (Thieme Medical Publishers Inc.: New York, 1992).
2. Alexander AA, Miller LS, Liu J-B, Feld RI, Goldberg BB, High resolution endoluminal sonography of the anal sphincter complex, *J Ultrasound Med* 1994; **13**:281–4.
3. Alexander A, The effect of endorectal ultrasound scanning on the preoperative staging of rectal cancer, *Surg Oncol Clin North Am* 1992; **1**:39–56.
4. Kimmey MB, Martin RW, Haggitt RC, Wang KY, Franklin DW, Silverstein FE, Histologic correlates of gastrointestinal ultrasound images, *Gastroenterology* 1989; **96**:433–41.
5. Boscaini M, Montori A, Transrectal ultrasonography:

interpretation of normal intestinal wall structure for the preoperative staging of rectal cancer, *Scand J Gastroenterol* 1986; **21**(Suppl 123):87–98.
6. Wang KY, Kimmey MB, Nyberg DA et al, Colorectal neoplasms: accuracy of US in demonstrating the depth of invasion, *Radiology* 1987; **165**:827–9.
7. Heintz A, Guess G, Frank K, Kuntz C, Strunck H, Junginger T, Endoluminal ultrasonic examination of sessile polyps and early carcinomas of the rectum, *Surg Endosc* 1989; **3**:92–5.
8. St Ville EW, Jafri SZH, Madrazo BL et al, Endorectal sonography in the evaluation of rectal and perirectal disease, *AJR* 1991; **157**:503–8.
9. Beynon J, Mortensen NJMcC, Foy DMA, Channer JL, Rigby H, Virjee J, The detection and evaluation of locally recurrent rectal cancer with rectal endosonography, *Dis Colon Rectum* 1989; **32**:509–17.
10. Zainea GG, Lee F, McLeary RD, Siders DB, Thieme ET, Transrectal ultrasonography in the evaluation of rectal and extrarectal disease, *Surg Obstet Gynecol* 1989; **169**:153–6.
11. Orrom WJ, Wong WD, Rothenberger DA, Jensen LL, Goldberg SM, Endorectal ultrasound in the preoperative staging of rectal tumors, *Dis Colon Rectum* 1990; **33**:654–9.
12. Hildebrandt U, Feifel G, Preoperative staging of rectal cancer by intra-rectal ultrasound, *Dis Colon Rectum* 1985; **28**:42–6.
13. Hildebrandt U, Feifel G, Schwarz HP, Scherr O, Endorectal ultrasound: instrumentation and clinical aspects, *Int J Colorect Dis* 1986; **1**:203–7.
14. Alexander AA, Liu J-B, Palazzo JP et al, Endorectal color and duplex imaging of the normal rectal wall and rectal masses, *J Ultrasound Med* 1994; **13**:509–15.
15. Jakab Z, Duliskovich T, Alexander AA, Lestar B, Ritter L, Initial experiences with color Doppler ultrasonography of rectal tumors, *Lege Artis Medicinae* 1994; **4(4)**:340–5
16. Lindmark G, Elvin A, Pahlman L, Glimelius B, The value of endosonography in preoperative staging of rectal cancer, *Int J Colorect Dis* 1992; **7**:162–6.
17. Tio TL, Tytgat GNJ, Endoscopic ultrasonography in analyzing peri-intestinal lymph node abnormality. Preliminary results of studies in vitro and in vivo, *Scand J Gastroenterol* 1986; **21**(Suppl 123):158–63.
18. Hildebrandt U, Klein T, Feifel G, Schwarz HP, Koch B, Schmidt RM, Endosonography of pararectal lymph nodes. In vitro and in vivo evaluation, *Dis Colon Rectum* 1990; **33**:863–8.
19. Glaser F, Layer G, Zuna I, van Knick G, Schlag P, Herfartl C, Praoperative beurteilung pararectaler lymphknoten durch ultraschall, *Chirurg* 1990; **61**:587–91.
20. Boring CC, Squires TS, Tong T, Montgomery S, Cancer statistics. *The American Cancer Society Department of Epidemiology and Statistics* (1994) 7–26.
21. DeCosse JJ, Tsioulias GJ, Jacobson JS, Colorectal cancer: detection, treatment and rehabilitation. *The American Cancer Society Department of Epidemiology and Statistics* (1994) 27–42.
22. Akasu T, Sunouchi K, Tsioulias GJ, Muto T, Morioka Y, Preoperative staging of rectal carcinoma: prospective comparison of transrectal ultrasonography and computed tomography, *Gastroenterology* 1990; **98**:268.
23. Baden R, Badea C, Philippi W, Dejica D, Bologa S, Cazacu M, Wert und grenzen der endorektalen sonographie in der praoperativen stadieneinteilung des rektumkarzinoms, *Ultraschall* 1988; **9**:265–9.
24. Boyce GA, Sivak MV, Lavery Fazio V et al, Endoscopic ultrasound in the preoperative staging of rectal cancer, *Gastrointest Endosc* 1991; **37**:269.
25 Cohen JL, Grotz RL, Welch JP, Deckers PJ, Intrarectal sonography: a new technique for the assessment of rectal tumors, *Am Surg* 1991; **57**:459–62.
26. Detry R, Gigot JF, Gerard R, Performance de l'echographie endorectale en pathologie tumorale du rectum, *Gastroenterol Clin Biol* 1988; **12**:810–13.
27. Dorner A, Kahl HJ, Petersen P, Reich P, Intrakavitare sonographie, *Rontgen-Bl* 1988; **41**:186–8.
28. Glaser F, Schlag P, Herrarth C, Endorectal ultrasonography for the assessment of invasion of rectal tumours and lymph node involvement, *Br J Surg* 1990; **77**:883–7.
29. Feifel G, Hildebrandt LI, Dhom G, Assessment of depth of invasion in rectal cancer by endosonography, *Endoscopy* 1987; **19**:64–7.
30. Heintz A, Buess G, Junginger T, Endorektale sonographie zur praoperativen beurteilung der infiltrationstiefe von rektumtumoren, *Dtsch Med Wschr* 1990; **115**:1083–7.
31. Herzog LI, Die endoluminale sonographie als praoperative staging-methode beim rektumkarzinom, *Schweiz Med Wschr* 1990; **120**:1439–45.
32. Konishi F, Ugajin H, Ito K, Kanazawa K, Endorectal ultrasonography with a 7.5 MHz linear array scanner for the assessment of invasion of rectal carcinoma, *Int J Colorect Dis* 1990; **5**:515–20.
33. Mosnier H, Guivarc'h M, Barbagelata M, L'echographie endorectale: appreciation de l'extension loco-regionale des cancers du rectum, *Gastroenterol Clin Biol* 1987; **11**:307–11.
34. Napoleon B, Pujol B, Berger F, Valette PJ, Gerard JP, Souque JC, Accuracy of endosonography in the staging of rectal cancer treated by radiotherapy, *Br J Surg* 1991; **78**:785–8.
35. Rifkin MD, McGlynn ET, Marks G, Endorectal sonography: prospective staging of rectal cancer, *Scand J Gastroenterol* 1986; **21**(Suppl 123):99–103.
36. Pappalardo G, Reggio D, Frattaroli FM et al, The value of endoluminal ultrasonography and computed tomography in the staging of rectal cancer: a preliminary study, *J Surg Oncol* 1990; **43**:219–22.
37. Romano G, de Rosa P, Vallone G, Rotondo A, Grassi R, Santangelo ML, Intrarectal ultrasound and computed tomography in the pre- and post-operative assessment of patients with rectal cancer, *Br J Surg* 1985; **72**(suppl):S117–19.
38. Roseau G, Palazzo L, Amouyal P et al, Resultats de l'echoendoscopie dans le bilan preoperative du cancer de rectum, *Ann Chir* 1990; **44**:527–30.
39. Rotte KH, Kluhs L, Kleinau H, Kreidemann E, Computed tomography and endosonography in the preoperative staging of rectal carcinoma, *Eur J Radiol* 1989; **9**:187–90.
40. Ruf G, Kohlberger E, Radecke J, Lausen M, Wimmer B, Kirchner R, Praoperatives staging des rektumcarcinoms: endosonographie versus computer tomographie, *Langenbecks Arch Chir* 1989; **374**:164–8.
41. Sacco S, Arienti V, Cancelliere A, Gasbarrini G, Cola B, Die transrektale ultrasonographie beim praoperativen staging von rektumtumoren, *Colo-proctology* 1989; **5**:305–8.
42. Tio TL, Coene PPLO, van Delden OM, Tytgat GNJ, Colorectal carcinoma: preoperative TNM classification with endosonography, *Radiology* 1991; **179**:165–70.

43. Truong S, Hartung R, Rohrmann D, Praoperatives staging und verlaufskontrolle bei rektumkarzinomen mittels endorektaler sonographie, *Zentbl Chir* 1986; **111**:333–8.
44. Yamashita Y, Machi J, Shirouzu K, Morotomi T, Isomoto H, Kakegawa T, Evaluation of endorectal ultrasound for the assessment of wall invasion of rectal cancer, *Dis Colon Rectum* 1988; **31**:617–23.
45. Zerhouni EA, Arbor A, CT and MR imaging in the staging of colorectal carcinoma: report of the radiologic diagnostic group 2 trial, *Radiology* 1991; **181**(P):109.
46. Thaler W, Watzka S, Martin F et al, Preoperative staging of rectal cancer by endoluminal ultrasound vs magnetic resonance imaging. Preliminary results of a prospective, comparative study, *Dis Colon Rectum* 1994; **37**:1189–93.
47. Deen KI, Madoff RD, Belmonte C, Wong WD, Preoperative staging of rectal neoplasms with endorectal ultrasonography, *Semin Colon Rectal Surg* 1995; **6**:78–85.
48. Roubein LD, David C, DuBrow R et al, Endoscopic ultrasonography in staging rectal cancer, *Am J Gastroenterol* 1990; **85**:1391–4.
49. Shimizu S, Yada M, Kawai K. Use of endoscopic ultrasonography for the diagnosis of colorectal tumors, *Endoscopy* 1990; **22**:31–4.
50. Glaser F, Kuntz C, Schlag P, Herfarth C, Endorectal ultrasound for control of preoperative radiotherapy of rectal cancer, *Ann Surg* 1992; **217**:64–71.
51. Napoleon B, Pujol B, Berger F, Valette PJ, Gerard JP, Souquet JC, Accuracy of endosonography in the staging of rectal cancer treated by radiotherapy, *Br J Surg* 1991; **78**:785–8.
52. Zainea GG, Lee F, McLeary RD, Siders DB, Thieme ET, Transrectal ultrasonography in the evaluation of rectal and extrarectal disease, *Surgery* 1989; **169**:153–6.
53. Horn A, Morild I, Dahl O, Tumour shrinkage and down staging after preoperative radiation of rectal adenocarcinomas, *Radiother Oncol* 1990; **18**:19–28.
54. Hulsmans FH, Tio TL, Mathus-Vliegen EMH, Bosma A, Tytgat GNJ, Colorectal villous adenoma: transrectal US in screening for invasive malignancy, *Radiology* 1992; **185**:193–6.
55. Detry RJ, Kartheuser A, Cessions PJ, Endorectal ultrasonography for staging small rectal tumours: technique and contribution to treatment, *World J Surg* 1993; **17**:271–6.
56. Hulsmans FJH, Mathus-Vliegen LMH, Bosman S, Bosma A, Tytgat GNJ, Colorectal adenomas: inflammatory changes that simulate malignancy after laser coagulation-evaluation with transrectal US, *Radiology* 1993; **187**:367–71.
57. Soga J, Carcinoids of the rectum, tumours of the carcinoid family endocrinomas, *Acta Med Biol* 1982; **29**:157–201.
58. Shimizu S, Tada M, Kawai K, The value of endoscopic ultrasonography in the assessment of inflammatory bowel diseases, *Endoscopy* 1992; **24**(Suppl 1):354–8
59. Schratter-Sehn AU, Lochs H, Handl-Zeller L, Tscholakoff D, Schratter M, Endosonographic features of the lower pelvic region in Crohn's disease, *Am J Gastroenterol* 1993; **88**:1054–7.
60. Cataldo PA, Senagore A, Martin MS, Luchtefeld MA, Intrarectal ultrasound in the evaluation of perirectal abscesses, *Dis Colon Rectum* 1993; **36**:554–8.
61. Tio TL, Mulder CJJ, Wijers OB, Sars PRA, Tytgat GNJ, Endosonography of peri-anal and peri-colorectal fistula and/or abscess in Crohn's disease, *Gastrointest Endosc* 1990; **36**:331–6.
62. Williams JG, Anal ultrasonography in the diagnosis and management of abscess and fistula disease of the anorectum, *Semin Colon Rectal Surg* 1995; **6**:105–13.
63. Wiersema MJ, Kochman ML, Cramer CA, Kesler KA, Real-time endoscopic ultrasound-guided fine needle aspiration of a mediastinal lymph node, *Gastrointest Endosc* 1993; **39**:429–31.
64. Giovannini M, Seitz FJ, Perrier H, Monges G, Endosonography-guided fine-needle aspiration biopsy in submucosal and extrinsic tumours of the gastrointestinal tract: preliminary results in 31 patients, *Gastroenterology* 1993; **104**:405A.
65. Alexander AA, Eschelman DJ, Nazarian LN, Bonn J, Transrectal sonographically guided drainage of deep pelvic abscesses, *AJR* 1994; **162**:1227–30.
66. Nielsen MB, Pedersen JF, Hauge C, Rasmussen OO, Christiansen J, Endosonography of the anal sphincter: findings in healthy volunteers, *AJR* 1991; **157**:1199–202.
67. Rasmussen OO, Anorectal function, *Dis Colon Rectum* 1994; **37**:386–403.
68. Senagore AJ, Intrarectal and intra-anal ultrasonography in the evaluation of colorectal pathology, *Surg Clin North Am* 1994; **74**:1465–73.
69. Law PJ, Bartram CI, Anal endosonography: technique and normal anatomy, *Gastrointest Radiol* 1989; **14**:349–53.
70. Schafer A, Enck P, Furst G, Kahn Th, Frieling T, Lubke HJ, Anatomy of the anal sphincters. Comparison of anal endosonography to magnetic resonance imaging, *Dis Colon Rectum* 1994; **37**:777–81.
71. Tjandra JJ, Milsom JW, Stolfi VM, et al, Endoluminal ultrasound defines anatomy of the anal canal and pelvic floor, *Dis Colon Rectum* 1992; **35**:465–70.
72. Burnett SJ, Bartram CI, Endosonographic variations in the normal internal anal sphincter, *Int J Colorect Dis* 1991; **6**:2–4.
73. Sultan AH, Loder PB, Bartram CI, Kamm MA, Hudson CN, Vaginal endosonography. New approach to image the undisturbed anal sphincter, *Dis Colon Rectum* 1994; **37**:1296–9.
74. Alexander AA, Liu JB, Merton DA, Nagle DA. Fecal incontinence: transvaginal evaluation of the anatomic causes. *Radiology* 1996; **199**:529–32.
75. Blatchford GJ, Anal ultrasonography in the evaluation of fecal incontinence, *Semin Colon Rectal Surg* 1995; **6**:99–104.
76. Emblem R, Dhaenens G, Stien R, Morkrid L, Aasen AO, Bergan A, The importance of anal endosonography in the evaluation of idiopathic fecal incontinence, *Dis Colon Rectum* 1994; **37**:42–8.
77. Felt-Bersma RJF, van Baren R, Koorevaar M, Strijers RL, Cuesta MA, Unsuspected sphincter defects shown by anal endosonography after anorectal surgery. A prospective study, *Dis Colon Rectum* 1995; **38**:249–53.
78. Nielsen MB, Hauge C, Pedersen JF, Christiansen J, Endosonographic evaluation of patients with anal incontinence: findings and influence on surgical management, *AJR* 1993; **160**:771–5.
79. Sultan AH, Kamm MA, Hudson CN, Chir M, Thomas JM, Bartram CI, Anal-sphincter disruption during vaginal delivery, *N Engl J Med* 1993; **329**:1905–11.
80. Hill J, Corson RJ, Brandon H, Redford J, Faragher EB, Kiff ES, History and examination in the assessment of patients with idiopathic fecal incontinence, *Dis Colon Rectum* 1994; **37**:473–7.

81. Sultan AH, Kamm MA, Bartram CI, Hudson CN, Anal sphincter trauma during instrumental delivery, *Int J Gynecol Obstet* 1993; **43**:263–70.
82. Falk PM, Blatchford GJ, Cali RL, Christensen MA, Thorson AG, Transanal ultrasound and manometry in the evaluation of fecal incontinence, *Dis Colon Rectum* 1994; **37**:468–72.
83. Morgado PJ Jr, Wexner SD, Jorge JMN, Discrepancies in anal manometric pressure measurement-important or inconsequential? *Dis Colon Rectum* 1994; **37**:820–3.
84. Nielsen MB, Dammegaard L, Pedersen JF, Endosonographic assessment of the anal sphincter after surgical reconstruction, *Dis Colon Rectum* 1994; **37**:434–8.
85. Law OJ, Talbot RW, Bartram CI, Northover JMA, Anal endosonography in the evaluation of perianal sepsis and fistula in ano, *Br J Surg* 1989; **76**:752–5.
86. Solomon MJ, McLeon RS, Cohen EK, Zohen Z, Anal wall thickness under normal and inflammatory conditions of the anorectum as determined by endoluminal ultrasonography, *Am J Gastroenterol* 1995; **90**:574–8.
87. Finne CO, The role of endorectal sonography in the follow-up of malignant disease of the anorectum, *Semin Colon Rectal Surg* 1995; **6**:86–93.
88. Goldman S, Glimelius B, Norming U, Pahlman L, Seligson U, Transanorectal ultrasonography in anal carcinoma. A prospective study of 21 patients, *Acta Radiol* 1988; **29**:337–41.
89. Goldman S, Norming U, Svensson C, Glimelius B, Transanorectal ultrasonography in the staging of anal epidermoid carcinoma, *Int J Colorect Dis* 1991; **6**:152–7.
90. Rankin RN, Fenster A, Downey DB, Munk PL, Levin MF, Vellett AD, Three-dimensional sonographic reconstruction: techniques and diagnostic applications, *AJR* 1993; **161**:695–702.
91. Littrup JP, The development of a three-dimensional prostate model, *Prog Clin Biol Res* 1987; **237**:213–18.
92. Richard WD, Grimmell CK, Bedigian K, Frank KJ, A method for three-dimensional prostate imaging using transrectal ultrasound, *Comput Med Imag Graphics* 1993; **17**:73–9.
93. Sehgal CM, Broderick GA, Whittington R, Gorniak R, Arger PH, Three-dimensional US and volumetric assessment of the prostate. *Radiology* 1994; **192**:274–8.
94. Kallimans G, Garra BS, Tio TH et al, The feasibility of three-dimensional ultrasonography: a preliminary report, *Gastrointest Endosc* 1995; **41**:235–9.
95. Miller LS, Liu JB, Colizzo FP et al, Correlation of high-frequency esophageal ultrasonography and manometry in the study of esophageal motility, *Gastroenterology* 1995; **109**:832–7.

Chapter 8 Pancreaticobiliary tract

Larry S Miller, Thomas D Schiano and Ji-Bin Liu

INTRODUCTION

Endoscopic ultrasound (EUS) was initially developed to overcome many of the limitations of transabdominal ultrasound. EUS using 7.5- and 12-MHz dedicated echoendoscopes has become a useful tool in the evaluation of patients with diseases of the pancreaticobiliary system. The normal echo-anatomy for the pancreas, ampulla of Vater, portal vasculature and bile ducts has long since been delineated, allowing for the diagnostic usage of EUS in an ever-increasing number of disease processes.[1] Newer higher-frequency catheter-based ultrasound probes with greater resolution are now being used during standard endoscopy (EGD) and endoscopic retrograde cholangiopancreatography (ERCP) to better evaluate the actual histologic layers of the pancreatic and bile ducts and sphincter of Oddi. We will summarize the many roles that EUS plays in the evaluation of the pancreas and biliary system and then review the latest developments in the use of high-frequency endoluminal sonographic (HRES) probes in studying the biliary tract.

ANATOMY OF PANCREATICOBILIARY TRACT

The pancreas is divided into three portions: the head, which lies in the concavity of the duodenum; the neck, which overlies the portal vein; and the body, which tapers to form the tail towards the spleen. The uncinate process is the portion of the head that curves back towards the spleen under the mesenteric vessels. The pancreatic ductal system is formed by fusion of the duct of Santorini in the dorsal pancreatic anlage with Wirsung's duct in the ventral anlage. The minor papilla drains Santorini's duct, while the major papilla represents the common termination of Wirsung's duct and the bile duct (Fig. 8.1).

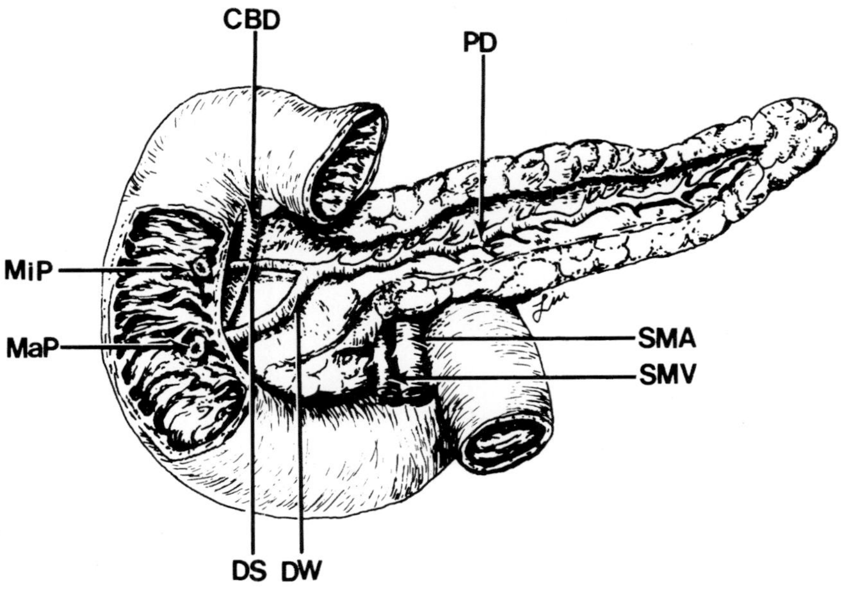

Figure 8.1 *Diagrammatic representation of pancreaticobiliary system. CBD, common bile duct; PD, pancreatic duct; SMA, superior mesenteric artery; SMV, superior mesenteric vein; DS, duct of Santorini (accessory pancreatic duct); DW, duct of Wirsung (principal pancreatic duct); MiP, minor papilla; MaP, major papilla.*

The gallbladder lies on the inferior surface of the liver in a fossa marking the division of the liver into its anatomic right and left lobes. The cystic duct runs beside the hepatic duct before actually opening into it. The extrahepatic biliary tree arises from the liver as the left and right hepatic ducts, each of which drains a hepatic lobe. The common hepatic duct is formed by the junction of these two ducts. In the liver hilum, the bile ducts are generally ventral to the portal vein and hepatic artery. The common hepatic duct lies along the anterolateral aspect of the portal vein. The common bile duct, formed by the union of the cystic and common hepatic ducts, is a direct continuation of the common hepatic duct. It passes behind the first portion of the duodenum and through the pancreatic head to enter the descending portion of the duodenum (Fig. 8.2).

The duodenum is divided into four portions: the bulb, the second (directly posteriorly), the third (descending to form the C-loop) and the fourth (transverse from the C-loop to the ligament of Treitz). The arterial supply to the proximal duodenum is from the branches of the gastroduodenal artery via the common hepatic artery, the most prominent of which is the superior pancreaticoduodenal artery. The distal duodenum is supplied by the inferior pancreaticoduodenal artery via the superior mesenteric artery (SMA). These two vessels form an arcade along the inner aspect of the duodenal C-loop supplying the duodenum, with small branches laterally to the right, and the pancreatic head with small branches medially to the left. Venous drainage parallels the arterial supply, ultimately forming the superior mesenteric vein (SMV).

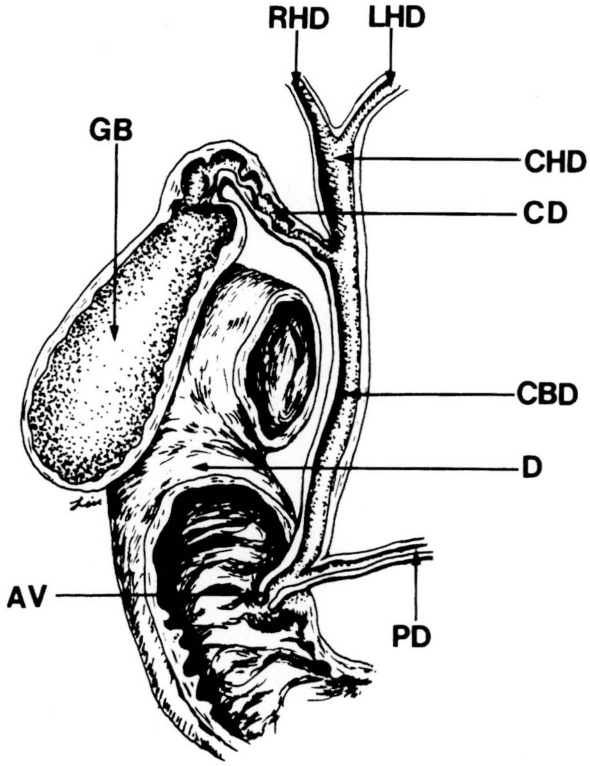

Figure 8.2 *Diagrammatic representation of biliary tract. RHD, right hepatic duct; LHD, left hepatic duct; CHD, common hepatic duct; CD, cystic duct; GB, gallbladder; CBD, common bile duct; D, duodenum; PD, pancreatic duct; AV, ampulla of Vater.*

TECHNICAL CONSIDERATIONS

To adequately image the pancreatiobiliary system, the tip of the echoendoscope is first placed into the third portion of the duodenum. Controlled withdrawal of the instrument allows imaging of the uncinate process, distal common bile duct, ampulla, ventral pancreas, superior mesenteric and portal veins and occasionally the right kidney. Continued withdrawal into the bulb affords imaging of the pancreatic head with its upper border delineated by the gastroduodenal artery. The gallbladder, portal vein, hepatic artery and inferior vena cava are also imaged from this position. Further imaging of the pancreatic body, gallbladder and splenic and portal veins is performed in the gastric antrum. The pancreatic tail, the spleen and its hilar vessels and occasionally the left kidney are imaged from the gastric fundus. Technical limitations include a small field of view and operator dependency in maneuvering the scope into the appropriate imaging position.[2–8]

The entire pancreas can be imaged in more than 95% of patients. The normal main bile duct is visualized in 80–90% of cases, while a dilated common duct is almost always seen endosonographically. The liver hilum with the hepatic branches is more difficult to delineate, with success being achieved only 50–60% of the time. Because only small parts of the left lobe and none of the right lobe of the liver can be visualized, systematic examination of the intrahepatic bile ducts is not possible.[2–8]

ENDOSONOGRAPHIC ANATOMY OF THE PANCREATICOBILIARY TRACT

While imaging the duodenum, the aorta should be placed at 5 o'clock and the vena cava at the 7 o'clock position, with the anechoic spine being visualized between these two great vessels. The SMA can often be seen branching from the aorta in the direction of the transducer. The SMV or splenic vein is immediately ventral to the SMA. These mesenteric vessels are located to the left of the aorta. The gastroduodenal artery, which originates from the hepatic artery, can be imaged between the duodenum and ventral pancreas in close proximity to the common bile duct. The uncinate process is localized between the aorta and mesenteric vessels. The branch of the pancreatic duct that drains the uncinate process is found ventrally from the superior mesenteric vein or splenic vein. The main pancreatic duct is ventral to the aorta and vena cava. The bifurcation created by the portal and splenic veins and the SMV can often be visualized. The common bile and common hepatic ducts are imaged using the portal vein as a guide. The bile duct is parallel to the portal vein and adjacent to the duodenum. The cystic duct and gallbladder are variable in location, with the former often being found close to the ampulla or adjacent to the hilum. The papilla is visualized as a raised area in the duodenal wall containing the common bile and pancreatic ducts. The common channel connecting the two can often be delineated.[2–8]

The pancreatic body and tail are located adjacent to the posterior stomach with the echoendoscope within the stomach; the left hepatic lobe and portal vein are used as landmarks for imaging. The splenic vein is found as a continuity of the portal vein. If the gastric lumen is filled with water, the spleen can also be used as a landmark. It is distinguished from the liver by the absence of the intrahepatic branches of the portal vein, and the spleen's proximity to the pancreatic tail and left kidney. The splenic vein and artery course together into the splenic hilum. The splenic vein is located on the immediately dorsal aspect of the pancreas, continuing along the pancreatic body and tail into the hilum. The main pancreatic duct is found ventral to the splenic vein.[2–8]

ENDOSCOPIC ULTRASOUND OF THE PANCREATICOBILIARY TRACT

PANCREAS

Using EUS, the pancreatic parenchyma is characterized by a uniform echo pattern bounded by the duodenal wall, the gastroduodenal artery, and the portal vein (Fig. 8.3).[2] Differentiation between the echogenic dorsal segment and the poorly echogenic ventral pancreatic segment, and identification of the pancreatic ductal system, can almost always be achieved. This difference in echogenicity is felt to be due to the significant quantity of fat contained in the dorsal segment within interlobular septae and acinar cell fat vacuoles. Clear visualization of this differential echogenicity is a strong indicator of

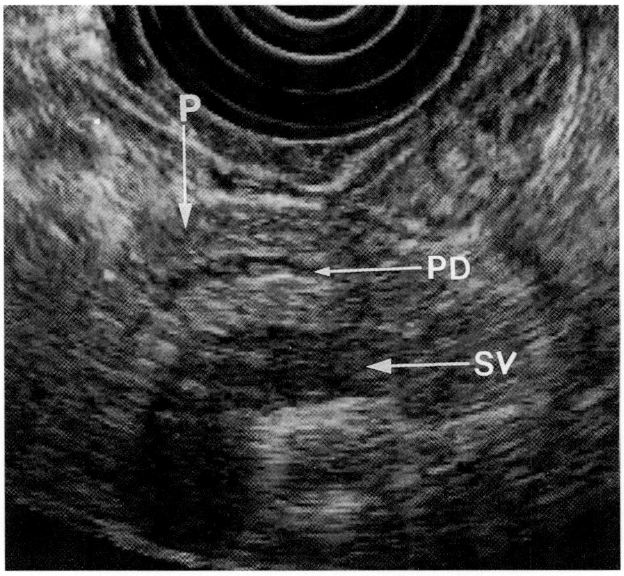

Figure 8.3 *An EUS image of the pancreatic body through the posterior wall of the stomach. Note the uniform echo pattern of the pancreas (P). The splenic vein (SV) posterior to the body of the pancreas is used as a landmark to identify the pancreas. The thin hypoechoic structure running through the body of the pancreas (PD) represents the pancreatic duct.*

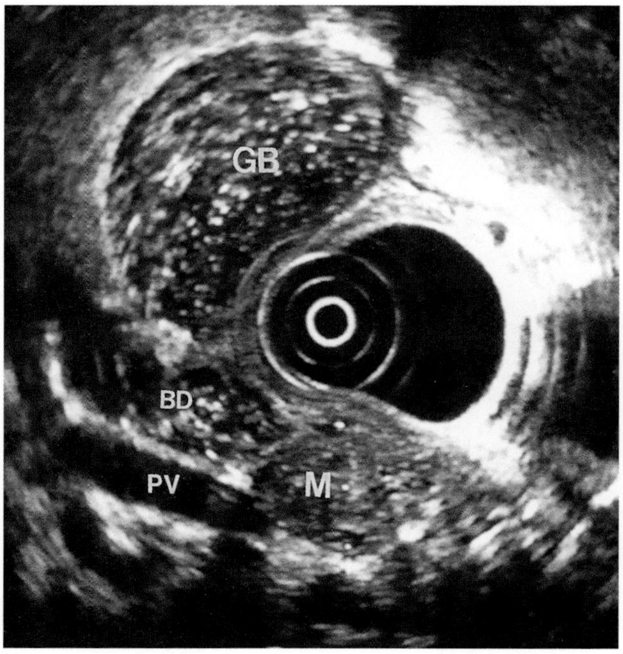

Figure 8.4 *A hypoechoic mass (M) in the head of the pancreas is seen obstructing the common bile duct (BD). The dilated common bile duct and gallbladder (GB) are filled with sludge. PV, portal vein.*

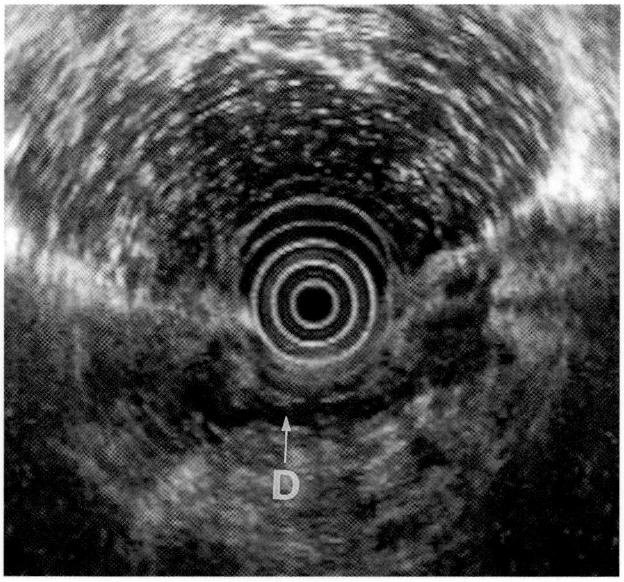

Figure 8.6 *In a patient with chronic pancreatitis, EUS shows a heterogeneous pancreas with a dilated pancreatic duct (D).*

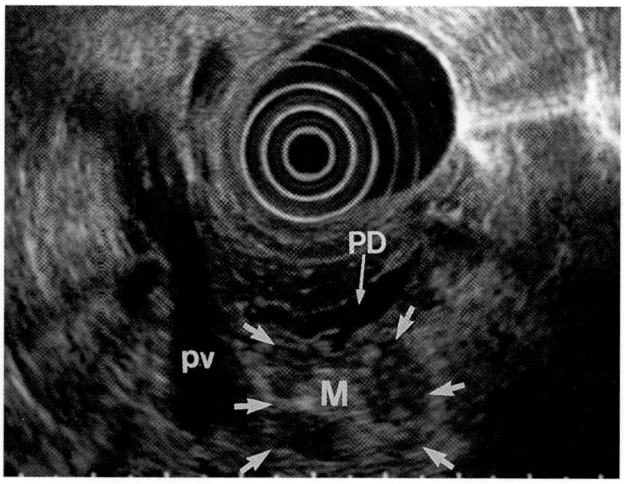

Figure 8.5 *A hypoechoic mass (M) with irregular borders (arrows) is seen within the head of the pancreas. The pancreatic duct (PD) appears dilated due to post-stenotic changes. PV, portal vein.*

normalcy, usually excluding an inflammatory process.[2]

EUS has become an important modality in the diagnosis and staging of pancreatic exocrine tumors. On EUS, pancreatic cancer presents as a distinct mass, clearly demarcated from the more homogeneous echo pattern of the organ itself. Echo-free areas within the tumor probably represent focal areas of necrosis. The echo pattern of pancreatic neoplasms is highly variable with irregular or indistinct imaging in most cases (Fig. 8.4). Smaller lesions tend to be more homogeneous with smoother margins. When the mass is large, the outer borders are difficult to delineate because of the short depth of penetration of the ultrasound beam. Thus, small lesions are better demonstrated than larger masses.[3,4] Pancreatic carcinoma and neoplasms of the pancreatic head may lead to post-stenotic dilation of the main pancreatic duct and narrowing of the common bile duct, both of which can also be noted on EUS (Figs 8.4 and 8.5).

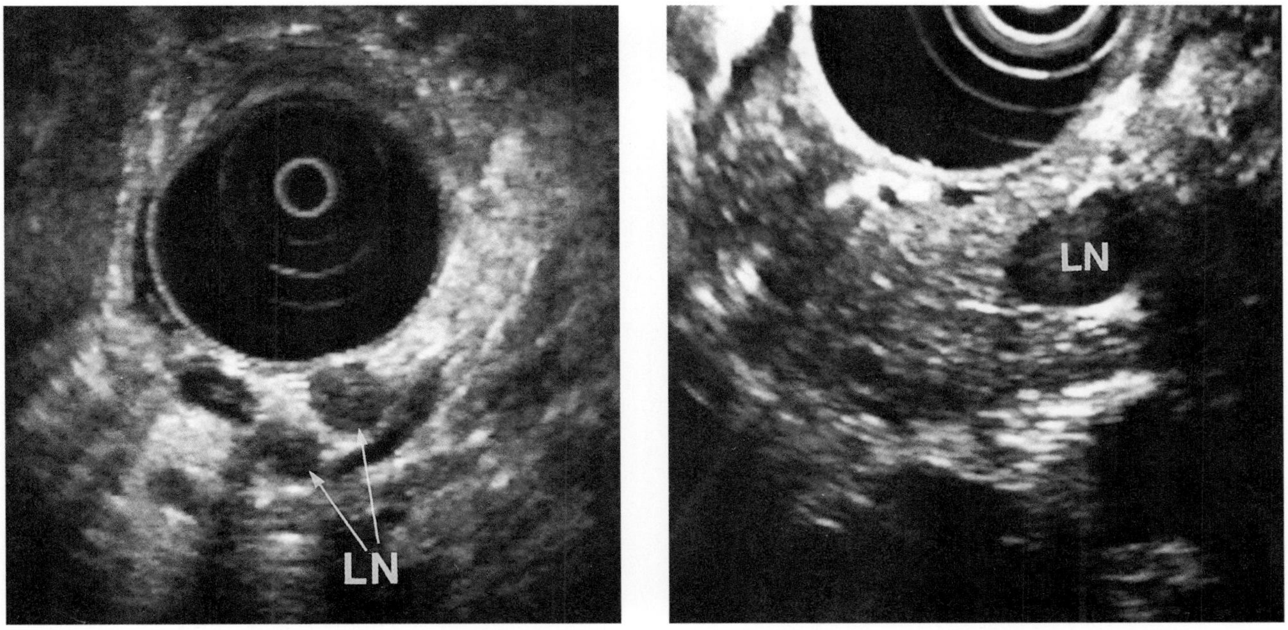

a *b*

Figure 8.7 *These malignant lymph nodes (LN) are imaged in different patients with pancreatic carcinoma. Note that these lymph nodes are round, echopoor and well demarcated, which is characteristic of the malignant involvement.*

When a mass has been identified in the pancreas, the main problem is the differential diagnosis between cancer and focal nodular pancreatitis. EUS has been found superior to transabdominal ultrasound, equal to CT and inferior to ERCP in this respect; it cannot, however, routinely differentiate cancer from focal pancreatitis (Fig. 8.6).[2–4] Establishment of a diagnosis differentiating between the different forms of pancreatic malignancy is also not possible by means of EUS.[5]

Apart from the tumor itself, adjacent viscera and vascular structures can also be well visualized by EUS.[6] Infiltration of the gastric or duodenal wall, distal common bile duct, liver or spleen can be demonstrated. The most important criterion for assessment of local tumor spread, and thus resectability is involvement of the parapancreatic vasculature.[2–4] EUS appears to be superior to transabdominal ultrasound, CT, and even angiography, in staging and in the evaluation of the invasion of the veins, though less so in the staging of arterial invasion.[7,8] Peritumorous lymph node metastasis can also be identified by means of EUS, using the criteria of size (10 mm or more) and/or certain qualitative echo features; malignant lymph nodes are reported to be echopoor, roundish, and well demarcated (Fig. 8.7).[2–4]

EUS has been found to be highly accurate in the staging of pancreatic carcinoma, being superior to standard transabdominal ultrasound and CT.[9,10] It has also been shown to be more precise than transabdominal ultrasound and CT in determining actual tumor size when correlated with pathologic TNM stage of the resected specimen.[11] In addition, EUS can provide information on tumor size and shape that is not provided by even ERCP.[9,10]

Pancreatic cancer has recently been included in the TNM staging system as follows. The TNM classification corresponds to the criteria published by The American Joint Committee on Cancer.

T: Primary tumor
T_1: Tumor limited to pancreas
T_{1a}: Tumor 2 cm or less at greatest dimension
T_{1b}: Tumor more than 2 cm at greatest dimension
T_2: Tumor extending directly into duodenum, bile duct or peripancreatic tissue
T_3 Tumor extending directly into stomach, spleen, colon or adjacent large blood vessels
Tx: Primary tumor cannot be assessed

N: Regional lymph nodes
N_0: No regional lymph nodes
N_1: Regional lymph node metastasis
Nx: Regional lymph nodes cannot be assessed

M: Distant metastasis
M_0: No distant metastasis
M: Distant metastasis; hepatic metastasis, peritoneal dissemination
Mx: Distant metastasis cannot be assessed

In clinical practice, EUS has become an important diagnostic modality in selecting the appropriate patient for surgery and in defining nonresectable cases of pancreatic carcinoma.[9,10] In performing local tumor resection, preoperative staging with EUS is mandatory. EUS-guided biopsy and cytology aspiration is now being used to obtain a tissue diagnosis at the time of the initial examination.[12]

Yasuda reported that 50 cases of pancreatic carcinoma were examined by EUS before surgery. Histologic confirmation of EUS findings were obtained in all patients of at least 50 lesions. Ten were studied with catheter-based miniprobes. The diagnostic accuracy for T stage was 70% with the miniprobe and 92% with EUS. The sensitivity and specificity for the diagnosis of metastatic lymph nodes were 40% and 100%, respectively, with the miniprobe, and 53% and 90%, respectively, with EUS. The staging of pancreatic carcinoma by means of the miniprobe was, therefore, less accurate than when using EUS.[13]

Gress et al have evaluated EUS and criteria for determining vascular invasion and unresectability in pancreatic carcinoma. EUS is highly accurate in detecting vascular invasion, either as direct tumor invasion of the portal vein, SMV, or as loss of vascular interface. Gress et al prospectively analyzed the significance of tumor abutment of the portal vein, SMA or SMV in predicting resectability, to determine if tumors in close proximity to these vessels are equivalent to direct vascular invasion. Patients in whom the mass closely abuts, but does not invade, the portal vein, SMA and SMV made up the study group. The distance between the mass and the vessel's hyperechoic border and the length of tumor abutment along the vessel for each case were measured. EUS findings were correlated with surgical pathology in 10 patients. Eight patients were found to be unresectable, based on the vascular encasement. In two patients undergoing resection, tumor was unable to be completely removed from the portal vein and the margin of the resection was positive. EUS staging and prediction of vascular involvement and resectability based on the criteria of tumor abutment is highly accurate. This finding may imply that patients with tumor that closely abuts the portal vein, SMV or SMA are probably unresectable, because of the adherence of tumor to the vessel.[14]

In another study by Brugge et al, three EUS criteria—irregular venous wall, loss of inner space and proximity—were tested against results of surgically defined vascular staging using both the Olympus EUS20 and the Pentax FG32 UA EUS scopes. The EUS criterion of irregular venous wall—had the greatest overall accuracy rate (85–90%) for linear and radial EUS, with a high specificity rate (100–94%); however, it suffered from a lower sensitivity rate (42–50%). The other EUS criteria were less accurate because of low sensitivity and specificity rates. The use of the criteria of irregular venous wall and bi-linear and radial EUS enables the prediction of portal venous system invasion with high accuracy.[15]

In a report by Bhutani et al, fine needle aspiration was performed in 21 lesions in 20 patients to evaluate pancreatic masses. EUS and fine needle aspiration accurately detects pancreatic masses and stages pancreatic malignancy. Ultrasound-directed fine needle aspiration has a 90% accuracy in detecting cancer. If EUS is used in the initial workup, the patients with suspected pancreatic malignancy can avoid unnecessary ERCP or surgical exploration.[16]

EUS has become the technique of choice to detect very small islet cell endocrine tumors of the pancreas.[17] These neoplasms usually manifest as echopoor, homogeneous, smoothly demarcated lesions, within the pancreas; specific echo patterns do not exist for the different histologic tumor types (Fig. 8.8). Orientation is achieved in relation to the adjacent large vessels, pancreatic duct and other landmarks.[2–4,18] Initial diagnosis of these endocrine tumors is made on the basis of laboratory tests or upon clinical suspicion; localization has previously been difficult using CT, transabdominal ultrasound, angiography and venous sampling, and may fail in up to 40–60% of cases.[2,3,17,18] Differentiation from

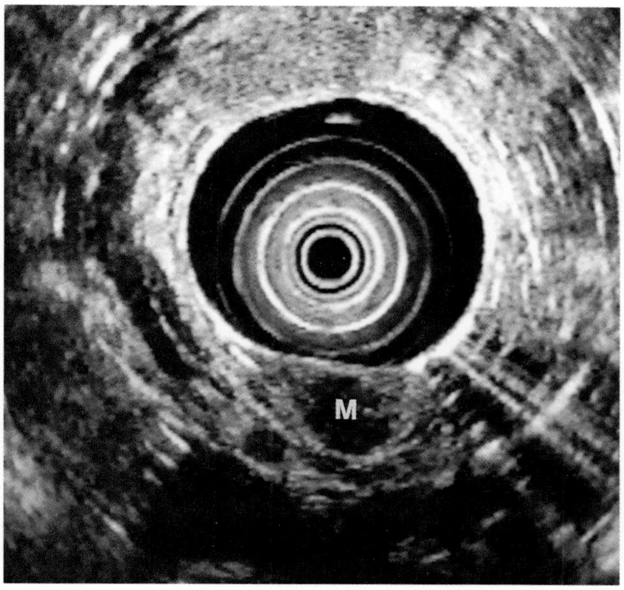

Figure 8.8 *A hypoechoic mass (M) is seen within the head of the pancreas. Pathologic examination proved this to be an islet cell tumor.*

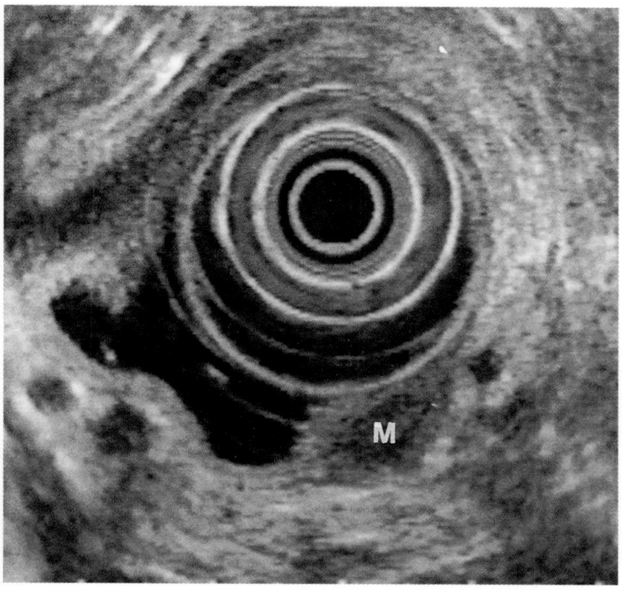

Figure 8.9 *EUS image shows a hyperechoic mass (M) arising from the wall of the duodenum. The gastronoma was confirmed by surgical pathology.*

parapancreatic lymphadenopathy can occasionally be difficult in small tumors at the border of the pancreas. Extrapancreatic sites of endocrine tumors (such as gastrinomas) may be visualized by EUS (Fig. 8.9), but with much less sensitivity.[2,3] Despite these shortcomings, EUS appears to be the most accurate modality for preoperative localization of pancreatic endocrine tumors, even when transabdominal ultrasound and CT are negative. Generally, the rate of false-positive findings is very low.[17,18]

The features of chronic pancreatitis on EUS vary according to the severity of the disease. Such features mainly represent changes readily recognizable on transabdominal ultrasound, but EUS provides considerably better image resolution. The pancreas may be enlarged, shrunken, or normal in size. The echo pattern may be irregular and have a speckled or mottled appearance.[2,3] Intraparenchymal calcifications are seen as strong echogenic foci with acoustic shadowing. Multiple calcifications may hamper proper visualization of the rest of the pancreas and the main pancreatic duct. Focal areas of hypodensity may also occur; the pancreatic duct may be dilated and irregular with hyperechoic foci (intraductal lithiasis) within it.[2,3,19]

EUS may be useful in chronic pancreatitis for establishing the initial diagnosis, for differentiating between inflammation and malignancy in focal masses, and for making decisions concerning treatment, in which case precise determination of the location and extent of ductal change and cysts is necessary.[2,3,19,20] Diagnosis of advanced chronic pancreatitis is possible with a high degree of accuracy via EUS, but these causes can also be readily diagnosed via ERCP, transabdominal ultrasound and CT. EUS may complement ERCP in diagnosing chronic pancreatitis and clarifying equivocal findings of ductal stenosis or obstruction. It can also readily identify ductal stones as the cause of obstruction.

AMPULLA OF VATER

The ampulla of Vater is generally a difficult region to image. Transabdominal ultrasound and CT are not well suited for the evaluation of this area.[4,6] This is compounded by the fact that the clinical presentation is usually nonspecific, making it difficult to differentiate between an ampullary tumor, an impacted stone and a papillary stenosis. Though ERCP is the gold standard, EUS may yield additional information in both diagnosis and subsequently in staging, if a malignancy is discovered.

Ampullary tumors present as localized duodenal wall thickening at the level of the papilla. In most cases the dilated distal common bile duct can be traced up to its entry into the tumor, with extension often present into the distal lumen (Fig. 8.10).[4,6,8,21] Differential diagnosis between ampullary carcinoma and a pancreatic cancer invading the ampulla is based upon the connecting angulation between the tumor and the duodenal wall (more acute in the former, and obtuse in the latter), but remains difficult. Transducer's balloon overfilling in the case of smaller lesions may cause compression of the tumor, resulting in overstaging. Smaller tumors are usually homogeneous in their echo pattern and are echo-poor; heterogeneous internal echoes occur more frequently with increasing tumor size.[4,6,8,21] Though EUS is very sensitive in detecting tumors of the papilla and periampullary region, it cannot confidently differentiate between an adenoma or villous adenoma and an early carcinoma. Differentiation of a small localized tumor of the ampulla of Vater from papillitis after stone passage or sphincterotomy is also difficult using EUS. EUS plays no role in the diagnosis of biliary dyskinesia.

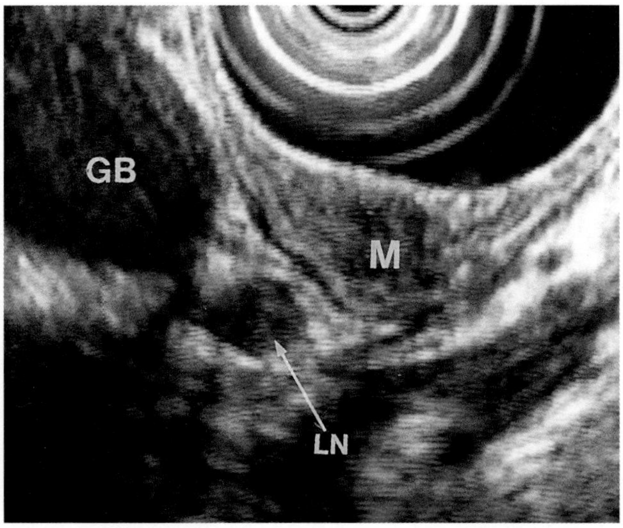

Figure 8.10 *A hypoechoic mass (M) arising from the ampulla of the duodenum, corresponding with ampullary carcinoma. Note the dilated gallbladder (GB) and a lymph node (LN) adjacent to the mass.*

Despite these shortcomings, EUS has proven invaluable in the staging of ampullary tumors. It can be quite precise in assessing the depth of tumor invasion and in detecting lymph node metastases. CT and transabdominal ultrasound play a role only in the detection of distant metastases and in delineating gross pancreatic involvement.[4,6,8]

The TNM staging system is being used to classify cancers in the ampulla of Vater as follows:

T: Primary tumor
T_0: No tumor assessable
T_1: Tumor limited to ampulla of Vater
T_2: Tumor invading duodenal wall, in particular the muscularis of the duodenum
T_3: Tumor invading 2 cm or less into pancreas
T_4: Tumor invading more than 2 cm into pancreas or other adjacent organs, in particular the major blood vessels
Tx: Primary tumor cannot be assessed

N: Regional lymph nodes
N_0: No regional lymph node metastasis
N_1: Regional lymph node metastasis
Nx: Regional lymph node cannot be assessed

M: Distant metastasis
M_0: No distant metastasis
M_1: Distant metastasis; hepatic metastasis, peritoneal dissemination, lymph node metastasis along the splenic vein or at the splenic hilum
Mx: Distant metastasis cannot be assessed

Because the muscularis can be clearly distinguished, EUS is highly accurate for the staging of ampullary tumor. The differentiation between T_3 and T_4 is made according to the depth of tumor invasion into the pancreas.

BILE DUCTS

In experienced hands, a normal common bile duct is seen with EUS in 80–90% of cases, while a dilated duct can be seen in 100% of cases.[3,4] The hilum of the liver with the hepatic branches is more difficult to delineate, with a success rate of 50–60%. Because only small parts of the liver can be viewed by EUS, an adequate assessment of intrahepatic bile ducts cannot be performed. The normal common bile duct appears as an anechoic tubular structure lined by a three-layered wall consisting of a major central echo-poor layer bordered by a slim echogenic band on each side (Fig. 8.11).[3,4,22]

Bile duct carcinoma is characterized on EUS by a variable but mostly hypoechoic and irregular echo pattern with intraductal or transductal growth (Fig. 8.12).[3,4,22,23] EUS is helpful in determining tumor size and infiltration into neighboring structures, such as the duodenal wall and adjacent vessels. Distinction between metastatically involved or inflamed lymph nodes is difficult. Despite this, EUS is considered a standard diagnostic imaging modality in the staging of common bile duct and extrahepatic bile duct cancer. In the detection of smaller common bile duct tumors, EUS appears to be equal to ERCP but far superior to transabdominal ultrasound, CT and angiography.[3,4,22,23] In more proximal tumors, the EUS penetration depth is not sufficient in all cases to reveal infiltration of a tumor into the hepatic ducts or to delineate portal venous involvement in the proximal duct. Tio et al have found that EUS could be used to predict tumor resectability with an accuracy of 80% in distal and proximal bile duct carcinoma.[24]

The TNM staging of extrahepatic bile duct cancer is as follows:

T: Primary tumor
T_1: Tumor invading mucosa or muscle layer of the bile duct wall
T_{1a}: Tumor invading mucosa
T_{1b}: Tumor invading muscle layer
T_2: Tumor invading perimuscular connective tissue
T_3: Tumor invading adjacent structures: liver, pancreas, duodenum, gallbladder, colon, or stomach

N: Regional lymph nodes
N_0: No regional lymph node metastasis
N_1: Regional lymph node metastasis
N_{1a}: Lymph node along the common bile duct or cystic duct and in the liver hilum

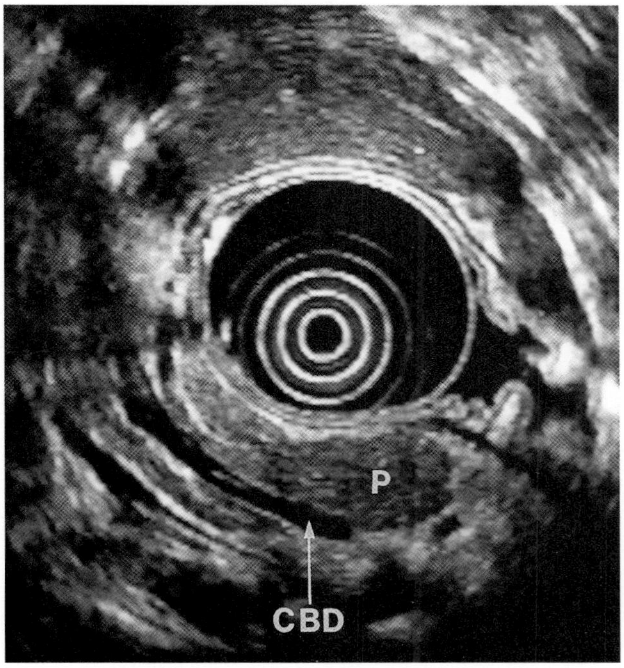

Figure 8.11 *EUS image shows the distal segment of the normal common bile duct (CBD) passing through the head of the pancreas (P).*

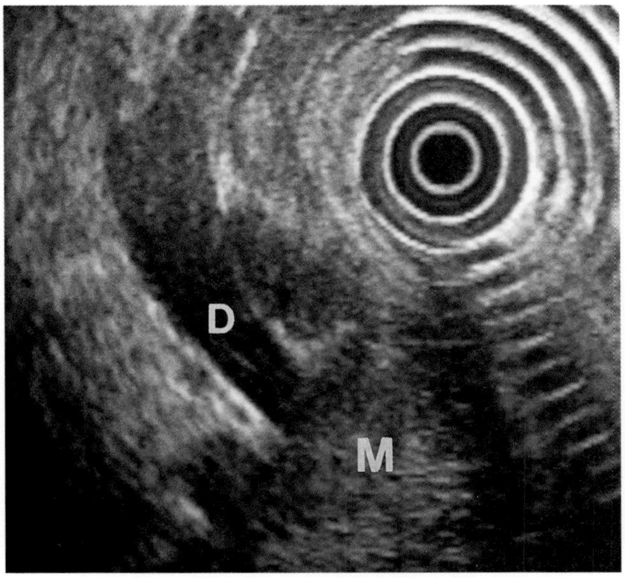

Figure 8.12 *EUS shows a hypoechoic mass (M) arising from the distal common bile duct with ductal dilation (D). Biopsy of the mass shows a cholangiocarcinoma.*

N_{1b}: Periduodenal, periportal, adjacent to the celiac trunk, and mesenteric blood vessels

M: Distant metastasis
M_0: No distant metastasis
M_1: Distant metastasis; peritoneal dissemination, hepatic metastasis, or perigastric lymph nodes

At present, EUS should be used as a complementary method in the evaluation of bile duct abnormalities after transabdominal ultrasound, CT and ERCP have been performed. All common bile duct strictures of unknown etiology should be further investigated by EUS, though differentiation between benign and malignant strictures, especially in flat, spreading carcinomas, is extremely difficult.[3,4,22] EUS has not been used in the evaluation of cholangitis but has recently been shown to be the most reliable pre-therapeutic diagnostic tool for choledocholithiasis compared with transabdominal ultrasound and CT (Fig. 8.13).[25] It can accurately estimate common bile duct diameter, stone number and location. In a majority of cases, EUS can lead to diagnostic certainty about the presence or absence of choledocholithiasis in pre- and post-cholecystectomy patients with suspected biliary obstruction.[25] Overall, however, it is still somewhat less sensitive than ERCP. Additionally, EUS can demonstrate anomalous connections within the pancreatiobiliary duct, which are known to cause cholangitis and be associated with the development of cholangiocarcinoma.[22,26] A preliminary study has shown that sonographic features of pancreatic duct stones might predict the feasibility of their removal during ERCP.[27]

The sensitivity of transabdominal ultrasound for common bile duct stones is between 22%[28] and 70%.[29] Choledocholithiasis is diagnosed at EUS by findings of reproducible hyperechoic focus in the bile duct with associated posterior acoustic shadowing.[30] EUS can also demonstrate wall thickening of the bile duct corresponding to thickened, inflamed pseudomembranous ductal walls, which may be caused by inflammation from gallstone migration.[31] In one retrospective series of 15 patients it gave a correct diagnosis in 73%, compared with only 33% by transabdominal ultrasound and 23% by CT scan.[32] There have been several prospective and retrospective studies demonstrating the performance of EUS in evaluating common bile duct stones. Edmundowicz[33] evaluated 20 patients by EUS and ERCP. EUS correctly diagnosed three of these patients, transabdominal ultrasound correctly diagnosed two of these patients, and EUS correctly excluded choledocholithiasis in all 16 patients without common bile duct stones. Amouyal et al[31] reported on 62 patients, in which EUS missed 1 of 32 patients, with a sensitivity and specificity of 97% and 100% respectively. EUS and cholangiography were compared in 64 patients pre- and post-cholecystectomy. The overall accuracies of EUS and ERCP for the diagnosis of choledocolithiasis were 92% and 97%, respectively.[34]

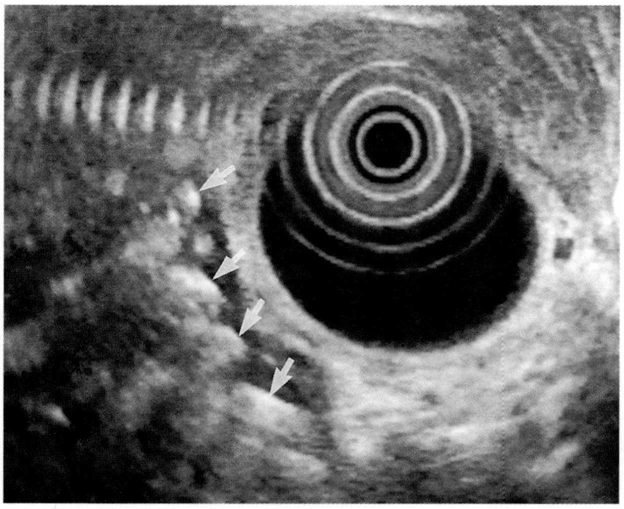

Figure 8.13 *Multiple hyperechoic reflectors (arrows) with acoustic shadowings are seen within the common bile duct, corresponding with choledocholithiasis.*

EUS sensitivity for common bile duct stones may equal[31,34,35] or exceed that of direct cholangiography (ERCP or intraoperative), thereby avoiding unnecessary diagnostic ERCPs or intraoperative cholangiograms. ERCP has high, overall positive (94%) and negative predictive values (93%); therefore EUS has the potential to replace diagnostic ERCP on non-high-risk patients who have a 0–25% risk of stones.[34]

EUS may have a potential role in evaluating and following patients with a history of gallstones, suspected choledocholithiasis and negative ultrasound, in patients with contraindications to ERCP (such as contrast allergy or pregnancy), in patients with histories of unsuccessful ERCP, in patients with histories of post-ERCP pancreatitis, in non-high-risk patients with elevated liver function tests minimal to non-dilation or remote history of jaundice of pancreatitis, and in patients with idiopathic acute pancreatitis.[34]

GALLBLADDER

EUS provides excellent images of the gallbladder with the probe in the pre-pyloric or post-bulbar region. With EUS, the normal wall of the gallbladder is imaged as three echo layers.[22,36] A hypoechoic central layer best corresponds to the gallbladder's muscular core, while the inner and outer hyperechoic layers represent mucosal and subserosal/serosal surfaces, respectively.

Gallstones are seen as echogenic foci within the gallbladder lumen with posterior acoustic shadowing (Fig. 8.14). Microlithiasis and gallbladder sludge is imaged as 0.5–2-mm hyperechoic foci without acoustic shadowing Gallbladder carcinoma presents as a polypoid, intraluminal mass of varying echodensity and irregularity with progressive wall destruction and liver infiltration, depending on the tumor state. The crucial EUS feature of malignancy is transmural tumor growth with an irregular outer lining or protruding tumor.[22,36,37] Mitake et al. performed preoperative EUS in patients with gallbladder carcinoma and compared the EUS findings with the histology of the resection specimens. Carcinomas without lymph node metastasis were correctly diagnosed by EUS in 87.5% of cases. In 79.5% of cases, a differentiation between early and advanced cancer was possible with EUS. EUS assessment of lymph node metastasis reached a sensitivity of 82% and a specificity of 93%.[37] Thus, EUS may be useful in the staging of gallbladder cancer.

The depth of invasion of gallbladder cancer is clearly defined by the TNM classification as follows:

T: Primary tumor
T_1: Tumor limited to the mucosa of the gallbladder without penetration into the muscularis
T_2: Tumor invading muscularis of the gallbladder
T_3: Tumor invading adjacent structures such as duodenum, liver, or major blood vessels

N: Regional lymph nodes
N_0: No regional lymph node metastasis
N_1: Regional lymph node metastasis
Nx: Regional lymph node metastasis cannot be assessed

M: Distant metastasis
M_0: No distant metastasis
M_1: Distant metastasis; hepatic metastasis, peritoneal dissemination
Mx: Distant metastasis cannot be assessed

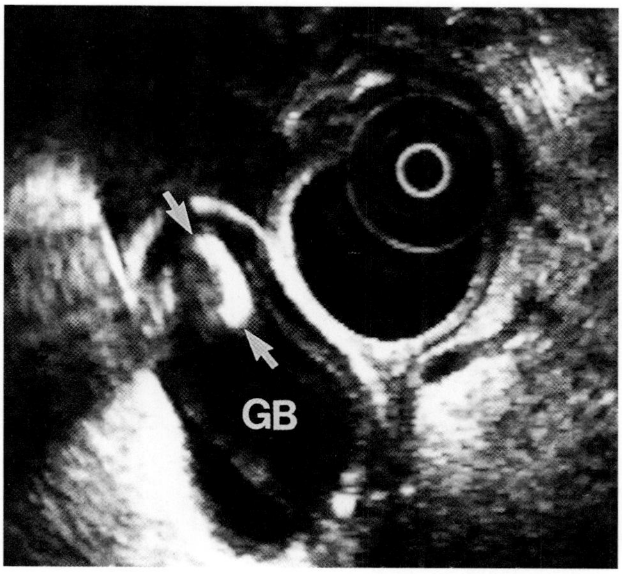

Figure 8.14 *A gallstone (arrows) is seen within the gallbladder (GB). The stone appears as an echogenic focus with posterior acoustic shadowing.*

Other gallbladder diseases have also been imaged by EUS. Imaging of adenomyomatosis has shown thickening of the muscular and serosal layers of the gallbladder wall; small cystic areas within the wall correspond to dilated sinuses.[22,36] Cholesterol polyps show a granular echo pattern with multiple hypoechoic spots. Thus, it may be possible to differentiate cholesterol polyps from gallbladder cancer, which transabdominal ultrasound is unable to do (Fig. 8.15).[22,36]

Dahon et al evaluated patients with acute pancreatitis and biliary colic who had normal transabdominal ultrasound findings. EUS found gallstones, sludge or minilithiasis in two-thirds of the patients, with a sensitivity of 100% and a specificity of 81%.[38] Dill et al used a linear-array endoscopic ultrasound transducer to diagnose chronic cholecystitis in patients with negative transabdominal ultrasound.[39] In another study, 21 patients with biliary pain and negative transabdominal ultrasound were imaged with EUS. EUS diagnosed gallbladder sludge in 95% of these patients in whom chronic choleycystitis was confirmed after cholecystectomy.[40] Limited follow-up

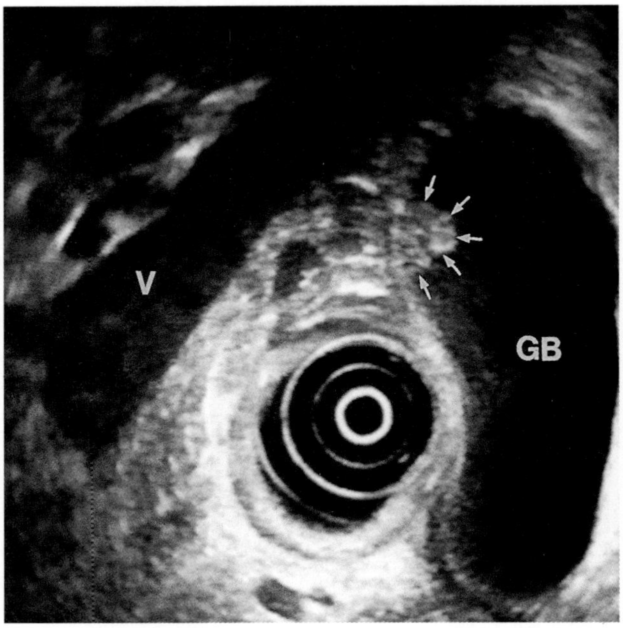

Figure 8.15 *A polyp (arrows) attached to the posterior wall of the gallbladder is imaged. V, vessel; GB, gallbladder.*

showed resolution of pain in 18 of 20 patients. Amouyal et al[41] evaluated 44 patients with non-alcoholic acute pancreatitis and no gallstones by transabdominal ultrasound. EUS provided the biliary origin of acute pancreatitis in 28 of 38 patients by demonstrating the presence of minilithiasis or common bile duct stones. The sensitivity and specificity of EUS for biliary lithiasis in the setting of acute pancreatitis were 97% and 75%, respectively.[11]

CATHETER-BASED ENDOLUMINAL ULTRASOUND OF PANCREATICOBILIARY TRACT

Over the last several years, high-frequency (12.5 to 30-MHz) catheter-based ultrasound transducers (4.8 to 9 Fr), originally designed with intravascular imaging in mind, have found application in the evaluation of the human biliary tract.[42,43] These catheter-based ultrasound transducers differ from dedicated echoendoscopes in a number of ways. Because of their small size, they can easily fit through the biopsy channel of a conventional endoscope or be inserted into the bile and pancreatic ducts via ERCP or through surgically created openings in the biliary tract. In addition, their small size allows them to be inserted through strictured areas where the dedicated scopes cannot be placed. An operating frequency of 20 MHz results in an axial resolution to 0.1 mm. Despite the greater axial resolution, however, the penetration of the ultrasound waves is limited by their higher frequency to about 2 cm. Because these transducers are not surrounded by a water-filled balloon, there is much less distortion of most mural structures. HRES examination can be performed during routine ERCP without the need to perform endoscopic papillotomy.[20]

Furukawa et al used a 30-MHz transducer with an axial resolution of 0.07 mm and a lateral resolution of 0.18 mm to assess the normal anatomy of the common bile duct and pancreatic duct from human autopsy specimens, and then compared endoluminal ultrasound images with corresponding histologic sections.[44] They also studied five patients with biliary disease (three with cholangiocarcinoma, one with choledocholithiasis and one with a congenital choledochal cyst) and four patients with pancreatic disease (two with chronic pancreatitis and two with mucin-producing tumors) using a similar transducer inserted through an endoscope into the ducts via the major papilla. Acoustic echoes were found between the transducer and mucosa interface, the mucosa and fibromuscular layer, and the fibromuscular layer and adventitia interface in the biliary intraductal examination. In examining the pancreatic duct, imaging interfaces were found between the transducer and mucosa, the mucosa and connective tissue, and the connective tissue and pancreatic parenchyma.[44]

The ductal walls were imaged and found to have three layers (an outer echogenic layer, a middle hypoechoic layer, and an inner echogenic layer) (Fig. 8.16). Histopathologic sectioning revealed a mucosal, a fibromuscular and an adventitial layer. The thickness of the first layer tended to overestimate that of the histologic correlate. The in vivo examination revealed a similar three layers in the choledocholithiasis patient; instead of a three-layered appearance, however, a hypoechoic mass was seen on HRES in the case of carcinoma. HRES of the pancreatic parenchyma demonstrated a fine reticular pattern (Fig. 8.17). Imaging of the

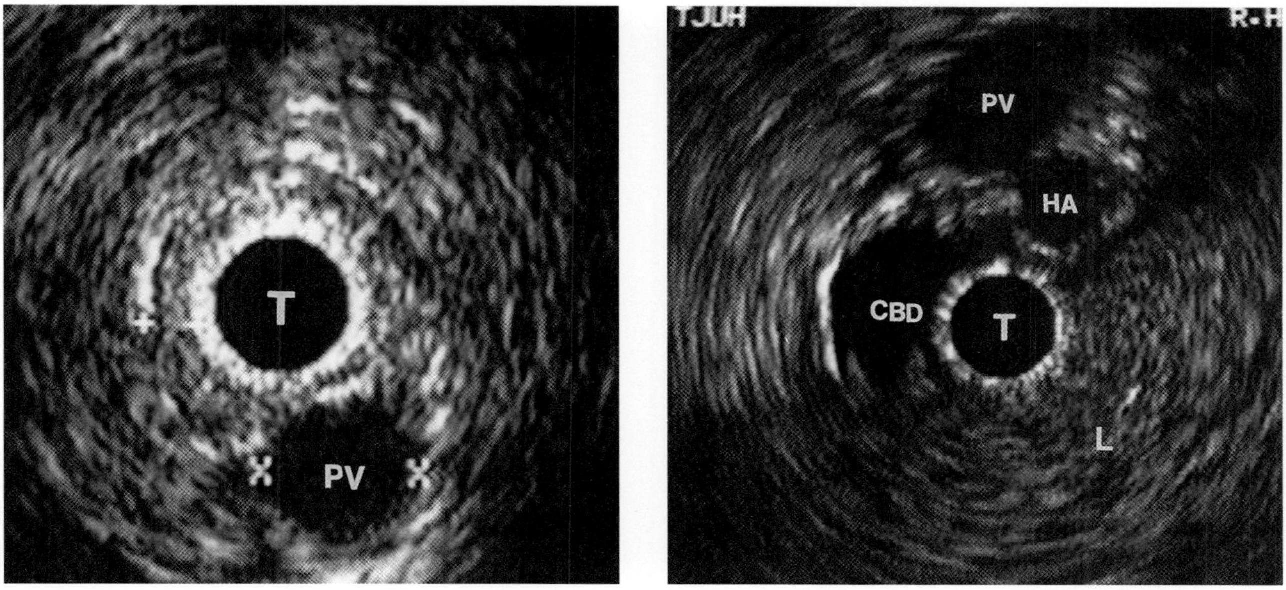

Figure 8.16 *(a) The 20-MHz ultrasound transducer (T) is within the intrapancreatic portion of the common bile duct. The pancreatic parenchyma is seen as the fine reticulated echotexture pattern. The adjacent structures, such as the portal vein (PV), can be seen. (b) With the transducer (T) positioned at the level of the intrahepatic portion of the common bile duct (CBD), the hepatic parenchymal (L) and surrounding strictures are demonstrated. PV, portal vein; HA, hepatic artery.*

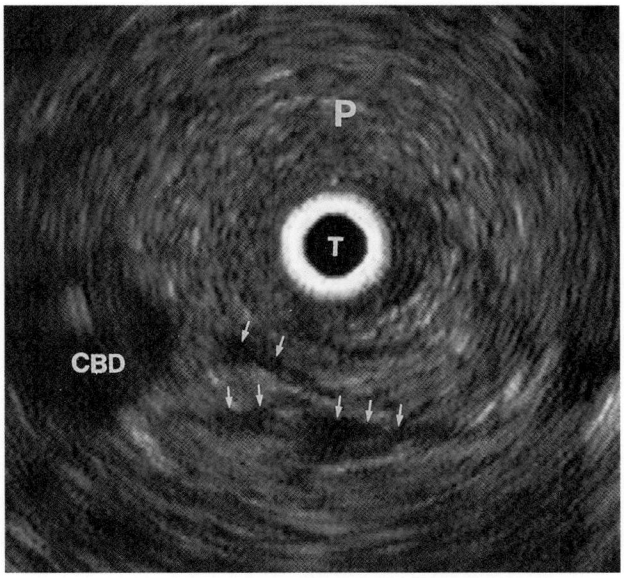

Figure 8.17 *The 20-MHz sonographic image obtained from within the pancreatic duct shows the uniform pancreatic parenchyma (P). The adjacent common bile duct (CBD) and branches of pancreatic ducts (arrows) are also seen. T, transducer.*

pancreatic parenchyma in chronic pancreatitis revealed a slightly inhomogeneous echopoor layer with a fine reticular pattern.[20,44]

Yasuda performed intraductal scanning in 141 patients. The procedures were performed to assess the extent of tumor and the nature of the cystic lesions and to evaluate the degree of ductal and parenchymal changes in chronic pancreatitis.[13] Intraductal scanning in the biliary tract is not difficult. Determination of the extent of biliary tumor is the primary indication. Eighteen lesions were examined by intraductal miniprobe scanning. Tumor invasion and lymph node status were assessed according to the TNM classification. The accuracy rates for assessment of T stage by the miniprobe were 70% (EUS, 70%) in cancer of the papilla of Vater, and 83% (EUS, 75%) in carcinoma of the extrahepatic bile duct. The sensitivity and specificity of N staging (lymph node metastasis) by the miniprobe were 57% and 82%, respectively. These results suggest that the additional examination of these tumors with the miniprobe increases the accuracy of TNM staging.[13]

We have used a 6.2 Fr, 200-cm catheter housing a 20-MHz ultrasound transducer to evaluate the human

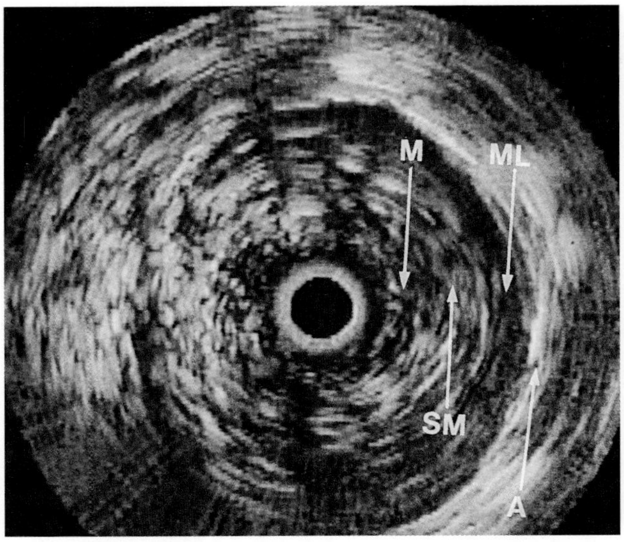

Figure 8.18 *The 20-MHz sonographic image of the sphincter of Oddi while the ultrasound catheter is within the common bile duct. The hypoechoic bands represent the muscle layers (ML) of the sphincter of Oddi. M, mucosa; SM, submucosa, A, adventitia.*

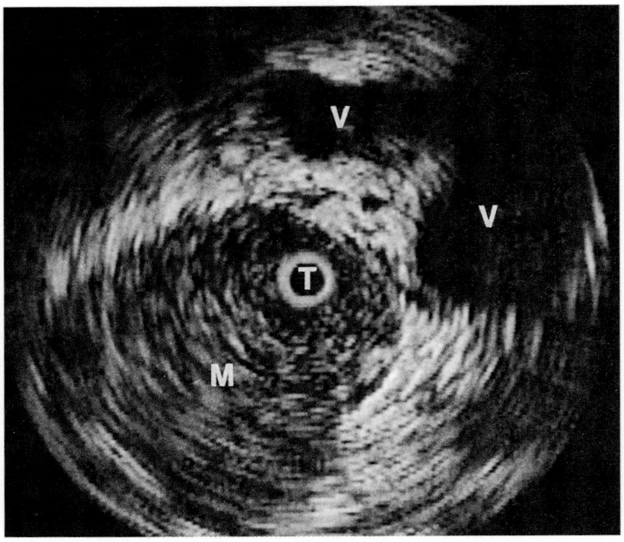

Figure 8.19 *A tumor in the area of the sphincter of Oddi is seen as a hypoechoic mass (M) surrounding the 20-MHz ultrasound transducer (T). The individual layers of the sphincter of Oddi are no longer identified. V, vessel.*

sphincter of Oddi during ERCP. This transducer is small and flexible enough to pass through the biopsy channel of a 34 Fr side-viewing ERCP endoscope and, over a guidewire, be passed high into the common bile duct through the ampulla. The sphincter of Oddi was found to consist of two hypoechoic layers separated by a thin hyperechoic layer (Fig. 8.18). Correlation of HRES with the histologic sections taken during an autopsy demonstrated that the inner hypoechoic layer corresponded to the circular smooth muscle, the outer hypoechoic layer to the longitudinal smooth muscle, and the hyperechoic layer between the two muscle layers to an intermuscular connective tissue component. The circular smooth muscle was significantly thicker than the longitudinal smooth muscle in the sphincter of Oddi.

Though the sphincter of Oddi has been imaged with lower-frequency dedicated echoendoscopies, it had not previously been possible to do detailed imaging of its individual muscle layers. As biliary manometry is the only other dynamic noninvasive means of evaluating the sphincter of Oddi, HRES may ultimately be used to evaluate patients with biliary dyskinesia (sphincter of Oddi dysfunction), ampullitis, papillary stenosis or tumor of Oddi's sphincter (Fig 8.19).

Cushing et al used a different catheter-based ultrasound transducer with an outside diameter of 1.6–2.6 mm to evaluate the biliary and pancreatic ductal system in two patients undergoing ERCP.[45] The transducer contained a fixed ceramic piezoelectric crystal, a center frequency in the range of 20–30 MHz, and a high-speed rotating mirror that produced a cross-sectional image orthogonal to the catheter axis. The catheters were 2.2 mm in diameter and 190 cm long. The catheter was passed to the hepatic duct bifurcation and beyond into the intrahepatic ducts under fluoroscopic guidance. In one patient the catheter was passed into the distal pancreatic duct to the point where a large stone obstructed the lumen. Imaging of the extrahepatic bile ducts revealed an inner hyperechoic layer and a second discontinuous hypoechoic layer. Comparison with histologic sections suggested that this second layer might represent discontinuous bands of smooth muscle.

Surrounding connective tissue appeared to create bright echoes and a third ultrasound layer. Structures deep to the bile duct wall, including the pancreas, cystic duct, and near the edge of the gallbladder, could also be seen. HRES penetration was nearly 1 cm with the 30-MHz transducer and up to 2 cm with the 20-MHz catheter.[46] In the first patient, HRES also revealed a distal common bile duct stricture, seen as a hyperechoic intraluminal filling defect. The HRES cross-section demonstrated an irregular border of the histologically benign stricture and eccentric encroachment of the lumen, not evident on concurrent cholangiography. The stricture could be clearly seen to be confined to the duct wall without apparent invasion into surrounding tissue structures.[45]

Using 15–20-MHz ultrasound probes inserted into the bile duct during percutaneous transhepatic biliary drainage and cholangioscopy, Tamada et al preoperatively staged extrahepatic bile duct cancers and compared the diagnostic accuracy of intraductal HRES with that of conventional transabdominal ultrasound, CT, angiography, ERCP and standard EUS.[46] In the study, CT did not demonstrate the tumor adequately, and transabdominal ultrasound detected middle and inferior bile duct cancers in only 57% of cases because of interference from bowel gas. Angiography was able to assess tumor invasion of the portal vein or hepatic artery but could not adequately assess less advanced cancers. EUS successfully assessed serosal and portal vein invasion and epicholedochal lymph node metastases but could not adequately evaluate tumor located at the hepatic hilum. In comparison, intra-bile duct HRES was very sensitive in assessing the hepatic hilum and for portal vein and right hepatic artery invasion. Diagnosis of right hepatic artery invasion is very important in planning therapeutic treatment of cancer of the hepatic hilum. HRES, however, could not assess tumor invasion of the SMV or hepatic artery or vessel invasion outside the hepatoduodenal ligament because of echo attenuation, and was only partially successful in detecting lymph node metastases. HRES was very sensitive, however, in detecting pancreatic parenchymal invasion, the presence of which is important in deciding between a pancreatoduodenectomy with or one without an attempt at curative bile duct resection. The investigators felt that HRES was proven to be essential in the preoperative staging of extrahepatic bile duct cancer when used in conjunction with other diagnostic modalities, like angiography.[46]

HRES probes have also been used to demonstrate the presence and extent of cholangiocarcinoma and to evaluate the effectiveness of biliary stents (Figs 8.20–8.22). Elfant et al have used HRES probes in evaluating biliary strictures with regard to their benign or malignant nature.[47] A blinded investigator noted irregular/ulcerated mucosa in seven of seven patients with histologically proven malignant strictures and in none of two with benign strictures. Abnormal lymph nodes were noted in five of seven malignant strictures and in one of two benign ones. Common bile duct stones were characterized by typical acoustic shadowing (Fig. 8.23). Malignant strictures were correctly identified in eight of nine patients. The presence of irregular/ulcerated mucosa was the most predictive indicator of malignant disease.[47]

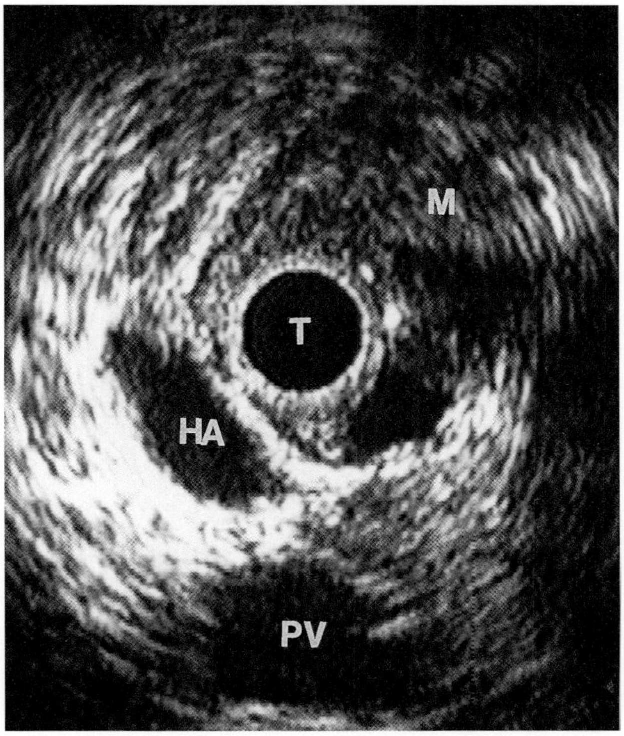

Figure 8.20 *A malignant structure is seen as a hypoechoic mass (M) within the bile duct. The normal portion of the bile duct can still be appreciated by its hyperechoic borders from 4 to 11 o'clock. HA, hepatic artery; PV, portal vein. T, transducer.*

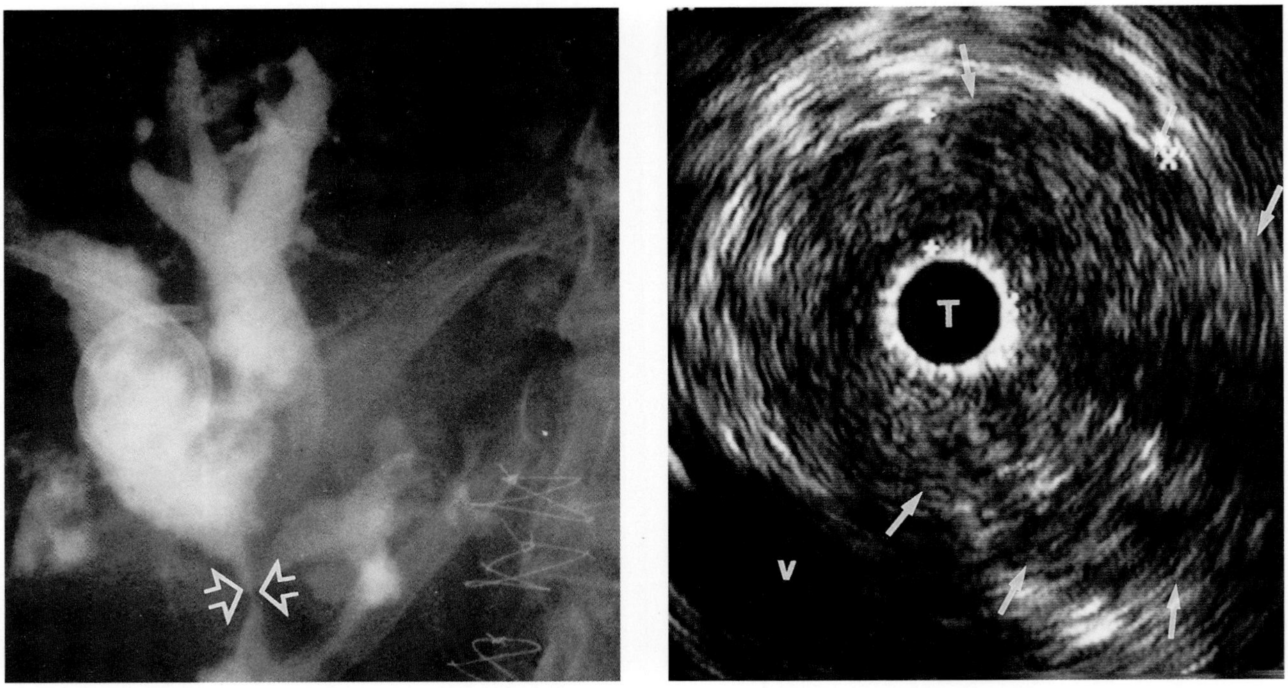

a *b*

Figure 8.21 *(a) In a patient with jaundice and fever, the cholangiogram shows partial obstruction of the biliary tract (arrows). (b) A large hypoechoic mass (arrows) within the common bile duct is seen compatible with cholangiocarcinoma. V, vessel; T, transducer.*

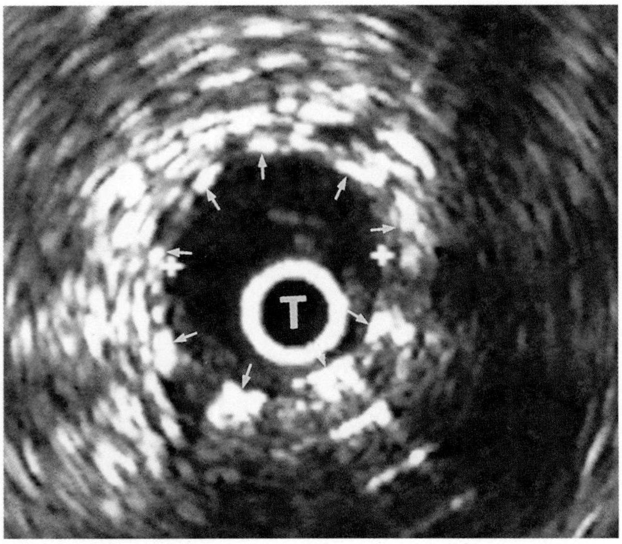

Figure 8.22 *The catheter transducer (T) is seen within the common bile duct surrounded by a metallic stent. The wires of the metallic stent appear as a hyperechoic (arrows) pattern with reverberation artifact.*

The most common abnormality of the common bile duct that can be delineated by HRES is wall thickening and mass effects that are due to either primary cholangiocarcinoma or extrinsic tumor involving adjacent structures, such as the liver, pancreas, or lymph nodes. Limited penetration of the ultrasound beam precludes adequate staging of cancer, however, and complementary diagnostic modalities, like ERCP, are almost always necessary when other noninvasive testing does not provide adequate delineation of a bile duct process.[20] HRES probes may provide additional information in the work-up of these patients.

Furukawa et al used a somewhat higher-frequency HRES probe (30 MHz) inserted via the papilla into the main pancreatic duct in 20 patients with pancreatic cancer.[48] Owing to its high frequency, the probe only allowed visualization of the ductal wall and the immediate periductal area. In 15 of 20 patients the tumors were surgically resected and similar HRES imaging was performed in vitro on the resection specimens. Of these 15 patients, 13 were found to have

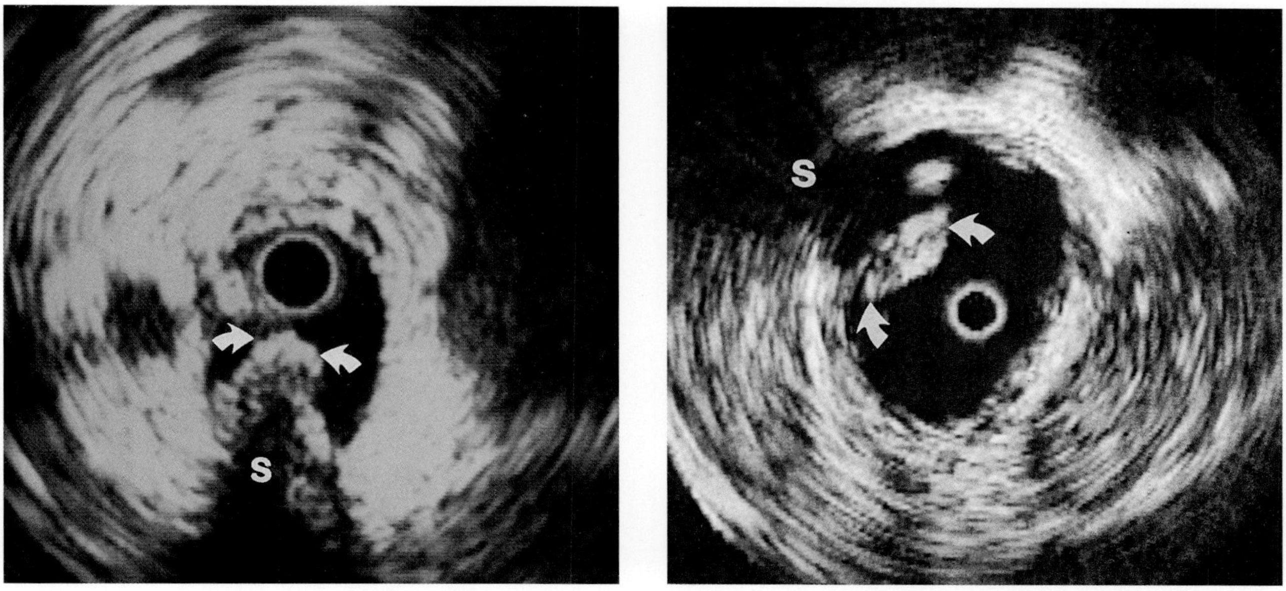

a *b*

Figure 8.23 *(a,b) In different cases, intraductal ultrasound identified stones (arrows) in the common bile duct as hyperechoic structures with typical acoustic shadowing (S).*

ductal adenocarcinomas, with all but one being successfully diagnosed by transabdominal ultrasound, CT, ERCP or standard EUS. HRES imaging demonstrated an echorich area (corresponding to neoplastic canaliculi on histopathologic examination) surrounded by an echopoor area (abundant stroma). In two patients found to have intraductal papillary carcinomas in whom a conclusive diagnosis was not established by conventional modalities, HRES demonstrated tumor with an inhomogeneous echo pattern within or outside the pancreatic duct.[22,48] Thus, HRES may be used to complement transabdominal ultrasound, CT, ERCP and 7–12-MHz EUS in differentiating intraductal papillary carcinomas from pancreatic adenocarcinomas, which is especially important as the former usually carry a much more favorable prognosis.

Similar HRES probes have also been used to visualize the pancreatic duct at the time of surgery. They can be inserted either through the ampulla of Vater by opening the duodenum or by direct insertion into the surgically exposed pancreatic duct. This approach may prove useful in assessing the extent of a pancreatic neoplasm that is to be resected (Fig. 8.24). In addition to evaluating tumors, HRES has also been used to demonstrate the presence of calcification in patients with chronic pancreatitis and in identifying pancreatic duct stones (Fig. 8.25).[20,49]

Kuroiwa et al have evaluated intraductal ultrasound for preoperative diagnosis of bile duct carcinoma in 42 cases. The depth of invasion of the bile duct carcinoma was diagnosed with a 93% accuracy rate. The tumor infiltration into the surrounding organs was clearly visualized by intraductal ultrasound, with an accuracy of 100% in the right hepatic artery, 93% in the portal vein, and 93% in the pancreas. However, the accuracy rates for CT were 60%, 67%, and 80%, and for angiography were 87%, 80% and 88%. The authors feel that intraductal ultrasound should be further studied as a diagnostic modality for staging malignancy in the biliary field.[50]

Van Sonnenberg et al have used this technology to evaluate the gallbladder and bile ducts in 22 patients with gallstone disease, bile duct malignancies and strictures.[51] Studies were performed via percutaneous

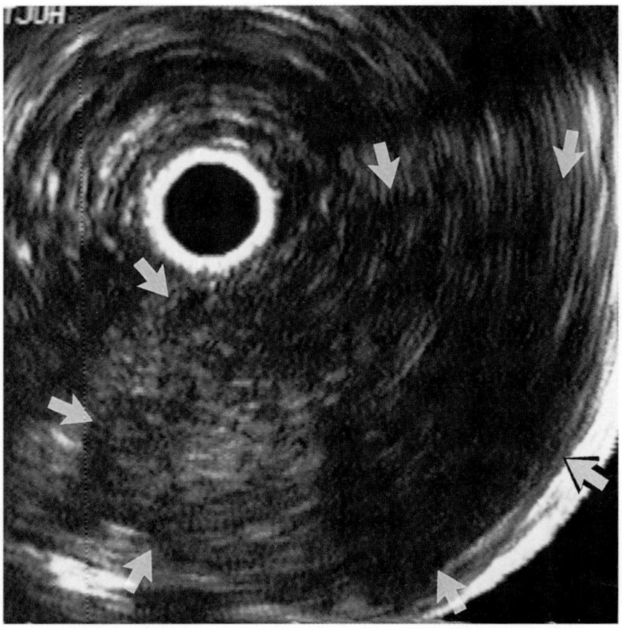

a

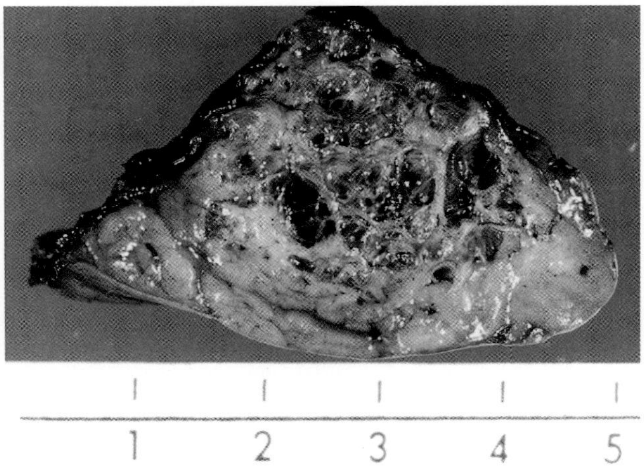

b

Figure 8.24 *(a) The ultrasound catheter located within the pancreatic duct. A pancreatic neoplasm is imaged as a complex mass with multiple septations extending from the 3 o'clock to the 8 o'clock position. (b) The ultrasound findings correlate with the pathologic diagnosis of microcystic adenocarcinoma.*

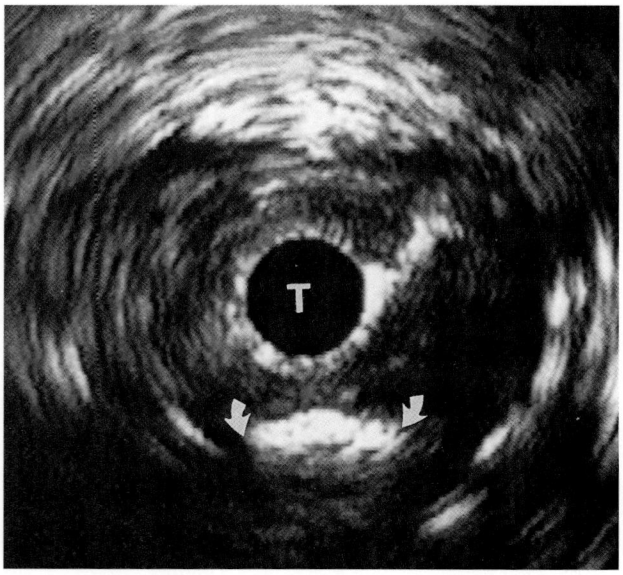

Figure 8.25 *The catheter transducer (T) within the pancreatic duct in a patient with chronic pancreatitis. The pancreatic parenchyma appears as a heterogeneous pattern. A stone (arrows) within the pancreatic duct is seen at the 6 o'clock position and appears as a hyperechoic area.*

radiographic tracts and via laparoscopy in an additional four patients. These percutaneous tracts had been previously created to treat stones, tumors or strictures. Patients were undergoing solvent dissolution of gallstones, percutaneous gallstone extraction and percutaneous drainage proximal to an obstruction.

The technique is straightforward, once typical access to the gallbladder or bile ducts is established. A rotating radial 20-MHz transducer at the terminus of a metallic shaft and housed and bathed in saline for acoustic coupling is utilized. The shaft is inserted into a 6 Fr guiding catheter with the capability to be inserted over a guidewire. The depth of penetration of the ultrasound beam is approximately 2 cm. An 8 Fr or larger sheath is inserted over a guidewire through the percutaneous tract into the bile duct or gallbladder. A safety guidewire is also placed to maintain access. The ultrasound catheter is inserted, with its position monitored by both ultrasound and periodic fluoroscopy after injection of contrast. At the time of laparoscopic cholecystectomy, the percutaneous catheter and transducer can be inserted through a trocar and positioned within the cystic duct through a small slit and maneuvered into the bile duct under visual laparoscopic guidance. Significant speckled artifact and loss of contrast may be a problem because of electrical devices in close proximity, such as cautery instruments. Studies usually last 15–20 min.[51]

Stones were visualized in the gallbladder, intra- and extrahepatic bile ducts and cystic duct. Debris was observed in the bile ducts, the gallbladder and cystic duct and within a metallic stent. Tumor was visualized in the intra- and extrahepatic ducts, but adjacent lymph nodes could not be identified with certainty. Portal vein branches and the hepatic artery were noted in their characteristic location. Wall thickening was seen with sclerosing cholangitis and benign strictures. Stones appeared as highly echogenic foci with radial acoustic shadowing. Debris (sludge) was noted as moderately echogenic material without posterior shadowing. Evaluation of metallic biliary stents demonstrated a circumferential echogenicity; one stent was seen to be flattened and distorted by an adjacent periductal tumor.[51]

Compared with fluoroscopy after injection of contrast material, percutaneously introduced HRES offered the following additional information: gallbladder wall thickening, differentiation of stone from debris or clot within a metallic stent, presence of cystic duct stones when the duct was not seen fluoroscopically, and demonstration and differentiation of stones in the common bile duct from debris and air bubbles at laparoscopic cholecystectomy.[51] Similar findings can be expected with the future use of longer HRES probes advanced through the sphincter of Oddi into the biliary system at the time of ERCP.

NEW TECHNIQUES

Although EUS provides detailed imaging of the biliary tract, histology and tissue sampling is still required to confirm the diagnosis. Sampling of subepithelial lesions and extrinsic masses is now possible with use of the Pentax FG-32UA probe in conjunction with a flexible small-gauge biopsy needle.[52] After localization of the area to be biopsied with the Pentax system, a fine needle aspiration catheter is advanced into it under EUS visualization. The curvilinear arrangement of the transducer scan plane and biopsy channel permits continuous imaging of the needle, which is not possible with radially scanning probes.[53] The maximum penetration depth depends on needle length (up to 35 mm).

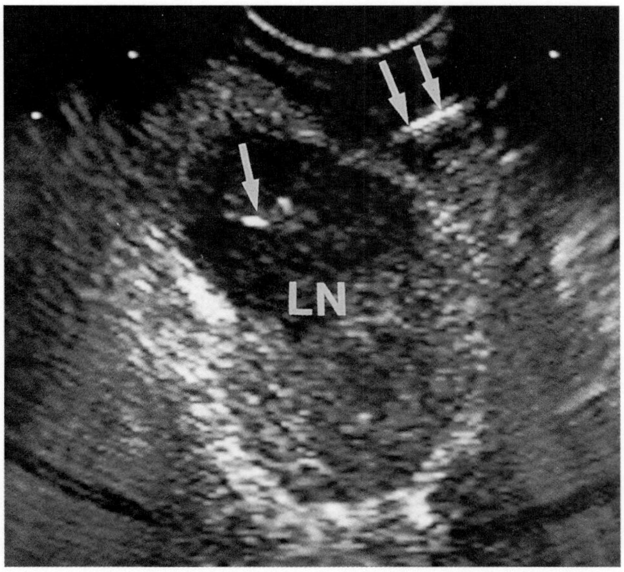

Figure 8.26 *This is a large, hyperechoic perigastric lymph node (LN) being biopsied through the Pentax ultrasound scope. The biopsy needle is seen as a hyperechoic reflection (arrows) just outside and within the hypoechoic node.*

This improvement in diagnostic sensitivity is offset by the invasive nature of the procedure; the requirement for sedation during EGD may make it less attractive than percutaneous techniques in certain patients.[52] However, as more experience is gained with the technique of EUS-guided biopsy, it may ultimately play as important a role as laparoscopy or percutaneous biopsy in obtaining tissue for histologic diagnosis in certain neoplasms (Fig. 8.26). In addition, the new Pentax EUS system has both spectral and color Doppler capabilities, which is very useful in differentiating blood vessels from nonvascular structures (Fig. 8.27).

Wiersema et al[54] employed a Pentax FG32UA echoendoscope in conjunction with a 22- or 23-gauge 4-cm needle catheter to perform endosonographically directed cholangiopancreatography. The needle was advanced when the needle was identified within the common bile duct by endosonography, and contrast was injected. Fluoroscopy confirmed the

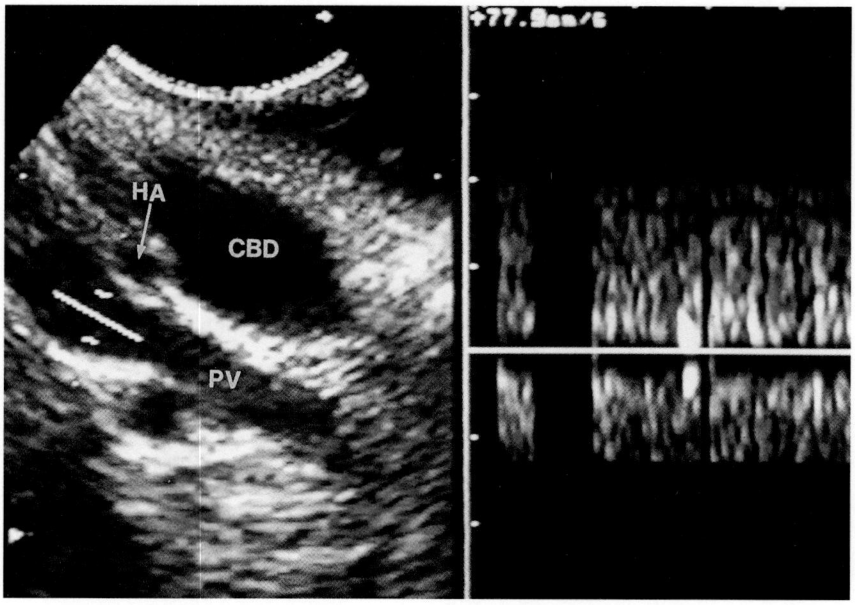

Figure 8.27 *The EUS image using the Pentax probe shows the structures of the porta hepatis with the spectral Doppler display of the flow information in the portal vein (PV). HA, hepatic artery; CBD, common bile duct.*

ductal nature of the injection. If adequate ductography was not achieved, the needle was repositioned slightly under ultrasound visualization. Of 205 patients undergoing ERCP, complete ductography was not possible in 11. This ultrasound system was employed to perform transduodenal cholangiography in 10 of the 11 patients and transgastric pancreatography in one of the patients. Successful ductography was possible in 8 of 11 patients. In five patients, abnormalities identified with endoscopically guided cholangiopancreatography led to repeat ERCP without precut sphincterotomy. In all of the cases, 100% agreement was found between endosonographically guided cholangiopancreatography and ERCP findings. They concluded that endosonographically guided cholangiopancreatography provides an alternative method for obtaining cholangiopancreatographs in those patients in whom ERCP is unsuccessful.[54]

For several years, real-time intraoperative ultrasound has been effectively used during surgery, to detect lesions too small to be visualized with other imaging modalities.[55] Conventional ultrasound probes, however, cannot be employed through the small puncture ports used during laparoscopic surgery. Liu et al have recently used a newly developed laparoscopic probe with color and spectral Doppler capabilities during laparoscopic surgery.[56] The semi-flexible ultrasound probe, which is 9.6 mm in diameter and 35 cm long, contains a multifrequency (5.0, 6.5 and 7.5 MHz) convex-array transducer with a maximum penetration of 13 cm and a sector scanning angle of 60°, allowing the imaging of structures deep within the liver or retroperitoneum. The transducer located on a flexible tip can pass through a 10-mm-diameter trocar.

In a study of 25 patients undergoing laparoscopy for abnormalities, this miniature ultrasound probe was able to delineate normal structures, such as blood vessels, allowing the surgeon the optimal approach for dissection. The color and spectral Doppler capabilities proved especially useful in differentiating vascular from nonvascular structures. The presence or absence of stones within the gallbladder and common bile duct was readily determined. It was possible to detect masses and to provide guidance for biopsy within abdominal viscera. In 10 cases, laparoscopic ultrasound imaging altered the planned surgical approach (i.e. identifying choledocholithiasis during laparoscopic cholecystectomy, not previously identified by transabdominal ultrasound). In many cases, the additional information provided by laparoscopic ultrasound could not have been obtained with conventional imaging techniques.

Other investigators have used laparoscopic ultrasound in the detection of small metastases not found by other conventional imaging techniques,[57] and in guiding percutaneous liver biopsy.[58] In the future, it may be used to image areas not readily reached by an EUS beam, like the right lobe of the liver. As more experience is gained with the use of these probes, they will probably be used during other diagnostic procedures, allowing for even greater diagnostic capabilities with less invasive procedures.[59]

CONCLUSION

HRES has to date found utility in the diagnosis and staging of certain biliary neoplasms and in the evaluation of bile duct strictures and pancreaticobiliary ductal lithiasis. The use of longer HRES probes will make it possible to image any part of the intrahepatic ductal system and even the cystic duct and gallbladder. This technology may ultimately find a role in detecting choledocholithiasis when both EUS and cholangiography are equivocal. HRES may also prove invaluable in evaluating biliary stents; for instance, to discern whether a stent occlusion is secondary to debris or to tumor ingrowth. Further technical developments may allow these miniature probes to image at lower frequencies, giving them both the ability to be placed in usually inaccessible places and greater imaging penetration, to better stage malignant processes. Intraoperative and/or laparoscopic use of similar HRES probes may also prove helpful in evaluating lesions for their malignant potential. HRES may prove invaluable when other more conventional imaging techniques cannot make a definitive diagnosis.

REFERENCES

1. Kimmey MB, Martin RW, Haggitt RC, Wang KY, Franklin DW, Silverstein FE, Histologic correlates of gastrointestinal ultrasound images, *Gastroenterology* 1989; **96**:433–41.
2. Lees WR, The pancreas: differential diagnosis and pancreatitis, *Gastrointest Endosc Clin North Am* 1992; **2**:657–71.
3. Rösch T, Classen M, *Gastroenterologic Endosonography* (Thieme Medical Publishers, Inc.: New York, 1992).
4. Napoleon B, Souquet JC, Pujol B, Ponchon T, Pancreas and ampulla of Vater. In: Dubbins PA, Joseph AEA, eds. *Ultrasound in Gastroenterology* (Churchill Livingstone: New York, 1994).
5. Snady H, Cooperman A, Siegel J, EUS compared with computed tomography with ERCP in patients with obstructive jaundice or small pancreatic mass, *Gastrointest Endosc* 1992; **38**:27–34.
6. Rösch T, Braig C, Gain T et al, Staging of pancreatic and ampullary carcinoma by endoscopic ultrasonography: comparison with conventional sonography, computed tomography and angiography, *Gastroenterology* 1992; **102**:188–99.
7. Kaufman AR, Sivak MV Jr, Endoscopic ultrasonography in the differential diagnosis of pancreatic disease, *Gastrointest Endosc* 1989; **35**:214–19.
8. Tio TL, Endosonography in diagnosing and staging of pancreatic and ampullary cancer, *Gastrointest Endosc Clin North Am* 1992; **2**:673–84.
9. Rösch T, Classen M, Preoperative localization of endoscopic tumors of the pancreas, *Gastrointest Endosc Clin North Am* 1992; **2**:685–96.
10. Yasuda K, Mukai H, Fujimoto S, Nakajima M, Kawai K, The diagnosis of pancreatic cancer by endoscopic ultrasonography, *Gastrointest Endosc* 1988; **34**:1–8.
11. Hayashi Y, Nakazawa S, Kimoto E, Naito Y, Morita K, Clinicopathological analysis of endoscopic ultrasonograms in pancreatic mass lesions, *Endoscopy* 1989; **21**:121–5.
12. Vilmann P, Jacobson GK, Henriksen FW, Hancke S, Endoscopic ultrasonography with guided fine needle aspiration biopsy in pancreatic disease. *Gastrointest Endosc* 1992; **38**:172–4.
13. Yasuda K, Ultrasonic probes for pancreaticobiliary strictures, *Gastrointest Endosc* 1996; **43**(2):S35–8.
14. Gress F, Savides T, Ikenberry S, Hawes R, Improved endoscopic ultrasound (EUS) criteria for determining vascular invasion (VI) and unresectability in pancreatic cancer (PCa), *Gastrointest Endosc* 1996; **43**(2):S56.
15. Brugge WR, Lee MJ, Warshaw AL, EUS methods for the staging of pancreatic cancer, *Gastrointest Endosc* 1996; **43**(2):S57.
16. Bhutani MS, Hawes RH, Baron PL, van Velse A, Sanders-Cliette A, Hoffman BJ, Utility of endoscopic ultrasound (EUS) guided fine needle aspiration (FNA) in the evaluation of pancreatic masses, *Gastrointest Endosc* 1996; **43**(2):S61.
17. Rösch T, Lightdale CJ, Botet JF et al, Endosonographic localization of pancreatic endocrine tumors, *N Engl J Med* 1992; **326**:1721–6.
18. Lightdale CJ, Botet JF, Woodruff JM, Brennan MF, Localization of endocrine tumors of the pancreas with endoscopic ultrasound, *Cancer* 1991; **68**:1815–20.
19. Zuccaro G Jr, Sivak MV Jr, Endoscopic ultrasonography in the diagnosis of chronic pancreatitis, *Endoscopy* 1992; **24**:347–9.
20. Liu JB, Miller LS, Goldberg BB, Endoluminal ultrasound in gastroenterology: application of new technology. In: Dubbins PA, Joseph AEA, eds. *Ultrasound in Gastroenterology* (Churchill Livingstone: New York, 1994).
21. Yasuda K, Mukai H, Cho E, Nakajima M, Kawai K, The use of endoscopic ultrasonography in the diagnosis and staging of carcinoma of the papilla of Vater, *Endoscopy* 1988; **20**:218–22.
22. Dancygier H, Endosonographic evaluation of biliary tract disease, *Gastrointest Endosc Clin North Am* 1992; **2**:697–713.

23. Yasuda K, Nakajima M, Kawai K, Technical aspects of endoscopic ultrasonography of the biliary system, *Scand J Gastroenterol* 1986; **21**(Suppl 123):143–50.
24. Tio TL, Cheng J, Wijers OB, Sars PRA, Tytgat GNJ, Endosonographic TNM staging of extrahepatic bile duct cancer: comparison with pathological staging, *Gastroenterology* 1991; **100**:1351–61.
25. Amouyal P, Amouyal G, Levy P et al, Diagnosis of choledocholithiasis by endoscopic ultrasonography, *Gastroenterology* 1994; **106**:1062–7.
26. Mitake M, Nakazawa S, Naitoh Y et al, Value of endoscopic ultrasonography in the detection of anomalous connections of the pancreatobiliary duct, *Endoscopy* 1991; **23**:117–20.
27. Bhutani M, Hoffman B, Hawer R, Tarnasky P, Cunningham J, Cotton P, Can endoscopic ultrasound (EUS) features of pancreatic duct (PD) predict removal at initial ERCP? *Gastrointest Endosc* 1995; **41**:A298.
28. Pasanen P, Partane K, Pikkarainen P et al, Ultrasonography, CT, and ERCP in the diagnosis of choledochal stones, *Acta Radiol* 1992; **33**:53–6.
29. Birkigt HG, Lossner C, Buhtz C, Winckelmann B, Preoperative ultrasonic of common bile stones and its importance to surgical management—result of a prospective controlled trial, *Acta Chir Hung* 1989; **30**:171–7.
30. Canto M, Endoscopic ultrasonography and gallstone disease, *Gastrointest Endosc* 1996; **43**(2):S37–47.
31. Amouyal P, Amouyal G, Levy P et al, Diagnosis of choledecholithiasis by endoscopic ultrasonography, *Gastroenterology* 1994; **106**:1062–67.
32. Sakai K, Nasu T, Tanabe Y et al, Evaluation of endoscopic ultrasound in the diagnosis of choledocholithiasis, *Gastroenterology* 1991; **100**:A388.
33. Edmundowicz SA, Aliperti G, Middleton WD, Preliminary experience using endoscopic ultrasonography in the diagnosis of choledocholithiasis, *Endoscopy* 1992; **24**:774–8.
34. Canto M, Chak A, Sivak MV et al, Endoscopic ultrasonography (EUS) versus cholangiography for diagnosing extrahepatic biliary stones: a prospective blinded study in pre- and post-cholecystectomy patients, *Gastrointest Endosc,* 1995; **41**:391.
35. Amouyal P, Amouyal G, Mompoint D et al, Endosonography: promising method for diagnosis of extrahepatic cholestasis, *Lancet* 1989; **ii**:1195–8.
36. Morita K, Nakazawa S, Kimoto E, Yamao K, Hayashi Y, Gallbladder diseases. In Kawai K, ed. *Endoscopic Ultrasonography in Gastroenterology* (Igaku-Shoin: New York, 1988).
37. Mitake M, Nakazawa S, Naitoh Y et al, Endoscopic ultrasonography in diagnosis of the extent of gallbladder carcinoma, *Gastrointest Endosc* 1990; **36**:562–6.
38. Dahan P, Amouyal P, Amouyal G et al, Is endoscopic ultrasonography (EUS) helpful in patients with suspicion of complicated gallstones and normal ultrasonography? *Gastroenterology* 1993; **104**:A358.
39. Dill J, Callis J, Hill S, Evans P, Combined endoscopic ultrasound and endoscopic Meltzer-Lyon testing in the diagnosis of cholelithiasis, *Am J Gastroenterol* 1994; **89**:956–7.
40. Dill J, Combined endoscopic ultrasound and stimulated biliary drainage in the diagnosis of cholecystitis and microlithiasis, *Endoscopy* 1995; **27**:218.
41. Amouyal G, Amouyal P, Levy P et al, Value of endoscopic ultrasonography in the diagnosis of idiopathic acute pancreatitis, *Gastroenterology* 1994; **106**:A283.
42. Shapiro MJ, Bonn J, Sullivan KL et al, Endoluminal biliary ultrasound: initial clinical experience, *J Vasc Intervent Radiol* 1991; **2**:11–12.
43. Goldberg BB, Liu JB, Merton DA et al, Sonographically guided laparoscopy and mediastinoscopy using miniature catheter-based transducers, *J Ultrasound Med* 1993; **12**:49–54.
44. Furukawa T, Naitoh Y, Tsukamoto Y et al, New technique using intraductal ultrasonography for the diagnosis of diseases of the pancreatobiliary system, *J Ultrasound Med* 1992; **11**:607–12.
45. Cushing GL, Fitzgerald PJ, Bommer WJ et al, Intraluminal ultrasonography during ERCP with high frequency ultrasound catheters, *Gastrointest Endosc* 1993; **39**:432–5.
46. Tamada K, Ido K, Ueno N, Kimura K, Ichiyama M, Tomiyama T, Preoperative staging of extrahepatic bile duct cancer with intraductal ultrasonography, *Am J Gastroenterol* 1995; **90**:239–46.
47. Elfant AB, Miller LS, Sarrazin J et al, Endoluminal ultrasonography (EU) for evaluation of biliary strictures: a single-blinded study, in press.
48. Furukawa T, Tsukamoto Y, Naitoh Y, Hirooka Y, Katoh T, Evaluation of intraductal ultrasonography in the diagnosis of pancreatic cancer, *Endoscopy* 1993; **25**:577–81.
49. Engstrom CF, Wiechel KL, Endoluminal ultrasound of the bile ducts, *Surg Endosc* 1990; **4**:187–90.
50. Kuroiwa M, Tsukamoto Y, Naitoh Y, Hirooka Y, Furukawa T, Katou T, New technique using intraductal ultrasonography for the diagnosis of bile duct cancer, *J Ultrasound Med* 1994; **13**:189–95.
51. van Sonnenberg E, D'Agostino HB, Sanchez RL et al, Percutaneous intraluminal US in the gallbladder and bile ducts, *Radiology* 1992; **182**:693–6.
52. Giovanni M, Seitz JF, Perrier H, Monges G, Endosonography-guided fine needle aspiration biopsy in submucosal and extrinsic tumors of the gastrointestinal tract. Preliminary results in 31 patients, *Gastroenterology* 1993; **104**:A405.
53. Tio TL, Sie LH, Tutgat GNJ, Endosonography and cytology in diagnosing and staging pancreatic body and tail carcinoma, *Dig Dis Sci* 1993; **38**:59–64.
54. Wiersema MJ, Sandusky D, Carr R, Wiersema LM, Erdel WC, Frederick PK, Endosonography-guided cholangiopancreatography, *Gastrointest Endosc* 1996; **43**:102–6.
55. Machi J, Sigel B. Overview of benefits of operative ultrasonography during a ten-year period, *J Ultrasound Med* 1989; **8**:547–52.
56. Liu JB, Feld RI, Goldberg BB et al, Laparoscopic gray-scale and color doppler US: preliminary animal and clinical studies, *Radiology* 1995; **194**:851–7.
57. Okita K, Kodama T, Oda M et al, Laparoscopic ultrasonography: diagnosis of liver and pancreatic cancer, *Scand J Gastroenterol* 1984; **19** (Suppl 94):91–100.
58. Fornari F, Civardi G, Cavanna L et al, Laparoscopic ultrasonography in the study of liver diseases, *Surg Endosc* 1989; **3**:33–7.
59. Goldberg BB, Liu JB, Merton DA et al, Sonography guided laparoscopy and mediastinoscopy using miniature catheter-based transducers, *J Ultrasound Med* 1993; **12**:49–54.

Chapter 9 Lungs and mediastinum

Robert M Steiner, Heinrich D Becker, Ji-Bin Liu and Barry B Goldberg

INTRODUCTION

Designed by Iketa in 1967, flexible video-assisted fiberoptic bronchoscopy is the procedure of choice for the direct investigation of the tracheobronchial tree.[1,2] Major indications for the use of fiberoptic bronchoscopy include examination for the underlying causes of hemoptysis, pneumonia, interstitial lung disease and atelectasis, and for the diagnosis of endobronchial neoplasm.[2–10]

Fiberoptic bronchoscopy is accurate for the diagnosis of central pulmonary neoplasms in 80–97% of patients.[7,8] On the other hand, the positive yield of fiberoptic bronchoscopy for the diagnosis of peripheral neoplasms lying beyond the tip of the bronchoscope may be as low as 33%. This is particularly true for small lesions under 2 cm in diameter.[6–8] The relatively low diagnostic yield in peripheral neoplasms occurs in spite of the use of C-arm or biplane fluoroscopic guidance during the procedure as well as the availability of pre-procedural chest radiographs and CT for lesion localization.[10–13] Because the endoscopist's field of view is restricted to the inner surface of the airways, the exact site of peripheral intraluminal and both peripheral and central extraluminal masses may not be evident.[9] As a result, fiberoptic bronchoscopy-guided needle and brush biopsies may not yield useful or diagnostic information.[10–14] If a pulmonary neoplasm or an involved lymph node outgrows its blood supply and is necrotic, or if there are large vascular structures in the region of the mass, a biopsy may also be unrewarding.

The major complications of bronchoscopy include bleeding (0.04–0.12%) and pneumothorax (1.8–2.9%).[3,7] Other complications of fiberoptic bronchoscopy are unusual. However, improvement in the visualization of the peribronchial structures means that biopsy of the normal lung, or necrotic areas within a tumor or surrounding vascular structures, may be avoided, and complications such as bleeding can be minimized. Ultrasound-assisted fiberoptic bronchoscopy was evaluated in our institutions because of these technical limitations of fiberoptic bronchoscopy and the likelihood that ultrasound could clearly visualize the extraluminal anatomy.[9]

The use of ultrasound for the diagnosis of thoracic disease is not new. For many years transthoracic ultrasound has been used for the diagnosis of lung, mediastinal, subpleural, pleural and soft-tissue masses.[15–21] A recently developed technique, transesophageal echocardiography, is useful not only for cardiovascular imaging but also for the definition of mediastinal lymph nodes and periesophageal masses.[22,23] Transesophageal echocardiography is also helpful in guiding fine needle aspiration biopsy in patients with mediastinal disease who cannot undergo biopsy under fluoroscopy or with CT guidance.[24]

Endoluminal ultrasound examination of the esophagus using high-frequency catheter-based transducers is a promising imaging technique for the study of esophageal pathology, including scleroderma, varices, achalasia, esophagitis and tumor, and for the characterization of surrounding lymph nodes.[25–28] The genitourinary tract, the biliary system and now the tracheobronchial tree have also been studied with similar catheter-based transducers.[29–36]

Hürter and Hanrath first described the use of catheter-based ultrasound transducers in 1990 for the examination of the tracheobronchial tree during bronchoscopy.[33,34] In 1991, Goldberg, Steiner and Liu began a collaborative project with members of the Thomas Jefferson University Hospital's (TJUH) Division of Pulmonary Medicine and Critical Care to assess the role of ultrasound guidance during routine fiberoptic bronchoscopy for central, and then later peripheral, lesions.[36] Since this study began, 50 patients with central and/or peripheral neoplasms have been examined.[9] More recently, Becker, Ono and others described their experience with the use of ultrasound-guided bronchoscopy for both diagnosis and treatment.[32,37–39]

In this chapter we discuss our experience with transbronchoscopic, transmediastinoscopic and transthoracoscopic ultrasound. We also speculate on future enhancements needed to optimize these techniques.

TRANSBRONCHOSCOPIC ULTRASOUND

TECHNICAL CONSIDERATIONS

At TJUH, video-assisted fiberoptic bronchoscopy is performed using a 60-cm-long bronchoscope designed by the Pentax Precision Instruments Corporation (Orangeburg, New York). This instrument has an external diameter of 4.9 mm and a biopsy channel of 2.3 mm. The biopsy port or working channel accepts a flexible 6.2 Fr (2.2 mm in diameter) catheter, 95 cm in length, integrated with a single-element rotating ultrasound transducer (Sonicath, Medi-Tech, Boston Scientific Corp., Natick, MA) (Fig. 9.1). It has a frequency of either 20 MHz or 12.5 MHz. The transducer is connected to an ultrasound machine (IVUS, Diasonics, Santa Clara, CA). The ultrasound motor rotates 360° at 10° off right angles to the long axis of the catheter, producing a real-time cross-sectional image with a radius of 20 mm and an axial resolution of 0.1 mm. Sterile water (0.5–1.0 ml) is injected into the chamber between the transducer and the catheter to eliminate air which may interfere with ultrasound transmission (Fig 9.2). After exclusion of air from the catheter system, the miniature transducer-containing catheter

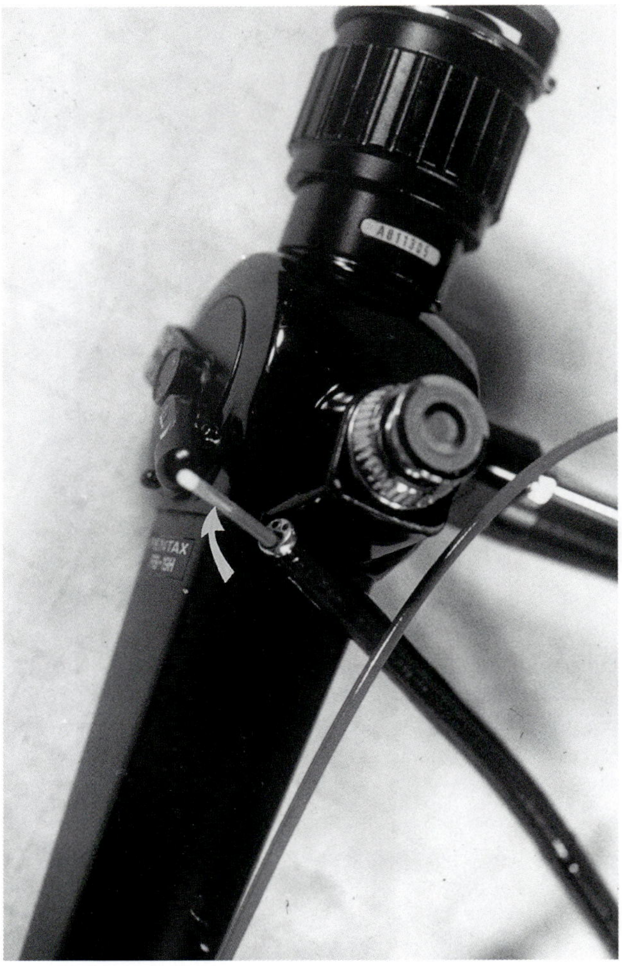

Figure 9.1 *The catheter-based ultrasound transducer (arrow) is passed through the working channel of the fiberoptic bronchoscope.*

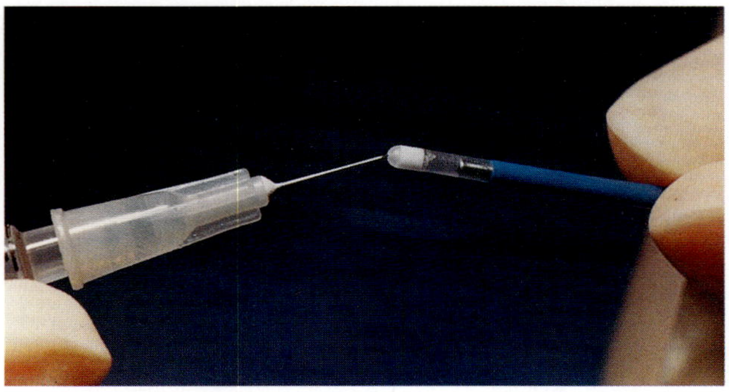

Figure 9.2 *The miniaturized ultrasound transducer is mounted on the tip of a wire core housed in a 6.2 Fr (2.2 mm) catheter. Preparation of the catheter transducer requires introduction of 0.5–1.0 ml of sterile water using a 27-gauge needle into the reservoir at the sealed tip of the catheter to eliminate air around the transducer. (Reproduced with permission from Liu et al.[25]).*

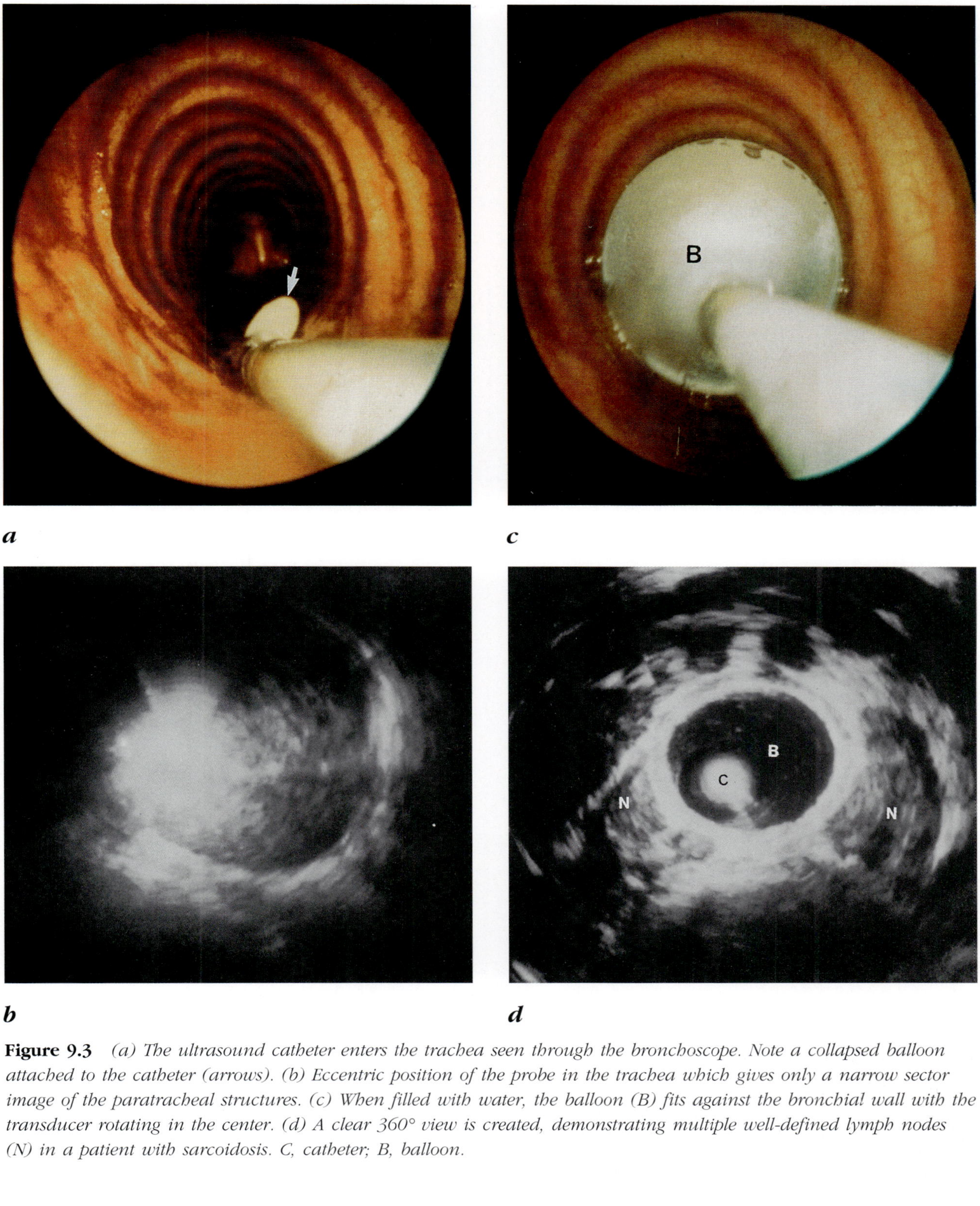

Figure 9.3 *(a) The ultrasound catheter enters the trachea seen through the bronchoscope. Note a collapsed balloon attached to the catheter (arrows). (b) Eccentric position of the probe in the trachea which gives only a narrow sector image of the paratracheal structures. (c) When filled with water, the balloon (B) fits against the bronchial wall with the transducer rotating in the center. (d) A clear 360° view is created, demonstrating multiple well-defined lymph nodes (N) in a patient with sarcoidosis. C, catheter; B, balloon.*

is inserted into a cup filled with water to test the quality of the ultrasound image.

Another approach to the application of ultrasound for imaging of the tracheobronchial tree is the use of a dedicated ultrasound-fitted bronchoscope with a maximum diameter of 6.3 mm and with a curvilinear transducer on one side of the bronchoscope tip.[32] Becker tested several intravascular ultrasound–catheter systems for their applicability and found the Olympus ultrasound probe and the Sonotron® CVIS instrument to be most suitable. Both include an ultrasound processor and miniaturized probes with single element transducers at the tips of the probes.

The Olympus ultrasound probe has an outer diameter of 2 mm, a single-element 20 MHz transducer rotating 360° at 400 rev/min, and a metallic guidance sheath. For improved contact and 360° of visualization the probe is equipped with a plastic introducer sheath with a balloon at its tip. Without the sheath, it can be passed through the instrument channel of a flexible bronchoscope. If the catheter probe with the introducer sheath in place is used, it is advisable to use a rigid large caliber bronchoscope or a dual channel fibroscope.[32]

A newer version of the CVIS ultrasound catheter has an outer diameter of 8 Fr (12 MHz) or 10 Fr (20 MHz), an axial resolution of 0.12 mm, and a lateral resolution of 0.23 mm. This catheter system can be introduced into a fiberoptic endoscope with a working channel 2.8 mm in diameter (Fig. 9.3). To date, it has not been possible to equip the CVIS catheter probe with a suitable balloon system.

At TJUH, the CT examination is performed with a third-generation 9800 Quick scanner (GE Medical Systems, Milwaukee, Wisconsin) or with a spiral GE scanner with or without contrast enhancement. CT scans 5–10 mm thick are performed through the chest and upper abdomen from the apex to the adrenal glands. Additional 5-mm-thick scans are performed through the hila, and 1-mm high-resolution thin-cut scans are performed at predesignated levels throughout the chest.

After review of the pre-procedure radiographic images, the fiberoptic bronchoscope is inserted into the tracheobronchial tree and passed to the bronchial branch of interest under fluoroscopic control and/or direct vision through the fiberoptic bronchoscope. The transducer-containing catheter is then advanced through the working channel of the bronchoscope to a position beyond the end of the instrument. The tip of the catheter is monitored with the C-arm portable fluoroscope (Fig. 9.4). The side of the distal end of the catheter containing the rotating transducer is placed against the tracheobronchial mucosa in the region of the suspected abnormality (Fig. 9.5). In most cases, bronchial secretions are sufficient to produce acoustic coupling and transmit the ultrasound beam into the adjacent tracheal or bronchial tissues. However, as acoustic coupling between the wall of the airway and the probe occurs only in the

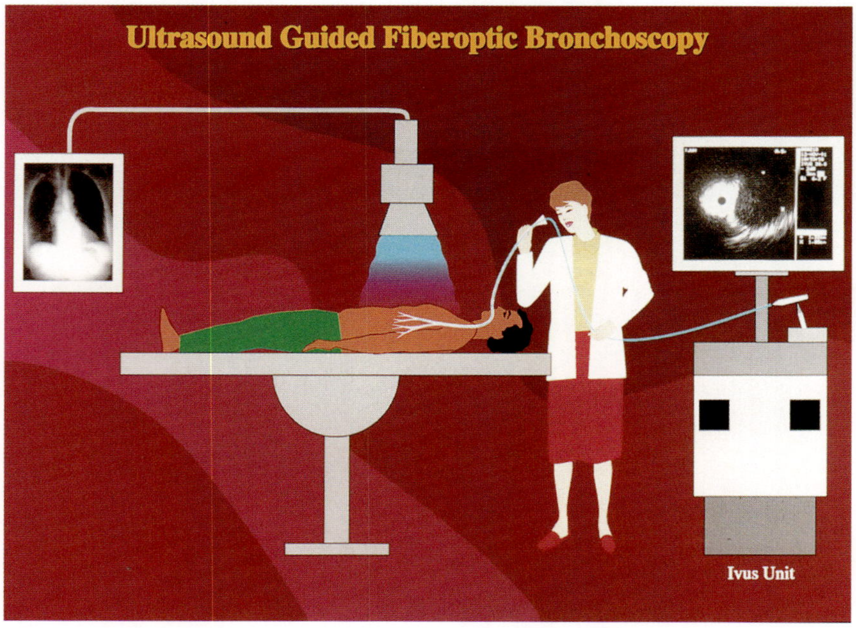

Figure 9.4 *An illustration of the procedure shows real-time viewing of the ultrasound image with fluoroscopic monitoring.*

area of direct contact, a limited imaging sector is produced in a large-diameter airway.

When the lesion in question is in the periphery of the lung, well beyond the tip of the fiberoptic bronchoscope, an ultrasound catheter without a balloon can be passed into a bronchial segment within or adjacent to the peripheral mass with the aid of fluoroscopy. In the periphery of the lung a full 360° image can be obtained because of the similarity in size of the outer diameter of the catheter to the inner diameter of the 3rd- to 5th-order bronchi. In the trachea and proximal bronchi, only a wedge of information can be obtained, limited to the region where the balloon-free catheter is in direct contact with the tracheobronchial mucosa.

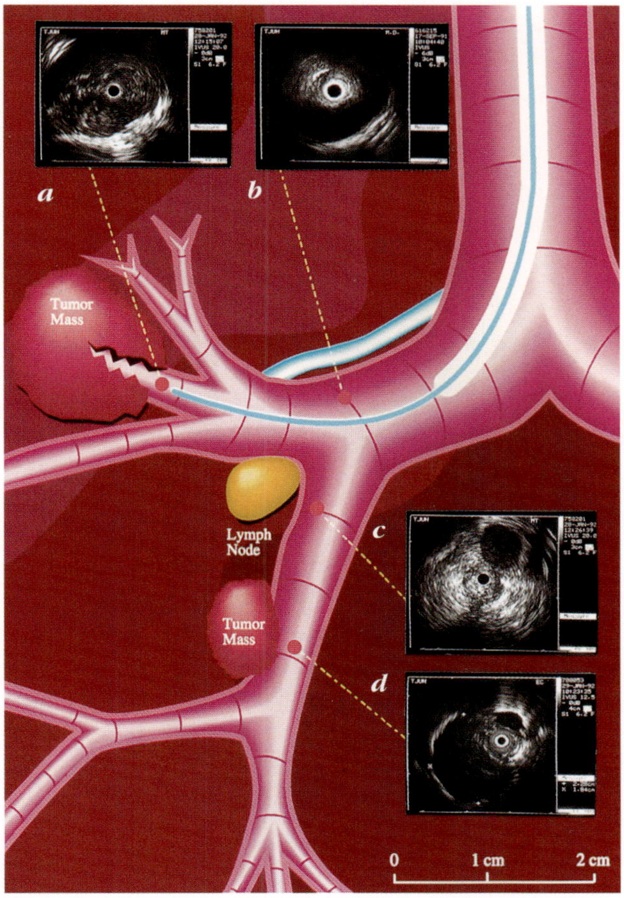

Figure 9.5 *Schematic demonstration of the catheter-based transducer in the right bronchus with four ultrasound images illustrating: (a) a large vessel adjacent to the right main stem bronchus; (b) Neoplasm surrounding an encased bronchial lumen; (c) a well-defined lymph node at the bifurcation of the right upper lobe bronchus and the bronchus intermedius; (d) eccentric tumor mass adjacent to the bronchial lumen.*

When a single-channel fiberoptic bronchoscope is used and the exact site for biopsy is determined, the ultrasound catheter is removed and the biopsy or brush instrument is introduced to the fiberoptic bronchoscope and passed to the same location where the ultrasound catheter was placed. Because localizing information may be lost when the catheters are exchanged, it is helpful instead to use a dual-channel fiberoptic bronchoscope to place both the biopsy instrument and the ultrasound catheter into the same location simultaneously (Fig 9.6). In this way a transbronchial biopsy will be obtained with the confidence that the tissue is from the same site visualized by ultrasound.

The ultrasound images can be viewed in several formats. These include real-time viewing on the IVUS monitor, and review of individual freeze-frame images stored in the digital imaging disk system (3M Medical Imaging Systems, St Louis, MO) or recorded on videotape for later review.

SONOGRAPHIC ANATOMY OF THE THORAX

Tracheobronchial Tree

With a high-resolution imaging system, a three-layered sonographic image of the trachea and main stem bronchus is produced in vivo, consisting of a hyperechoic mucosa/submucosa, a hypoechoic muscularis and a hyperechoic adventitia (Fig 9.7).[32,37] Resected tracheal specimens studied by Becker produced a sonographic pattern of two double-layer rings. Each ring is composed of tissue of low echogenicity underlying an echodense superficial mucosa on the inner side and an echodense adventitia on the external side of the tracheal wall. These two double-layer rings cover a three-layered central slab of tissue composed of two echodense layers separated by an echo-poor central ring.

On examination of tracheal cartilage devoid of its mucosal and adventitial covering, only the central three-layered slab of tissue was seen. Since the tracheal cartilage has the same appearance as the inter-cartilagenous connective tissue in vivo, it is apparent that cartilage cannot be differentiated from non-cartilagenous tissue by this ultrasound method.[32,37]

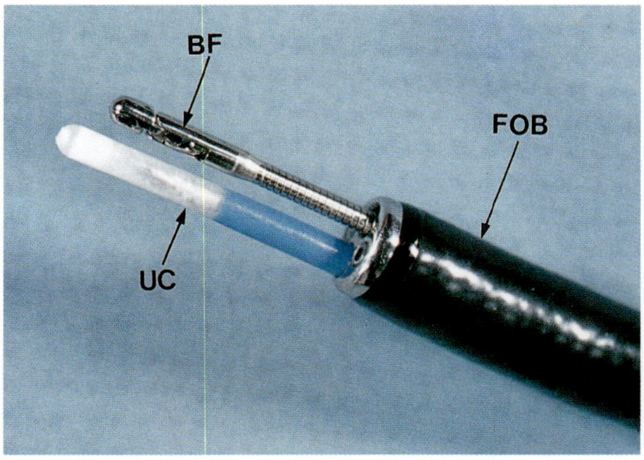

a

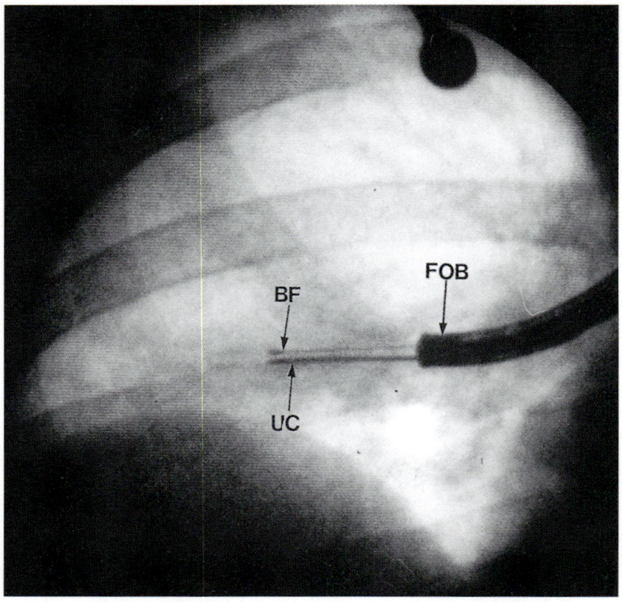

b

Figure 9.6 *(a) The biopsy forceps (BF) and ultrasound catheter (UC) lie beyond the tip of a dual-channel fiberoptic bronchoscope (FOB). (b) A fluoroscopic image shows both the ultrasound catheter (UC) and a bronchoscopic biopsy forceps (BF) in the right middle lobe bronchus beyond the tip of a dual-channel fiberoptic bronchoscope (FOB).*

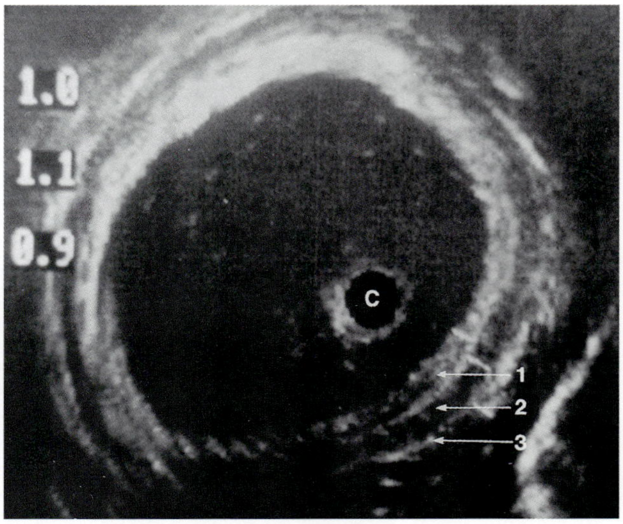

Figure 9.7 *The three major layers of the bronchial wall are demonstrated in this in vivo ultrasound image. The echo-rich mucosa and submucosa (1), the hypoechoic muscularis (2) and the hyperechoic adventitia (3) are demonstrated. C, ultrasound catheter.*

The echotexture of normal lung is generally different from that of abnormal structures. The normal air-filled lung presents as a dense pattern of reflections due to a multitude of air–soft-tissue interfaces. On the other hand, tumors and lymph nodes exhibit hypo- or mixed echogenicity and may be separated from normal structures by a well-defined interface (Fig. 9.8). When the tracheal or bronchial wall is invaded, the normal multi-layered circular pattern of the wall is lost.[32,37] In cases of complete airway occlusion by tumor, it may be possible to image the distal edge of the endoluminal mass and identify a patent airway distal to the mass. Potentially, this could be helpful in planning palliative interventional procedures such as laser therapy.[40]

Mediastinum

The correlative anatomy of the mediastinum imaged with ultrasound is difficult to appreciate, especially when compared with CT, because of the unique oblique planes created by the variable orientation of the ultrasound beam and by respiratory and cardiac motion artifact. Within these imaging planes, hilar and mediastinal vascular structures may be identified by their low amount of echogenic flow information and characteristic pulsations.[41] Even with the addition of echographic contrast media, separation of the

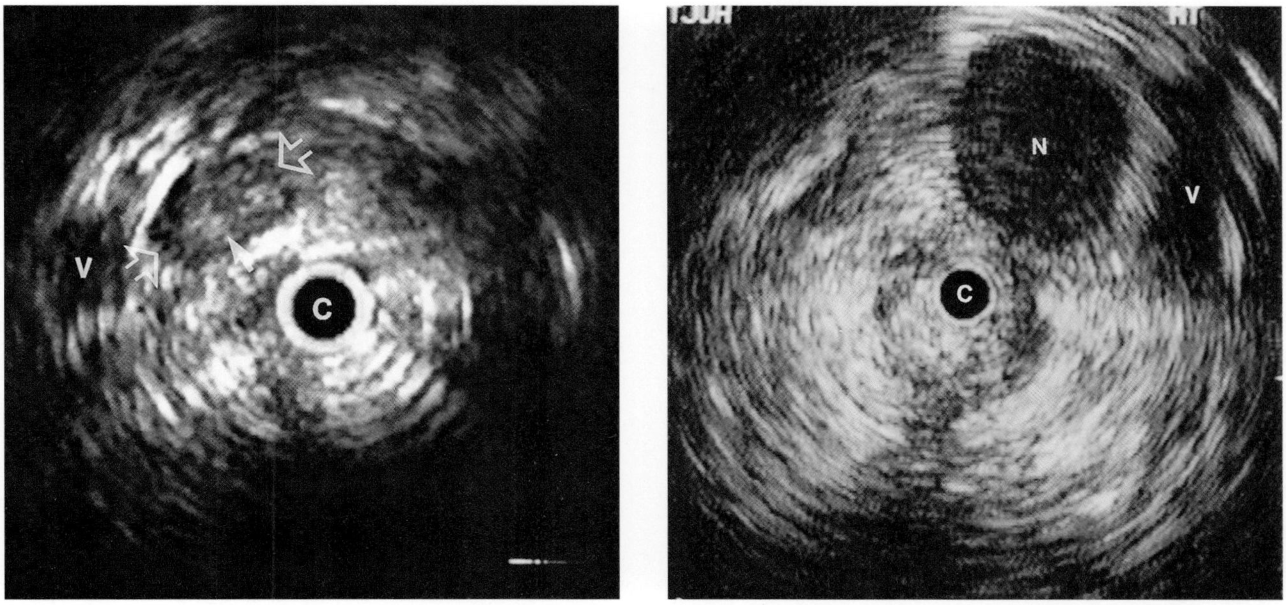

a ***b***

Figure 9.8 *(a) A normal-sized lymph node (open arrows) characterized by an ovoid shape and a hyperechoic central reflection from an intact fatty nodal hilum (arrow). V, vessel; C, ultrasound catheter. (b) Endoluminal ultrasound image demonstrated a round-shaped hypoechoic lymph node (N) with well-defined margin. The normal air-filled lung appears as a dense pattern of reflections. C, catheter; V, vessel.*

pulmonary arteries from the pulmonary veins may be difficult, because of variations in branching. However, mediastinal and hilar lymph nodes as small as a few millimeters may be easily detected, especially with a high-resolution ultrasound transducer via bronchoscopy and mediastinoscopy[36,37–39,42]

When the water-filled balloon located just proximal to the tip of the probe is inflated, the field of view is widened to a full 360° and the depth of penetration is increased to as much as 5 cm (Fig 9.3). The atrioventricular cardiac valves are often visible from the left or right main stem bronchi. With the probe at the tracheal bifurcation, the ascending aorta, the main pulmonary artery, the left and right pulmonary artery branches and intervening mediastinal tissue are clearly discerned (Figs 9.9–9.11).[32,37]

When the inflated balloon-tipped catheter is placed along the right tracheal wall, the right paratracheal region, including the superior vena cava and azygos vein, may be identified. The esophagus and the descending aorta are clear ultrasound landmarks posterior to the azygos vein. Imaging of the aorticopulmonary window from the trachea itself is usually not possible; but access to the aorticopulmonary

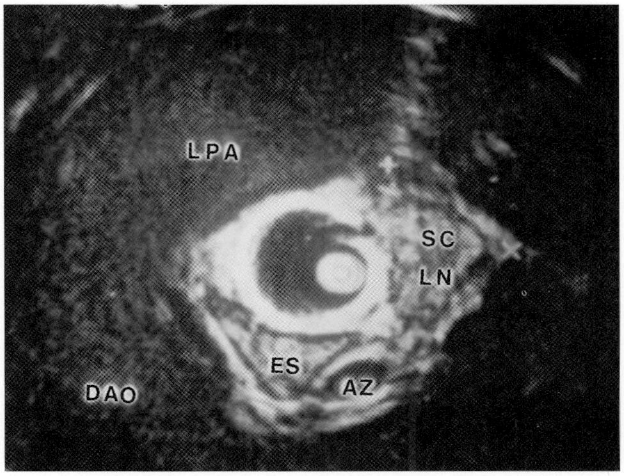

Figure 9.9 *Sonographic image from the left main bronchus showing the azygos vein (AZ), esophagus (ES), left pulmonary artery (LPA), and descending aorta (DAO). Adjacent to the medial wall of the bronchus is a 2-cm-diameter lymph node representing a metastasis from a small cell carcinoma of the right lower lobe (SCLN).*

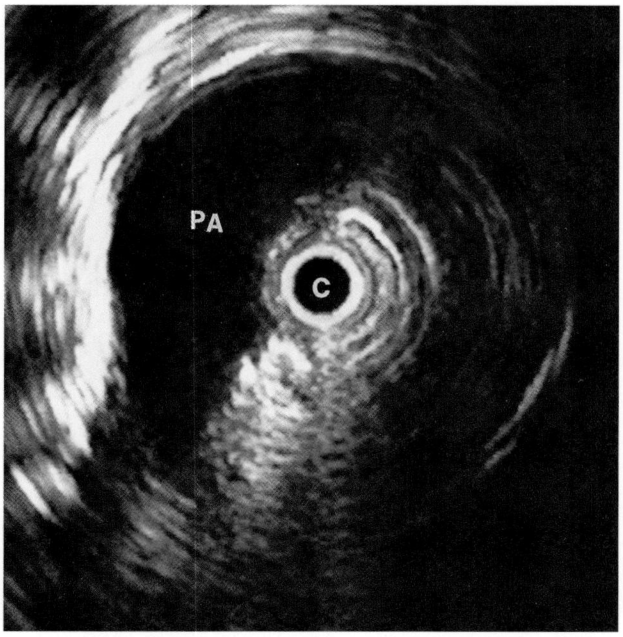

Figure 9.10 *Endoluminal ultrasound image shows a pulsating vessel adjacent to the trachea representing the main pulmonary artery (PA). C, ultrasound catheter.*

window is available from the left mainstem or from the left upper lobe bronchus adjacent to the mediastinal pleura (Fig. 9.12). Imaging of the mediastinum is usually not feasible when the transducer-containing catheter lies within a peripheral bronchus, because of the poor ultrasound conduction of the surrounding air-filled lung.

During the procedure, anatomic structures other than the mass in question are identified and recorded. The bronchial wall and nearby lymph nodes can be identified in many patients. The mediastinal lymph and peribronchial nodes are round, elliptical or oval hypoechoic structures (Figs 9.13 and 9.14). Frequently, an echo-rich zone will be identified in the center of the lymph node due to fat within the nodal hilus (Fig. 9.15). This pattern suggests that, at least in the area of the hilum, the architecture is normal.[9,35,36]

Vascular structures are identified by their echo-free or hypoechoic patterns of flowing blood. Arteries, because of their vigorous pulsations, may be clearly separated from venous structures. Veins, with their more sluggish pulsatile motion, emit streams of reflections due to slow-moving red blood cells (Fig. 9.16).[41]

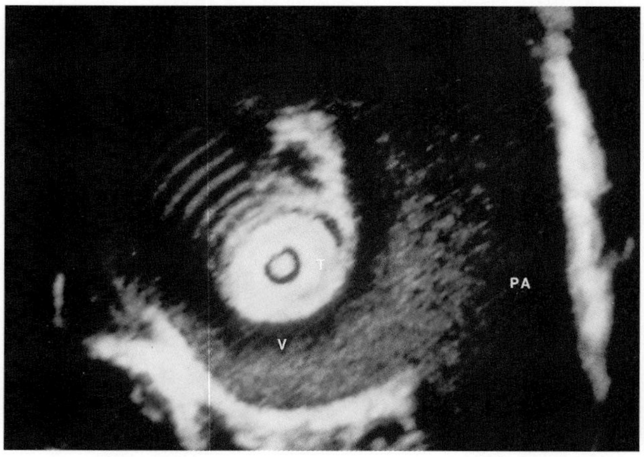

a

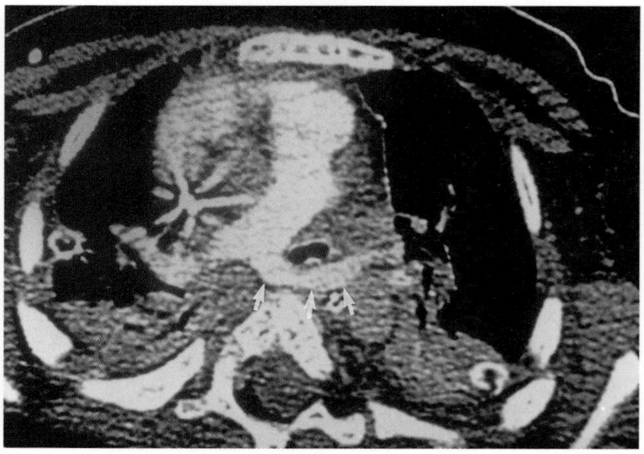

b

Figure 9.11 *(a) Endoluminal ultrasound demonstrates an atypical vessel (V) arising from the right pulmonary artery (PA) passing behind the trachea (T) to the left side and causing the typical pulmonary sling syndrome. (b) A contrast-enhanced CT scan confirmed the abnormal crossing vessel (arrows), which could be successfully repaired by surgery.*

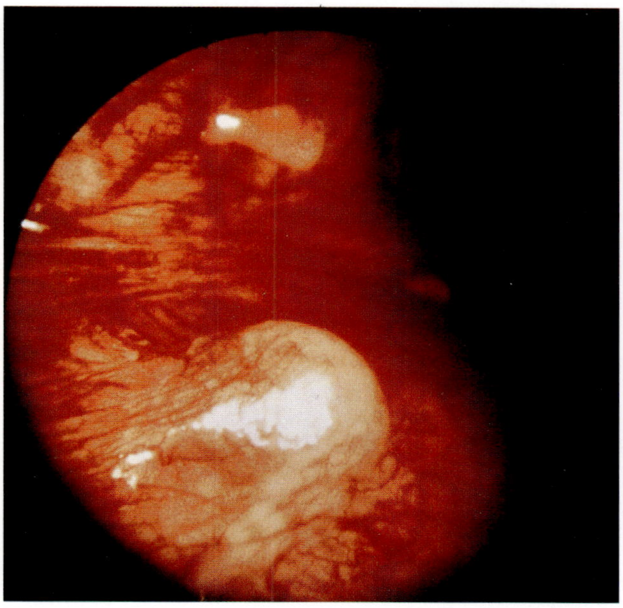

a

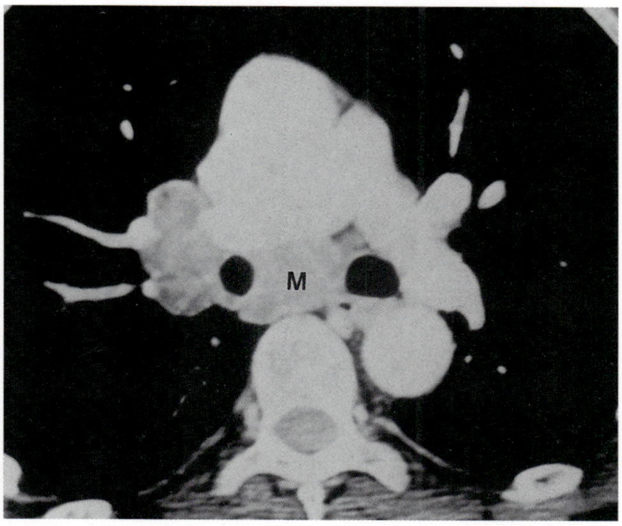

b

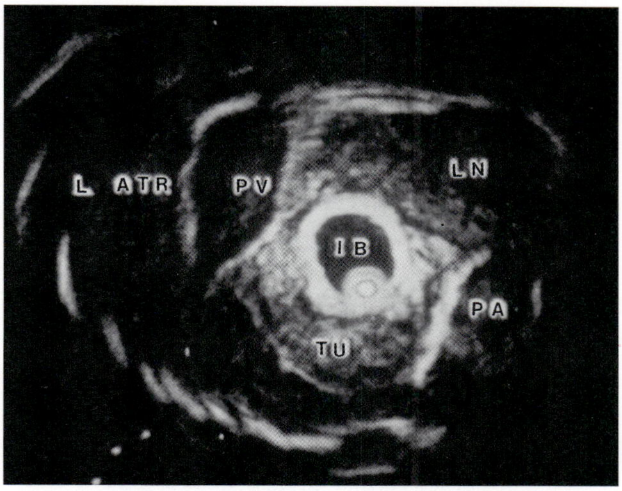

c

Figure 9.12 *(a) A bronchoscopic view at the level of the dorsal wall of the bronchus intermedius. Vascular engorgement suggested a submucosal tumor. (b) CT scan at the same level demonstrates a subcarinal and right hilar mass (M) encasing the bronchus intermedius. (c) The tumor (TU) lies dorsal to the bronchus intermedius (IB). It has infiltrated the bronchial wall and extends across the midline. A large lymph node (LN) is anterior in position. The pulmonary artery (PA), the pulmonary vein (PV) and the left atrium (LATR) are not invaded.*

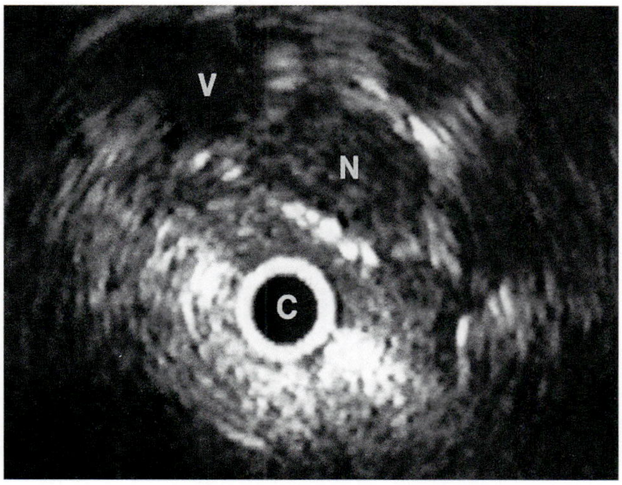

Figure 9.13. *A normal-sized oval hypoechoic lymph node (N) is shown adjacent to a vessel (V). C, ultrasound catheter.*

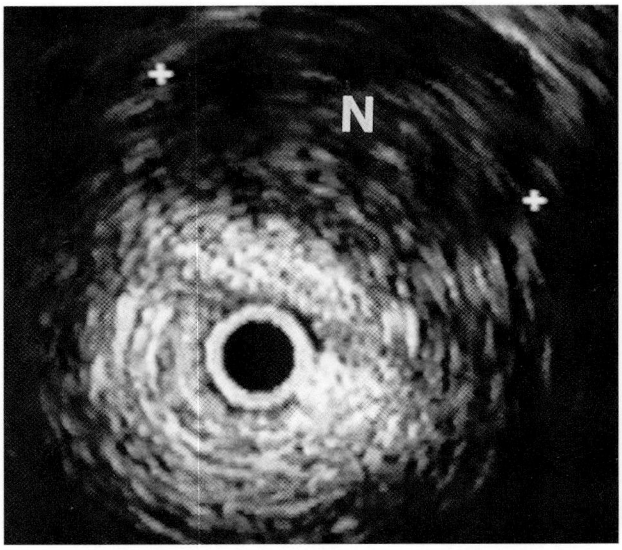

Figure 9.14. *A hypoechoic peribronchial node (N) measuring of 0.9 × 0.6 cm is demonstrated. Transbronchoscopic biopsy was performed and there was no evidence of tumor involvement. P, probe.*

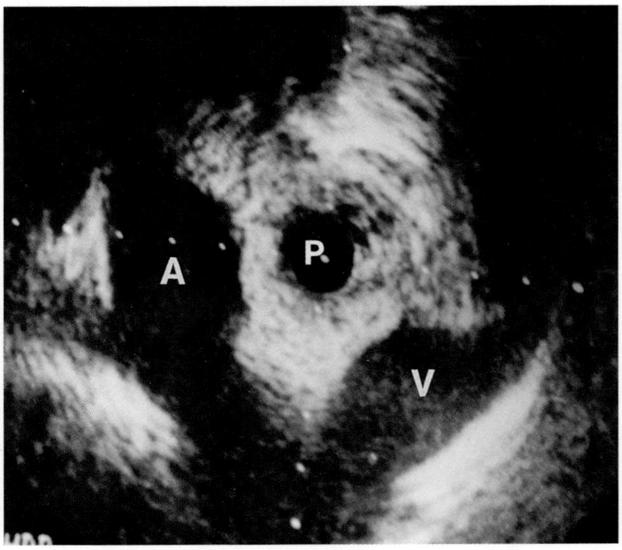

Figure 9.16 *Endoluminal ultrasound demonstrates the vascular structures adjacent to the bronchial wall. The artery (A) is characterized by an echo-free pattern with vigorous pulsations, and the vein (V) has the slow-flow reflections from red blood cells in real time. P, probe.*

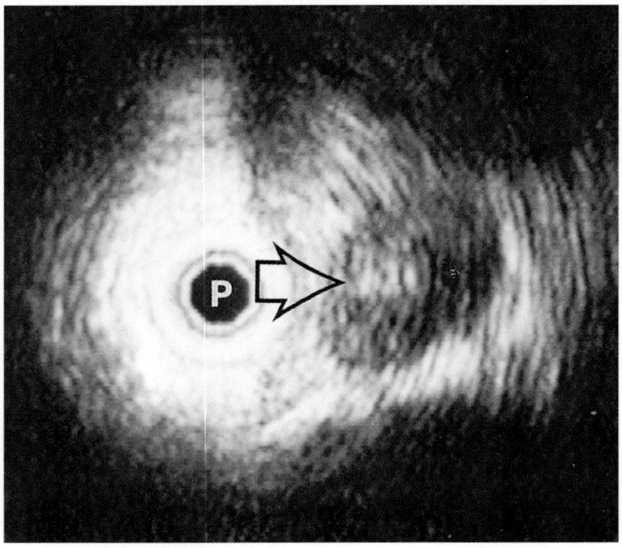

Figure 9.15 *A normal-appearing lymph node characterized by oval shape and central reflections from an intact hilus (arrow). P, probe.*

SONOGRAPHIC CHARACTERISTICS OF LUNG AND MEDIASTINAL PATHOLOGY

Both central and peripheral neoplasms were hypoechoic compared with the surrounding lungs (Fig. 9.17). However, in several patients the echotexture was complex because of regions of increased or decreased aeration or areas of necrosis and hemorrhage (Fig. 9.18). In a certain type of the tumor the lesion may have a unique sonographic appearance (Fig. 9.19). In addition to simply identifying the lesion in question, dimensions of the mass could also be delineated up to 2 cm from the bronchial wall with ultrasound imaging. This limitation was not considered serious, because the size of the tumor was usually appreciated from inspection of the previously obtained chest radiograph or CT scan. More importantly, the location of the lesion in relation to the bronchus and vital structures in which the transducer was located could be determined. In some cases, tumors were found to be eccentric, with their surface abutting only

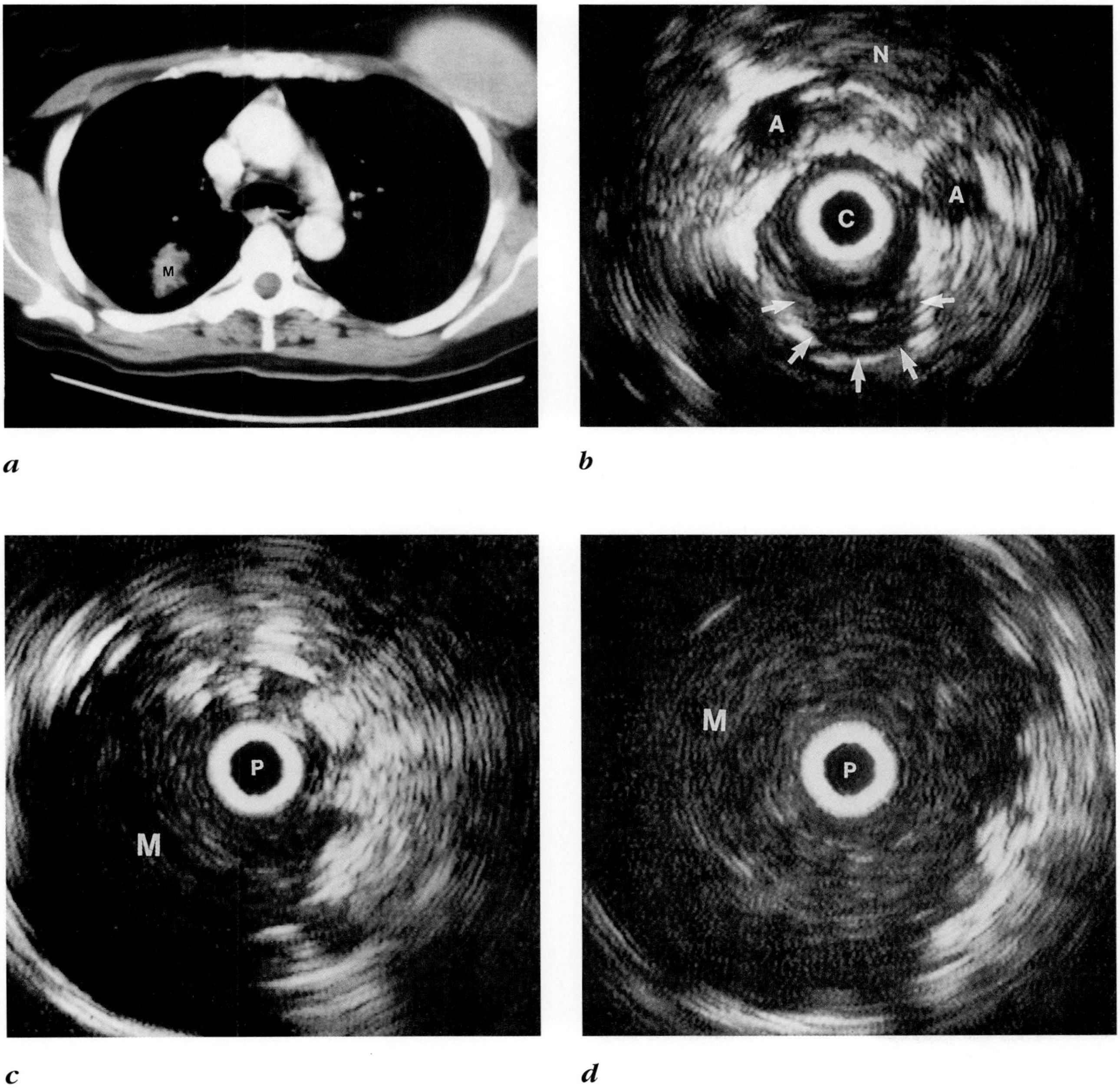

Figure 9.17 *Peripheral neoplasm. A 53-year-old woman presented with a 2 × 3 cm solitary right lower lobe pulmonary nodule. (a) CT scan demonstrated an irregular mass (M) in the superior segment of the right lower lobe. There was no mediastinal adenopathy. (b) With the transbronchoscopic ultrasound catheter (C) in the right main stem bronchus, a lymph node was identified anteriorly (N) and two small arterial vessels (A) characterized by brisk pulsations were seen anterior to the transducer. The upper portion of the mass (arrows) encroached on the bronchus posteriorly. (c, d) Beyond the right main stem bronchus, the catheter-based transducer (P) lay within a bronchus surrounded by the mass (M). The walls of the bronchus are not visible because of tumor involvement. Biopsy at this level demonstrated poorly differentiated non-small cell carcinoma. (Reproduced with permission from Goldberg et al.[36])*

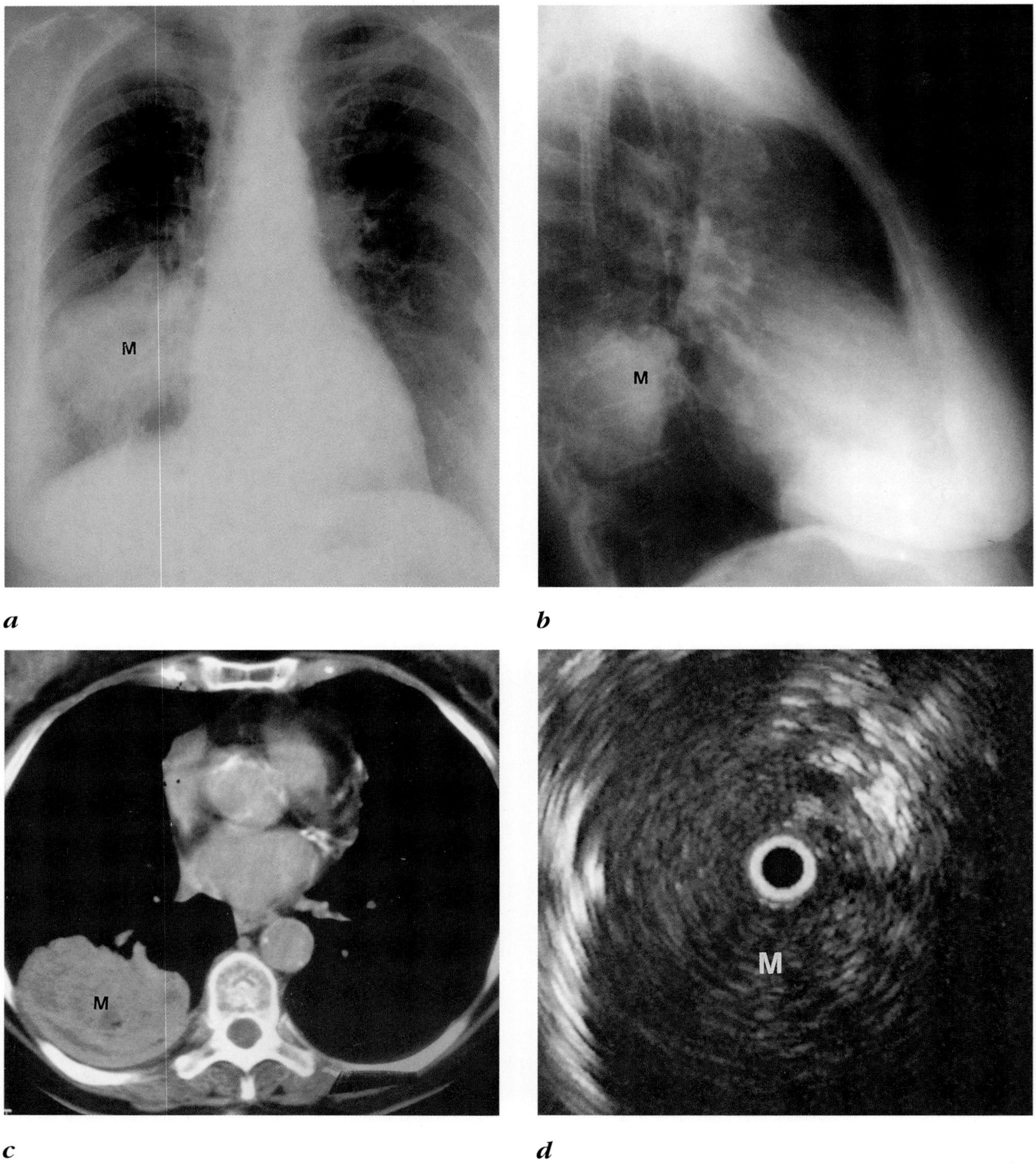

Figure 9.18 *A 76-year-old woman was found to have a large posterior basal segment right lower lobe mass (M) on a posterior-anterior (a) and lateral (b) chest films. (c) CT scan demonstrated a large pleural-based heterogeneous mass (M) without mediastinal involvement. (d) Although peripheral, the mass (M) was easily biopsied using endoluminal ultrasound guidance. The complex ultrasound pattern is due to areas of necrosis within the mass. Cytology showed squamous cell carcinoma. (Reproduced with permission from Steiner et al.*[9]*)*

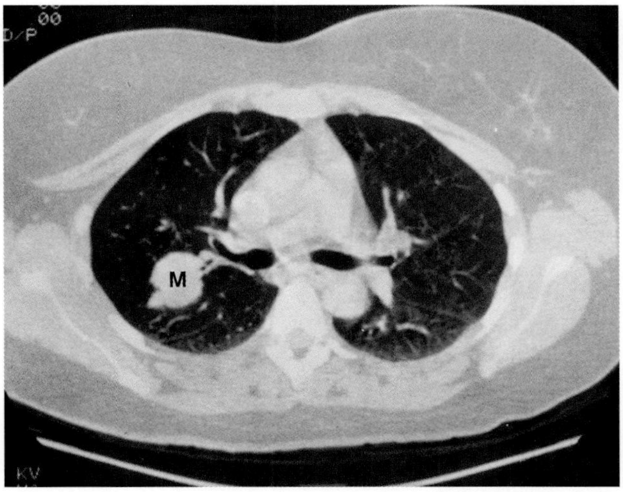

a

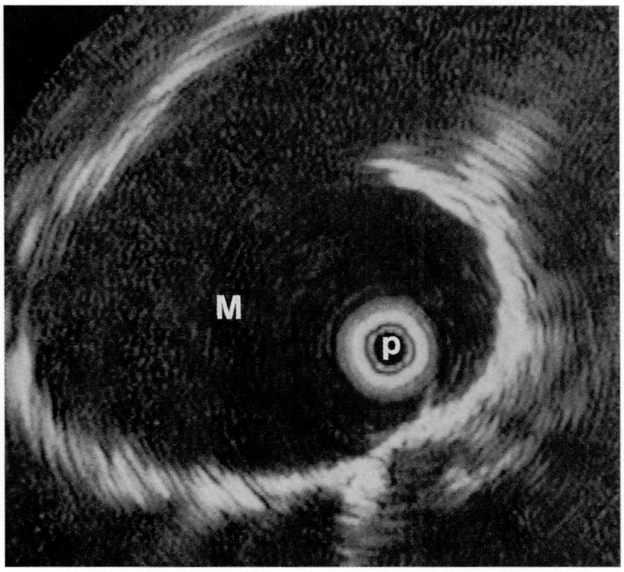

b

Figure 9.19 *A 45-year-old woman underwent bronchoscopy for a peripheral mass in the right upper lobe. (a) A well-demarcated round mass (M) of increased attenuation was seen on the CT scan. (b) Endoluminal ultrasound image showed a 3.3 × 3.3 cm uniformly hypoechoic mass (M) with highly reflective margins. Ultrasound information was used to select the biopsy site. T, transducer. (c) Pathologic examination demonstrated a uniformly cellular pattern consistent with spindle cell carcinoma. (Reproduced with permission from Goldberg et al.[36])*

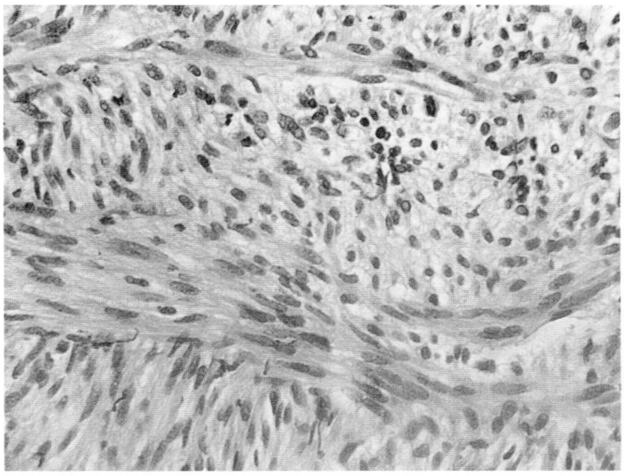

c

a small portion of the bronchus, whereas in others the masses were seen to completely surround the bronchus (Figs 9.17–9.21). Although the tracheal and bronchial mucosa were normally hyperechoic, when the tumor invaded the bronchial wall this pattern disappeared and the bronchial wall tended to blend in with the adjacent hypoechogenic tumor.

As the transducer moved along the surface of the bronchus or trachea, the extent of the tumor and its maximum depth could be demonstrated. This was most dramatically seen in cases of peripheral lesions, in which the relatively small bronchus permitted complete contact with the ultrasound catheter, resulting in a 360° cross-sectional image (Fig. 9.17). The peripheral masses were more sharply defined than central masses, because of the contrast between the highly reflective surrounding lung and the hypoechoic mass (Figs 9.20 and 9.21). Areas of atelectasis were usually more reflective than the tumor itself, owing to the multiple interfaces produced by the airless lung parenchyma mixed with alveolar secretions in residual air-filled spaces.

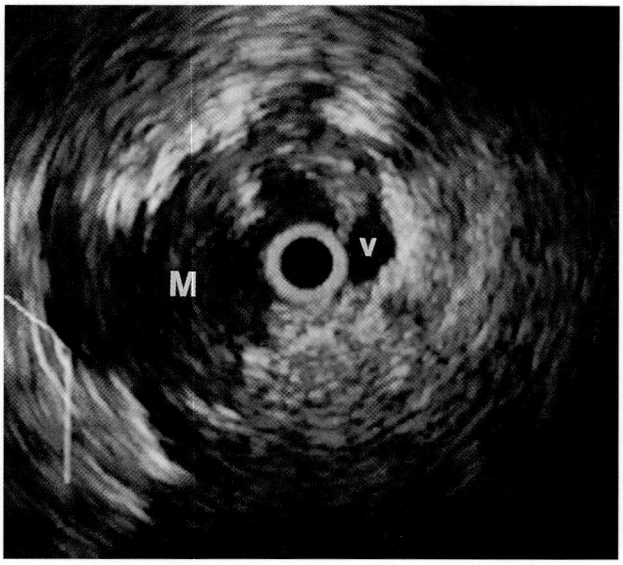

Figure 9.20 *An irregular hypoechoic mass (M) with a sharply defined margin arising from the peripheral lung is demonstrated. A small vessel (V) adjacent to the bronchial wall is also seen.*

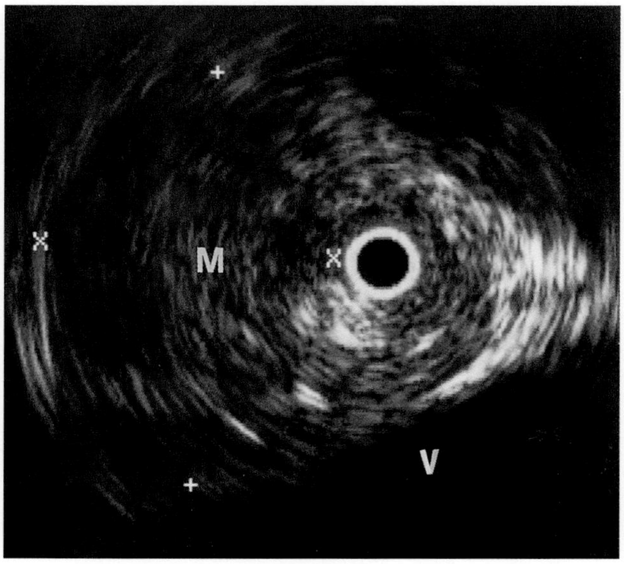

Figure 9.21 *Endoluminal ultrasound image obtained from the trachea shows a hypoechoic mass (M) with poorly defined margins and a large vessel (V) passing behind the lesion.*

Lymph nodes were well-marginated hypo- or mixed echogenic structures with discrete edges (Figs 9.13–9.15). Since the distance between lymph nodes and the tracheobronchial wall may be calculated with ultrasound, transtracheal node biopsy is feasible for peribronchial nodes which lie 1–2 cm away from the bronchial wall. In cases of central lesions, both the tumor and lymph nodes can be successfully sampled under ultrasound guidance.

Blood vessels were demonstrated as anechoic tubular or oval structures. The diameters of the blood vessels could be measured and their positions relative to the bronchus, tumor or lymph nodes could be demonstrated. With this information, it was possible to avoid puncturing blood vessels by choosing a site for transbronchoscopic biopsy away from these vital structures (Fig. 9.22).

For the most part, ultrasound penetration of the aerated lung parenchyma is suboptimal and as a result ultrasound plays only a minor role in the investigation of intrapulmonary lesions compared with other imaging procedures. Only in selected cases can atelectasis due to bronchial obstruction be differentiated from passive atelectasis adjacent to pleural effusion. In these patients, pleural masses may be visualized because of the acoustic window available through the pleural effusion.

Endobronchial ultrasound has proved to be extremely useful for the detection of central airway invasion by surrounding tumor, including carcinoma of the esophagus. In such cases the ultrasound probe can be simultaneously placed inside the esophagus and in the bronchus to assess the extent of tumor infiltration and fistula formation caused by laser resection in combination with rotational radiotherapy.[43]

CLINICAL FEASIBILITY STUDIES

We performed a prospective study of ultrasound-guided video-assisted fiberoptic bronchoscopy to evaluate the efficacy of this technique for localizing and biopsying abnormal structures compared to bronchoscopy without ultrasound guidance.[9] The criteria for patient acceptance into the study group included a clinical history and prebronchoscopic imaging findings suggestive of a peripheral or central

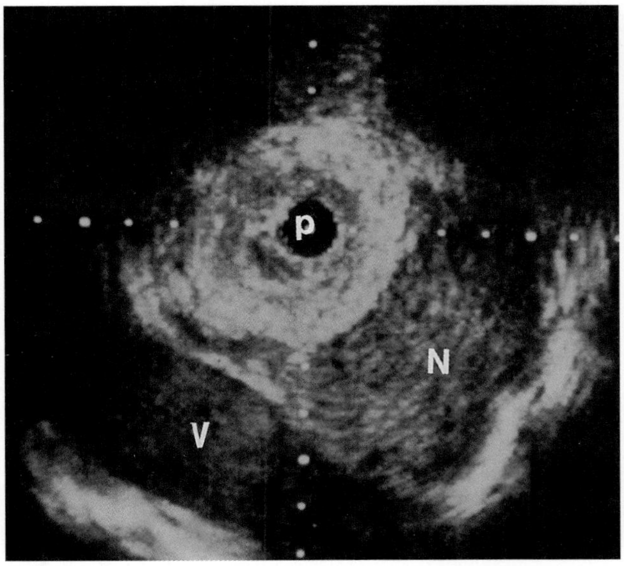

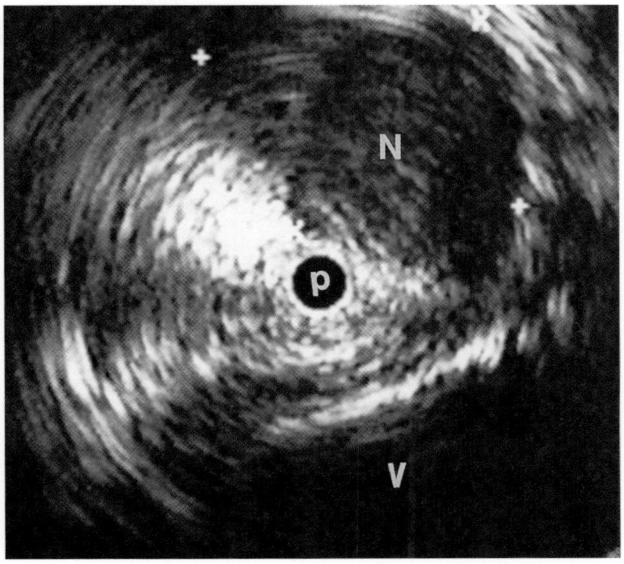

a *b*

Figure 9.22 *(a, b) Endoluminal ultrasound images obtained from different cases demonstrated enlarged lymph nodes (N) adjacent to blood vessels (V). The ultrasound information was used to avoid puncturing these vessels during the biopsy procedures. P, probe.*

thoracic mass as well as a commitment from the bronchoscopist to permit the use of ultrasound before biopsy or brushing of the lesion. Those patients excluded were either thought to be uncooperative or had acute respiratory distress which might be affected by the length of the procedure, which is increased by approximately 10 min when ultrasound is added. The additional time needed for ultrasound guidance is related to manipulation of the imaging catheter and the time required to identify anatomic structures.

Three categories of patients were evaluated separately: they were (1) those with central lesions, (2) those with peripheral lesions, and (3) those with both central and peripheral lesions. In addition to the location of the mass itself, the size, sonographic tissue characteristics (e.g. homo- or heterogeneous, hypo- or hyperechogenicity) and the presence or absence of vascular structures and lymph nodes were tabulated. A radiologist and a bronchoscopist together determined the diagnostic value of the ultrasound information obtained using a four-point rating scale of 0–3.[9,36]

Category 0 included those patients who underwent a technically inadequate ultrasound examination which did not contribute to the performance of the fiberoptic bronchoscopy study.

Category 1 included those patients in whom the abnormality was demonstrated but ultrasound guidance did not aid in the localization of the mass for biopsy.

Category 2 included those patients in whom ultrasound was helpful in the separation of blood vessels, lymph nodes or masses, but did not alter the site of biopsy.

Category 3 included those patients in whom ultrasound was useful in altering biopsy site to a location in which the abnormality was seen to better advantage or which was helpful in preventing puncture of a major blood vessel.

Of 44 patients in the TJUH study, 16 were male and 28 were female.[36] There were 22 peripheral masses measuring from 1 to 3 cm in diameter. Four lesions were large and ill-defined, and their outer margins lay beyond the 2-cm limit of the ultrasound image. Lymph nodes were identified in 16 of 22 patients in this series, and major arteries and veins were visualized in 16 patients. In an overlapping group of 22 patients, 16 (73%) had a confirmed

Table 9.1 US guidance for fiberoptic bronchoscope: results in 44 patients.

Site	*Number*	*Positive biopsy*	*Negative biopsy*	*Vessels*	*Lymph nodes*	*Mass identified*
Central	15	15	0	8	12	15
Peripheral	22	20	2	16	16	20
Central and peripheral	7	7	0	5	7	7

diagnosis of malignancy or inflammatory disease. In addition, one patient yielded a histologic specimen suspicious for malignancy. Of these 17 patients, four had metastatic disease, six had squamous cell carcinoma, three had adenocarcinoma, two had small cell carcinoma and two had unclassified inflammatory disease[36] (Table 9.1).

The four-point efficacy scale used to measure the 'success' of ultrasound guidance in 25 cases demonstrated that 12 (48%) of peripheral lesions were considered category 3; that is, ultrasound helped to determine the site of biopsy. Six were category 2, five were category 1 and two were category 0; that is, studies that were technically unsatisfactorily for adequate interpretation[36] (Table 9.2).

Fifteen patients underwent ultrasound-guided bronchoscopy and biopsy of a central mass initially identified by chest X-ray or CT. These masses were adjacent to or within the trachea or main stem bronchi. Twelve (80%) of the masses were neoplastic, including one with metastatic carcinoma, one with squamous cell carcinoma, two with small cell carcinoma, one with non-small cell carcinoma and seven with adenocarcinoma. In addition, three (20%) had a non-neoplastic inflammatory process. When ultrasound-guided bronchoscopy was performed in patients with central masses, four patients were given a rating category of 3, six patients a rating of 2, and five patients a rating of 1; there were no patients with a rating of category 0.[36]

The third group consisted of seven patients with both central and peripheral lesions. Six were positive for malignancy (83%), including five primary adenocarcinomas and one non-small cell carcinoma. One additional specimen was suspicious for neoplasm. In this group, lymph nodes were identified in six patients and major blood vessels in five patients. Of those patients with central and peripheral masses, four of seven were rated as category 3, two were

Table 9.2 Value of US guidance using efficacy score in 25 patients.

Value rating	*Number of cases*	*%*
0	2	8
+1	5	20
+2	6	24
+3	12	48

0 = no help, technical difficulties.
+1 = identified adnormal anatomic structures.
+2 = somewhat helpful, but did not significantly alter the biopsy procedure.
+3 = very helpful, altered course of biopsy procedure.

rated as category 2, one was rated as category 1 and none were rated 0.[36]

There were no complications referable to the ultrasound portion of the bronchoscopic procedure. While endoluminal ultrasound added approximately 10 min to the length of the procedure, the information elicited from ultrasound guidance often shortened the procedure by obviating the need for additional biopsies, as the bronchoscopist was comfortable that a satisfactory biopsy was obtained from the area of concern.[36]

A control group of 25 patients underwent fiberoptic bronchoscopy without ultrasound assistance. Eighteen peripheral and seven central lesions were identified prior to bronchoscopy. Of 18 patients with peripheral lesions, 11 (62%) were found to have a neoplasm. Four (57%) of the central masses were positive for tumor.[9]

In another study, transbronchial ultrasound was used in approximately 600 (6%) of 11 000 consecutive bronchoscopies at the ThoraxClinic in Heidelberg, Germany from 1993 to 1995 whenever it was determined that additional information would be obtained by this technique.[32,37] To minimize the cost of the procedure, the transducers were resterilized and reused as long as they would stand up to the mechanical stress of the procedure. In this study, the ability of bronchoscopic ultrasound to stage bronchogenic carcinoma was compared to that of standard imaging studies. The appearance of regional nodes and the bronchial wall and evidence of invasion from nearby vessels were examined.

In this series the depth of ultrasound penetration was insufficient to detect mediastinal masses and lymph nodes in the retrosternal region. On the other hand, mediastinal cysts in close proximity to the tracheobronchial wall were easily diagnosed by their central echo-free character and in some cases by internal septations.[32,37] Encroachment on the upper trachea by a retrosternal goiter was identified by tissue inhomogenicity and clear delineation of the mass from the tracheal lumen. Invasion by thyroid carcinoma could also be assessed if the tracheal wall was infiltrated by tumor.[32,37]

Airway compression by an aortic aneurysm or displacement of the airway by kyphoscoliosis was diagnosed by endoluminal ultrasound and was confirmed by surgery in several cases when conventional procedures such as angiography were unable to establish a diagnosis. In one patient with severe hemoptysis, rupture of a surgical patch was demonstrated at the site of aortic hypoplasia and pseudoaneurysm was later confirmed by surgery. Angiography in this case was considered normal.[32,37]

Hürter and Hanrath used an ultrasound transducer-containing catheter similar to ours.[33,34] Their study cohort included 58 patients, and the procedure was successfully performed in 50. Neoplastic tissue was not obtained in five patients with small peripheral lesions, and in three the probe could not be passed through the tumor. Three of their patients had tumor not seen by fiberoptic bronchoscopy but recognized by endoluminal ultrasound either within the bronchial wall or surrounding the bronchus.[33,34]

In a separate in vitro study of 84 lymph nodes from 15 patients recovered by systematic lymph node dissection at surgery, the nodes were evaluated by ultrasound criteria that assessed malignant involvement, including nodal size echodensity, tissue homogenicity and demarcation from surrounding structures.[37] In this study it was not possible to determine malignant involvement by any of the criteria examined in spite of an image resolution of less than 0.1 mm.[37] This may be due to the nonspecific reaction of the hilar and mediastinal nodes to a variety of pathologic conditions, including pneumonia, pneumoconiosis and granulomatous disease, as well as neoplasms that cause irregularities of nodal contour and inhomogenicity of the nodal sonographic pattern.[37]

Finally, in a recent study of 80 patients with mediastinal adenopathy who had ultrasound-guided fiberoptic bronchoscopy, a comparison with conventional fiberoptic bronchoscopy was made. There were no significant differences between the biopsy results of ultrasound-guided fiberoptic bronchoscopy and those of conventional fiberoptic bronchoscopy. The specificity (100% versus 100%), sensitivity (82.6% versus 90.5%) and accuracy (86.7% versus 91.7%) were also similar, but there was a significant decrease in the number of aspirations needed for successful lymph node sampling with ultrasound guidance.[35]

FUTURE DEVELOPMENTS

In order to make ultrasound-assisted fiberoptic bronchoscopy practical, limitations of this procedure need to be addressed. For example, the greater availability of inflatable fluid-filled balloons will aid in producing circumferential acoustic coupling of the transducer to the wall of the trachea and larger bronchi. Currently, balloon-tipped catheters are only selectively available for research investigators.[35,37–39] Similar inflatable balloon-tipped transducers incorporated into endoscopes are currently used for evaluation of the gastrointestinal tract and for intravascular use.

A bronchoscope with a dual working channel should be used for simultaneous advancement of both the biopsy forceps and the ultrasound catheter so that the biopsy will be performed directly under ultrasound control (Fig. 9.6). On-line confirmation of the biopsy site eliminates the need for fluoroscopy, which is now used to confirm the position of the transducer and biopsy catheter. Compatibility between the size of the bronchoscope's working channel and the ultrasound catheter probe is needed, particularly when the bronchoscope is dual channel. To achieve compatibility, further miniaturization of the currently available balloon catheters is necessary to permit their introduction into the biopsy port of a conventional single- or dual-channel fiberoptic bronchoscope.

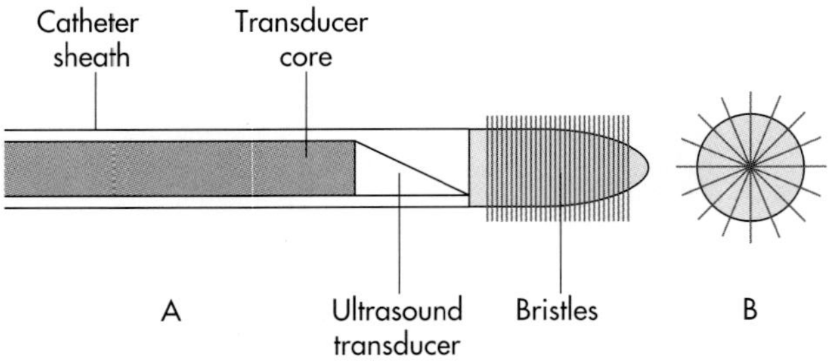

Figure 9.23 *An illustration of the biopsy brush for cytology to be incorporated into the tip of the transducer catheter for simultaneous ultrasound imaging and biopsy (patented). This instrument should be useful for peripheral lung lesion biopsies. A, longitudinal view; B, transverse view.*

Recently, we developed a new brush-tipped transducer catheter (patented) for direct biopsy of the peripheral lesions under simultaneous ultrasound guidance (Fig. 9.23).[9,36] This new tool has promise and, like other enhancements, it needs to be brought to commercial production in order to make ultrasound-guided biopsy practical and widely available.

The use of Doppler ultrasound to improve discrimination of vascular structures may be an additional potential improvement. Color-coded tissue characterization of images based on vector quantitization algorithms may also be useful for tissue differentiation, resulting in improved sensitivity and specificity of diagnostic results.

SUMMARY

Improvements in fiberoptics and image acquisition technology, as well as biopsy equipment, have enhanced the capability of fiberoptic bronchoscopy so that today there is a positive yield in most patients with obstructing carcinoma. However, there are well-recognized limitations to the procedure. For example, it is often difficult to achieve useful diagnostic results in necrotic tumors or small submucosal neoplasms. Sampling tracheal lesions accurately can be difficult because of the angle of the biopsy needle in relation to the tracheal wall.

The rate of diagnostic retrieval of masses in the outer third of the lung with bronchoscopy is certainly lower than that of central lesions. Small peripheral tumors with diameters of 2 cm or less are particularly difficult to characterize.[7,8,11] In a lesion 2 cm or less in diameter, only one or two bronchi traverse the mass. Larger lesions may have three or more bronchi encased or invaded by the tumor, increasing the chance that the bronchoscope will locate a suitable site for biopsy. Before bronchoscopic biopsy of a peripheral mass is performed, supplementary imaging techniques, including C-arm or biplane fluoroscopy, will further localize the bronchi in the mass and increase the yield of the bronchoscopic procedure. On the other hand, fluoroscopy may show the relationship of the tip of the bronchoscope to the mass in the anterior–posterior projection, but the bronchoscope may actually lie in front or behind the mass, so that, in spite of fluoroscopy guidance, a biopsy may be unrewarding.

Ultrasound has a major advantage over fluoroscopy, because it can precisely locate a peripheral mass within or adjacent to the bronchus. The depth of the mass from the wall of the airway as well as the presence or absence of adjacent vessels or lymph nodes can also be demonstrated.

It is ironic that peripheral lesions are more consistently visualized with ultrasound imaging than are central lesions. This is because in the peripheral bronchus a full 360° cross-sectional image is obtained. Because of the wider luminal diameter of the trachea and major bronchi, a full cross-sectional image cannot be obtained without a liquid-filled balloon at the catheter tip.

TRANSMEDIASTINOSCOPIC ULTRASOUND

CT is the preferred imaging procedure for preoperative assessment of mediastinal lymph node status in bronchogenic cancer. However, a CT scan cannot distinguish malignant from benign lesions, Therefore, cervical mediastinoscopy in some situations is advisable to obtain lymph node tissue for histologic examination in the case of enlarged lymph nodes seen on CT scan.[44] On the other hand, during mediastinoscopy, direct palpation is not possible. Therefore, it is important to find another method to determine what structures lie beneath the visualized surface.

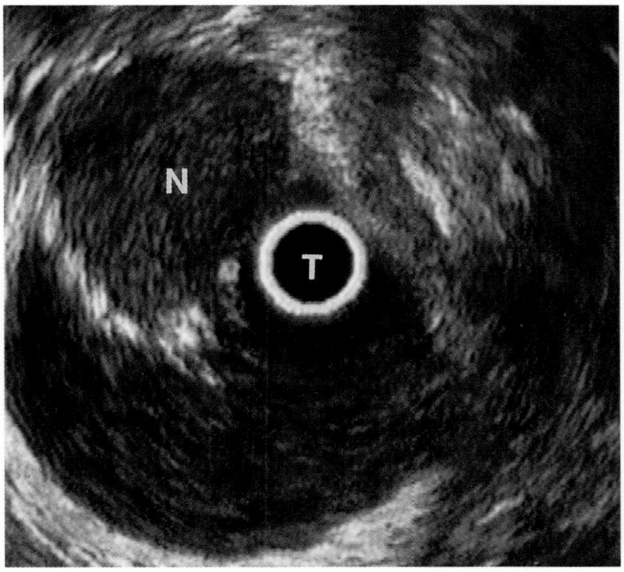

Figure 9.24 *The miniature ultrasound transducer (T), which has been inserted through a mediastinoscope into the mediastinum, shows the presence of a hypoechoic lymph node (N).*

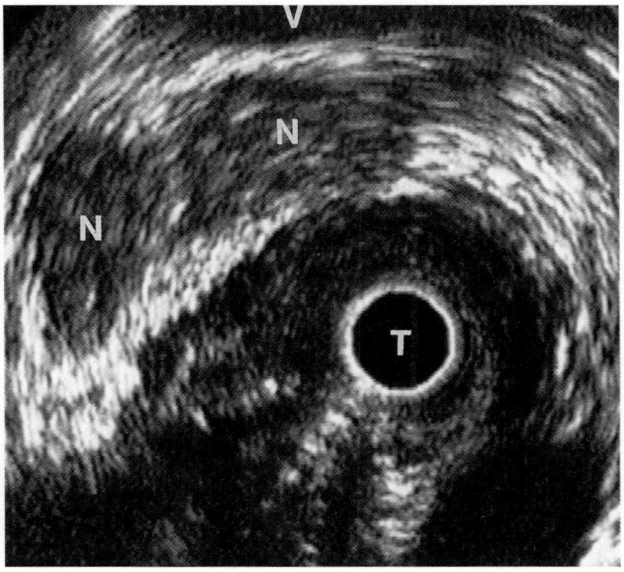

Figure 9.25 *Endoluminal ultrasound transducer (T) was placed in the mediastinal space through mediastinoscope. Two lymph nodes (N) adjacent to a vessel (V) were detected that were not seen with the mediastinoscope. They were subsequently removed under ultrasound guidance and the pathologic examination confirmed the presence of metastases.*

Miniature ultrasound transducer-containing catheters (6.2 or 9 Fr) have been advanced through positioned mediastinoscopes to evaluate a variety of normal and abnormal mediastinal structures in patients undergoing staging of lung tumors.[42] Using either a 12.5- or 20-MHz transducer producing a real-time cross-sectional image, it is possible to image normal mediastinal structures (such as blood vessels and trachea) as well as to locate enlarged lymph nodes for biopsy (Fig. 9.24). Whereas the surgeon is able to see some lymph nodes by direct observation, ultrasound is able to image additional lymph nodes located beneath the exposed surface (Fig. 9.25). With this approach, the surgeon is able to avoid dissection in those areas where no enlarged lymph nodes or masses are present. The relationship of the lymph nodes to adjacent blood vessels can be demonstrated (Fig. 9.26). The additional information provided by these endoluminal ultrasound images reduces the time required for mediastinal lymph node dissection or mass biopsy. This approach increases the confidence of the surgeon that no further lymph nodes or masses are hidden behind other structures.

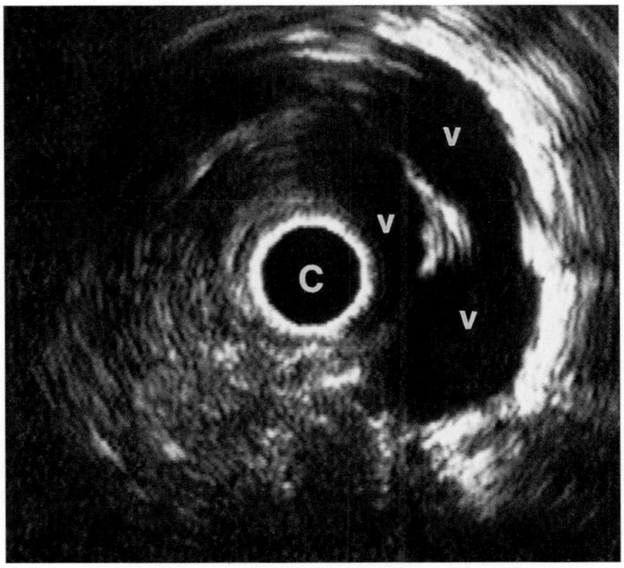

Figure 9.26 *The ultrasound catheter (C) demonstrates the position of major blood vessels (V) within the mediastinum. It was not necessary to dissect behind these structures, as no lymph nodes could be identified.*

Transmediastinoscopic ultrasound provides information to the surgeon that was not previously available, thus reducing the chances of inadvertent trauma to vital structures as well as decreasing the time needed to perform the procedure.[42]

The relatively high-frequency (12.5-MHz) transducer allows for excellent resolution, with the capability of seeing small vessels and normal-sized lymph nodes; however, there is a relative lack of penetration of the ultrasound beam (radial depth of no more than 2–3 cm). Now, a new miniature transducer (9 Fr) with a frequency of 9 MHz is available that should overcome this limitation. It is envisioned that in the future a variety of miniature transducers of various sizes and frequencies, as well as with Doppler capability for the analysis of flow, will add to the usefulness of this approach.

TRANSTHORACOSCOPIC ULTRASOUND

An important recent development in thoracic surgery is the expanded use of video-assisted thoracoscopy for a wide range of indications, including diffuse pulmonary interstitial disease, mediastinal masses, pleural disease and small peripheral pulmonary nodules.[45–47] Indications for thoracoscopic resection of peripheral lung nodules include an inconclusive transbronchial or percutaneous biopsy procedure and nodules of less than 8 mm in diameter where fine needle aspiration biopsy is unlikely to be successful. Therapeutic resection of presumed metastases or a primary peripheral lung cancer are additional indications for thoracoscopy. For the resection of pulmonary nodules utilizing the thoracoscopic technique, nodules must be visible on the pleural surface or palpable with endoscopic forceps or by digital manipulation.[46]

The difficulty in evaluating lesions identified prior to thoracoscopy by CT, MRI, transesophageal echocardiography or plain film is caused by the fact that the position of the lesion is drastically changed by interoperative lung collapse.[44] For this reason, preoperative localization of peripheral pulmonary nodules can be critical for thoracoscopic excision.

Recently, spring-hook wires originally designed for mammographic biopsy guidance were adapted to localize peripheral pulmonary nodules for thoracoscopy.[48–50] Guidance with this technique has been successful. In a group of 32 patients studied by Shah et al, only three patients (9%) had unsuccessful thoracoscopic biopsy procedures.[50] However, complications of the localization procedure are not inconsiderable. In this series, pneumothorax occurred in 15 of 32 patients, two of whom required catheter drainage during localization. Parenchymal hemorrhage occurred in 11 patients, and severe pleuritic pain in two. If there is significant delay before surgery is performed, hemorrhage may obscure the borders of the nodule, or progressive pneumothorax may require tube placement.[50]

Recently, intraoperative ultrasound has been used during video-assisted thoracoscopic surgery in patients to determine whether localization of peripheral pulmonary nodules prior to wedge resection is feasible.[51] To perform this procedure a specially designed ultrasound probe with color and spectral Doppler capabilities (Flextip; Bruel&Kjaer Instruments, Marlborough, MA) was used. This probe is designed for use with the Bruel&Kjaer system 3535. The semi-flexible probe, which is 9.6 mm in diameter and 35 cm long, contains a multifrequency (5.0, 6.5 and 7.5 MHz) convex-array transducer with maximum penetration of 13 cm and a sector scanning angle of 60°. The transducer is located on a flexible tip that is steered by a controller and can move 90° up and 90° down from the 0° position (Fig. 9.27).

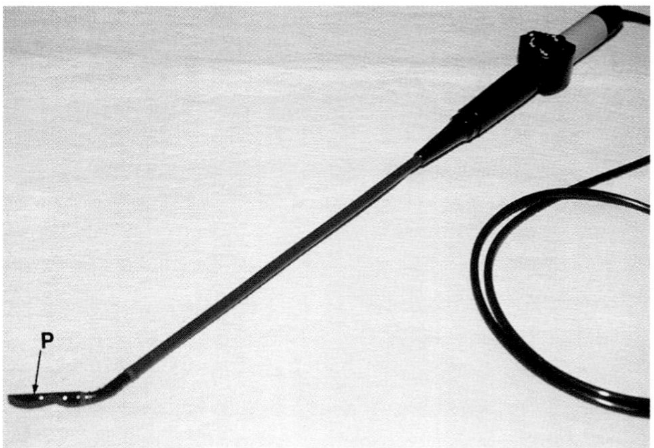

Figure 9.27 *An endoscopic ultrasound probe (P) with a flexible tip facilitates optimal contact with the lung surface. This probe has not only gray-scale imaging but also color and pulsed Doppler capabilities.*

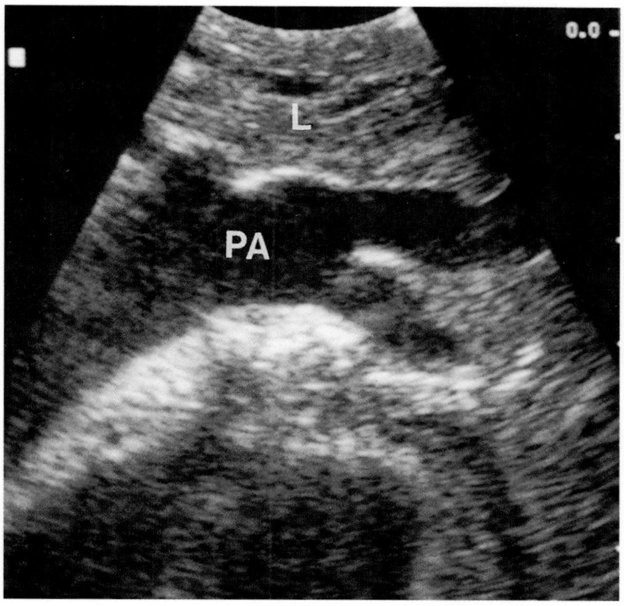

Figure 9.28 *Thoracoscopic ultrasound image shows the pulmonary artery (PA) and branches through the collapsed lung (L).*

The probe is covered by a sterile plastic sheath and introduced through a 10 mm diameter trocar during thoracoscopic surgery. It is placed directly on the collapsed lung in the area of the suspected nodule. The normal structures (such as blood vessels) can be seen through the collapsed lung tissue (Fig. 9.28). When the nodule was localized, a small needle or indicator dye was used to document the position of the nodule for the wedge resection. In addition to intraoperative localization of the pulmonary nodule, the size of the lesion and distance from the lung surface was determined to help plan the wedge resection (Fig 9.29). If a cystic lesion is considered, color and spectral Doppler imaging should be used for distinguishing the cystic lesion from the vascular structures (Fig. 9.30).

This procedure was successful in demonstrating the abnormality and permitting rapid and safe biopsy. The procedure required approximately 5–10 min of additional operating room time, and CT-guided hook-wire localization was not shown to be necessary prior to surgery. On the other hand, important pitfalls limit the value of ultrasound

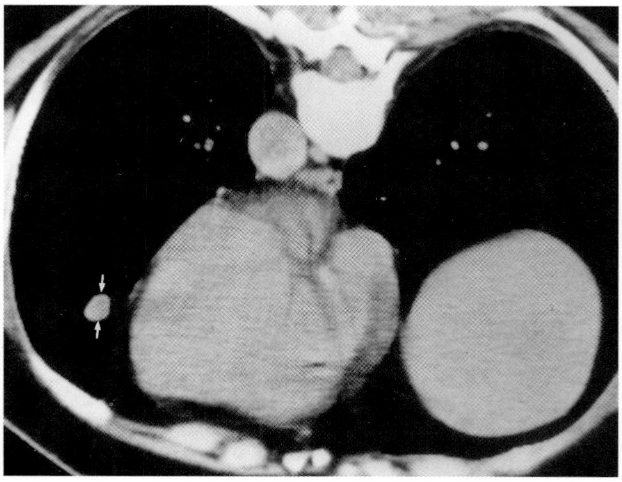

a

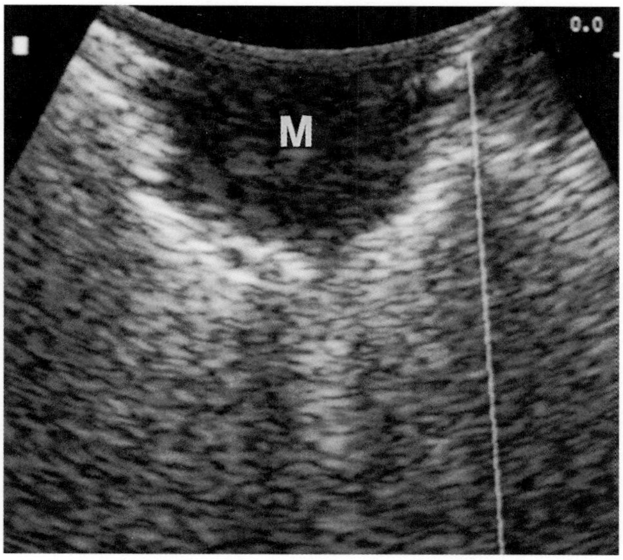

b

Figure 9.29 *(a) CT scan shows a small solitary pulmonary nodule (arrows) in the lingular segment of the left upper lung. (b) Ultrasound shows an oval, well-defined hypoechoic mass (M) compared with normal lung. The lesion was found to be a carcinoid tumor by histology.*

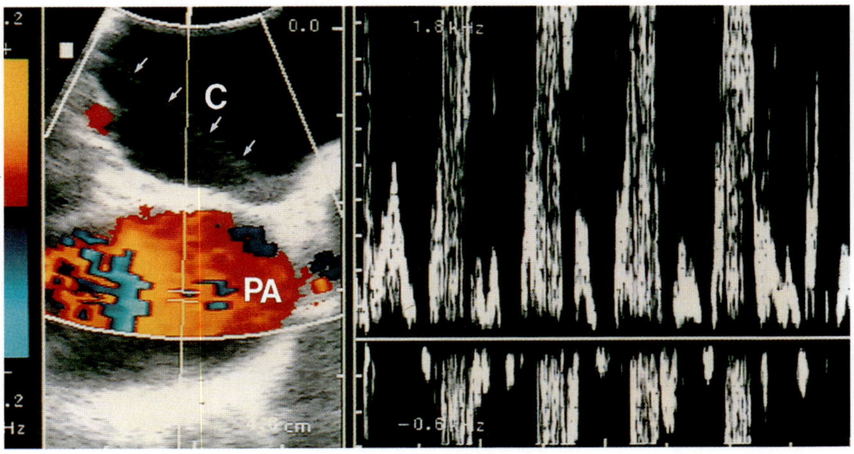

Figure 9.30 *The ultrasound probe demonstrated a cystic mass (C) with septations (arrows). The mass was located adjacent to the main pulmonary artery (PA). The Doppler spectral waveform demonstrates an arterial flow pattern. Pathology proved it to be a thymoma.*

assistance during thoracotomy. The presence of residual air within the lung during the procedure produces disturbing artifacts and limits the ability to identify the abnormality.

This new application of ultrasound in thoracic surgery should, in selected cases, eliminate the need for preoperative hook-wire needle localization and permit the surgeon to safely expand the use of thoracoscopy to areas adjacent to major blood vessels and other vital structures which can be demonstrated with ultrasound.

ACKNOWLEDGMENT

We wish to thank our associates for their suggestions and help with this project. They include: John Cohn MD, Antje L. Greenfield MD, Dan Merton RDMS, Sandra Weibel MD, Herbert Cohen MD, Krishna Mohan MD, Robert M. Solit MD, James Fish MD Nandkumar M. Rawool MD and Joseph Darby RDMS. We also thank Traci Marsden for her excellent secretarial assistance.

REFERENCES

1. Ikeda S, Flexible broncho-fiberoscopy, *Ann Otolaryngol Rhinol Laryngol* 1970; **79**:916–23.
2. Arrogliga AC, Matthay RA, The role of bronchoscopy in lung cancer, *Clin Chest Med* 1993; **14**:87.
3. Prakash UBS, Offord KP, Stubbs SE, Bronchoscopy in North America: The ACCP Survey, *Chest* 1991; **100**:1668–75.
4. Wang KP, Terry PB, Transbronchial needle aspiration in the diagnosis and staging of bronchogenic carcinoma, *Am Rev Respir Dis* 1983; **127**:344–7.
5. Zavana DC, Diagnostic fiberoptic bronchoscopy: technique and results of biopsy in 600 patients, *Chest* 1975; **68**:12–19.
6. Shure D, Fedullo PF, Transbronchial needle aspiration of peripheral masses, *Am Rev Respir Disease* 1983; **128**:1090–2.
7. Shure D, Fiberoptic bronchoscopy: diagnostic applications, *Clin Chest Med* 1987; **8**:1–12.
8. Fletcher EC, Levin DC, Flexible fiberoptic bronchoscopy and fluoroscopy guided transbronchial biopsy in the management of solitary pulmonary nodules, *West J Med* 1983; **138**:364–70.
9. Steiner RM, Liu JB, Goldberg BB, Cohn JR, The value of ultrasound-guided fiberoptic bronchoscopy, *Clin Chest Med* 1995; **16**:519–34.
10. Harrow E, Halber M, Hardy S, Haltemann W, Bronchoscopic and roentgenographic correlates of a positive transbronchial needle aspiration in the staging of lung cancer, *Chest* 1993; **100**:1592–6.
11. Shure D, Fedullo PF, Transbronchial needle aspiration of peripheral masses, *Am Rev Respir Dis* 1983; **128**:1090–2.
12. Radke JR, Conway WA, Eyler WR et al, Diagnostic accuracy in peripheral lung lesions. Factors predicting success with flexible fiberoptic bronchoscopy, *Chest* 1979; **76**:176–9.
13. Wernecke KP, Vassallo R, Pottee HG, Luckener PE, Mediastinal tumors: Sensitivity of detection with sonography compared with CT and radiography, *Radiology* 1990; **175**:137.
14. Shure D, Transbronchial needle aspiration: current status, *Mayo Clin Proc* 1989; **64**:251–4.

15. Izumi S, Tamaki S, Watori H, Kira S, Ultrasonically-guided aspiration needle biopsy in diseases of the chest, *Am Rev Respir Dis* 1982; **125**:460–4.
16. Mueller PR, Saini S, Simeone JF et al, Image-guided pleural biopsies: indications, technique, and results in 23 patients, *Radiology* 1988; **169**:1–4.
17. Pedersen OL, Aasen TB, Gulsvik A, Fine needle aspiration biopsy of mediastinal and peripheral pulmonary masses guided by real-time sonography, *Chest* 1986; **89**:504–8.
18. Saito T, Kobayashi H, Kitamura S, Ultrasonographic approach to the diagnosis of chest wall tumors, *Chest* 1968; **94**:1271–5.
19. Yang PC, Luh KT, Sheu JC, Kuo SH, Yang SP, Peripheral pulmonary lesions: ultrasonography and ultrasonically-guided aspiration biopsy, *Radiology* 1985; **155**:451–6.
20. Anderson T, Lindgren PG, Elvin A, Ultrasound guided tumor biopsy in the anterior mediastinum. An alternative to thoracotomy and mediastinoscopy, *ACTA Radiol* 1992; **33**:423–6.
21. Mathis G, Sutterlutti G, Ultrasound-guided fine needle biopsy of the peripheral pulmonary masses, *Radiology* 1990; **30**:214–6.
22. Kondo D, Imaizumi M, Abe T, Naruke T, Suemasu K, Endoscopic ultrasound examination for mediastinal and lymph node metastases of lung cancer, *Chest* 1990; **98**:586–93.
23. Rifkin MD, Gordon SJ, Goldberg BB, Sonographic examination of the mediastinum and upper abdomen by fiberoptic gastroscope, *Radiology* 1984; **151**:175–80.
24. Gardiner D, VanSonnenberg E, D'Agostino HB et al, CT-guided transthoracic needle biopsy, *Cardiovasc Interven Radiol* 1991; **14**:17–23.
25. Liu JB, Miller LS, Goldberg BB et al, Transnasal US of the esophagus: preliminary morphologic and function studies, *Radiology* 1992; **184**:721–7.
26. Liu JB, Miller LS, Feld RI, Barbarevech CA, Needleman L, Goldberg BB, Gastric and esophageal varices: 20-MHz transnasal endoluminal US, *Radiology* 1993; **187**:363–6.
27. Miller LS, Liu JB, Klenn PJ, Dhuria M, Feld RI, Goldberg BB, High-frequency endoluminal ultrasonography of the esophagus in human autopsy specimens, *J Ultrasound Med* 1993; **12**:563–6.
28. Miller LS, Liu JB, Klenn PJ et al, Endoluminal ultrasonography of the distal esophagus in systemic sclerosis, *Gastroenterology* 1993; **105**:31–9.
29. Goldberg BB, Liu JB, Merton DA, Kurtz AB, Endoluminal ultrasound: experiments with non-vascular uses in animals, *Radiology* 1990; **175**:39–43.
30. Goldberg BB, Bagley D, Liu JB, Merton DA, Alexander A, Kurtz AB, Endoluminal sonography of the urinary tract: preliminary observations, *AJR* 1991; **156**:99–103.
31. Rösch TH, Classen M, A new ultrasonic probe for endosonographic imaging of the upper GI tract, *Endoscopy* 1990; **22**:41–6.
32. Becker HD, Bronchoscopy for airway lesions. In: Wang KP, Mehta AC, eds, *Flexible Bronchoscopy.* (Blackwell Publishers: Cambridge, MA, 1995): 136–59.
33. Hürter TH, Hanrath P, Endobronchial sonography in the diagnosis of pulmonary mediastinal tumors, *Dtsch Med Wochenschr* 1990; **115**:1899–905.
34. Hürter TH, Hanrath P, Endobronchial sonography: feasibility and pulmonary results, *Thorax* 1992; **47**(7):565–7.
35. Shannon JJ, Bude RO, Orens JB et al, Endobronchial ultrasound-guided needle aspiration of mediastinal adenopathy, *Am J Resp Crit Care Med* 1996; **153**:1424–30.
36. Goldberg BB, Steiner RM, Liu J-B, Merton D, Articolo G, Cohn J, Ultrasound-assisted bronchoscopy with the use of miniature transducer containing catheters, *Radiology* 1994; **190**:233–8.
37. Becker HD. Endobronchialer ultraschall eine neue. Perspektive in der bronchologie, *Endoskopie Heute* 1995; **1**:55–6.
38. Ono R, Suemasu K, Matsunaka T, Bronchoscopic ultrasonography for diagnosis of lung cancer, *Jpn J Clin Oncol* 1993; **23**:34–40.
39. Ono R, Shirano H, Egawa S, Suemasu K. Bronchoscopic ultrasonography and brachytherapy in roentgenologically occult bronchogenic carcinoma, *J Bronchol* 1994; **1**:281–7.
40. Lewis JW, Pearlberg JL, Buete GH et al, Can computed tomography of the chest stage lung cancer? Yes and No, *Ann Thorac Surg* 1990; **49**:591–5.
41. Shung KK, Physics of blood echogenicity, *J Cardiovasc Ultrasound* 1991; **2**:401–6.
42. Goldberg BB, Liu JB, Merton DA et al, Sonographically guided laparoscopy and mediastinoscopy using miniature catheter-based transducers, *J Ultrasound Med* 1993; **12**:49–54.
43. Jakob H, Lorenz T, Clement N et al, Mediastinal lymph node staging with transesophageal echocardiography in cancer of the lung, *Eur J Cardiothorac Surg* 1990; **4**(8):355–8.
44. Patterson GA, Ginsberg RJ, Poon PY et al, A prospective evaluation of magnetic resonance imaging, computed tomography, and mediastinoscopy in the preoperative assessment of mediastinal node status in bronchogenic carcinoma, *J Thorac Cardiovasc Surg* 1987; **94**:679–84.
45. Wakabayashi A. Expanded applications of diagnostic and therapeutic thoracoscopy, *Thorac Cardiovasc Surg* 1991; **102**:721–3.
46. Catharp WH, Arnold JH, Alford WC, Videothoracoscopy: improved technique and expanded indications, *Ann Thorac Surg* 1992; **53**:776–9.
47. Lewis RJ, Caccavale RJ, Sisler GE, Imaged thorascopic lung biopsy, *Chest* 1992; **102**:60–2.
48. Finch IJ, Preoperative CT-guided percutaneous localization of small masses with a Kopans needle, *AJR* 1991; **157**:179–80.
49. Mack MJ, Gordon MJ, Postma TW, Percutaneous localization of pulmonary nodules for thoracoscopic lung resection, *Ann Thorac Surg* 1992; **53**: 1123–4.
50. Shah RM, Spirn PW, Salazar A et al, Localization of peripheral pulmonary nodules for thorascopic excision: value of CT-guided wire placement, *AJR* 1993; **161**:279–83.
51. Greenfield AL, Steiner RM, Liu JB et al, Sonographic guidance for the localization of peripheral pulmonary nodules during thoracoscopy, *AJR* 1997; **168**:1057–60.

Chapter 10 Reproductive tract

Barry B Goldberg, Anna S Lev-Toaff and Ji-Bin Liu

ENDOLUMINAL ULTRASOUND

The importance of ultrasound in the evaluation of a variety of gynecological abnormalities has been established. When the transabdominal approach is used, the ultrasound beam traverses a distended urinary bladder, allowing for the visualization of the uterus, ovaries and adjacent pelvic region. With the development of transvaginal probes, taking advantage of higher transducer frequencies and the closer proximity of the transducer to the uterus and ovaries, the capability of detecting smaller and subtler abnormalities has improved.[1] Presently, transvaginal ultrasound is considered by most authorities to be the approach of choice for evaluating the female pelvis.

The concept of using ultrasound to evaluate the endometrial canal goes back to the 1970s, when von Miscky developed an ultrasound transducer on the tip of a steel rod which could be inserted into the uterine cavity.[2] This rigid ultrasound transducer had limitations, including the need for cervical dilation prior to insertion. A similar type of probe was used in the 1980s by Hotzinger for the planning of radiation treatment for endometrial carcinoma.[3]

Flexible ultrasound transducer-containing catheters have now been developed for intravascular use to image atherosclerotic plaque and evaluate the results of intervention such as angioplasty and thrombectomy.[4–8] In the 1970s Bom developed the first real-time endoluminal transducer; however, it was not until several years ago that advances in instrumentation and catheter technology allowed for its commercial development.[9] We have used these intravascular ultrasound catheters in a variety of nonvascular lumina. Our initial work in animal models showed the feasibility of passing these catheters into the endometrial canal and fallopian tube.[10] It was hypothesized that this approach could be used to detect abnormalities of both the endometrium and adjacent myometrium.

INSTRUMENTATION AND TECHNIQUES

Ultrasound catheters, ranging in size from 6.2 to 9 Fr (2 mm and 3 mm in diameter, respectively), containing either a 20- or 12.5-MHz transducer, were utilized in our studies (Fig. 10.1). These catheters were developed by Boston Scientific (Sonicath™, Natick, MA) using ultrasound equipment by Diasonics (IVUS™, Santa Clara, CA). The transducer was offset at 10° from true perpendicular and revolved at 30 frames/s, producing 360° cross-sectional real-time ultrasound images. The sterile outer catheter sheath is disposable; the sterilized transducer core is reusable. Once the transducer core was inserted into the catheter, 1.0 ml of sterile water was injected, using a 27 gauge needle, through the sealed tip of the catheter. Water surrounding the transducer is the acoustic medium for ultrasound beam transmission. Care was taken to ensure that no air bubbles got inside the catheter tip.

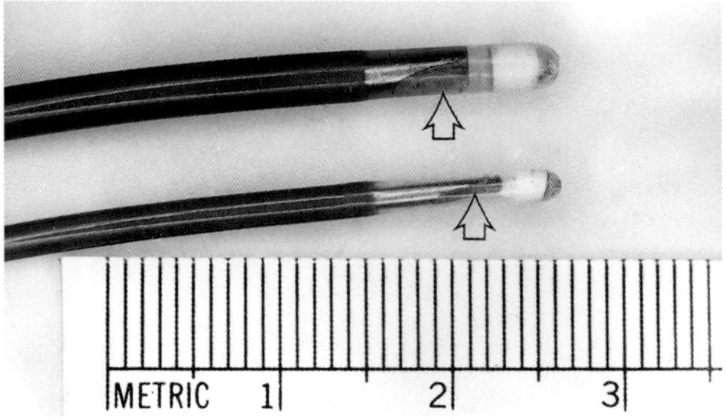

Figure 10.1 *Miniature catheter-based ultrasound transducers. Top, 9-Fr catheter housing a 12.5-MHz transducer (arrow); bottom, 6-Fr catheter containing a 20-MHz transducer (arrow). (Reproduced with permission from Goldberg et al.[19])*

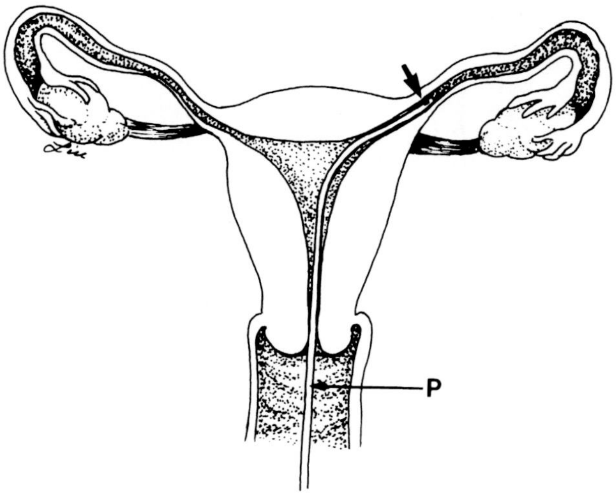

Figure 10.2 *A schematic representation of catheter-based ultrasound probe (P) passing transvaginally through the cervical canal into the endometrial canal and left fallopian tube. The distal tip of the probe is in the proximal tube (arrow).*

The procedures were performed in the operating room or in an ultrasound examination room with the patient placed in the dorsal lithotomy position. In each case a speculum was inserted into the vagina and a tenaculum was used to stabilize the cervix to facilitate passage of the catheter into the uterine cavity. The proximal catheter tip was coated with a small amount of sterile 2% lidocaine gel, which aided in the insertion of the catheter (Fig. 10.2). No cervical dilation was needed. The ultrasound images were monitored and recorded on videotape as the transducer was advanced in 3–5-mm increments until the fundus was reached. The ultrasound catheter was then withdrawn slowly. Under hysteroscopic guidance, the catheter was further advanced into the fallopian tubes. In some cases, transabdominal ultrasound examination was simultaneously carried out, resulting in the visualization of the catheter inside the endometrial canal.

ANIMAL STUDIES

As with any new technology, animal studies were initially carried out to test not only the instrument's feasibility but also its safety. In our initial animal research, we demonstrated the feasibility of using these catheter transducers in a variety of nonvascular lumina of the body.[10]

The ultrasound catheter was advanced through the cervix into the endometrial canal and then into the fallopian tubes in dog models. It was possible to obtain cross-sectional images of the uterus and fallopian tubes and to determine wall thickness and echotexture patterns (Fig. 10.3). In the fallopian tube, a pseudomass (a surgically created mucosal mass) was clearly imaged as a polyp-like protrusion (Fig. 10.4). To establish accuracy and reliability, multiple measurements of each structure seen sonographically were obtained and compared with measurements of autopsy specimens. Close correlation was found between these measurements and the cross-sectional anatomic specimens. The in vivo procedure caused no apparent intraluminal damage. No intimal flaps, lacerations or perforations were identified. This was confirmed at autopsy.

CLINICAL STUDIES

Evaluation of Vaginal Tumor in Children

Transabdominal and transperineal ultrasound have been used for initial diagnosis of vaginal tumors in young children. However, following response to chemotherapy and/or radiation treatment, these techniques proved limited for detailed evaluation of the vaginal wall to assess for residual or recurrent tumor. Transrectal ultrasound may be employed to examine the adjacent vaginal area and has been used to localize and guide transrectal needle biopsy in a child with a history of vaginal rhabdomyosarcoma and a recurrent vaginal mass.[11] There are inherent problems in examining the pediatric pelvis with this technique due to the relatively large size of the conventional endorectal probe. General anesthesia has been required to achieve adequate anal sphincter relaxation in order to accommodate the probe. Likewise, the size of the standard endovaginal probe prohibits the evaluation of the small pelvis of infants and children. We have assessed the usefulness and efficacy of endovaginal ultrasound using miniature catheter-based transducers (6.2 Fr, 20 MHz) for the evaluation of vaginal tumors in children.[12]

With use of the high-resolution miniature ultrasound transducer, it is feasible to demonstrate the normal vaginal wall in detail and to assess vaginal tumors. The layers of the vaginal wall and echotextures of each layer were imaged and measured (Fig. 10.5). The miniature ultrasound catheters (2 mm in

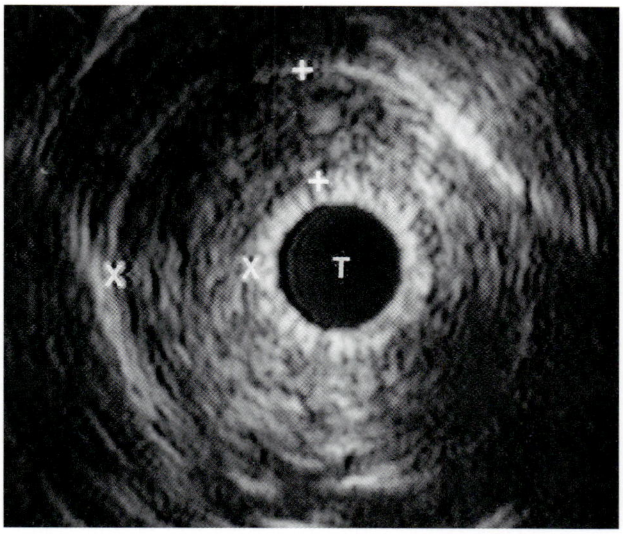

a

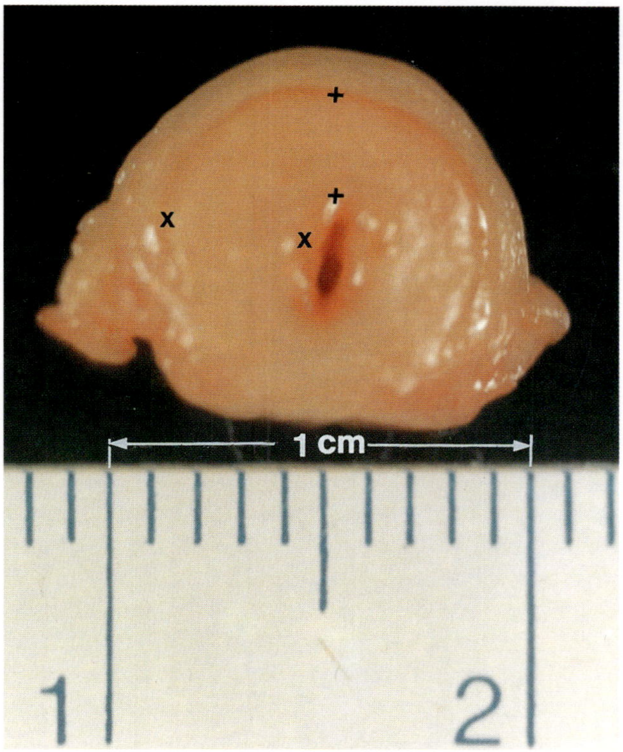

b

Figure 10.3 *(a) Cross-sectional sonogram of the uterus. The wall denoted by the calipers (+ and ×) measures 3.1–3.9 mm. T, transducer. (b) Corresponding image of the gross specimen demonstrates the close correlation between the ultrasound and anatomic measurements. Note the variation in thickness within the anatomic specimen, as also shown in the sonogram (+, anterior wall thickness; ×, right lateral wall thickness). (Reproduced with permission from Goldberg et al.[10])*

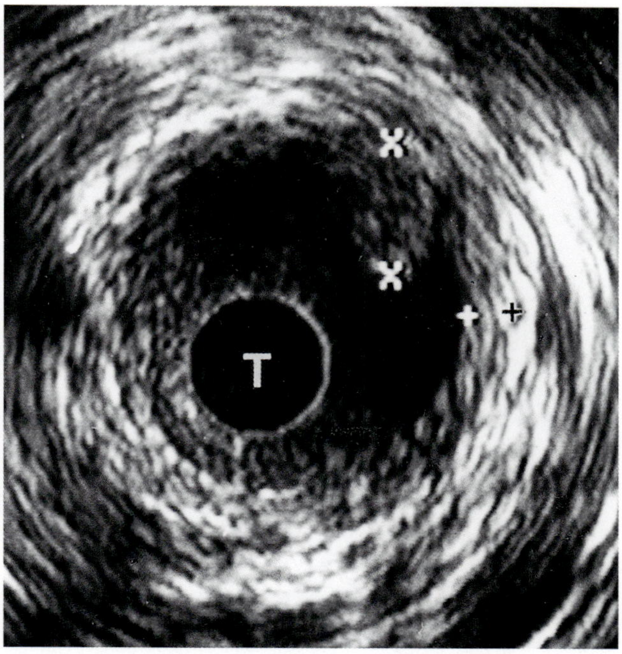

Figure 10.4 *The catheter-based ultrasound transducer (T) is located within the saline-distended fallopian tube. A polyp-like protrusion measuring 3.6 mm was clearly identified (between calipers, ×). The wall of the fallopian tube measured 1.2 mm (between calipers, +). (Reproduced with permission from Goldberg et al.[10])*

diameter) made it possible to examine the vagina via a transvaginal approach, which we found to be well tolerated by the young patients. If necessary, hydrosonovaginography can be employed simultaneously by utilizing a slender catheter alongside the transducer and injecting sterile water into the vagina.

For the evaluation of young children with vaginal tumors, routine transabdominal pelvic ultrasound is still the primary tool to rule out metastasis, lymphadenopathy and ascites. Based on our limited experience, we feel that endovaginal ultrasound using a catheter-based probe is feasible and reliable for following local tumor, residual or recurrent, in young girls treated for vaginal cancer, and may obviate the need for computed tomography (CT) and magnetic resonance imaging (MRI).

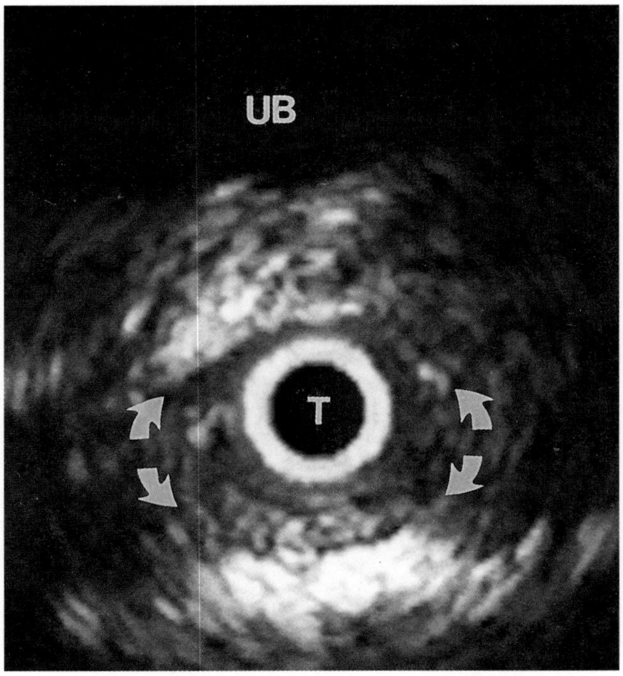

a

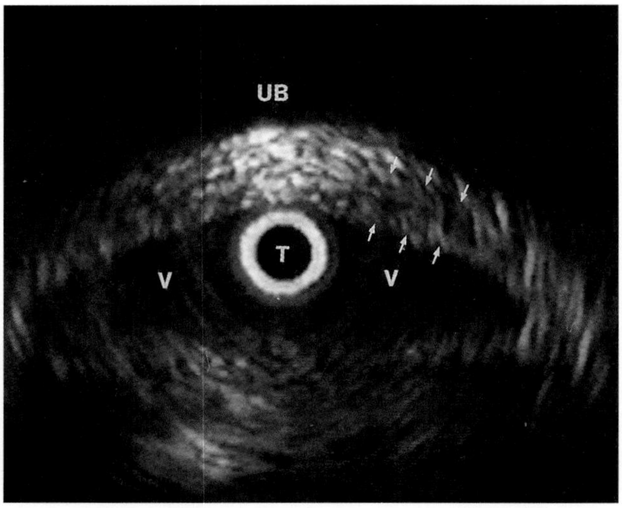

b

Figure 10.5 *(a) In a young child after radiation therapy for a rhabdomyosarcoma of the vagina, endoluminal ultrasound image of the vagina demonstrates the wall of the vagina (arrows) without focal mass or alteration of the echotexture to suggest tumor recurrence. (b) After instilling sterile water into the vagina (V) the layers of the vaginal wall (arrows) are more optimally imaged and discrete layers of the vaginal wall are demonstrated. T, transducer; UB, urinary bladder.*

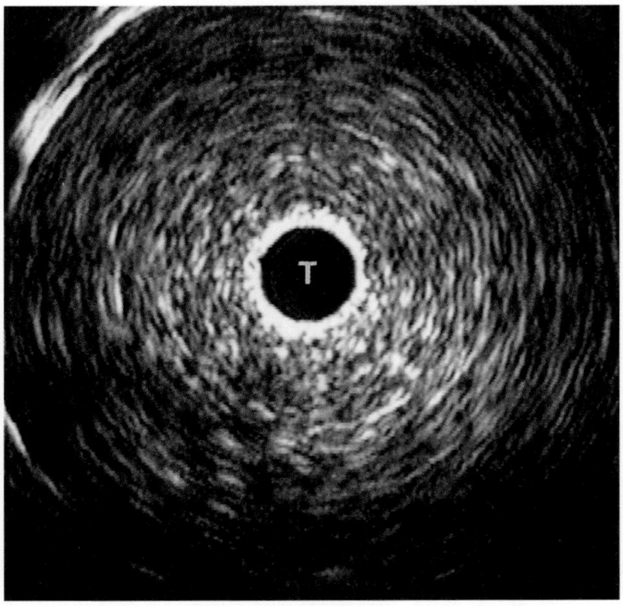

Figure 10.6 *20 MHz ultrasound image obtained from within the endometrial canal demonstrates the uniform echogenic texture of the normal uterus. This patient was at the beginning of her menstrual cycle and thus the endometrial lining is thin and not imaged separately from the homogeneous myometrium. T, transducer.*

Evaluation of Uterus and Fallopian Tubes

Patients presenting with a variety of symptoms, most commonly abnormal uterine bleeding, were evaluated by endoluminal ultrasound. It was possible to image the endometrium and adjacent myometrium (Fig. 10.6). Initial results have shown this method to be helpful in differentiating between various causes of abnormal bleeding. Endoluminal ultrasound has demonstrated submucosal or mural myomas and good correlation has been obtained with the cross-sectional pathologic specimens (Fig. 10.7). Myomas as small as 5 mm in diameter (Fig. 10.8) and cervical nabothian cysts (Fig. 10.9) have been identified. Endometrial hyperplasia has been identified and subsequently confirmed histologically following hysterectomy or hysteroscopy.

In a patient with abnormal uterine bleeding, transabdominal ultrasound demonstrated a thickened hyperechoic endometrium, but the nature of the lesion could not be determined (i.e. polyp versus

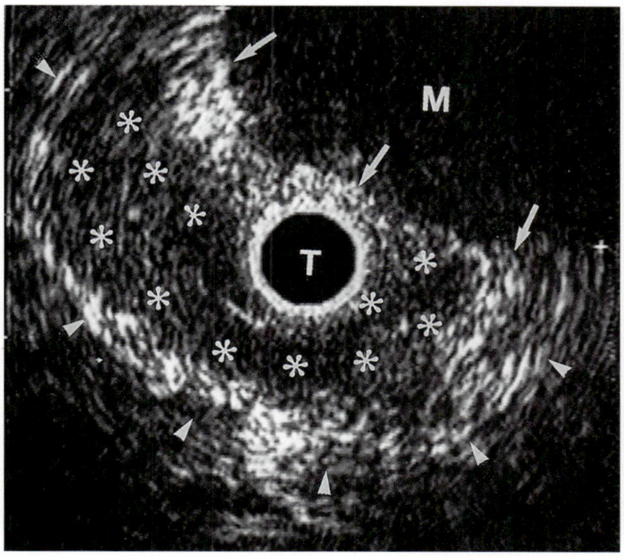

a

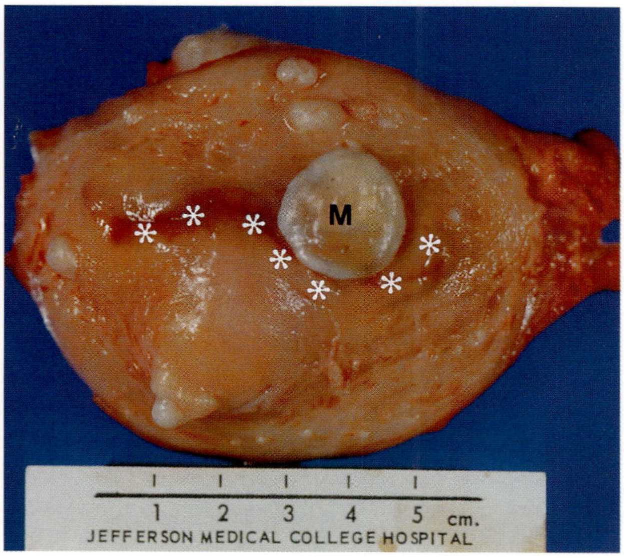

b

Figure 10.7 *(a) Cross-sectional ultrasound image obtained from within the endometrial canal (at the level of the uterine corpus) demonstrates a 1.8-cm hypoechoic submucous myoma (M) displacing the echogenic outer endometrial echoes (arrows). On this endoluminal sonogram at mid-cycle the endometrium has a striated appearance with an outer echogenic layer (arrowheads) and a thicker inner hypoechoic layer (asterisks). T, transducer. (b) Cross-sectional image of the specimen obtained at the same level as in (a) shows the submucosal myoma (M) impinging on the endometrial cavity (asterisks). (Reproduced with permission from Goldberg et al.[19])*

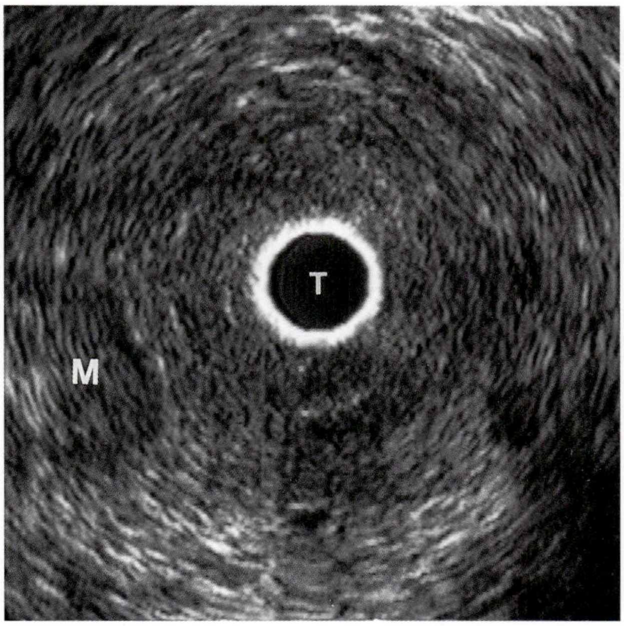

Figure 10.8 *Cross-sectional image of the uterus demonstrates a small hypoechoic mural myoma measuring 5 mm in diameter (M). T, transducer.*

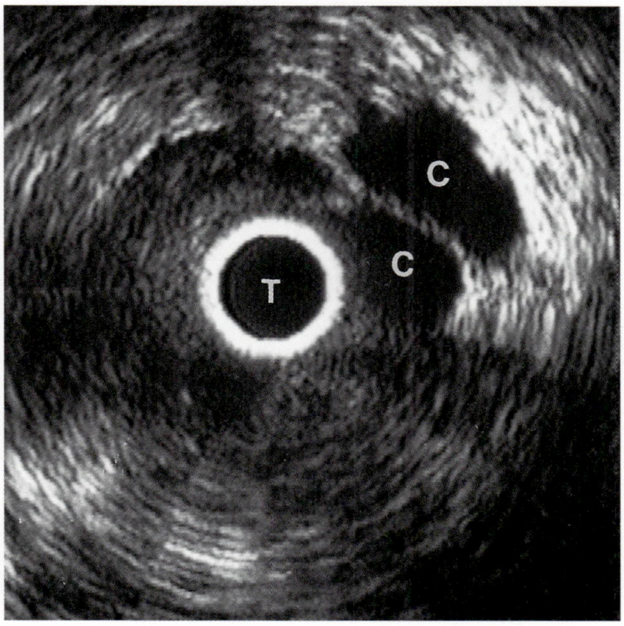

Figure 10.9 *Cross-sectional image obtained from the cervical region delineates two nabothian cysts (C) seen as echo free areas with distal enhancement. T, transducer. (Reproduced with permission from Goldberg et al.[19])*

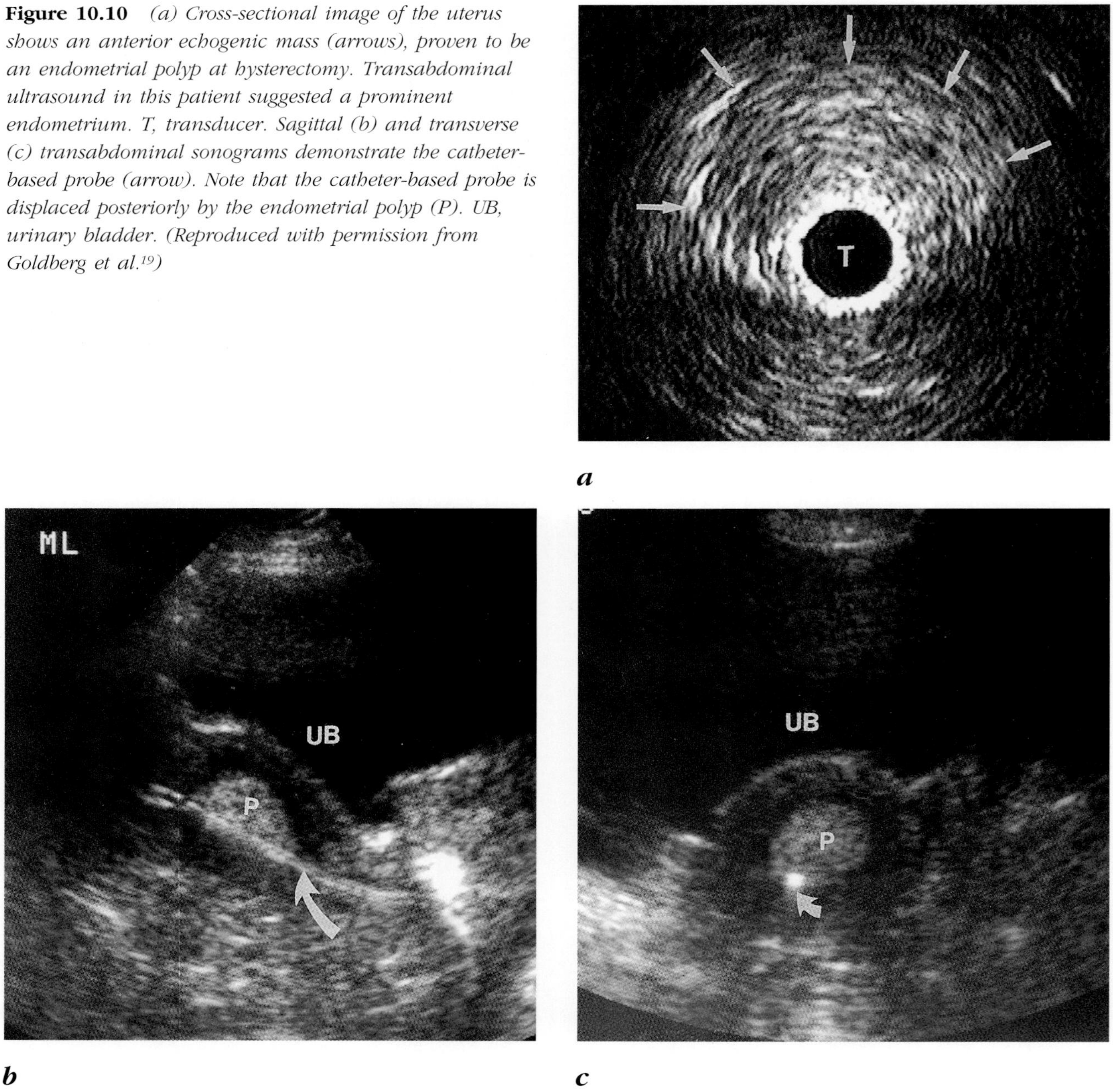

Figure 10.10 *(a) Cross-sectional image of the uterus shows an anterior echogenic mass (arrows), proven to be an endometrial polyp at hysterectomy. Transabdominal ultrasound in this patient suggested a prominent endometrium. T, transducer. Sagittal (b) and transverse (c) transabdominal sonograms demonstrate the catheter-based probe (arrow). Note that the catheter-based probe is displaced posteriorly by the endometrial polyp (P). UB, urinary bladder. (Reproduced with permission from Goldberg et al.[19])*

diffuse endometrial hyperplasia). The ultrasound catheter, when inserted into the endometrial canal, was displaced posteriorly by the hyperechoic mass. In diffuse endometrial hyperplasia, one would expect the catheter to be surrounded by the hyperechoic tissue. The relative positions of the catheter and this abnormal area were confirmed by transabdominal ultrasound (Fig. 10.10). At subsequent hysterectomy an anteriorly located endometrial polyp measuring 2.0×1.0 cm was identified. With the use of endoluminal ultrasound, synechiae were also identified within the endometrial canal and at the uterotubal junction (Fig. 10.11).

Carcinoma of the endometrium and cervix is the most common malignancy of the female reproductive tract.[13] A variety of imaging techniques are used to evaluate endometrial malignancy, including ultrasound, CT and MRI. However, microinvasive lesions

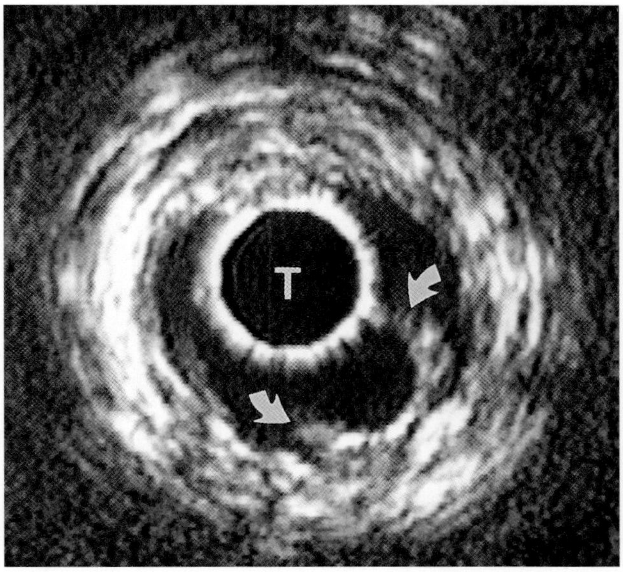

Figure 10.11 *Catheter-based transducer (T) was hysteroscopically placed into the proximal left fallopian tube, which was irrigated with saline. Note the synechia (arrows) at the uterotubal junction. (Reproduced with permission from Goldberg et al.[19])*

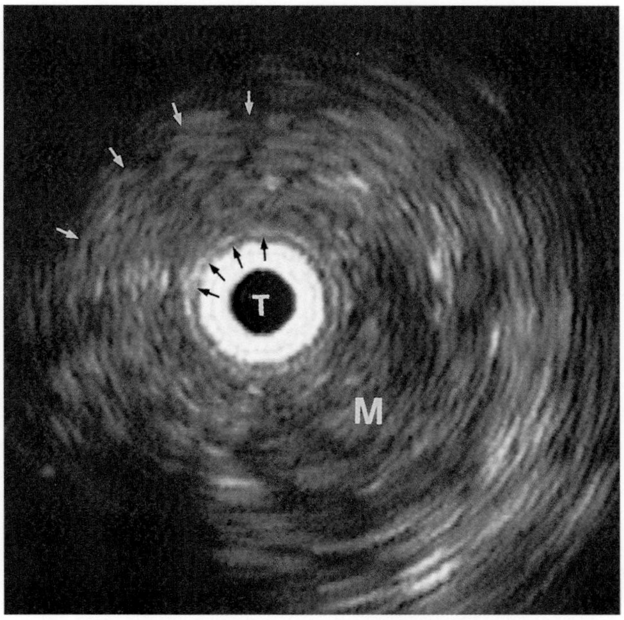

Figure 10.12 *Transcervical cross-sectional sonogram shows an irregular hypoechoic mass (M), proven at biopsy to be a cervical carcinoma. Note the more hyperechoic homogeneous echotexture of the normal cervical tissue (arrows). T, transducer.*

cannot be imaged with these conventional techniques. When lesions are below the resolution of these imaging techniques, hysterosalpingography, hysteroscopy, dilation and curettage (D&C) or endometrial biopsy can be used. The surgical approaches require the passage of an instrument into the endometrial canal after cervical dilation. Although hysterosalpingography visualizes the uterine cavity, the nature of intrauterine filling defects is more accurately revealed by hysteroscopy.[14] Although both of these methods can be used to visualize surface irregularities, they will not show changes beneath the endometrial surface. Conventional transabdominal and transvaginal ultrasound have been used to assess endometrial and cervical cancer invasion.[15,16]

Kikuchi et al have reported on the utility of intrauterine ultrasound with catheter-based high-frequency probes in the evaluation of myometrial invasion by endometrial carcinoma and endocervical invasion by cervical carcinoma.[17,18] They studied 48 patients with cervical carcinoma using both transvaginal and transcervical ultrasound and compared results with histologic and surgical findings. Intracervical ultrasound depicted the lesion in 8 of 16 patients (50%) in whom the depth of tumor invasion was less than or equal to 5 mm, whereas transvaginal ultrasound failed to depict the lesions in all patients. Intracervical ultrasound detected the lesions in all 19 patients with more than 5 mm tumor invasion, whereas transvaginal ultrasound was successful in only 14 cases (74%). However, because of the attenuation of the high-frequency ultrasound, intracervical ultrasound could not clearly demonstrate parametrial involvement.[17]

With the use of endoluminal ultrasound, we have studied patients with known cervical cancer and with suspected endometrial carcinoma to evaluate extent of tumor invasion.[19] In some cases, initial D&C confirmed the presence of malignant cells, but it was uncertain as to the exact location or extent of the cancer. The cervical tumors appear as irregular hyper- and hypoechoic areas, distinctly different from the normal cervix, which has a uniform echotexture (Fig. 10.12). In endometrial carcinoma, the ultrasound images showed relatively hypoechoic masses arising from the endometrium invading into the

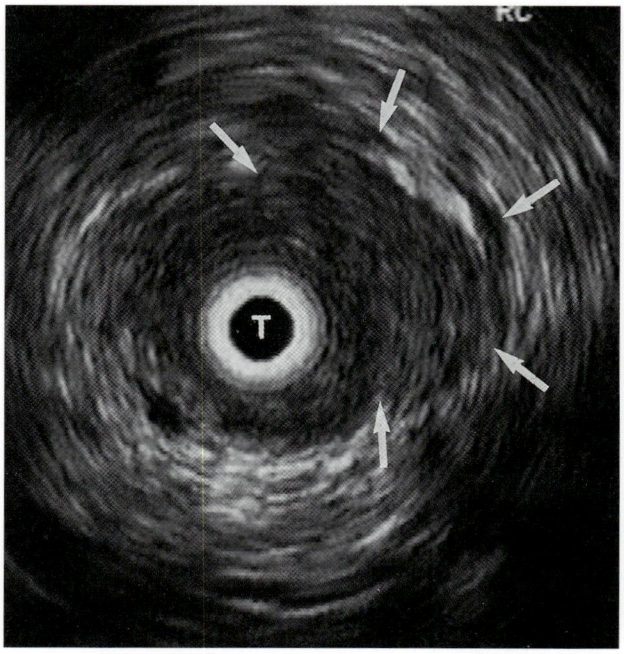

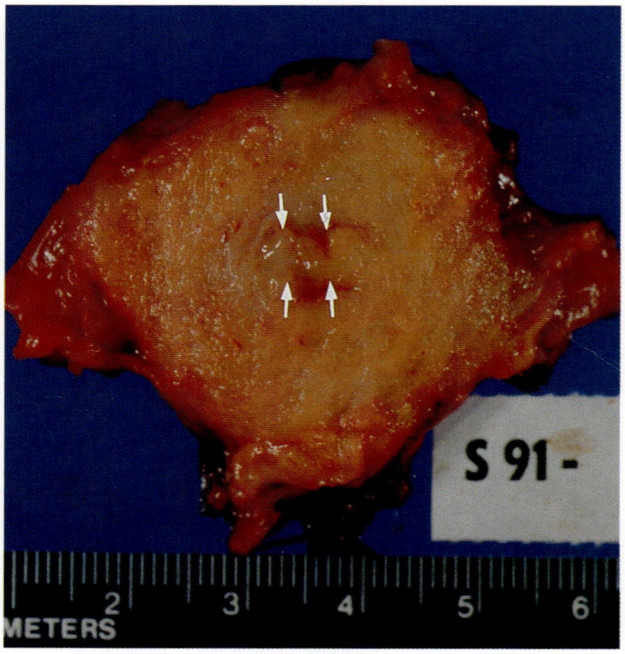

a *b*

Figure 10.13 *(a) Cross-sectional image obtained from the lower uterine segment reveals an eccentric irregular hypoechoic mass with focal invasion of the myometrium (arrows). (b) This was confirmed pathologically to be a stage I endometrial carcinoma (arrows) with focal invasion of only the inner one-third of the myometrium.*

myometrium (Fig. 10.13). Preliminary results suggest that transcervical and intrauterine ultrasound may be useful for evaluating invasion of cervical and endometrial carcinoma.[17–19]

Preliminary work has been carried out using these ultrasound catheters, inserted through a hysteroscope, for evaluation of the fallopian tube.[19,20] With this approach, it may be possible to detect a variety of abnormalities, such as masses blocking the tube. With insertion of these catheters through a laparoscope, external evaluation of fallopian tubes is also under investigation.[21] This approach (i.e. pelvic laparoscopic ultrasound) could prove helpful in the detection of small ovarian and tubal abnormalities, including early ectopic pregnancies and small tumors within normal-sized ovaries (Figs 10.14 and 10.15).[21]

Evaluation of the Embryo

As an investigational technique, ultrasound catheters have been inserted into the endometrial canal to image early gestations prior to voluntary termination of first-trimester pregnancy.[22,23] In none of the patients did the ultrasound catheter rupture the fluid-filled chorionic/amniotic cavity. Transcervical ultrasound was able to identify the yolk sac and embryonic structures, such as brain vesicles, heart, limb buds, liver, spinal canal, and umbilical cord with bloodflow at 5–8 weeks menstrual age (Fig. 10.16).[22,23] The neural tube is particularly suited for endoluminal ultrasound examination because of its fluid-filled structure. The information gleaned from such a study might facilitate the detection of a neural tube defect earlier than is possible at present. The initial results suggest that transcervical ultrasound may be used as an investigating tool to study the embryologic development of the human embryo.

Transcervical ultrasound is an invasive, investigational technique that offers a novel diagnostic approach to study the early human embryo. Unlike the safety of chorionic villus sampling, which has been well established,[24] the safety of transcervical ultrasound and its clinical applications is yet to be

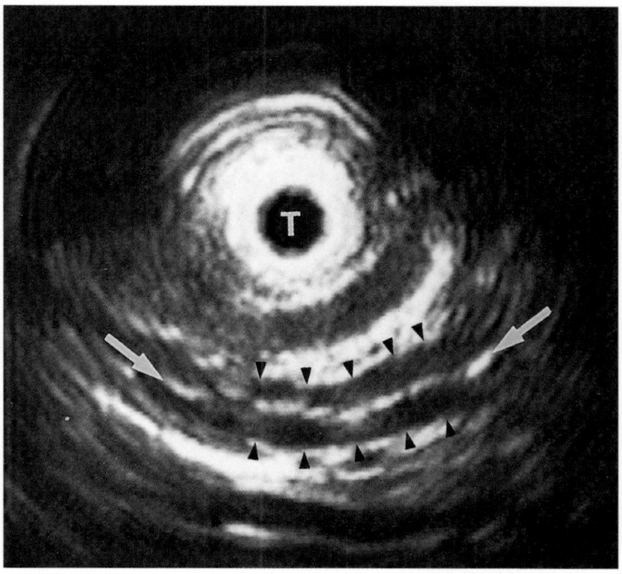

Figure 10.14 *Longitudinal sonogram of the fallopian tube obtained laparoscopically by the catheter-based transducer (T) delineates a central echogenic interface representing the tubal lumen (arrows) surrounded by hypoechoic muscular layers (arrowheads). (Reproduced with permission from Goldberg et al.[21])*

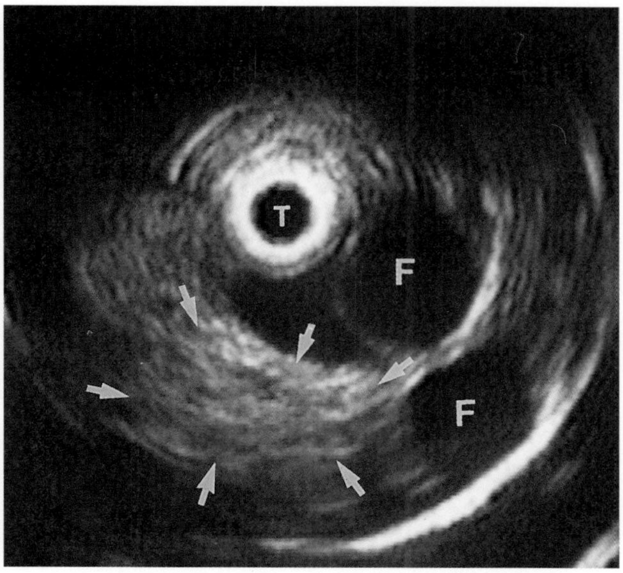

Figure 10.15 *Sonogram obtained at laparoscopy using the catheter-based transducer (T) demonstrates a hyperechoic mass (arrows) within a normal-sized ovary, representing an ovarian dermoid. The tumor was removed laparoscopically through a small incision in the ovary under ultrasound guidance. F, follicles.*

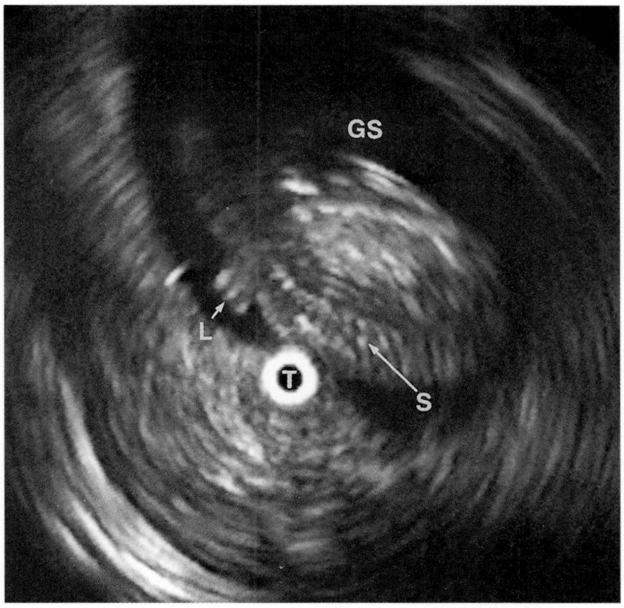

Figure 10.16 *Catheter-based transducer (T) is located within the endometrial canal posterior to an 8-week gestational sac (GS) just prior to elective abortion. Portions of the embryonic trunk are shown. L, limb bud; S, spine.*

defined. Therefore, it is stressed that until more data are available on the safety of this technique, particularly relating to the possibility of catheter-induced abortion, we do not recommend it for routine use in pregnancy.

POTENTIAL CLINICAL USES AND LIMITATIONS

Transvaginal ultrasound provides additional information compared to transabdominal ultrasound in up to 23% of the cases examined in one study.[25] The advantage of transvaginal ultrasound is the proximity of the probe to the area of interest, allowing utilization of a higher-frequency transducer, 5–7.5 MHz versus 3.5–5 MHz, for the abdominal approach. The same concept applies to the new endoluminal approach. However, since the transducer utilizes frequencies of either 12.5 or 20 MHz, its major limitation is its inability to penetrate beyond a radius of 2 cm when using the 20-MHz transducer and 3 cm when using the 12.5-MHz transducer. Thus, its usefulness is limited to abnormalities involving areas within or adjacent to the cervical, endometrial or fallopian tube lumina.

Its most practical use may be in the evaluation of dysfunctional uterine bleeding. The differential diagnosis includes submucosal myomas, polyps, hyperplasia, chronic endometritis, atrophic endometrium and endometrial or cervical carcinoma. While it has been shown that transvaginal and abdominal ultrasound can demonstrate some of these abnormalities, the cause of bleeding cannot be established sonographically in most cases. This new ultrasound approach shows promise as a technique able to differentiate among some of these conditions.

It has been reported that myomas are present in 22% of those cases in which the abdominal ultrasound examination is normal.[26] The ability to position the endoluminal high-frequency transducer closer to the area of interest improves our detection of small myomas, provided that they are adjacent to the endometrial canal. With this approach, myomas as small as 5 mm have been identified. With a larger myoma (>3 cm) only that portion adjacent to the canal is imaged. In addition, the location of the myomas relative to the endometrial canal is delineated.

Endometrial hyperplasia appears as a focal thickening of increased echogenicity within the endometrium. Endoluminal ultrasound also has the potential capability to identify synechiae and endometrial polyps.

This method should prove useful in the evaluation of foreign bodies, such as the location of intrauterine devices (IUDs) when they are completely or partially embedded in the uterine wall. The ability to locate embedded stones within the ureter and renal parenchyma has proven the feasibility of this approach.[27] Not only could the stone be identified, but also its exact depth beneath the surface measured. This information may aid the gynecologist in choosing the best approach for the retrieval of a lost IUD. Ultrasound guidance for IUD removal is possible for minimally embedded IUDs, whereas a hysteroscopic approach might be chosen for the more deeply embedded ones.

Clinically, the endometrial canal can be evaluated by such techniques as hysterosalpingography, hysteroscopy, endometrial biopsy and D&C. In the evaluation of the endometrial cavity, hysteroscopy can provide direct visualization of intrauterine abnormalities. It has proven particularly useful for submucosal myomas, polyps, and synechiae.[28] Endouterine ultrasound imaging has advantages over both hysteroscopy and hysterosalpingography in its ability to image beyond the mucosal surface. As an initial diagnostic procedure, it makes mechanical dilation of the cervix unnecessary and may provide direction for choosing the next diagnostic or therapeutic step. D&C may miss small lesions or endometrial polyps.[29] In addition, because ultrasound avoids ionizing radiation it has inherent advantages over hysterosalpingography, which requires both iodinated contrast material and fluoroscopy.

Both abdominal and transvaginal ultrasound have been used preoperatively to evaluate endometrial carcinoma. Myometrial invasion can be demonstrated with a sensitivity as high as 79%.[30] However, polypoid intraluminal growth is one of the most common factors confounding the ultrasound evaluation, probably due to the marked distortion of the uterine cavity filled by tumor.[31] Endoluminal ultrasound has demonstrated that invasive endometrial and cervical cancer disrupt the normal uniform echotexture of the uterus and cervix. Preliminary studies have shown the usefulness of endouterine ultrasound in the detection and staging of these tumors.[17–19] Further studies in a larger number of cases are needed before its full efficacy is established.

Transabdominal and transvaginal ultrasound are still the primary tools for the evaluation of a variety of gynecologic abnormalities. Preliminary studies using these specially developed ultrasound catheters in a variety of gynecologic cases suggest its potential as a new tool to supplement the established methods of transabdominal and transvaginal ultrasound.

TRANSVAGINAL SONOHYSTEROGRAPHY

Traditionally, imaging of the uterine cavity has been accomplished either indirectly by hysterosalpingography or directly by hysteroscopy. These techniques were reportedly more accurate than transabdominal ultrasound in the detection of intracavitary abnormalities.[32,33] Since the late 1980s, transvaginal ultrasound (TVU) has significantly improved the ability to evaluate the female pelvis. The value of TVU in the detection of abnormalities of the uterus and ovaries has been recognized.[25,34] Currently, TVU is the imaging method of choice for evaluating endometrial abnormalities, particularly in patients with abnormal vaginal bleeding.[35–40] This technique is highly sensitive for detecting small endometrial lesions, but is nonspecific. Recently, transvaginal sonohysterography, which is sonographic imaging of the uterus and uterine cavity distended with saline or contrast agents, has been reported to improve uterine imaging and to assist in the diagnosis of various uterine and fallopian tube abnormalities.[41–50]

TECHNIQUE CONSIDERATIONS

Most commercially available ultrasound systems have the capability of performing transvaginal examinations, and can be used for sonohysterography. The optimum transvaginal probe is a 3.5–7 MHz multifrequency transducer with color and pulsed Doppler capabilities. The following sterile instruments are needed for transvaginal sonohysterography: a single-hinged speculum, ring forceps, saline cup, cotton balls, antiseptic solution, 20-ml and 60-ml syringes, lubricating gel (use water instead of gel in infertility patients, because some gels have spermicidal properties), sound (to be used when there is difficulty passing the catheter), balloon-bearing catheters (5 or 7 Fr), and a light source.

In women with regular menstrual cycles, sonohysterography is best performed during the mid-follicular phase after cessation of menses. In women with irregular bleeding, the examination should be performed soon after cessation of bleeding. Initially, TVU should be performed to obtain a preliminary impression just before the procedure. With the patient in the dorsal lithotomy position, a single-hinged speculum is inserted vaginally, and the exocervix is exposed and cleansed with antiseptic solution. We use a 5 or 7 Fr balloon-bearing catheter (Ackrad Laboratories, Cranford, NJ) to inject saline or contrast medium into the uterine cavity (Fig. 10.17). Although some practitioners use catheters without balloons, we have found that the balloon assists in maintaining optimal distention of the uterine cavity during the examination and is well tolerated. The catheter should initially be flushed free of air with sterile saline and inserted into the lower uterine segment; the balloon is inflated with sterile saline (Fig. 10.18). After the speculum is removed, a condom-covered vaginal probe is inserted. The position of the catheter is first assessed. The catheter is then pulled back gently to the level of the internal os under real-time ultrasound monitoring (Fig. 10.19). The volume of the saline in the balloon may need to be adjusted under ultrasound visualization. Distention of the uterine cavity is accomplished by instillation of 20–40 ml of sterile saline during continuous real-time ultrasound examination. Both sagittal and coronal images of the uterus and ovaries should be obtained, using both gray-scale and color Doppler imaging. The study is recorded on videotape and hard copy film for later analysis and documentation. The entire procedure usually takes 10 min and no short- or long-term complications have been noted by us or reported by others. However, the potential

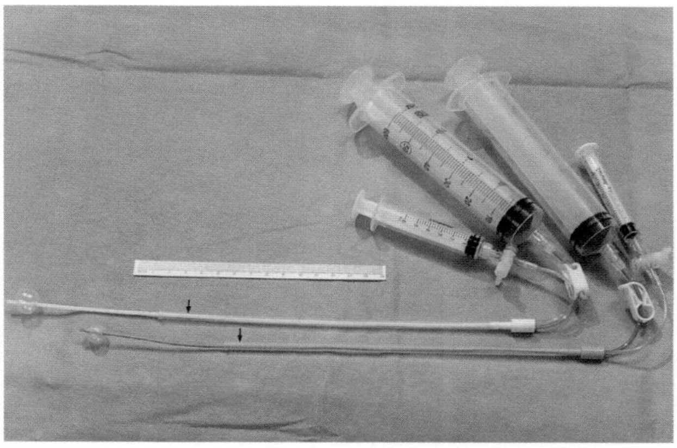

Figure 10.17 *Balloon-tipped catheters that we use for sonohysterography. The upper white catheter is 7 Fr and lower blue catheter is 5 Fr. Note that the rigid plastic tube (arrows) which houses the catheter allows the catheter to be advanced into the uterus without the use of a tenaculum. The outer plastic tube is positioned over the end of the catheter and placed against the external cervical os while the catheter is advanced.*

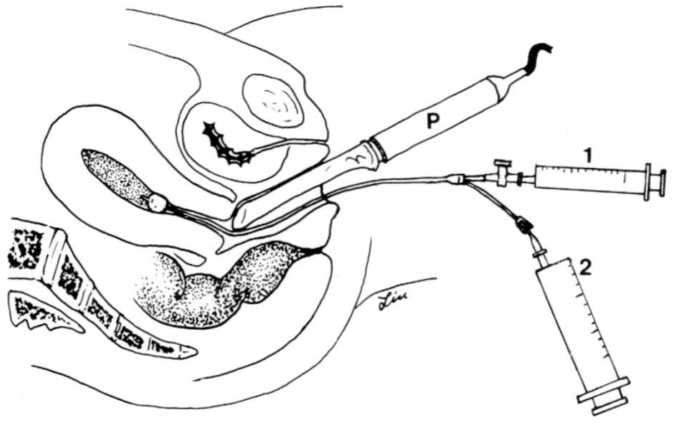

Figure 10.18 *A diagrammatic representation of transvaginal sonohysterography with a balloon-tipped catheter located in the lower uterine segment and the transvaginal probe in place. 1, balloon-inflating syringe; 2, contrast injection syringe; P, transvaginal probe.*

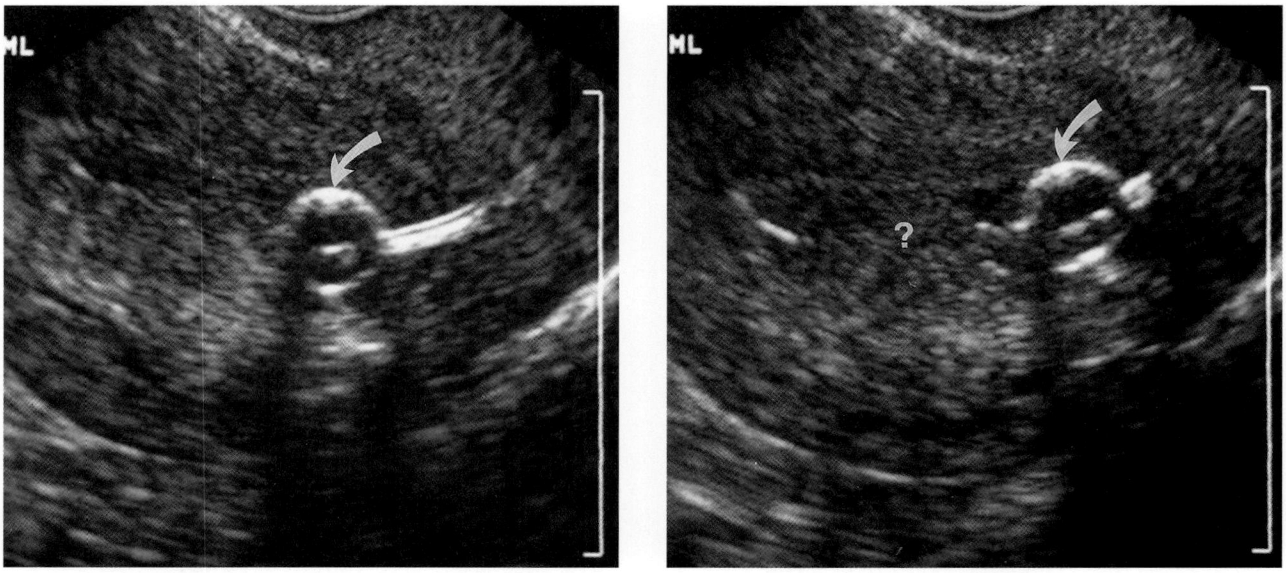

a *b*

Figure 10.19 *Optimal positioning of the balloon-tipped catheter in the lower segment of the uterus. (a) Initial image shows the catheter in the uterine corpus. (b) After pulling back gently, the catheter tip is now located in the lower uterine segment caudal to the abnormality (?) to be assessed.*

risks of sonohysterography are infection and perforation. Dissemination of an endometrial carcinoma is a theoretical risk, given the injection of fluid through the fallopian tubes. This concern (relating to X-ray hysterosalpingography and endometrial carcinoma) was addressed by Devore, who showed no difference in survival between two groups of patients with endometrial carcinoma (one with tubal patency and the other with tubal occlusion) who underwent hysterosalpingography.[51] Nontheless, it is recommended to avoid high-pressure injection when endometrial carcinoma is possible or suspected; sterile water instead of saline is used to cause lysis of any free neoplastic cells.

CLINICAL APPLICATIONS

Endometrial and Myometrial Abnormalities

Abnormal uterine bleeding is frequently caused by pathologic processes involving the endometrium (e.g. polyps, hyperplasia, atrophy, carcinoma) and the myometrium (e.g. fibroids). TVU is an effective imaging method for detecting small uterine masses and endometrial abnormalities. However, a major limitation of this technique is its inability to differentiate precisely between various types of endometrial abnormalities such as hyperplasia, polyp and carcinoma. In addition, the exact location of a lesion relative to the uterine cavity is often unclear. It is sometimes impossible to differentiate between a small central fibroid and an endometrial lesion. For example, a degenerated fibroid located centrally may mimic an endometrial abnormality. When a fibroid is located centrally and the endometrial echo complex is not well depicted, it is frequently difficult to define whether this is intracavitary, submucous or mural. These distinctions are clinically significant, since the surgical approach may vary depending on these factors.[52]

An abnormal TVU examination suggesting diffuse or focal endometrial thickening or irregularity or a centrally located fibroid, possibly submucous, is an indication for transvaginal sonohysterography. If the uterus is enlarged by multiple fibroids and the endometrial echo complex cannot be clearly delineated, sonohysterography may provide important information, especially if conservative uterine-sparing

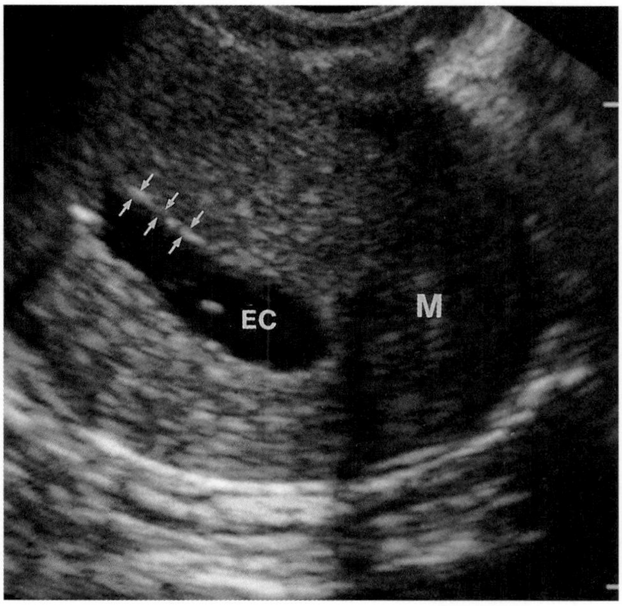

Figure 10.20 *Sagittal sonohysterogram in a retroverted uterus shows a normal thin endometrium (arrows). The endometrial cavity (EC) has a normal shape, unaffected by the small mural myoma (M).*

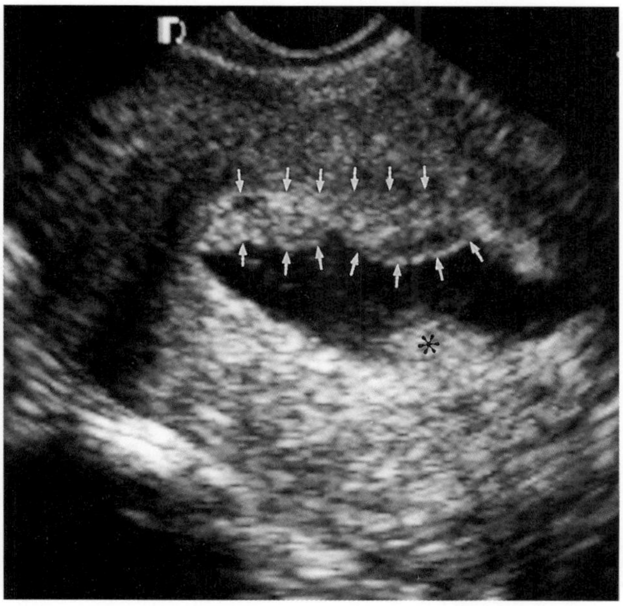

Figure 10.21 *Endometrial hyperplasia. Coronal sonohysterogram shows thick nodular endometrium anteriorly (arrows). Endometrial hyperplasia cannot be reliably distinguished from early endometrial carcinoma. Sonohysterography helps to direct the endometrial sampling to the area of abnormality. A polyp (asterisk) is also present.*

surgery is being considered. It should not be assumed in the presence of fibroids and abnormal bleeding that the fibroids are the etiology of the bleeding.[52] On multiple occasions we have identified endometrial polyps as the cause of bleeding in women with uterine fibroids. Other indications include evaluating the endometrial versus myometrial changes in women on tamoxifen, evaluation of uterine malformations, synechiae, and assessment of the uterine cavity after myomectomy, metroplasty, lysis of synechiae, etc. We have also used sonohysterography, instead of X-ray hysterosalpingography, in women who are allergic to iodinated contrast.

With the use of sonohysterography, normal endometrium (Fig. 10.20) and adjacent myometrium can be clearly imaged, and endometrial thickening (diffuse or focal) can be readily distinguished from other intracavitary pathologic conditions (Fig. 10.21). The normal thickness of the endometrium (double-layer thickness) in postmenopausal women without hormone replacement therapy is, according to many studies, 5 mm or less.[36,37,40,42,53–56] An endometrium more than 8 mm in thickness is indicative of possible hyperplasia, polyp or malignancy. If the endometrium measures more than 15 mm, biopsy, D&C or hysteroscopy is necessary regardless of symptoms or hormonal status. Endometrial carcinoma appears as irregularly thickened endometrium with variable echogenicity. The endometrium–myometrium junction may or may not be intact.[42] Careful examination of the myometrium for tumor invasion is necessary if the junction is not intact.

Endometrial polyps are a common lesion, encountered most frequently in women between the ages of 40 and 50. Abnormal bleeding is the most typical clinical presentation; polyps may also be the cause of infertility. Although the occurrence of carcinoma within a benign endometrial polyp is rare, Pettersson et al reported that endometrial polyps are associated

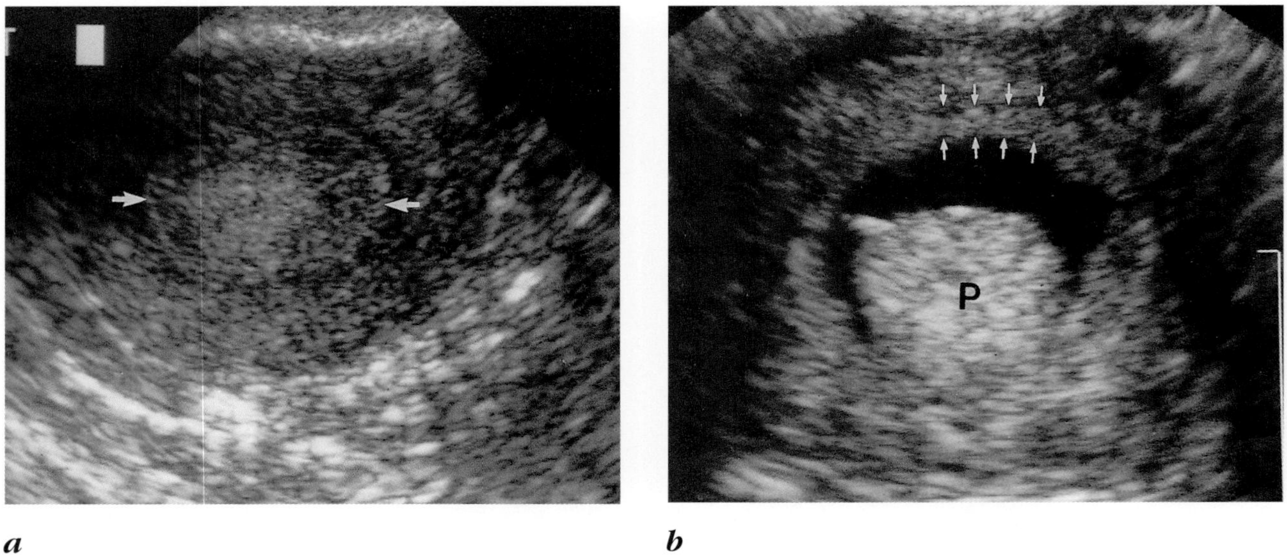

Figure 10.22 *Single endometrial polyp. (a) Preliminary transvaginal coronal image demonstrates a thick endometrial echo complex (arrows). (b) Coronal sonohysterogram shows a hyperechoic mass with smooth margins attached to the posterior wall of the uterus, consistent with an endometrial polyp (P). The endometrium is of normal thickness (arrows).*

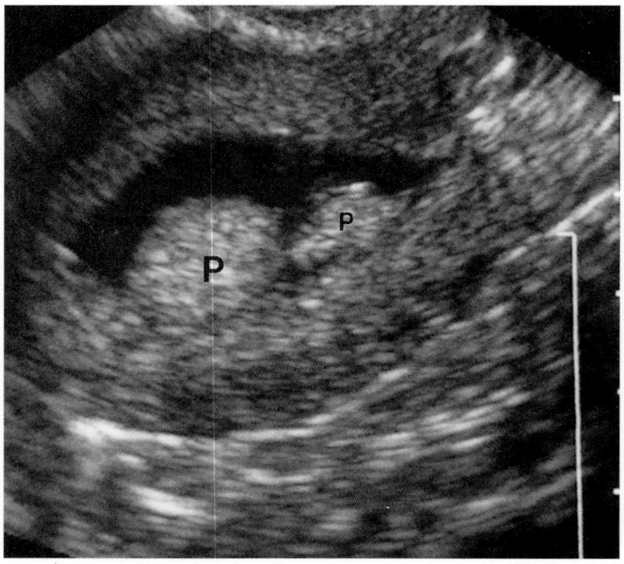

Figure 10.23 *Multiple endometrial polyps. Sagittal sonohysterogram shows two hyperechoic masses (P) attached to the posterior uterine wall.*

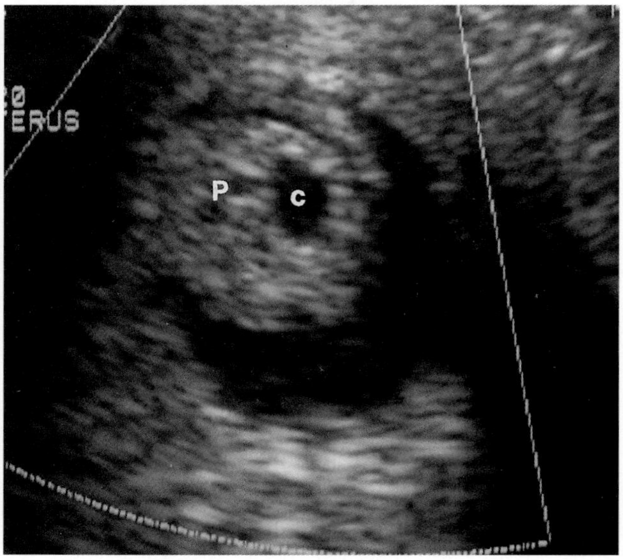

Figure 10.24 *Endometrial polyp associated with tamoxifen therapy. Coronal sonohysterogram shows a solitary polyp (P) with cystic changes (c).*

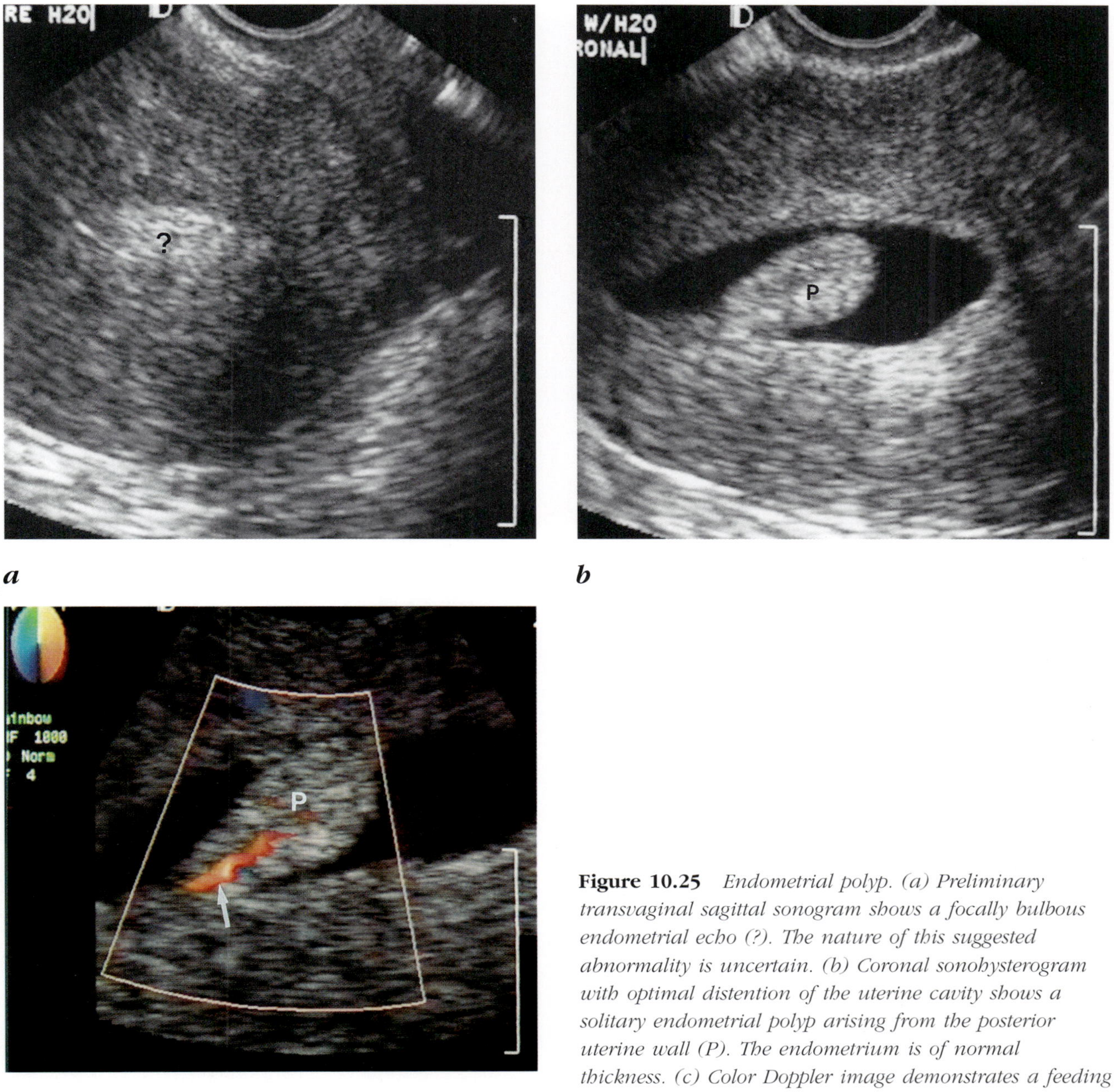

a *b* *c*

Figure 10.25 *Endometrial polyp. (a) Preliminary transvaginal sagittal sonogram shows a focally bulbous endometrial echo (?). The nature of this suggested abnormality is uncertain. (b) Coronal sonohysterogram with optimal distention of the uterine cavity shows a solitary endometrial polyp arising from the posterior uterine wall (P). The endometrium is of normal thickness. (c) Color Doppler image demonstrates a feeding vessel (arrow) at the base of the polyp.*

with a threefold increase in the incidence of endometrial carcinoma.[55] Endometrial polyps range in size from very small (mm) to large masses filling the entire endometrial cavity; they appear as smooth hyperechoic (usually homogeneous) masses with well-defined margins. They may be sessile or pedunculated; small cystic spaces are occasionally visible. In most cases a solitary polyp is found; in 20% of cases there are multiple polyps (Figs 10.22–10.24). A feeding vessel and small vessels within the polyp may be noted using color Doppler imaging (Fig. 10.25). This technique helps to assess the vascularity of a lesion and define the point of attachment of an intracavitary mass.

Fibroids, or leiomyomas, are the most common uterine neoplasm, occurring in 20–30% of women

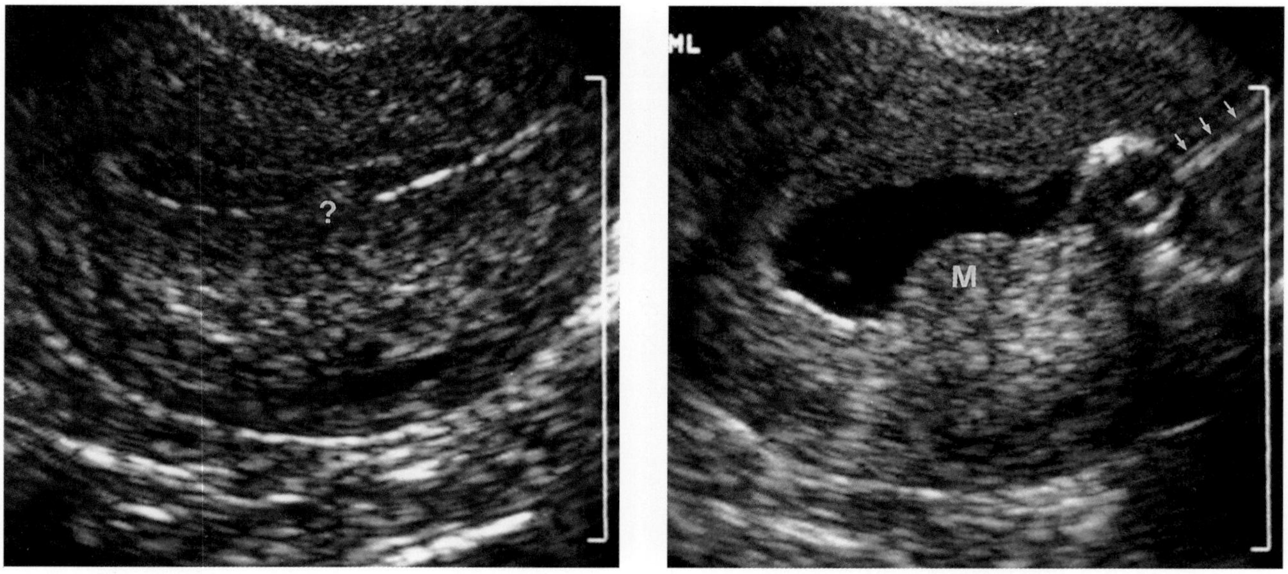

a *b*

Figure 10.26 *Small submucous fibroid. (a) Preliminary sagittal transvaginal sonogram reveals subtle focal interruption (?) of the endometrial echo complex. (b) Sonohysterogram in the sagittal plane demonstrates a very small submucous myoma (M) which is amenable to hysteroscopic resection in this young patient with multiple early pregnancy losses. Note that this mass is isoechoic with the myometrium. The balloon-tipped catheter is shown (arrows).*

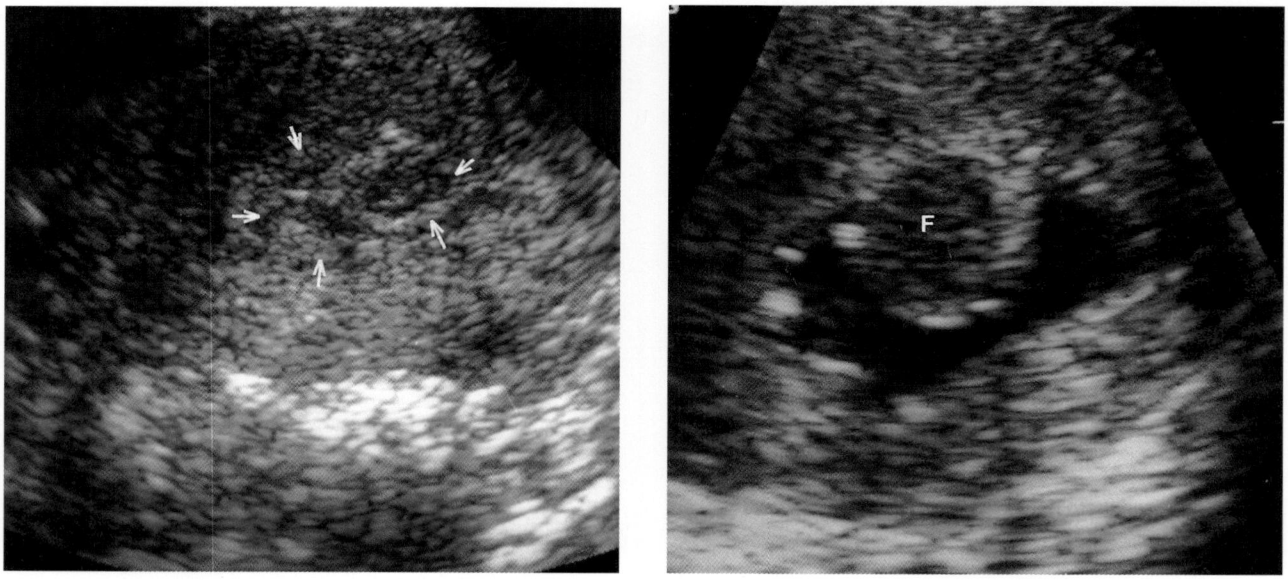

a *b*

Figure 10.27 *Intracavitary fibroid. (a) Preliminary transvaginal sonogram demonstrates an inhomogeneous endometrial echo complex (arrows); an endometrial abnormality was suspected in this patient with abnormal bleeding. (b) Sonohysterogram shows a small intracavitary fibroid (F) (isoechoic with the myometrium, smooth margins) which is amenable to hysteroscopic myomectomy. No endometrial abnormality is present.*

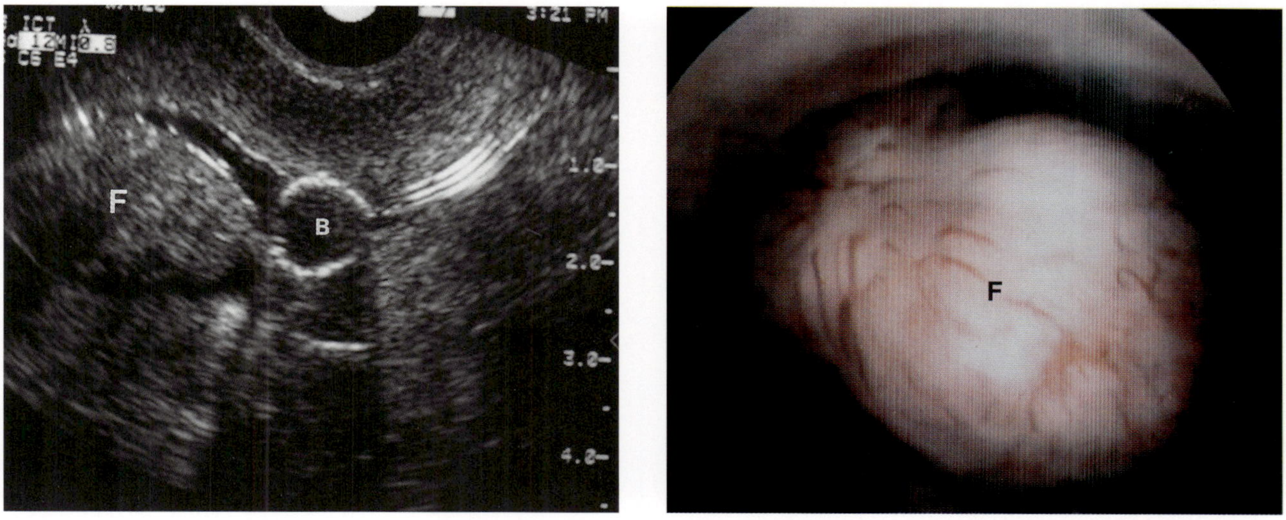

a *b*

Figure 10.28 *Large intracavitary fibroid. (a) Sagittal sonohysterogram in a patient with menorrhagia and a slightly enlarged uterus shows that a single large intracavitary fibroid (F) is the probable cause of bleeding. Hysteroscopic resection was deemed appropriate. B, catheter balloon. (b) Hysteroscopic view of the fibroid (F).*

older than 30 years of age. They are more common in black women than in white women. These tumors are usually found in middle-aged women; it appears that some fibroids regress after menopause, being less frequently found in older women. Fibroids are associated with diverse signs and symptoms, the most common being pain, pelvic pressure, and abnormal uterine bleeding. The size, location and number of lesions influence the clinical presentation. The location of fibroids is classified as subserosal (or pedunculated), mural or submucosal (including intracavitary), or a combination of these. Submucosal fibroids, even very small ones, can cause clinically significant bleeding, attributable to compression of the adjacent endometrium with resultant vascular compromise. Fibroids are also implicated as a cause of infertility.

On ultrasound, fibroids are more hypoechoic than polyps, usually isoechoic with the myometrium. They may have a heterogeneous echotexture if degenerative changes have occurred (Figs 10.26–10.28). The exact location and extent of any submucous element is important for planning the surgical approach for myomectomy. Even if an abdominal myomectomy is necessary because of multiple or large mural fibroids, it is still important to exclude the presence of a small intracavitary fibroid (Fig. 10.29). The latter would require the surgeon to explore the uterine cavity; otherwise a small, clinically significant, fibroid may be missed.[57]

In cases of Asherman's syndrome (traumatic hypomenorrhea/amenorrhea), the presence of amenorrhea or hypomenorrhea, as well as the extent of hypomenorrhea, is dependent on the location and severity of the intrauterine adhesions.[58] Sonohysterography can delineate the location and thickness of adhesions and demonstrate the degree of distortion or obliteration of the endometrial cavity (Fig. 10.30). In the presence of a cervical or isthmic adhesion, it may be necessary to gently introduce a sound past the adhesion, to allow the ready passage of fluid into the uterine cavity.

Clinical studies have shown that transvaginal sonohysterography is superior to conventional TVU in distinguishing endometrial thickening from endometrial polyps or fibroids in patients with bleeding.[40,48,50] By clearly delineating the type and location of a lesion, this technique helps to select the appropriate surgical approach.[43] A focal lesion such as a polyp or an intracavitary fibroid requires hysteroscopic resection, while a diffuse abnormality such as endometrial hyperplasia may be sampled reliably with a D&C.[50]

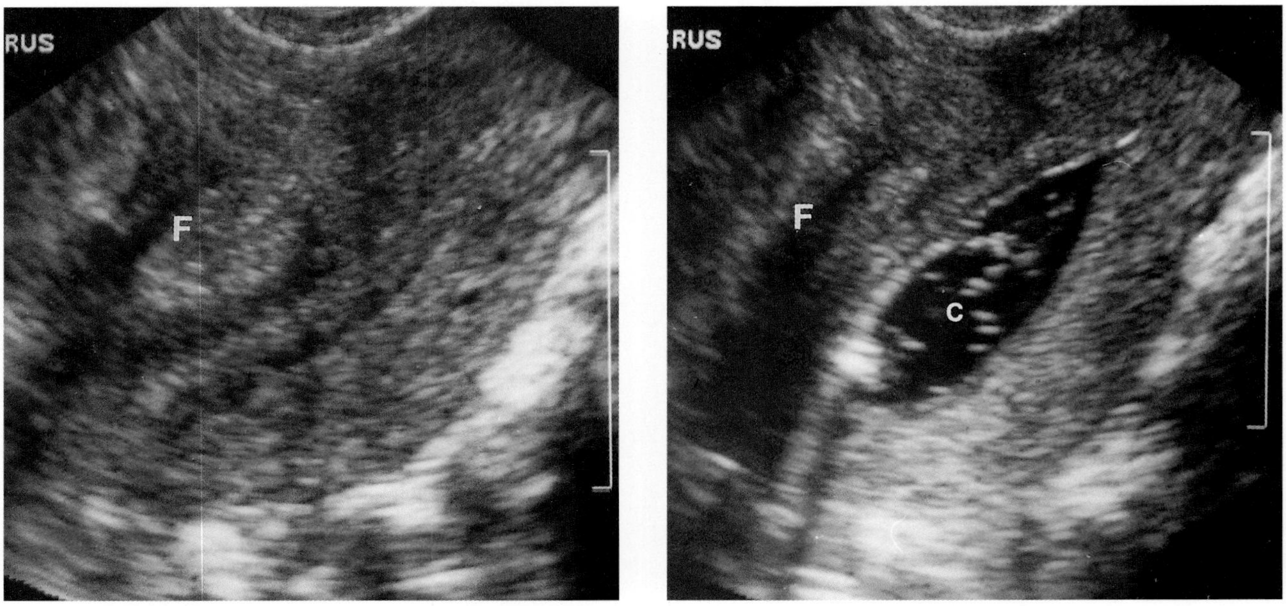

a *b*

Figure 10.29 *Large mural fibroid. (a) Preliminary transvaginal sonogram shows a large fibroid (F); the relationship to the endometrial cavity is uncertain. (b) Sagittal sonohysterogram demonstrates that the endometrial cavity (C) is displaced by the large mural fibroid (F), but otherwise intact. There is no evidence of a submucous component to the fibroid (F) or intracavitary lesion, so abdominal myomectomy (without exploration of the endometrial cavity) was deemed appropriate.*

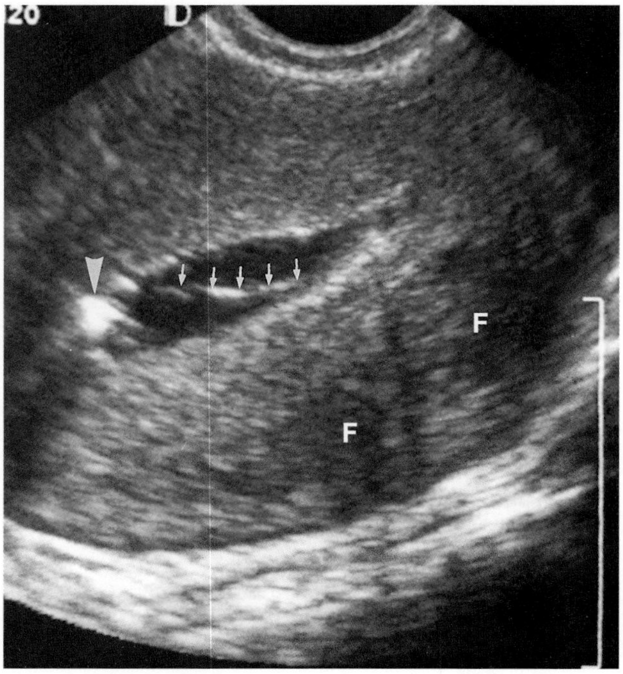

Figure 10.30 *Intrauterine synechiae. Sagittal sonohysterogram shows a single thin adhesion (arrows) crossing the endometrial cavity. A bubble of air is present (arrowhead). Small mural fibroids (F) are shown to be remote from the endometrial cavity and, therefore, of doubtful clinical significance in this patient with infertility.*

Sonohysterography has a promising role in the evaluation of patients with fibroids. By imaging the fluid-filled uterine cavity, it can define a fibroid as intracavitary, submucous or mural, or a combination of these. Therefore, preoperative sonohysterography is valuable in patient triage and surgical planning. In cases where bleeding is attributed to one or more submucous fibroids, sonohysterography can demonstrate the exact location of these fibroids as predominantly submucous (>50% volume projecting into the cavity) or predominantly mural.[50] This is important for surgical planning, since myomectomy (hysteroscopic and abdominal) requires special expertise beyond that required for hysterectomy or hysteroscopic polypectomy. In clinical practice, an intracavitary or predominantly submucous fibroid is usually amenable to hysteroscopic resection, while a fibroid which is predominantly mural (especially if it is large) may require an abdominal approach or a two-step hysteroscopic procedure.[59]

The incidence of endometrial carcinoma in women with postmenopausal bleeding was reported to range from 3.9% to 17.9%.[60] In patients with postmenopausal bleeding, endometrial carcinoma must be ruled out. Sonohysterography has been suggested as the imaging method of choice for evaluating and monitoring vaginal bleeding in postmenopausal women.[40,45,46] Although effective in distinguishing between diffuse endometrial changes and focal intracavitary masses, sonohysterography is unable to differentiate between endometrial hyperplasia and endometrial carcinoma. Therefore, evaluation of a diffuse endometrial abnormality requires tissue sampling by either D&C or endometrial biopsy for microscopic examination.

Infertility—The Fallopian Tube

Conventional X-ray hysterosalpingography and laparoscopy with chromopertubation are currently the primary methods for evaluating fallopian tube patency in women with infertility. TVU has been used as an important imaging modality for many aspects of infertility. However, this technique cannot provide any information about tubal patency, except for the demonstration of an hydrosalpinx. The injection of a contrast agent into the uterine cavity and tubes using TVU imaging is known as sonohysterosalpingography.

This technique is similar to transvaginal sonohysterography as described above (Fig. 10.31). The optimum time for evaluation of tubal patency is during the postmenstrual phase prior to ovulation (days 7–12) in order to avoid flushing an ovum or early conceptus out of the fallopian tube. The procedure can be performed in the ultrasound examination room.

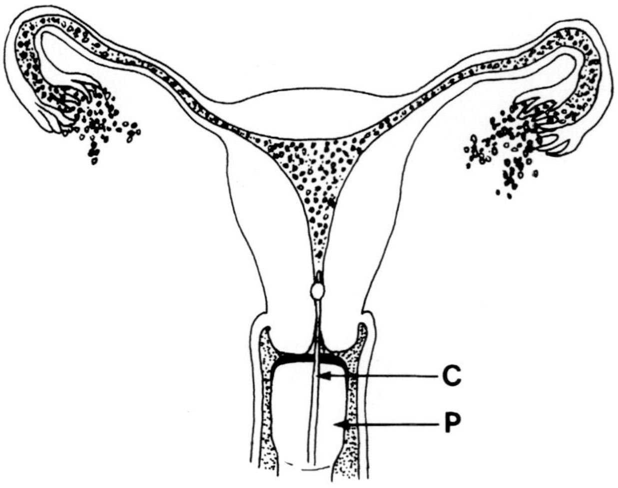

Figure 10.31 *Schematic representation, in the coronal plane, of transvaginal sonohysterosalpingography. C, balloon-tipped catheter; P, transvaginal ultrasound probe.*

Saline has been used as an echo-free contrast agent to visualize endometrial/myometrial pathology using transvaginal sonohysterography. In terms of tubal patency evaluation, some investigators have used saline to evaluate fallopian tubes with varying degrees of success.[44,61] The flow of saline could be seen only in the proximal part of the tubes. Although turbulence of echo-free fluid at the fimbria is the most reliable evidence of patency, in most cases the indirect diagnosis of tubal occlusion depends on demonstrating the presence of hydrosalpinges and/or a lack of fluid in the pouch of Douglas. We have used agitated saline as a contrast material, with variable success (Fig. 10.32).

Tufecki et al[62] reported their experience with saline injection using an 8-Fr Foley catheter in which 78% of cases had complete agreement between sonohysterosalpingography and laparoscopy, with the sensitivity of 76%, specificity of 94%, positive predictive value (PPV) of 84% and negative predictive value (NPV) of 90%. Allahbadia injected 20 ml of air and saline through an intrauterine 8-Fr. Foley catheter to

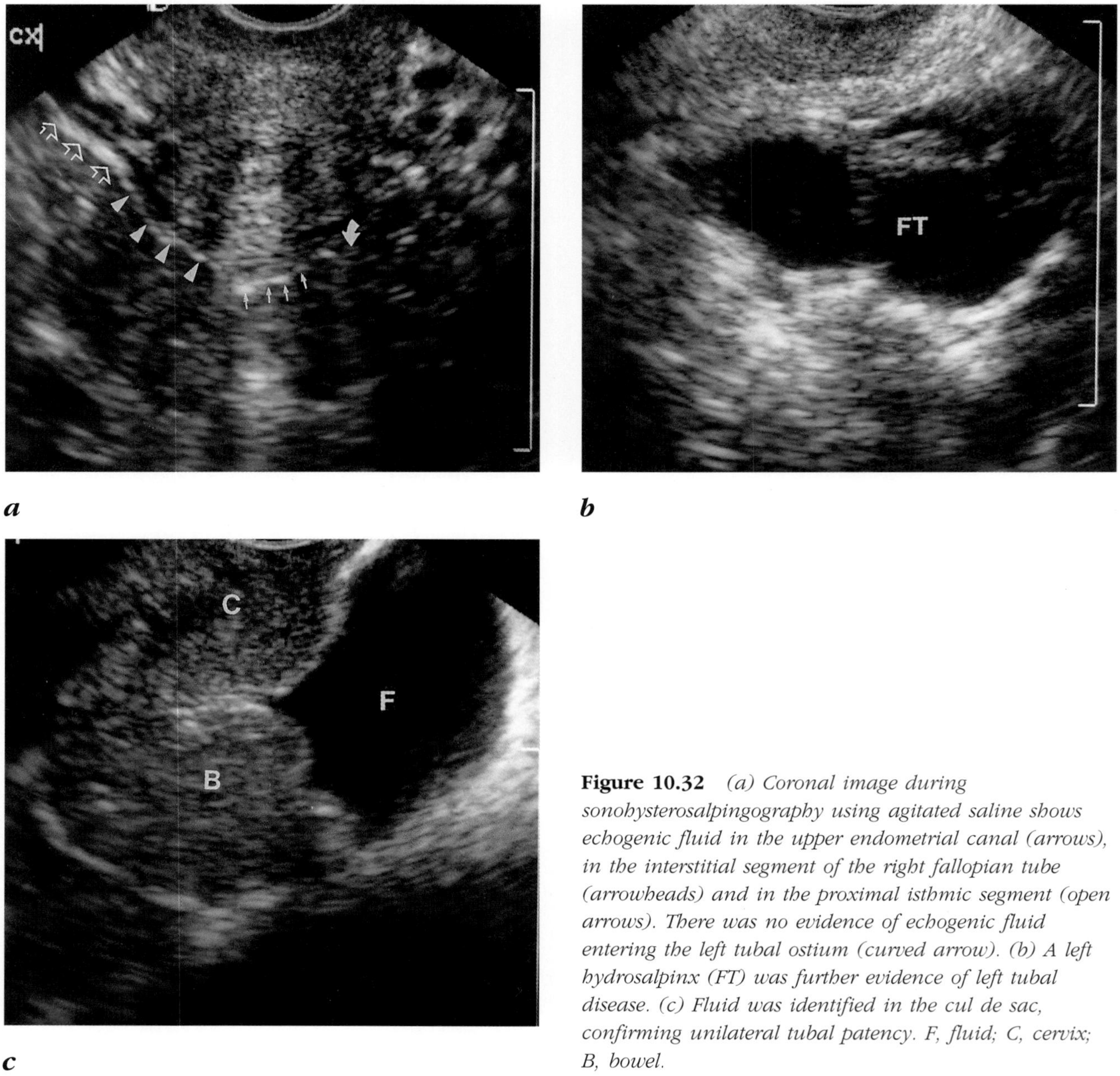

Figure 10.32 *(a) Coronal image during sonohysterosalpingography using agitated saline shows echogenic fluid in the upper endometrial canal (arrows), in the interstitial segment of the right fallopian tube (arrowheads) and in the proximal isthmic segment (open arrows). There was no evidence of echogenic fluid entering the left tubal ostium (curved arrow). (b) A left hydrosalpinx (FT) was further evidence of left tubal disease. (c) Fluid was identified in the cul de sac, confirming unilateral tubal patency. F, fluid; C, cervix; B, bowel.*

improve the visualization of the turbulence of flow. Patency status of the tubes was 91% concordant between ultrasound, hysterosalpingography and laparoscopy in 67 cases.[63]

Peters and Stern reported the results of hysterosalpingography with color Doppler ultrasound.[61,64] With color Doppler detection of interstitial flow or fimbrial expulsion, they found that this technique had 81% agreement with laparoscopy in 121 cases, with a sensitivity and specificity of 87%, a false-positive rate of 9%, and a false-negative rate of 20%. Although saline has been used to evaluate and improve the detectability of tubal patency, it is still not the ideal contrast agent.

During the past several years, investigators have developed a variety of ultrasound contrast agents which can enhance both gray-scale and Doppler signals, for both vascular and nonvascular applications.

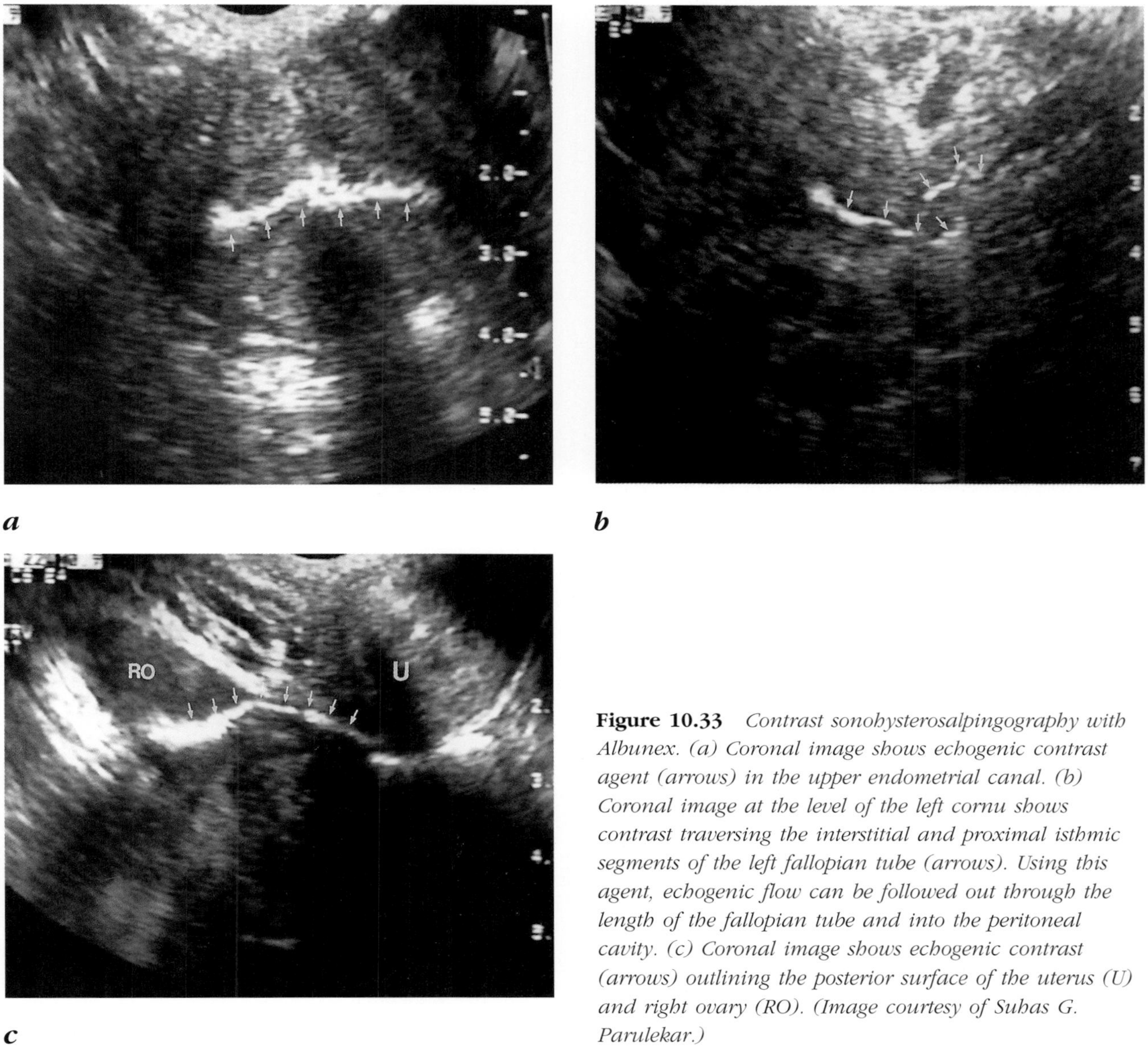

Figure 10.33 *Contrast sonohysterosalpingography with Albunex. (a) Coronal image shows echogenic contrast agent (arrows) in the upper endometrial canal. (b) Coronal image at the level of the left cornu shows contrast traversing the interstitial and proximal isthmic segments of the left fallopian tube (arrows). Using this agent, echogenic flow can be followed out through the length of the fallopian tube and into the peritoneal cavity. (c) Coronal image shows echogenic contrast (arrows) outlining the posterior surface of the uterus (U) and right ovary (RO). (Image courtesy of Suhas G. Parulekar.)*

Several of these contrast agents have been used to evaluate fallopian tube patency with sonohysterosalpingography in Europe. Deichert and Schlief[65,66] reported their investigations of sonohysterosalpingography with the use of Echovist in 120 patients and found it to be 100% predictive of patency with a sensitivity of 88% per tube, but a PPV of only 50% for tubal occlusion compared with laparoscopy. Standards for tubal patency included contrast agent flow to the isthmus lasting at least 10 seconds, visualization of contrast expulsion from the tube and around the ovary, and absence of hydrosalpinx. Although color Doppler imaging did not improve accuracy, the demonstration of isthmic flow by pulsed Doppler improved the accuracy to 100% in an additional 20 cases, which was confirmed by laparoscopy.

In over 600 European patients, sonohysterosalpingography with the use of Echovist had an

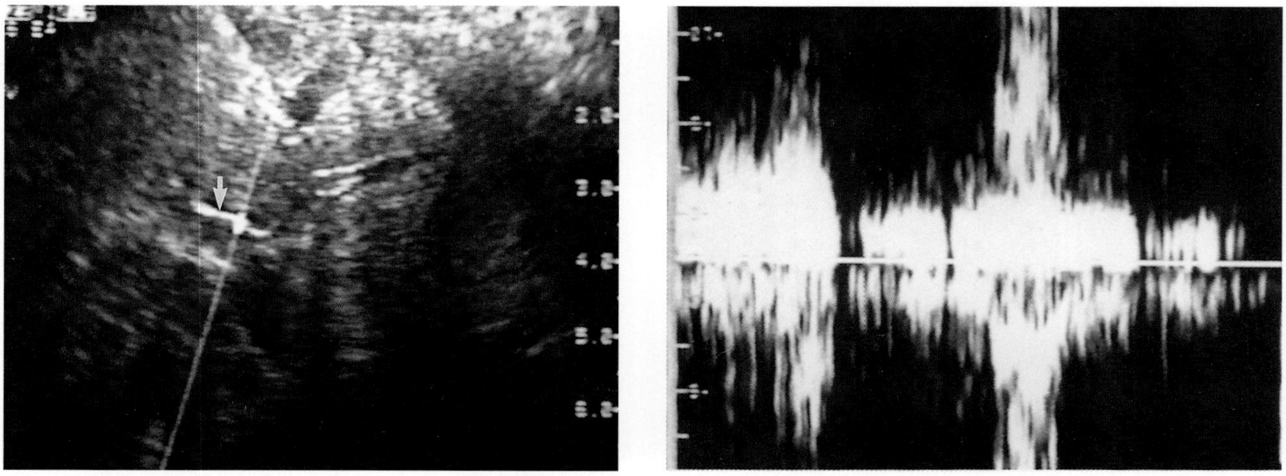

a *b*

Figure 10.34 *Sonohysterosalpingography with the assistance of spectral Doppler. (a) Coronal image shows location of sample gate at the right interstitial tubal segment (arrow). (b) Spectral tracing confirms flow through the patent fallopian tube. (Image courtesy of Subhas G. Parulekar.)*

84–91% concordance with conventional hysterosalpingography, and an 82–93% concordance with laparoscopy.[67] Contrast sonohysterosalpingography has also been used to investigate uterine abnormalities, which may be another cause of infertility. This technique proved to be a sensitive method for characterizing various types of uterine pathology, including arcuate, unicornuate, bicornuate and septate uteri.[66,68] These results indicate that this technique can give reliable and accurate information on tubal patency and should become a valuable outpatient procedure for the investigation of infertility. Another ultrasound contrast agent, 5% sonicated albumin (Albunex®, Malinckrodt Medical, Inc., St Louis, MO), has also be used, giving results which are similar to those found with Echovist (Fig. 10.33). Spectral Doppler may be used to confirm the motion of fluid through the fallopian tube (Fig. 10.34). Further investigations around the world are underway.[69]

Given the avoidance of ionizing radiation and general anesthesia, and with minimal discomfort and side-effects, contrast sonohysterosalpingography is a simple, accurate, well-tolerated and relatively inexpensive imaging technique for evaluating tubal patency in women with infertility.

REFERENCES

1. Mendelson EB, Bohm-Velez M, Joseph N et al, Gynecologic imaging: Comparison of transabdominal and transvaginal sonography, *Radiology* 1988; **166**:321–4.
2. von Micsky LI, Ultrasonic tomography in obstetrics and gynecology. In Grossman CC, eds, *Diagnostic Ultrasound*, (Plenum Press: New York, 1966) 348–68.
3. Hoetzinger H, Englmeier KH, Use of hysterosonography in the HDR afterloading treatment of endometrium cancer, *Sonderbande zur Strahlentherapie Onkologie* 1988; **82**:44–7.
4. Yock PG, Linker DT, Angelsen BA, Two-dimensional intravascular ultrasound: technical development and initial clinical experience, *J Am Soc Echocardiogr* 1989; **2**(4):296–304.
5. Meyer CR, Chiang EH, Fechner KP et al, Feasibility of high-resolution, intravascular ultrasonic imaging catheters, *Radiology* 1988; **168**:113–16.
6. Pandian NG, Kreis A, Brockway B et al, Ultrasound angioscopy: real-time, two-dimensional, intraluminal ultrasound imaging of blood vessels, *Am J Cardiol* 1988; **62**:493–4.

7. Mallery JA, Gregory K, Morcos NC et al, Evaluation of an ultrasound balloon dilatation imaging catheter, *Circulation* 1987; **76** (suppl IV):371.
8. Isner JM, Rosenfield K, Losordo DW et al, Percutaneous intravascular US as adjunct to catheter-based interventions: preliminary experience in patients with peripheral vascular disease, *Radiology* 1990; **175**:61–70.
9. Bom N, Lancee CT, van Egmond FC, An ultrasonic intracardiac scanner, *Ultrasonics* 1972; **10**:72–6.
10. Goldberg BB, Liu JB, Merton DA et al, Endoluminal US: experiments with nonvascular uses in animals, *Radiology* 1990; **175**:39–43.
11. Mandell MJ, Thieme GA, Eggli KD, Ballantine TVN, Transrectal ultrasound guided needle biopsy of recurrent vaginal mass in a 23 month old girl, *Pediatr. Radiol* 1989; **20**:120–1.
12. Rosenberg HK, Liu JB, Merton DA, Goldberg BB, Meadows AT, Endoluminal ultrasound using miniature high resolution transducer for evaluation of vaginal tumors in children: preliminary report, *Radiology* 1993; **189**(P):125.
13. Malignant tumors of the uterus. In: Mattingly RF, Thompson JD, eds, *Te Linde's Operative Gynecology* (Lippincott: Philadelphia, 1985) 845–76.
14. Fayez JA, Mutie G, Schneider PJ, The diagnostic value of hysterosalpingography and hysteroscopy in infertility investigation, *Am J Obstet Gynecol* 1987; **156**:558–60.
15. Lehtovirta P, Cacciatore B, Wahlstrom T, Ylostalo P, Ultrasonic assessment of endometrial cancer invasion, *J Clin Ultrasound* 1987; **5**:519–24.
16. Carter J, Carson LF, Elg S et al, Transvaginal sonography as an aid in the clinical staging of carcinoma of the cervix, *J Clin Ultrasound* 1992; **20**:283–7.
17. Kikuchi A, Okai T, Kobayashi K et al, Intracervical US with a high-frequency miniature probe: a method for diagnosing early invasive cervical cancer, *Radiology* 1996; **198**:411–13.
18. Kikuchi A, Okai T, Kobayashi K, Sakai M, Ryo E, Taketani Y, Intrauterine ultrasonography with a high-frequency probe: preliminary report, *Obstet Gynecol* 1995; **85**:457–61.
19. Goldberg BB, Liu JB, Kuhlman K, Merton DA, Kurtz AB, Endoluminal gynecologic ultrasound: preliminary results, *J Ultrasound Med* 1991; **10**:583–90.
20. Sohn C, Wallwiener D, Kaufmann M, Bastert G, Diagnosis of tubal function using intraluminal ultrasound: initial results, *Geburtshilfe Frauenheilkunde* 1992; **52**:663–6.
21. Goldberg BB, Liu JB, Merton DA et al, Sonographically guided laparoscopy and mediastinoscopy using miniature catheter-based transducers, *J Ultrasound Med* 1993; **12**:49–54.
22. Ragavendra N, McMahon JT, Perrella RR et al, Endoluminal catheter-assisted transcervical US of the human embryo, *Radiology* 1991; **181**:779–83.
23. Ragavendra N, Beall MH, McMahon JT, Bitonte RA, Grant EG, Transcervical sonography: an investigational technique for visualization of the embryo, *Obstet Gynecol* 1993; **81**:155–8.
24. Rhoades GG, Jackson LG, Schlesselman SE et al, The safety and efficacy of chorionic villus sampling for early prenatal diagnosis of cytogenetic abnormalities, *N Engl J Med* 1989; **320**:610–17.
25. Mendelson EB, Bohm-Velez M, Joseph N et al, Endometrial abnormalities: evaluation with transvaginal sonography, *AJR* 1988; **150**:139–42.
26. Gross BH, Silver TM, Jaffe MH, Sonographic features of uterine leiomyomas: analysis of 41 proven cases, *J Ultrasound Med* 1983; **2**:401–6.
27. Goldberg BB, Bagley D, Liu JB et al, Endoluminal sonography of the urinary tract: preliminary observations, *AJR* 1991; **156**:99–103.
28. Pellicer A, Hysteroscopy in the infertile woman, *Obstet Gynecol Clin North Am* 1988; **15**:99–105.
29. Loffer FD, Hysteroscopy with selective endometrial sampling compared with D&C for abnormal uterine bleeding: the value of a negative hysteroscopic view, *Obstet Gynecol* 1989; **73**:16–20.
30. Lehtovirta P, Cacciatore B, Wahlstrom T et al, Ultrasonic assessment of endometrial cancer invasion, *J Clin Ultrasound* 1987; **15**:519–24.
31. Cacciatore B, Lehtovirta P, Wahlstrom T et al, Preoperative sonographic evaluation of endometrial cancer, *Am J Obstet Gynecol* 1988; **160**:133–7.
32. Siegler AM, Hysterosalpingography, *Fertil Steril* 1983; **40**:139–42.
33. Wamsteker K, Hysteroscopy in the management of abnormal uterine bleeding in 199 patients. In: Siegler AM, Lindemann HJ, eds, *Hysteroscopy, Principles and Practice* (Lippincott: Philadelphia, 1984).
34. Coleman BG. Transvaginal sonography of adnexal masses, *Radiol Clin North Am* 1992; **30**:677–91.
35. Goldstein SR, Nachtigall M, Snyder JR et al, Endometrial assessment by vaginal ultrasonography before endometrial sampling in patients with postmenopausal bleeding, *Am J Obstet Gynecol* 1990; **163**:119–23.
36. Nasri MN, Coast GJ. Correlation of ultrasound findings and endometrial histopathology in postmenopausal women, *Br J Obstet Gynocol* 1989; **96**:1333–8.
37. Nasri MN, Shepherd JH, Setchell ME et al, Sonographic depiction of postmenopausal endometrium with transabdominal and transvaginal scanning, *Ultrasound Obstet Gynecol* 1991; **1**:279.
38. Varner RE, Sparks JM, Cameron DC et al, Transvaginal sonography of the endometrium in postmenopausal women, *Obstet Gynecol* 1991; **78**:195–9.
39. Fleischer AC, Mendelson EB, Bohm-Velez M et al, Transvaginal and transabdominal sonography of the endometrium, *Semin Ultrasound, CT MRI* 1988; **9**:81–101.
40. Sheth S, Hamper UM, Kurman R, Thickened endometrium in the postmenopausal woman: sonographic-pathologic correlation, *Radiology* 1991; **187**:135–9.
41. Randolph JF Jr, Ying YK, Amier DB et al, Comparison of real-time ultrasonography, hysterosalpingography, and laparoscopy/hysteroscopy in the evaluation of uterine abnormalities and tubal patency, *Fertil Steril* 1986; **49**:828–32.
42. Parsons AK, Lense JJ, Sonohysterography for endometrial abnormalities: preliminary results, *J Clin Ultrasound* 1993; **21**:87–95.
43. Cohen JR, Luxman D, Sagi J, Yovel I, Wolman, David MP, Sonohysterography for distinguishing endometrial thickening from endometrial polyps in postmenopausal women, *Ultrasound Obstet Gynecol* 1994; **4**:227–30.
44. Bonilla-Mausoles F, Simon C, Serra V et al, An assessment of hysterosalpingosonography (HSSG) as a diagnostic tool for uterine cavity defects and tubal patency, *J Clin Ultrasound* 1992; **20**:175–81.

45. Goldstein SR, Use of ultrasonohysterography for triage of perimenopausal patients with unexplained uterine bleeding, *Am J Obstet Gynecol* 1994; **170**:565–70.
46. Syrop CH, Sahakian V, Transvaginal sonographic detection of endometrial polyps with fluid contrast augmentation, *Obstet Gynecol* 1992; **79**:1041–3.
47. van Roessel J, Wamssteker K, Exalto N, Sonographic investigation of the uterus during artificial uterine cavity distention, *J Clin Ultrasound* 1987; **15**:439–50.
48. Dubinsky TJ, Parvey HR, Gormaz G, Maklad N, Transvaginal hysterosonography in the evaluation of small endoluminal masses, *J Ultrasound Med* 1995; **14**:1–6.
49. Achiron R, Lipitz S, Sivan E, Goldenberg M, Mashiach S, Sonohysterography for ultrasonographic evaluation of tamoxifen-associated cystic thickened endometrium, *J Ultrasound Med* 1995; **14**:685–8.
50. Lev-Toaff AS, Toaff ME, Liu JB, Merton DA, Goldberg BB, The value of sonohysterography in the diagnosis and management of abnormal uterine bleeding, *Radiology* 1996; **201**:179–84.
51. Devore GR, Schwartz PE, Morris J, Hysterography: a 5–year follow-up in patients with endometrial carcinoma, *Obstet Gynecol* 1982; **60**:369–72.
52. Fedele L, Bianchi S, Dorta M, Brioschi D, Zanotti F, Verchellini P, Transvaginal ultrasonography versus hysteroscopy in the diagnosis of uterine submucous myomas, *Obstet Gynecol* 1991; **77**:745–8.
53. Fleischer AC, Kalemeris GC, Machin JE et al, Sonographic depiction of normal and abnormal endometrium with histopathologic correlation, *J Ultrasound Med* 1986; **5**:446–52.
54. Granberg S, Wikland M, Karlsson B et al, Endometrial thickness as measured by endovaginal ultrasonography for identifying endometrial abnormality, *Am J Obstet Gynecol* 1991; **164**:47–52.
55. Pettersson B, Adami HO, Lindgren A et al, Endometrial polyps and hyperplasia as risk factors for endometrial cancer: a case control study of curettage specimens, *Acta Obstet Gynaecol Scand* 1985; **64**:653–9
56. Lin MC, Gosink B, Wilf S et al, Endometrial thickness after menopause: effect of hormone replacement, *Radiology* 1991; **180**:427–32.
57. Lev-Toaff AS, Karasick S, Toaff ME, Hysterosalpingography before and after myomectomy: clinical value and imaging findings, *AJR* 1993; **160**:803–7.
58. Toaff R, Ballas S, Traumatic hypomenorrhea-amenorrhea (Asherman's syndrome), *Fertil Steril* 1978; **30**:379–88.
59. Corson SL, Brooks PG, Resectoscopic myomectomy, *Fertil Steril* 1991; **55**:1041–4.
60. Merril JA, Management of postmenopausal bleeding, *Clin Obstet Gynecol* 1981; **24**:285–8.
61. Stern J, Peters AJ, Coulam CB, Colour Doppler ultrasonography assessment of tubal patency: a comparison study with traditional techniques, *Fertil Steril* 1992; **58**:897–900.
62. Tufecki EC, Girit S, Bayirli E et al, Evaluation of tubal patency by transvaginal sonosalpingography, *Fertil Steril* 1992; **57**:336–40.
63. Allahbadia GN, Fallopian tubes and ultrasonography: the Sion experience, *Fertil Steril* 1992; **58**:901–7.
64. Peters AJ, Coulam CB, Hysterosalpingography with color Doppler ultrasonography, *Am J Obstet Gynecol* 1991; **164**:1530–4.
65. Deichert U, van de Sandt M, Transvaginal hysterosalpingo-contrast-sonography (HyCoSy): the assessment of tubal patency and uterine abnormalities by contrast enhanced sonography. *Advances in echo-contrast.* (Lancaster, UK: Kluwer Medical Information Services, 1993) **2**:55–8.
66. Schlief R, Deichert U, Hysterosalpingo-contrast-sonography of the uterine and fallopian tubes: results of a clinical trial of a new contrast medium in 120 patients, *Radiology* 1991; **178**:213–15.
67. Campbell S, Bourne TH, Tan SL, Collins WP, Hysterosalpingo contrast sonography (HyCoSy) and its future role within the investigation of infertility in Europe, *Ultrasound Obstet Gynecol* 1994; **4**:245–53.
68. Deichert U, Schlief R, van de Sandt M, Juhnke I, Transvaginal hysterosalpingo-contrast-sonography (HyCoSy) compared with conventional tubal diagnostics, *Hum Reprod* 1989; **4**:418–24.
69. Parsons AK, Cullinan JA, Goldstein SR, Fleischer AC, Sonohysterography, sonosalpingography, and sonohysterosalpingography: a text-atlas of normal and abnormal findings. In: Fleischer AC, Manning FA, Jeanty P, Romero R, eds, *Sonography in Obstetrics and Gynecology-Principles and Practice*, 5th edn (Stamford, Connecticut: Appleton & Lange, 1996).

Chapter 11 Laparoscopic ultrasound of intra-abdominal organs

Ji-Bin Liu, Rick I Feld, Larry S Miller and Laurence Needleman

INTRODUCTION

Since the late 1980s, laparoscopy has become an increasingly important diagnostic and therapeutic tool for the surgeon in dealing with a variety of abdominal abnormalities.[1–4] This technique has obtained rapid and widespread acceptance among patients and surgeons. The introduction of video laparoscopy and the improvement in laparoscopic instruments have stimulated surgeons to use laparoscopy and develop new surgical procedures.

Intraoperative ultrasound has been used effectively during open surgery to evaluate a variety of abnormalities. It has become a important tool in intraoperative decision-making in abdominal surgery. With this technique, it has been possible to detect lesions too small to be visualized with transcutaneous ultrasound or other imaging modalities.[5–9] Parker et al[6] reported that intraoperative ultrasound influenced operative management in 49% of patients undergoing exploratory laparotomy for liver tumors, either primary or metastatic. Unlike conventional open surgery, standard ultrasound probes cannot be employed through laparoscopic ports to evaluate intracorporeal structures during laparoscopic surgery. Miniaturization of ultrasound transducers opened the way for the development of laparoscopic imaging. The combination of laparoscopic and ultrasound technology has expanded the potential for the clinical application of ultrasound in various laparoscopic surgical procedures.

Conventional transcutaneous ultrasonography has several shortcomings in terms of diagnosis of intra-abdominal abnormalities: (1) reflection artifact of the abdominal wall in the near-field image; (2) insufficient penetration in obese patients; (3) inability to detect small lesions; and (4) interference of imaging by intestinal gas or bone. On the other hand, laparoscopy is inherently limited as a diagnostic and staging tool, since the laparoscopic view of abdominal viscera is restricted to visible organ surfaces. Unlike with open surgery, palpable examination of suspicious abnormalities is not possible during a laparoscopic procedure. The external examination of the surface of abdominal organs laparoscopically can miss lesions in solid organs, hollow structures or the retroperitoneum. Laparoscopic ultrasound, which evolved from the concepts of endoscopic ultrasound and combined the techniques of diagnostic laparoscopy with intraoperative ultrasound, can overcome the limitations of both laparoscopy and transabdominal ultrasound.

HISTORICAL BACKGROUND

The concept of using ultrasound to image structures within the abdominal cavity through a laparoscopic opening was first described by Yamakawa et al in 1958.[10,11] Kratochwil used this approach in the 1970s to evaluate abnormalities within the female pelvis.[12] At that time, these investigators used rigid probes rather than flexible ones and produced only unidimensional A-mode echography to assess intra-abdominal organs and pathologies. Since then, many researchers have attempted to produce and utilize miniature ultrasound probes for laparoscopic applications. However, it was not until the early 1980s that the feasibility of gray-scale laparoscopic ultrasound scanning of abdominal structures was described by Japanese investigators.[13,14] In 1984, Fukuda et al reported the results of the use of a two-dimensional, real-time laparoscopic ultrasound system associated with a 10–12-mm-diameter rigid transducer and demonstrated intrahepatic lesions where external ultrasound imaging had failed.[15] Also in 1984, Okita et al tested 3.5- and 5-MHz real-time transducers, which they found had good penetration but poor resolution.[16] In 1985 Frank et al used a laparoscopic ultrasound probe that had some flexibility owing to an articulated shaft.[17] Fornari et al in 1989 described their preliminary experience using a sono-laparoscope in which a 7.5-MHz rotating transducer was fixed to the tip of a laparoscope to produce a 180° sector scan. They used laparoscopic ultrasound to guide the needle biopsy of the lesions concealed within the liver.[18] Some of the early prototype laparoscopic ultrasound transducers required insertion of large-diameter trocar ports.[16,19] On the other hand, prototype miniature transducers housed in 2–3-mm-diameter catheters have also been employed to evaluate hepatobiliary and pelvic structures during laparoscopic procedures and to detect lymph nodes during mediastinoscopy.[20,21] More recently, miniaturized laparoscopic ultrasound probes with both color and spectral Doppler capabilities have been developed and used in clinical practice. These transducers have higher resolution and better image quality than the previous generation of transducers.[22]

INSTRUMENTATION

There are several commercially available ultrasound systems which can be used with specially designed laparoscopic ultrasound probes. Generally, four different types of transducers, with rigid or flexible shafts, are used for real-time ultrasound imaging. They are: (1) linear-array transducers producing a rectangular image; (2) curvilinear-array transducers producing a fan-shaped image with a relatively large field of view; (3) electric sector scanners creating a pie-shaped image; and (4) mechanical rotating transducers displaying a 180° or 360° cross-sectional image (Fig. 11.1). In general, linear-array transducers are ideal for scanning widely exposed areas, whereas sector transducers, being small, are preferable for areas in which the exposure is limited or the region of interest is small. It is apparent that each type of laparoscopic ultrasound probe will possess its own advantages and disadvantages. Different probe configurations may be employed for various clinical applications.

Although transducers mounted on the tip of the rigid shaft are still used (Fig. 11.2), flexible probes are available in several ultrasound systems (Fig. 11.3). Since laparoscopic trocars are fixed in the abdominal wall, the probes with bendable tips give the operator more flexibility and control in scanning intra-abdominal organs, especially the dome of the liver and the pancreas. Newly developed transducers have color and spectral Doppler capabilities which have proven useful in differentiating vascular from nonvascular structures.

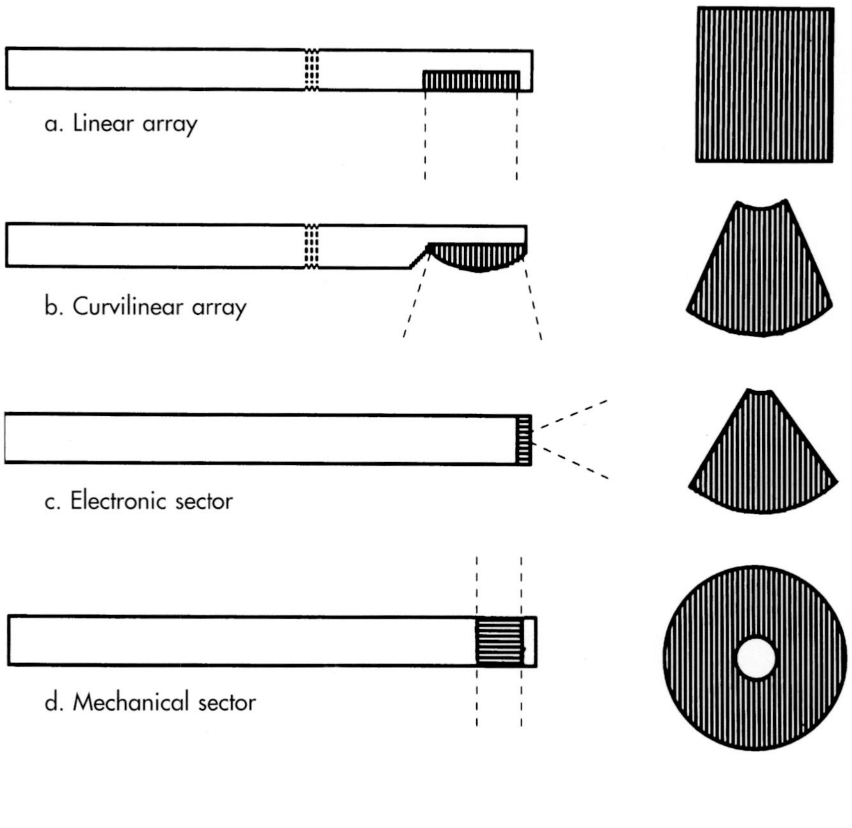

Figure 11.1 *A diagrammatic representation of four common configurations of the laparoscopic ultrasound probe and imaging displays: (a) linear-array transducer with or without the flexible tip; (b) curvilinear-array transducer with or without the flexible tip; (c) electronic sector transducer; (d) mechanical rotating sector transducer.*

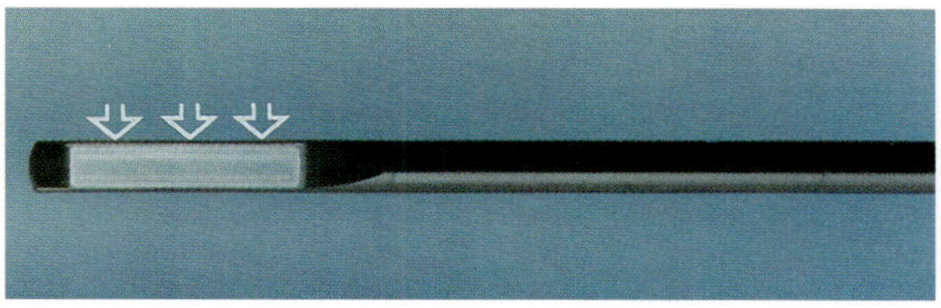

Figure 11.2 *An example of a laparoscopic ultrasound probe with a linear-array transducer (arrows) mounted on the tip of the rigid shaft.*

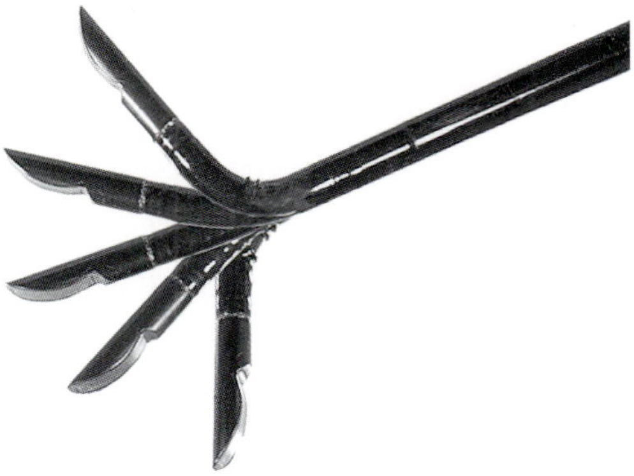

Figure 11.3 *An example of a laparoscopic ultrasound probe with a semi-flexible tip which allows the transducer to move up and down from the 0° position.*

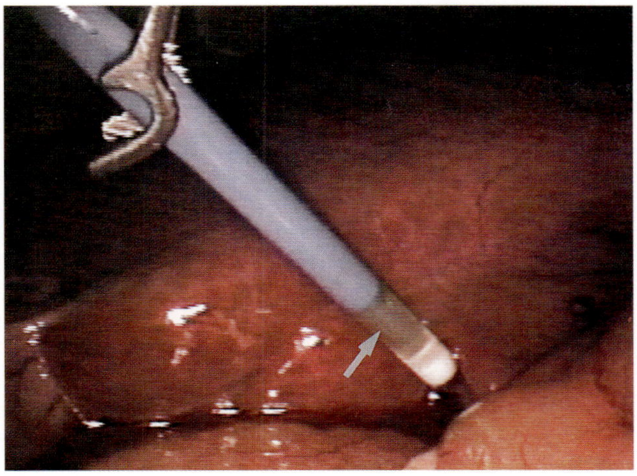

Figure 11.4 *The 20-MHz catheter-based transducer (arrow) has been inserted through a 5-mm laparoscopic trocar into the abdomen. An instrument is seen grasping the probe and directing its movement over the surface of the liver.*

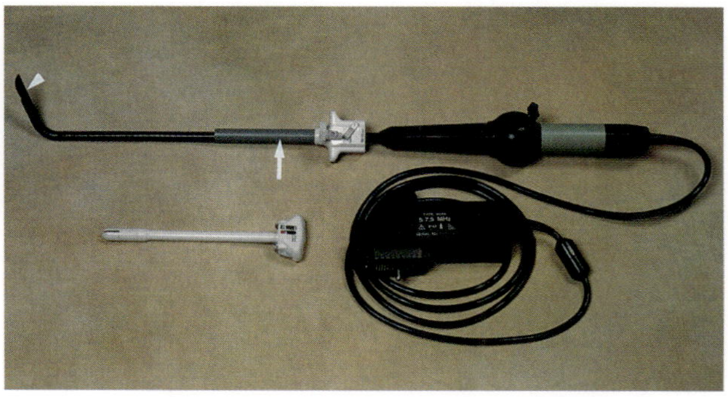

Figure 11.5 *The Brüel&Kjäer laparoscopic ultrasound probe containing a convex-array transducer passed through a 10/11-mm-diameter trocar (arrow). Note that the tip (arrowhead) of the probe was bent up 75°. (Reproduced with permission from Liu JB et al.[23])*

Most laparoscopic transducers are less than 10 mm in diameter. These transducers can readily pass through commonly used 10-mm-diameter trocars. In addition, the miniature catheter-based transducers (6.2–9 Fr) easily pass through a 5-mm-diameter laparoscopic trocar (Fig. 11.4).[19,20]

Ultrasonic frequency is important in determining the resolution of the imaging. Generally, the higher the frequency of the ultrasound beam, the better the resolution and the lower the depth of penetration. Therefore, the choice of transducers depends on the specific requirements of various operative sites. Because the transducer, during the laparoscopic procedure, comes in direct contact with the organ surface, acoustic interference caused by interposed tissues (i.e. skin and fat) is avoided. Higher-frequency ultrasound transducers should be used to provide high-resolution imaging, as in intraoperative ultrasound. The frequencies commonly used for laparoscopic transducers are 5 or 7.5 MHz, depending on the organ being scanned.

The laparoscopic ultrasound probe that we use is a convex-array transducer with color and spectral Doppler capabilities (Flextip™, Brüel&Kjäer Medical System, Inc., Marlborough, MA) (Fig. 11.5).[23] This probe is designed for use with the Diagnostic

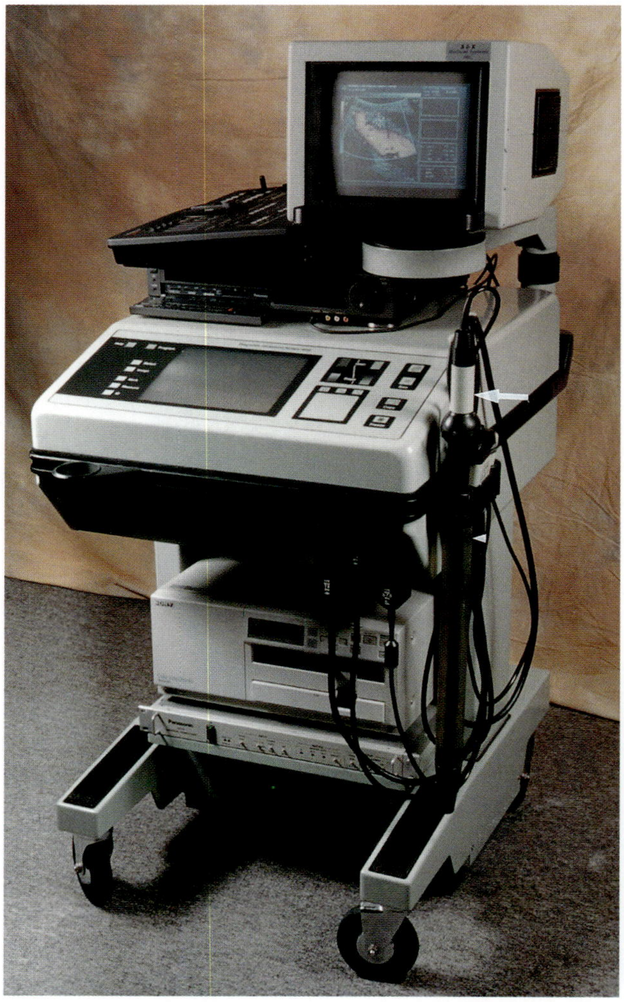

Figure 11.6 *The Brüel&Kjäer Diagnostic Ultrasound System 3535 with laparoscopic ultrasound probe (arrow) immersed within the Cidex-filled tube (arrowheads).*

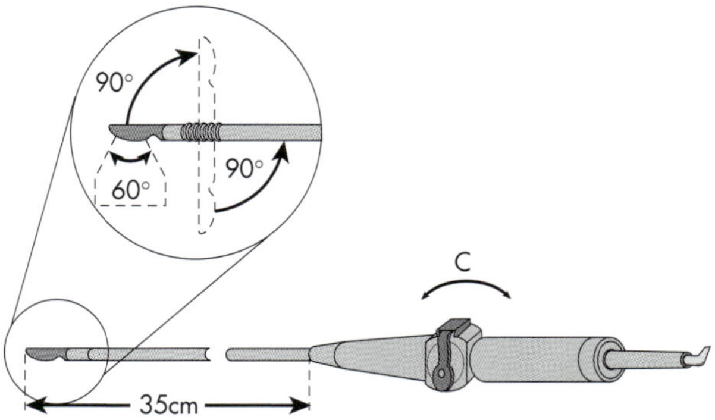

Figure 11.7 *A schematic representation shows the transducer steered by a controller (C) moving 90° up and 90° down from the 0° position. The scanning angle is up to 60°, with maximum penetration of 13 cm. (Reproduced with permission from the Liu et al.[22])*

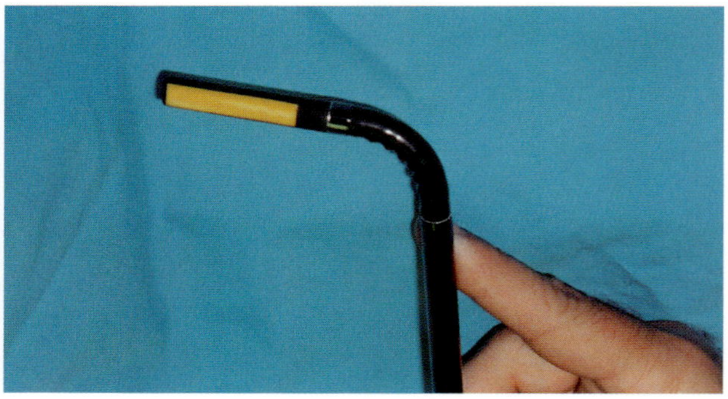

Figure 11.8 *The Toshiba laparoscopic ultrasound probe with four-directional flexible tip and 7.0/5.0-MHz dual-frequency linear-array transducer. This probe has both color and spectral Doppler capabilities.*

Ultrasound System 3535 (Brüel&Kjäer) (Fig. 11.6). The flexible-tipped probe measures 9.6 mm in diameter and 35 cm in length. It contains a multifrequency transducer (5.0, 6.5 and 7.5 MHz) with a maximum penetration of 13 cm and a sector scanning angle of 60°. The flexible tip can be steered by a controller and can be moved 90° up and 90° down from the horizontal plane (Fig. 11.7). The size of the probe allows for easy passage through a 10-mm-diameter trocar. Adjustment of the equipment is the same as that used for nonoperative ultrasound procedures. Parameter adjustments are made according to the size of the area being examined.[22]

Another laparoscopic ultrasound system we have experience with is the Toshiba SSH-140A unit associated with the PEF-704LA electronic linear-array laparoscopic probe (Fig. 11.8). The probe measures 10 mm in diameter and 40 cm in length of the insertion section, and the flexible tip can be moved in four directions (i.e. left, right, up and down 90° from

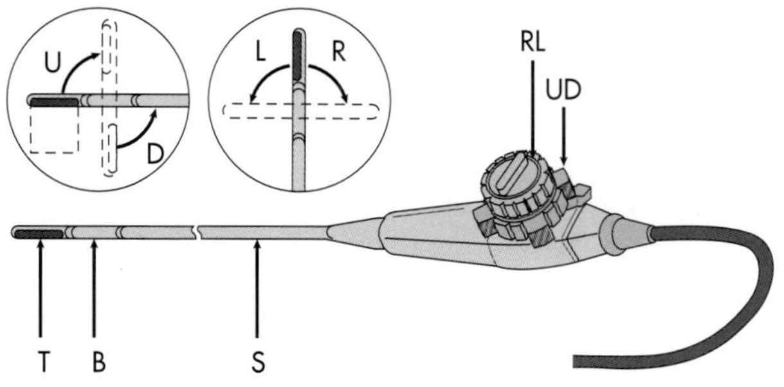

Figure 11.9 *A schematic representation of the Toshiba probe shows the transducer steered by two knobs allowing the transducer to move up, down, right and left 90° from the 0° position. T, transducer; B, bending section; S, shaft; RL, right and left angle knob; UD, up and down angle knob; U, up; D, down; L, left; R, right.*

the 0° position) (Fig. 11.9). The transducer has 7.0- and 5.0-MHz dual frequencies with both color and spectral Doppler capabilities.

TECHNIQUES

Prior to each examination, the laparoscopic ultrasound probe is disinfected by immersion in Cidex (Johnson & Jonhson Medical, Arlington, TX) for 30 min and, following removal from the Cidex bath, the probe is rinsed with sterile water. In the operating room, the probe is prepared in the following fashion. Using sterile technique, 3–5 ml of sterile water is placed into a special 15×350 mm sterile probe cover and the probe is inserted into this cover (Fig. 11.10a, b). The water acts as an acoustic couplant to displace any air located between the transducer surface and the sterile cover. To maintain the water at the tip, a sterile 2-0 silk suture is tied around the probe cover to fit in a notch proximal to the transducer tip (Fig. 11.10c). A sterile arthroscopic camera drape is advanced over the probe end to cover the probe handle and cable, while the shaft of the probe and probe tip are kept sterile by the special probe cover (Fig. 11.10d). The sterile ultrasound probe, guided by video laparoscopy, is inserted through a 10-mm-diameter trocar into the carbon dioxide-distended abdominal cavity.

In order to easily perform ultrasound scanning under direct laparoscopic view, the ultrasound system can be connected to the video display of the laparoscopic unit using a commercially available audiovisual mixture desk in order to obtain 'picture-in-picture' imaging on the same monitor (Fig. 11.11). Real-time ultrasound imaging can be recorded on videotape for documentation and later review. It is very important to perform scanning under the guidance of the laparoscopic video camera. The tip of the ultrasound transducer should always be kept within the field of laparoscopic view, avoiding injury to intra-abdominal organs.

There is a learning curve in the performance of laparoscopic ultrasound scanning. The major technical difference between laparoscopic and intraoperative ultrasound is the manipulation of the remote-controlled laparoscopic transducer as opposed to the direct manual-controlled conventional transducer. Surgeons and radiologists working as a team ensure the best use of this technique in performing the procedure and appropriately interpreting the ultrasound images. Sonographic findings can be interpreted on-line during real-time evaluation.

Depending upon the target organ to be scanned, the locations of trocar ports to be used should be carefully selected based on the lesion location, adjacent structures, scanning angle and imaging section desired. Under certain circumstances, a trocar port used for the ultrasound probe may have to switch with a port for laparoscopic camera. However, in most cases, only those openings already created for the planned laparoscopic procedure are used, and no additional ports are necessary. It is necessary to position the flexible probe in the 0° position when inserting and retracting it through the trocar.

For hepatobiliary examinations, the laparoscopic probe is placed systematically over the right and left lobes of the liver. Complete examination requires the identification of vascular landmarks, delineation of the various segments, and analysis of the parenchyma within each segment. The hepatic veins are first imaged at their confluence with the vena cava. The hilar area and the portal vein bifurcation are scanned next and followed intrahepatically. If necessary, an approach via the inferior surface of the liver should be utilized to evaluate areas of interest in the posterior right lobe and caudate lobe. Particular attention should be directed to the porta

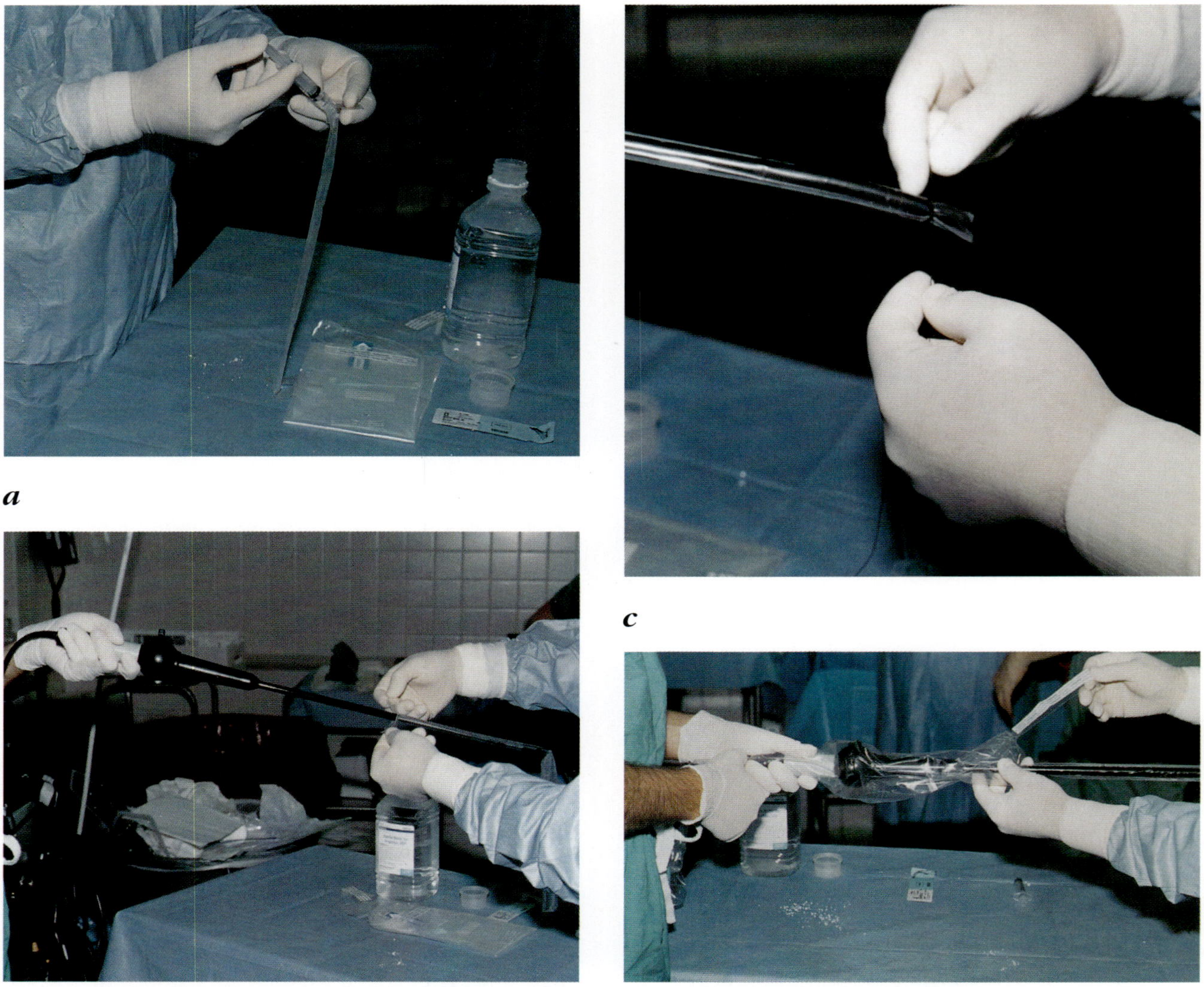

a *b* *c* *d*

Figure 11.10 *(a) Using sterile technique, 3–5 ml of sterile water is placed into a special 15×350 mm sterile probe cover, and (b) the probe is inserted into this cover. (c) To maintain the water at the tip, a sterile 2-0 silk suture is tied around the probe cover to fit in a notch proximal to the tip. (d) The probe handle and cable was covered by a sterile drape. ((b) and (c) reproduced with permission from Feld et al[26])*

hepatis for signs of possible portal lymphadenopathy. Color Doppler imaging is useful to determine the relationship of focal masses to regional vascular structures.

Laparoscopic ultrasound localization of liver lesions permits guided biopsies of deep parenchymal lesions. This is particularly important in patients with metastatic liver disease, since it may alter the surgical management of their disease either by demonstrating nonresectable disease or by modifying the amount of surgery necessary. For laparoscopic ultrasound-guided biopsies, it is very important to plan the needle approaches prior to the actual biopsy. In most situations, the transabdominal wall approach is required for liver biopsy, using the ASAP automatic 18-gauge core biopsy device (Microvasive, Boston

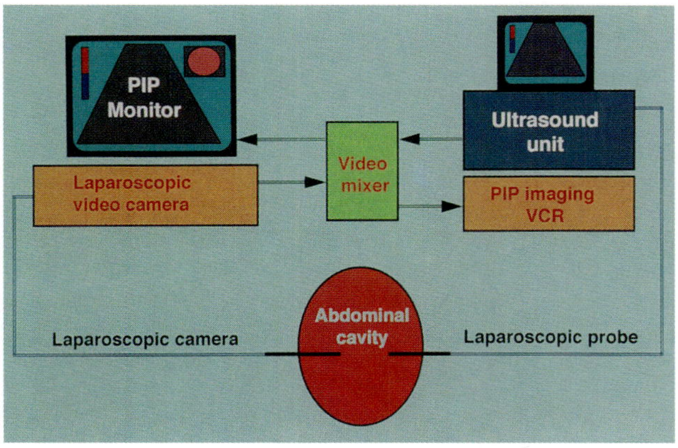

Figure 11.11 *Diagrammatic demonstration of the ultrasound system connected with a laparoscopic unit to obtain simultaneously a laparoscopic picture in the ultrasound imaging display. (Reproduced with permission from Liu JB et al.[23])*

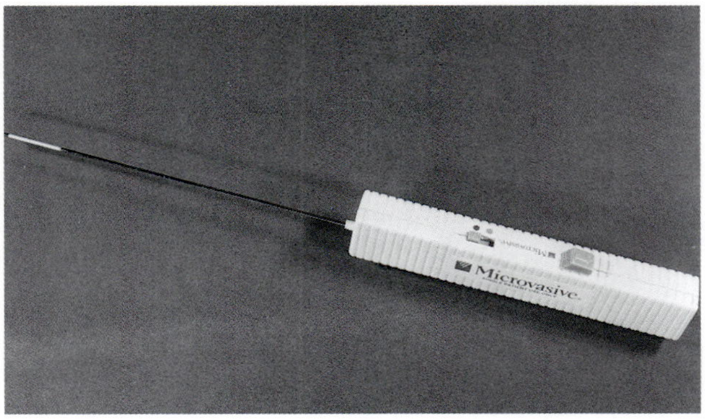

Figure 11.12 *The Microvasive core biopsy device is used for percutaneous tissue sampling under laparoscopic ultrasound guidance.*

Scientific Corporation, Natick MA) (Fig. 11.12). Unlike with open intraoperative biopsy, there are many factors which affect biopsy accuracy. Needle positions, angles and directions as well as the relationship to transducer scanning sections must be taken into consideration. Continuous laparoscopic ultrasound guidance should be used to monitor the position of the needle relative to the target.

ANIMAL STUDIES

Animal studies were initially performed to establish methods for the use of laparoscopic ultrasound probes. Miniature swine were used as animal models for laparoscopic ultrasound procedures. After these animals were placed under general anesthesia, the ultrasound probe was inserted into the carbon dioxide-insufflated abdominal cavity through a 10-mm trocar. Gray-scale and color Doppler images were obtained by direct contact of the transducer with a variety of intra-abdominal structures. The procedure was monitored by a miniature laparoscopic video camera.

With use of the laparoscopic ultrasound probe in animal models, it was possible to image normal anatomic structures in the abdominal cavity. Color and spectral Doppler imaging proved useful in identifying and differentiating blood vessels from bile ducts and other nonvascular structures. The arteries and veins could be easily distinguished by their color flow and duplex Doppler spectral waveforms. As the transducer was manipulated over the surface of solid and fluid-filled structures, the ultrasound images clearly demonstrated internal details of structures in organs such as the liver, gallbladder, spleen and kidneys (Fig. 11.13), as well as the multiple layers of the stomach and small bowel walls (Fig. 11.14). The relationship between the bile duct, portal vein and hepatic artery was easily delineated by real-time gray-scale and color flow imaging. At autopsy, no trauma was detected in any of the structures examined with the transducer.[22] Thus, these initial animal studies suggested that this technique would prove to be useful and safe in humans.

CLINICAL APPLICATIONS

Although transabdominal ultrasound, CT and MRI often do not detect masses less than 1 cm in diameter, laparoscopy can visualize metastases as small as 1 mm in diameter on the peritoneal surface.[23] In addition, biopsy under direct laparoscopic guidance is safer with more accurate tissue sampling than with percutaneous biopsy.[24] However, laparoscopy is inherently limited as a staging tool, since lesions located beyond the surface of the abdominal viscera are not able to be visualized by this technique. The combination of laparoscopy with intraoperative ultra-

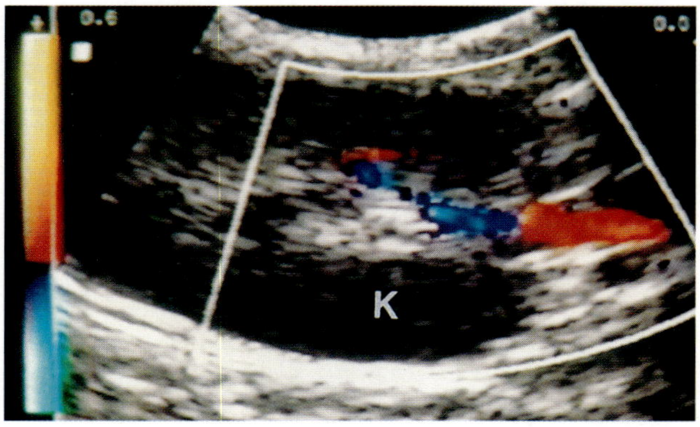

Figure 11.13 *Laparoscopic ultrasound image in a swine model demonstrating normal right kidney (K) with renal vessels shown in color.*

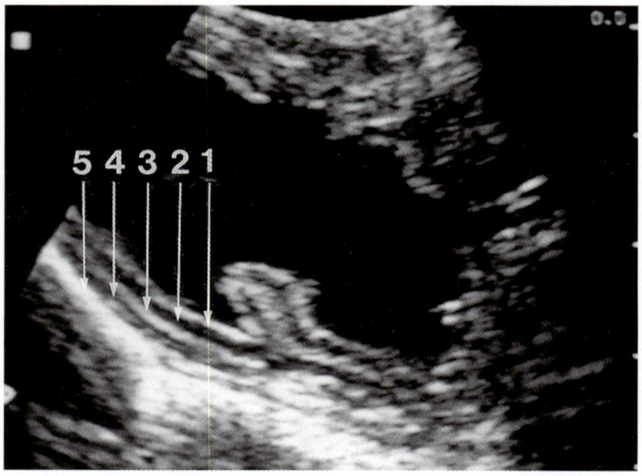

Figure 11.14 *Laparoscopic ultrasound image in a swine model clearly showing the multiple layers of the gastric wall: 1, mucosa; 2, deep mucosa and muscular mucosae: 3, submucosa; 4, muscularis propria; 5, adventitia.*

sound allows a significant improvement in the assessment of intra-abdominal structures for tumor staging. To make surgical decisions concerning liver resection, a surgeon often asks the following questions: What is the nature of the lesion? Are there additional lesions not detected preoperatively? Is the lesion close to major vessels? Is resection feasible? What should be the extent of the resection? Laparoscopic ultrasound seems to be able to answer these questions and help with surgical decision-making.

NORMAL STRUCTURES

With the use of high-resolution laparoscopic ultrasound, it is possible to demonstrate the detailed normal anatomy of intra-abdominal organs, including the liver, pancreas, spleen, kidney, adrenal gland and reptroperitoneum, as well as vascular structures adjacent to these organs (Figs 11.15–11.18). Although intra-abdominal vascular structures could be visualized by using gray-scale imaging, spectral and color Doppler ultrasound provide important information on characteristics of bloodflow (Figs 11.19 and 11.20). In addition, Doppler imaging proved especially useful in differentiating vascular from nonvascular structures (Fig. 11.21).

The ultrasound probe we used has a maximum penetration of 13 cm, which makes it possible to image structures deep within the liver or retroperitoneum. The semi-flexible probe allows for easier positioning and scanning within the abdomen. In addition, its color and spectral Doppler capabilities allow for evaluation of vessels. When using this technique, it has been possible to determine the best surgical approach for visualizing the precise location, size and characteristics of masses and establishing their relationship to normal structures.

FOCAL LIVER MASSES

A study by John et al reported on the use of laparoscopic ultrasound to stage potentially resectable liver tumors. In 33% of patients laparoscopic ultrasound showed liver tumors that had not been detectable by laparoscopic inspection alone. Seven of 43 patients (16%), for whom preceding investigations (including laparoscopy) had not shown any contraindications to operation, were shown by laparoscopic ultrasound alone to have unresectable disease. Laparoscopic ultrasound provided staging information in addition to that derived from laparoscopy alone in 18 of 43 patients (42%).[25]

To evaluate the ability of laparoscopy and laparoscopic ultrasound to determine resectability of hepatic masses, we have shown that laparoscopic ultrasound has a sensitivity of 100%, a specificity of 75% and a positive predictive value of 85%. Laparoscopy alone has a sensitivity of 100%, a specificity of 40% and a positive predictive value of 68%.

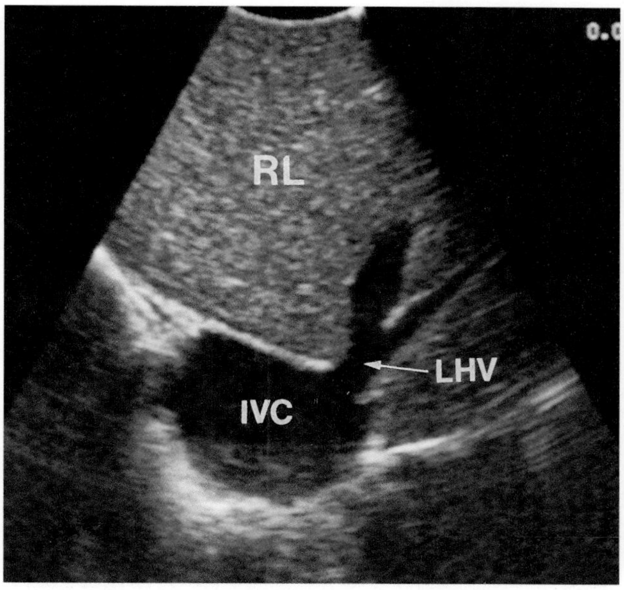

Figure 11.15 *Laparoscopic ultrasound image obtained from the dome of the liver showing normal right lobe of the liver (RL) and left hepatic vein (LHV) into the inferior vena cava (IVC).*

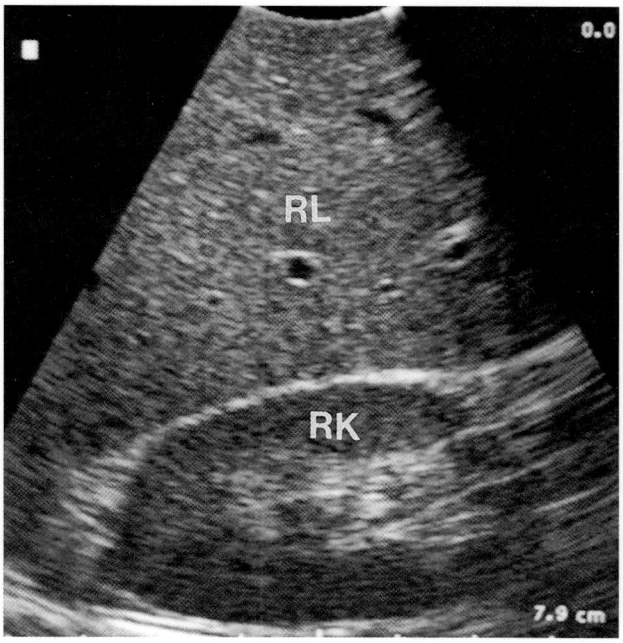

Figure 11.16 *High-resolution ultrasound image of the normal right kidney (RK) and right lobe of the liver (RL) is shown via the laparoscopic approach.*

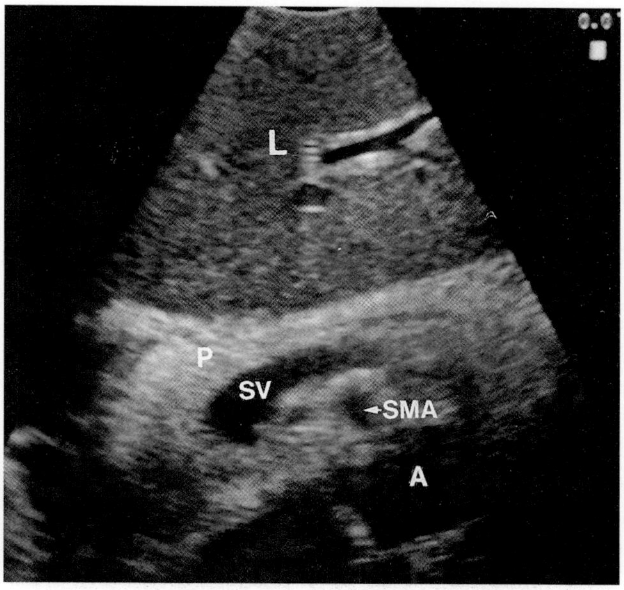

Figure 11.17 *Laparoscopic ultrasound image showing normal pancreas (P) and adjacent vascular structures. SV, splenic vein; SMA, superior mesenteric artery; A, aorta, L, liver.*

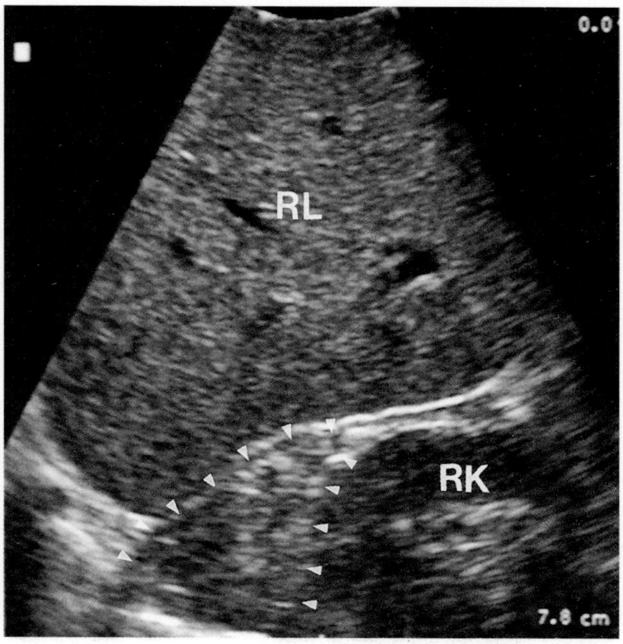

Figure 11.18 *Laparoscopic ultrasound image showing a normal right adrenal gland (arrowheads) located between the right lobe of the liver (RL) and the right kidney (RK).*

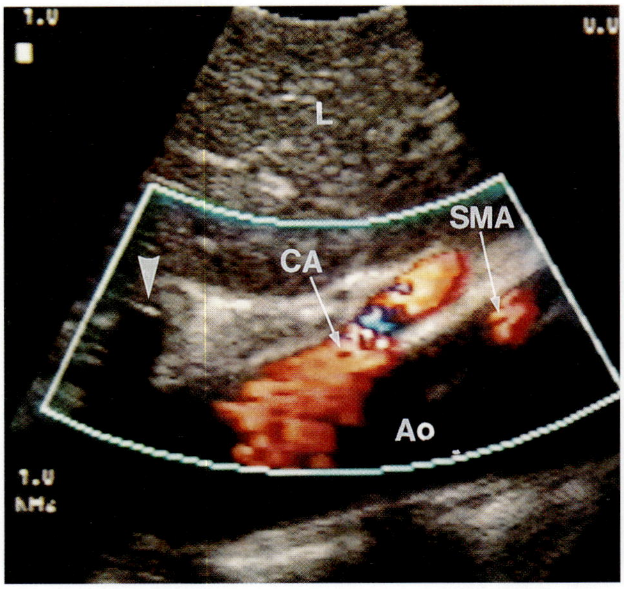

Figure 11.19 *Sagittal laparoscopic ultrasound image with color Doppler display showing a normal segment of abdominal aorta (Ao) and its branches, i.e. celiac artery (CA) and superior mesenteric artery (SMA). Note a nasogastric tube (arrowhead) with acoustic shadowing located at the gastroesophageal junction. L, liver.*

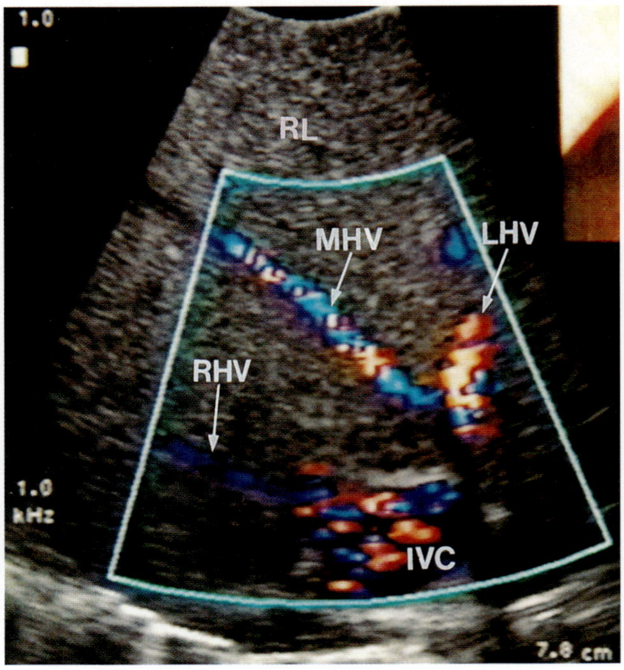

Figure 11.20 *Color Doppler image obtained from the right lobe of the liver (RL) demonstrating flow information for the inferior vena cava (IVC) and its confluence with the hepatic veins. RHV, right hepatic vein; MHV, middle hepatic vein; LHV, left hepatic vein.*

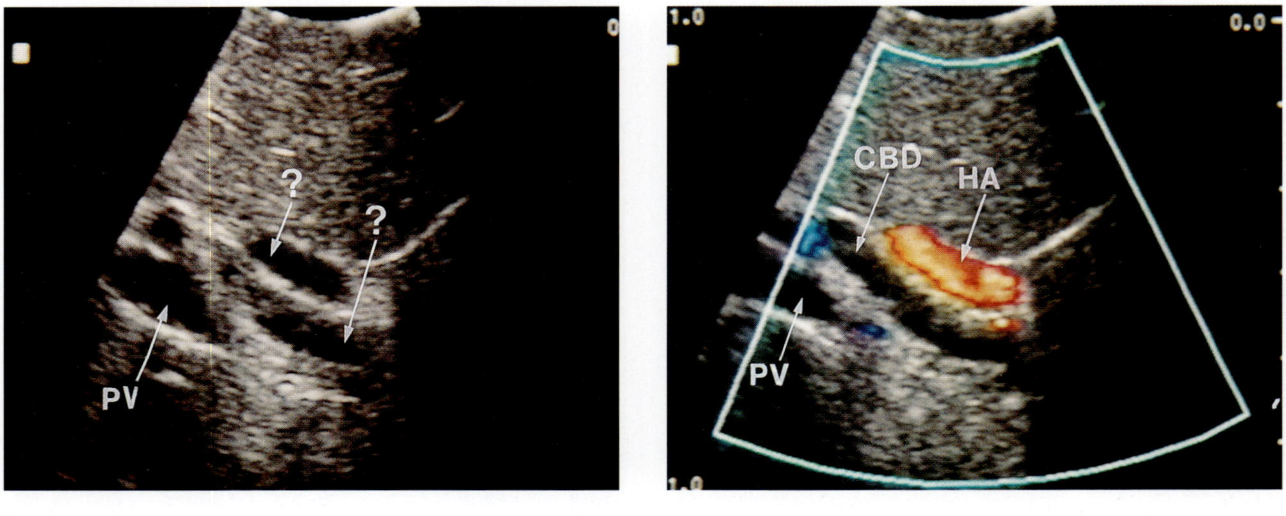

a ***b***

Figure 11.21 *(a) A gray-scale laparoscopic sonogram obtained at the porta hepatis showing three tubular structures corresponding with the portal vein, hepatic artery, and common bile duct. However, it is difficult to differentiate the hepatic artery from the common bile duct. (b) With the use of color Doppler imaging, vascular structures are easily distinguished from the nonvascular structures. In this case, the anatomic variation of the common bile duct (CBD) and the hepatic artery (HA) is clearly demonstrated. PV, portal vein.*

Intraoperative laparoscopic ultrasound saved unnecessary laparotomy in six of eight patients (75%) who were found to be unresectable. In four patients, intraoperative laparoscopic ultrasound verified the preoperative studies and the planned resection was performed without modification (26%). In 13 of the remaining 15 patients (86%), the surgical plan was altered by intraoperative laparoscopic ultrasound and laparoscopic findings being viewed together. In 11 of 15 patients (73%), the preoperative plan was changed based solely on intraoperative laparoscopic ultrasound findings. Two patients (10%) had tumors, that precluded resection and which were diagnosed at laparotomy missed on both laparoscopy and laparoscopic ultrasound. Considered together, laparoscopy and laparoscopic ultrasound saved needless laparotomy incisions in 7 of 11 patients (64%) found unresectable. This preliminary study suggests that laparoscopic ultrasound is an important addition to laparoscopy in staging hepatic tumors.[26]

Laparoscopic ultrasound provided important information which directly influenced surgical decision-making and changed surgical management in 40% of our cases. In 42% of cases, ultrasound provided anatomic information, demonstrated various lesions and/or was used to guide the biopsy of masses. In 8 of 11 cases, in which resection of a liver mass was planned, laparoscopic ultrasound showed additional

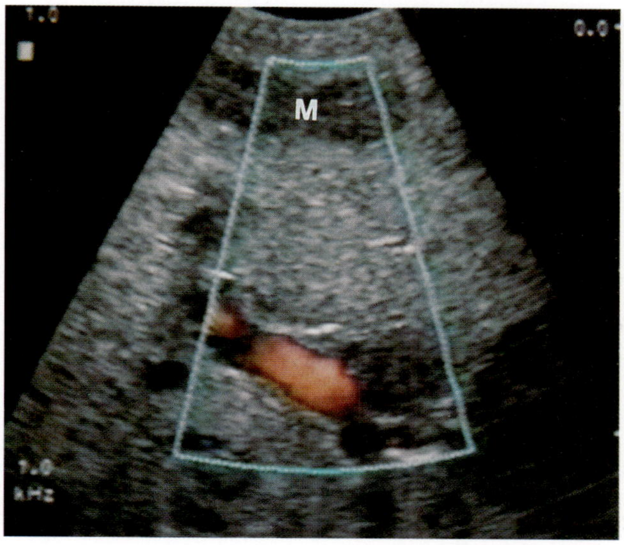

Figure 11.22 *In a patient with colon carcinoma, preoperative MRI had shown right and left medial masses and no evidence of masses in the left lateral segment. A right lobectomy and left medial segmentectomy was planned. Laparoscopic ultrasound demonstrated not only right and left medial lesions but also a lateral segmental mass (M). Laparoscopic ultrasound-guided biopsy of the mass demonstrated metastatic carcinoma, and the open surgery was aborted based on the laparoscopic ultrasound findings.*

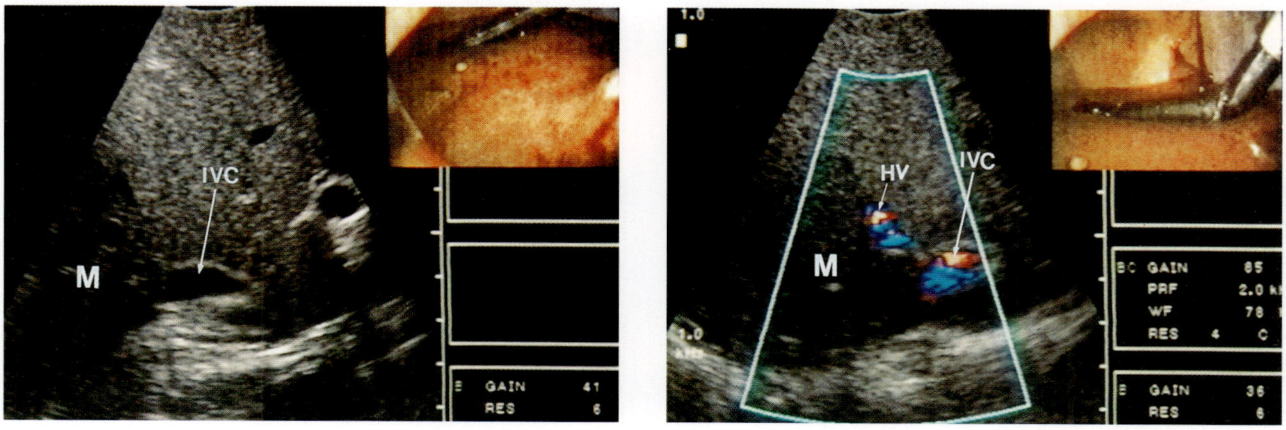

a *b*

Figure 11.23 *(a) Transverse laparoscopic sonogram demonstrating a large hepatic mass (M) adjacent to the inferior vena cava (IVC). (b) Color Doppler imaging clearly delineating the inferior vena cava (IVC) and hepatic vein (HV) invaded by the mass. The open surgery for resection of this mass was precluded based on the laparoscopic ultrasound findings.*

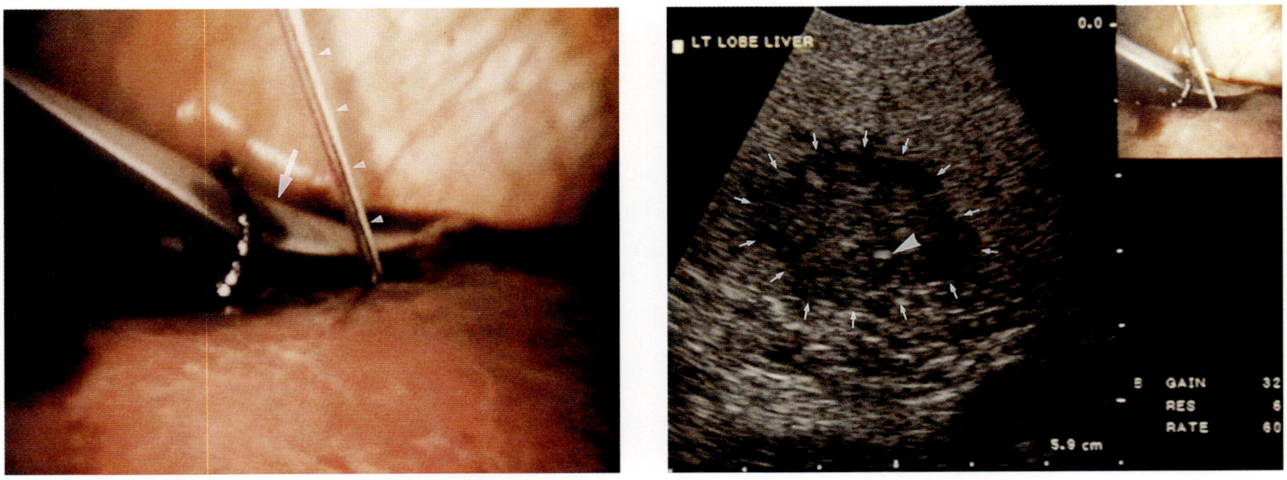

a *b*

Figure 11.24 *(a) An 18-gauge biopsy needle (arrowheads) which has been positioned through the abdominal wall is seen entering the anterior surface of the liver. The adjacent laparoscopic ultrasound transducer (arrow) has been placed in such a way as to guide the needle towards the previously identified hepatic lesion. (b) A reflector arising from the needle tip (arrowhead) has been seen within the solid mass (arrows).*

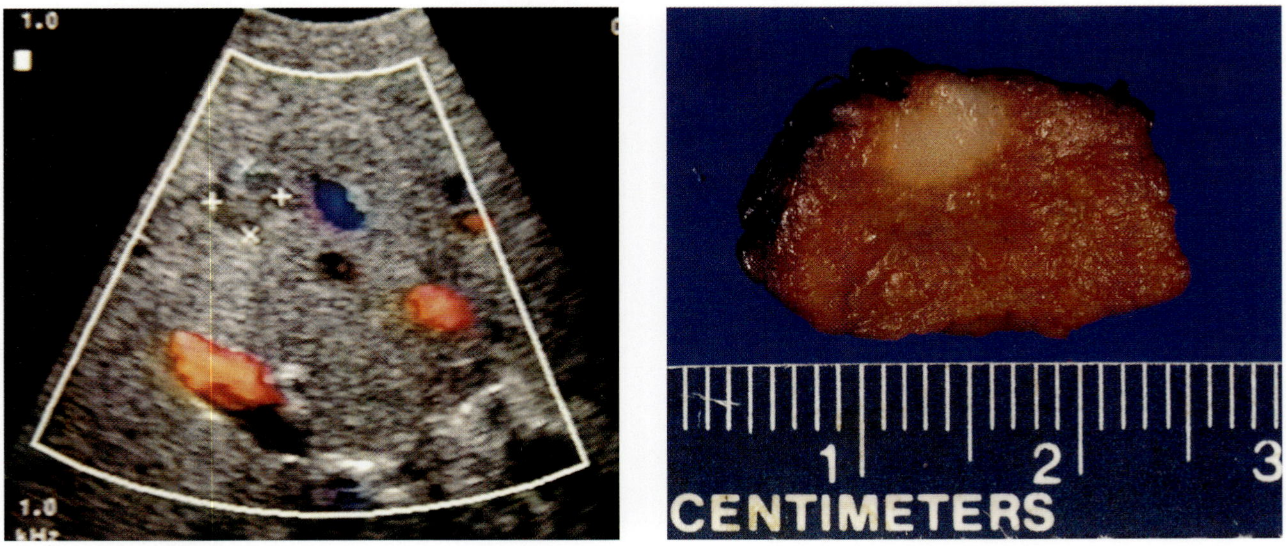

a *b*

Figure 11.25 *(a) In a patient with hepatic metastases, this laparoscopic ultrasound image demonstrates a large mass in the right lobe of the liver (not shown on this image) and a 5-mm mass (cursors) within the left lobe. (b) Pathologic examination of the resected specimen revealed the small tumor measuring 5 mm, corresponding with laparoscopic ultrasound findings.*

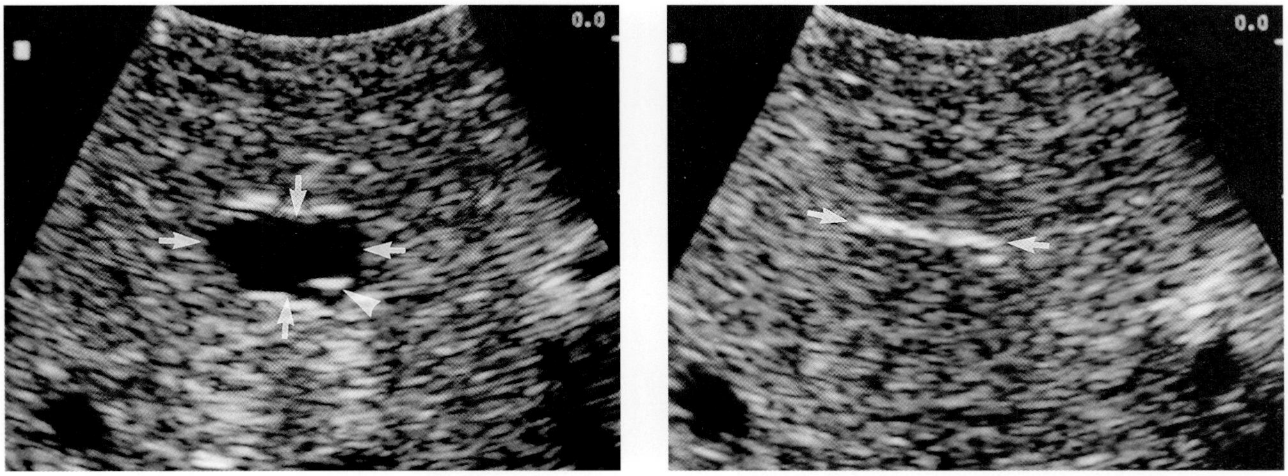

a *b*

Figure 11.26 *(a) A cystic mass (arrows) was identified beneath the surface of the right lobe of the liver. A needle has been directed into the mass guided by continuous laparoscopic ultrasound imaging. A strong reflection of the needle tip (arrowhead) was clearly identified within the cystic mass. (b) Aspiration of the cystic lesion could be monitored by laparoscopic ultrasound, and only a collapsed cystic wall remains following aspiration (arrows). (Reproduced with permission from Liu et al.[22])*

masses, and/or lymphadenopathy or masses immediately adjacent to vascular structures precluding resection; therefore, no further surgery was performed (Figs 11.22 and 11.23).[22] We compared laparoscopic ultrasound with CT portography in evaluating focal liver masses and found that laparoscopic ultrasound directly influenced the surgical management in 4 of 13 (31%) cases.[27] Its major limitation in focal liver disease is in visualization of abnormalities at the dome of the liver, due to the geometry of the probe on the curved surface.

Biopsy under laparoscopic ultrasound guidance was performed when histologic diagnosis was needed to confirm malignancy to help in deciding whether surgical resection could be performed. Laparoscopic ultrasound can be used as a guide for biopsy and is a very effective and safe procedure (Fig. 11.24). While the laparoscopic procedure time was lengthened by the utilization of ultrasound, in many cases the identification of masses within the liver or the imaging of abnormal lymph nodes provided important additional information, allowing more definitive surgical management decisions. In some cases, based on the laparoscopic ultrasound information, it was considered impossible to successfully resect liver tumors. A tumor as small as 5 mm in diameter in the liver was successfully imaged and resected (Fig. 11.25). This mass was not seen on a prior CT and transabdominal ultrasound. In order to rule out the possibility of malignancy, a hepatic cystic lesion was imaged and aspirated under real-time ultrasound guidance (Fig. 11.26). Laparoscopic ultrasound was also able to demonstrate enlarged lymph nodes in the retroperitoneal region which in some cases were not seen with transabdominal ultrasound and CT (Fig. 11.27).

Hepatic vein confluence or main portal vein involvement will alter the feasibility and extent of resection. The relationship of hepatic masses to major vessels can be clearly delineated with laparoscopic ultrasound (Figs 11.28 and 11.29). The criterion that our surgeons use for nonresectability is less than 1 cm of normal tissue between a major vessel (such as the hepatic vein–vena cava confluence) and the mass.

Many patients with hepatocellular carcinoma have intrahepatic metastasis from the primary

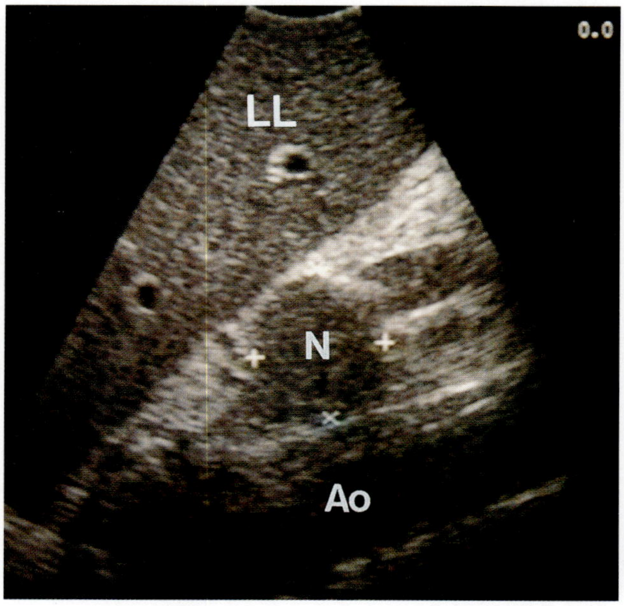

a

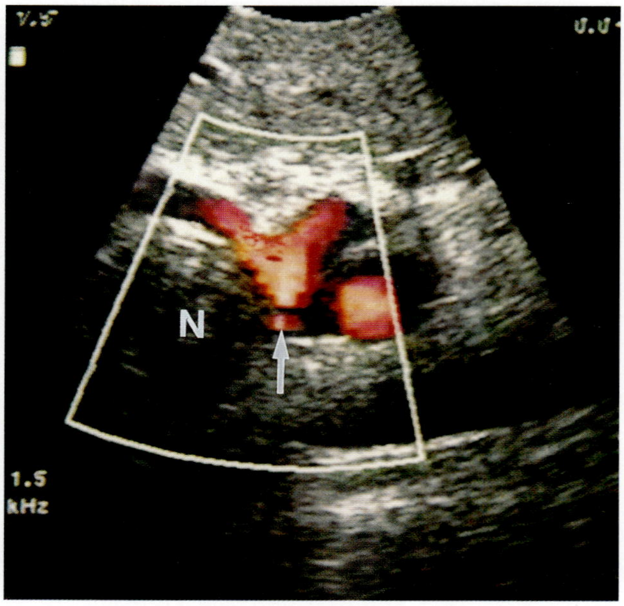

b

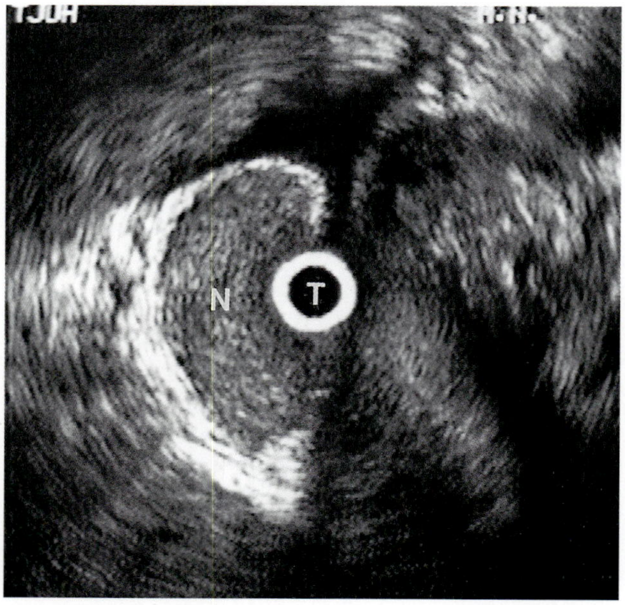

c

Figure 11.27 *(a) Laparoscopic ultrasound image showing a round hypoechoic lymph node (N) located in the para-aortic region which is not detected with transabdominal ultrasound. Ao, aorta; LL, left lobe of the liver. (b) Transverse laparoscopic ultrasound image showing an enlarged lymph node (N) adjacent to the celiac artery (arrow). (c) Laparoscopic ultrasound image obtained by using a catheter-based 20-MHz ultrasound probe delineating an enlarged lymph node (N) that was biopsied under ultrasound guidance. T, transducer.*

tumor, so-called satellite lesions or daughter nodules. The sensitivity of intraoperative ultrasound in detecting these metastatic lesions is significantly greater than that of preoperative modalities.[28] Detection of intravascular tumor thrombi, present in 10–20% of hepatomas, is best done with intraoperative ultrasound.[28] Once the tumor thrombus is found in the portal bifurcation, the tumor is unresectable, since spread to other areas within the liver is usually present at this stage.[29,30] Laparoscopy with laparoscopic ultrasound has been used in oncologic patients to screen for small metastases.[22,31–33] With gray-scale, color and spectral Doppler imaging, occlusion or tumor embolus in the portal veins and the inferior vena cava can be demonstrated (Fig. 11.30).[22]

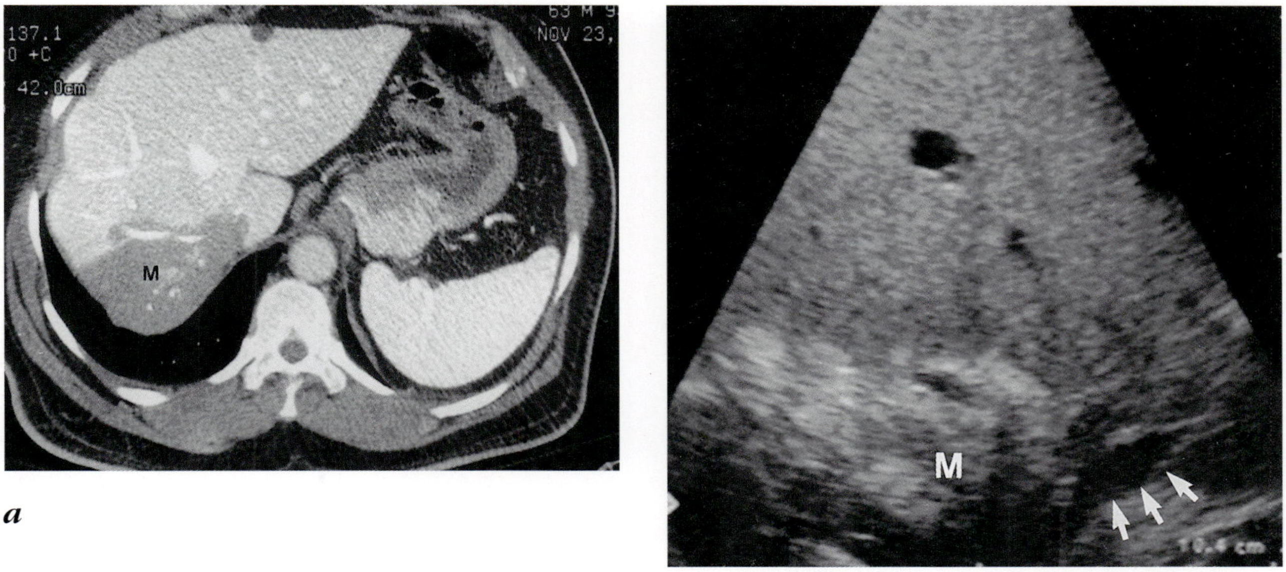

a *b*

Figure 11.28 *(a) Contrast-enhanced CT scan demonstrating a calcified mass (M) in the posterior segment of the right lobe of the liver. However, involvement of the inferior vena cava could not be excluded. (b) Laparoscopic ultrasound demonstrating the hyperechoic mass (M) in the posterior segment of the right lobe of the liver compressing the inferior vena cava wall (arrows). Lobectomy was aborted owing to the proximity of the tumor to this vessel. (Reproduced with permission from Liu et al.[22])*

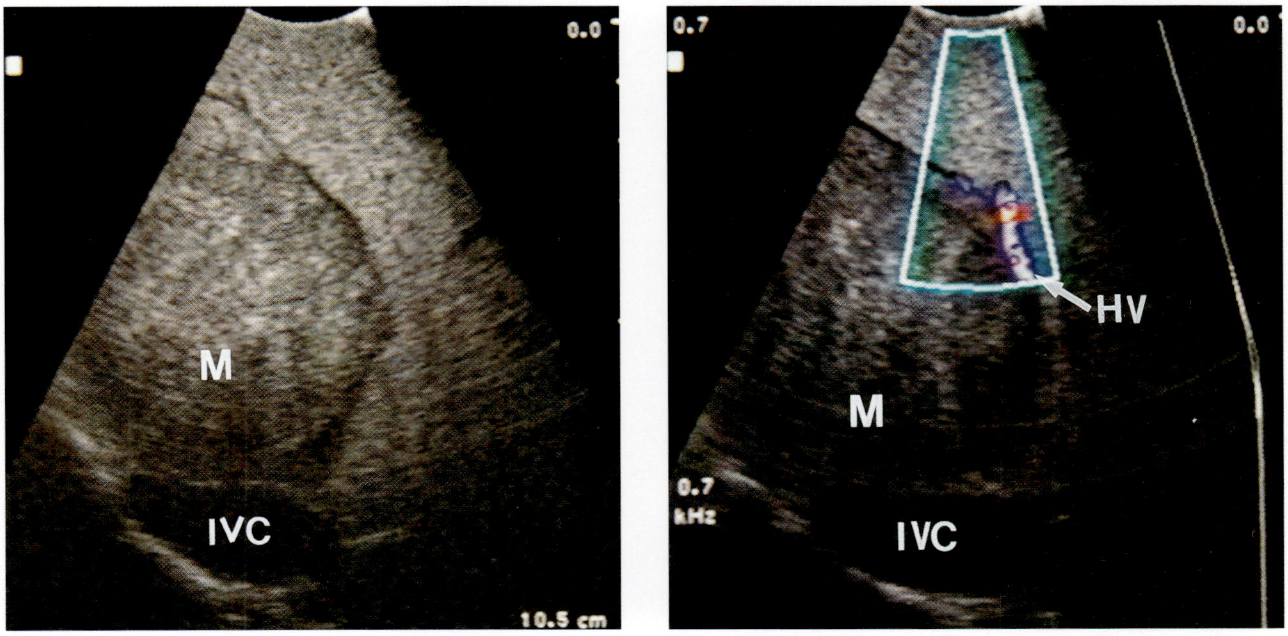

a *b*

Figure 11.29 *(a) In a patient with colon cancer, the gray-scale ultrasound image shows a mass (M) adjacent to the hepatic vein–vena cava confluence. (b) Color Doppler imaging confirmed the gray-scale sonographic findings. Because of the major vascular involvement, no further open surgery was performed. IVC, inferior vena cava; HV, hepatic vein.*

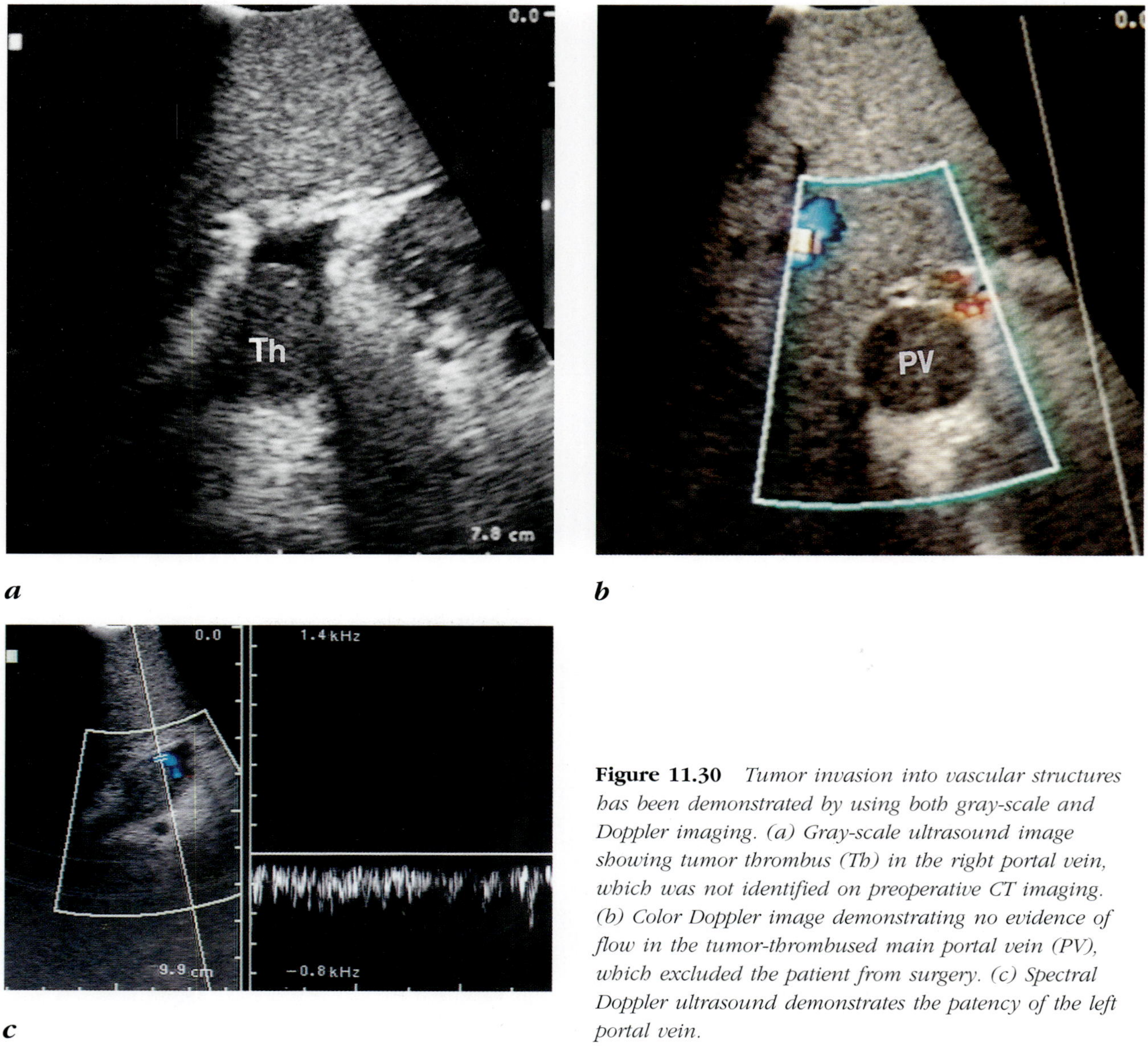

Figure 11.30 *Tumor invasion into vascular structures has been demonstrated by using both gray-scale and Doppler imaging. (a) Gray-scale ultrasound image showing tumor thrombus (Th) in the right portal vein, which was not identified on preoperative CT imaging. (b) Color Doppler image demonstrating no evidence of flow in the tumor-thrombused main portal vein (PV), which excluded the patient from surgery. (c) Spectral Doppler ultrasound demonstrates the patency of the left portal vein.*

PANCREATIC CANCER

Okita et al[16] and Murugiah et al,[34] respectively, reported their initial experience with laparoscopic ultrasound in the early detection and the preoperative staging of patients with carcinoma of the pancreas and periampullary region. Laparoscopic ultrasound was able to assess tumor size, peripancreatic lymphadenopathy and adjacent vascular involvement. It was also able to demonstrate occult hepatic metastases and was used for biopsy guidance.

In a study by Hann et al,[35] laparoscopic ultrasound was used to examine 20 patients with suspected pancreatic carcinoma. In 17 of 20 patients (85%), the vasculature was adequately visualized. Vascular encasement was identified in 12 of 20 patients (60%). Enlarged nodes were present in 12 of 20 cases (60%); nine were node positive for malignancy on laparoscopic ultrasound biopsy. Liver masses were noted in 5 of 20 patients (25%); four were malignant by laparoscopic ultrasound. Ten patients were deemed resectable by laparoscopic ultrasound.

In a study by Machi et al,[36] laparoscopic ultrasound was performed during 36 laparoscopies, including for gallbladder diseases, liver tumors, pancreatic tumors and splenic diseases. Laparoscopic ultrasound, provided beneficial information regarding the characteristics of disease and the stage and resectability of malignancy in 26 operations (72.2%). Based on beneficial findings by laparoscopic ultrasound, the previously planned subsequent operations were altered in 10 cases (27.8%). The authors concluded that laparoscopic ultrasound provides otherwise unobtainable valuable information, particularly in determining the extent of malignant disease, during exploratory laparoscopy.

Kane et al[37] assessed the results of laparoscopic ultrasound, in comparison to preoperative imaging and intraoperative ultrasound, and evaluated the impact of laparoscopic ultrasound on surgical decision-making. Seven of 18 patients (40%) with liver tumors had additional lesions demonstrated on laparoscopic ultrasound. Surgical resection was cancelled in five of these patients. Laparoscopic ultrasound demonstrated three patients with lymphadenopathy and showed evidence of unresectablity in two patients with pancreatic carcinoma. The authors concluded that laparoscopic ultrasound provided important additional information in patients with hepatic, pancreatic and biliary tumors, thereby positively affecting surgical decision-making.

Pietrabissa et al[38] used laparoscopic ultrasound to evaluate 25 patients with suspected pancreatic cancer. Ultrasound examination of the primary tumor can be performed by placing the probe on the region of interest, with interposition of the empty stomach or duodenum. However, an accurate assessment of the local extension of the tumor is best obtained after creation of a wide access, visual and ultrasonographic, to the lesser sac. Results of the study showed that metastatic disease precluding resection was detected in nine instances. Distant spread of the tumor was found in the liver in four patients, and superior mesenteric or portal vein invasion was found in five patients. Staging laparoscopy combined with laparoscopic ultrasound can provide a safe and accurate preoperative assessment of patients with pancreatic cancer.

LAPAROSCOPIC CHOLECYSTECTOMY

Gallbladder disease is very prevalent in the USA, with over 500 000 cholecystectomies being performed annually. Alternatives to open cholecystectomy have been proposed, including lithotripsy, percutaneous stone extraction, percutaneous dissolution of stones, cholecystomy, and percutaneous ablation of the gallbladder. None of these methods has been entirely adequate. However, laparoscopic cholecystectomy has offered a minimally invasive alternative to the open procedure. Laparoscopic cholecystectomy offers several advantages over the open procedure: (1) improved cosmetic results; (2) less postoperative pain; (3) fewer complications; and (4) reduced hospital stay and faster return to work. Laparoscopic cholecystectomy has gained widespread acceptance as the therapeutic choice for cholelithiasis.[1,4]

On the other hand, laparoscopic cholecystectomy has some disadvantages and limitations. With the laparoscopic approach for cholecystectomy, it is not possible for the surgeon to evaluate the distal and intrahepatic portions of the bile ducts. The common bile duct can be mistaken for the cystic duct, and the cystic duct can be inadequately clipped. Unsuspected stones in the bile duct may be present in 5–10% of patients with cholelithiasis.[39] When present, stones will change the surgical management to an open procedure, and it is, therefore, important to recognize them in patients undergoing laparoscopic cholecystectomy. Clinically, preoperative endoscopic retrograde cholangiography (ERCP) is very sensitive but is invasive, expensive and impractical as a routine procedure for the evaluation of biliary calculi. In addition, stones may migrate from the gallbladder into the common bile duct during laparoscopic manipulations.

Operative imaging is an important aspect of laparoscopic cholecystectomy, to reduce the risk of injury to structures in the hepatoduodenal ligament and to screen the bile ducts for stones. Currently, intraoperative cholangiography is the only imaging modality for delineating biliary anatomy and excluding retained common bile duct stones during laparoscopic cholecystectomy. Some investigators have advocated routine cholangiography during laparoscopic cholecystectomy, whereas others suggest performing it only on selected cases.[40,41] However, this approach is time-consuming, requires catheterization of the common bile duct, and may result in leakage of contrast material and/or bile. In addition, the introduction of gas bubbles into the bile ducts during the procedure can cause problems in image interpretation. Furthermore, contrast cholangiography does not image blood vessels in close proximity to bile ducts, such as the portal vein and hepatic artery.

Intracorporeal ultrasonography has been used as a new technique to examine the bile ducts and related structures during laparoscopic cholecystectomy.[22,42–47] Yamashita et al[43] and Jakimowize et al[44] reported the use of laparoscopic ultrasound for evaluation of the biliary system during laparoscopic cholecystectomy. Their results indicated that the entire common bile duct could be visualized in most cases, and that the presence or absence of biliary duct calculi was accurately determined.

John et al have prospectively evaluated laparoscopic ultrasound during elective laparoscopic cholecystectomy in 60 patients, and identified bile duct stones in nine patients, with one false positive and one false negative. Preoperative unsuspected duct stones were delineated in three out of four patients. The suprapancreatic, intrapancreatic and pancreatic ducts were identified in 100%, 80% and 85% of the patients.[45]

A prospective study comparing laparoscopic ultrasound and intraoperative cholangiography in 100 patients by Rothlin et al has shown that sensitivities and specificities for the detection of bile duct calculi were 100% and 98% respectively by laparoscopic ultrasound, and 75% and 99% respectively by intraoperative cholangiography. The time required for laparoscopic ultrasound averaged 5.4 min (range 2–12 min), compared to 16.4 min for intraoperative cholangiography (range 4–37 min).[46]

Another study by Teefey et al[47] reported that common duct stones were detected by laparoscopic ultrasound in 13% (12/90) of cases and by laparoscopic cholangiography in 6% (5/90) of cases. Laparoscopic sonography altered operative management in 2 of 93 patients. The time required to complete laparoscopic sonography ranged from 3 to 18 min, and that required to complete laparoscopic cholangiography ranged from 5–28 min.

Merlino et al[48] studied 123 patients with laparoscopic ultrasound. Eighty-five of these patients were undergoing laparoscopic cholecystectomy. Laparoscopic ultrasound adequately showed the gallbladder wall and contents in all cases and visualized the main bile duct in 93.5% of cases; stones in the common bile duct or cystic duct were demonstrated in three cases. In addition, the liver was examined in 24 patients and secondary lesions were identified in three cases, while benign lesions were seen in six cases. In patients operated on for laparoscopic colonic resection, laparoscopic ultrasound was successfully used to evaluate safely margins for the surgical excision. In six patients with pancreatic and/or extrapancreatic neuroendocrine tumors, laparoscopic ultrasound was useful for lesion identification and biopsy.

In our experience, laparoscopic ultrasound is suitable for imaging both intra- and extrahepatic bile ducts and gallbladder (Figs 11.31 and 11.32). The anatomic variation of the biliary system in the porta hepatus can also be identified (Fig. 11.21). The portal vein and hepatic artery can be identified by their pulsatility and/or color Doppler imaging (Fig. 11.33). In most cases the portion of the distal common bile duct within the head of the pancreas could be imaged (Fig. 11.34).[22]

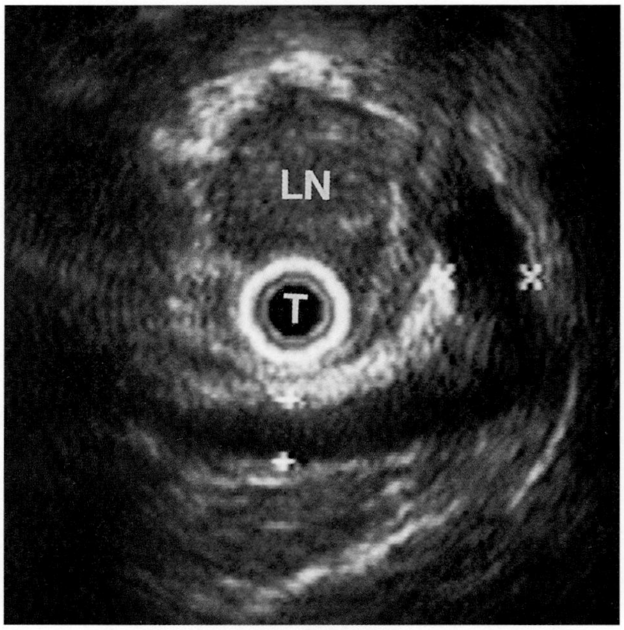

Figure 11.31 *Laparoscopic ultrasound image obtained by using a 20-MHz catheter-based probe (P) demonstrating the confluence of cystic (+) and common bile (×) ducts. A normal-sized lymph node (LN) is clearly delineated adjacent to the duct. T, transducer. (Reproduced with permission from Goldberg et al.[20])*

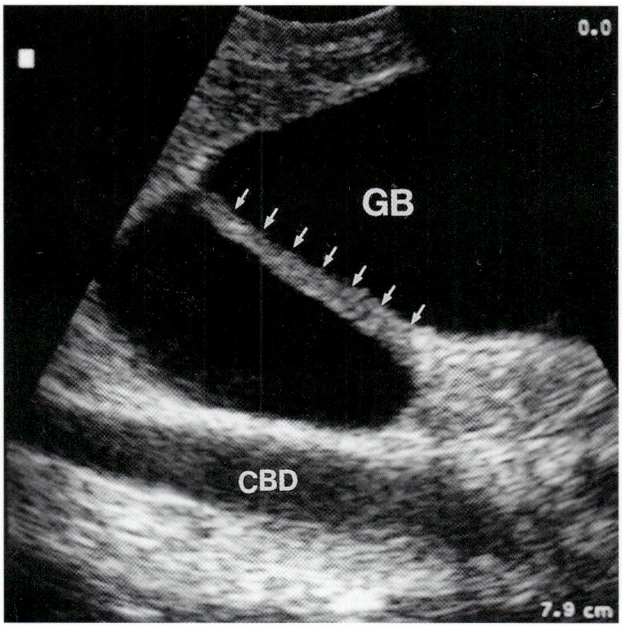

Figure 11.32 *Laparoscopic ultrasound image showing common bile duct (CBD) and a bile-filled gallbladder (GB) with a septum (arrows), which is a normal anatomic variation.*

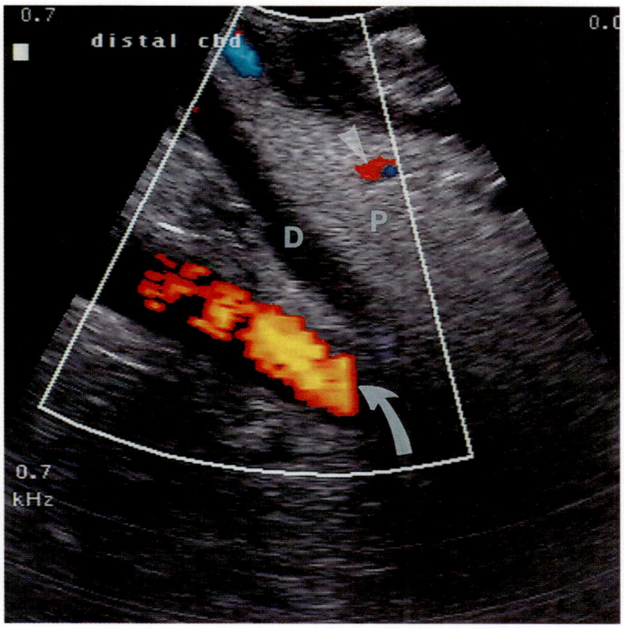

Figure 11.34 *Laparoscopic ultrasound imaging delineated the distal common bile duct (D) at the level of the head of the pancreas (P). The portal vein (arrow) and pancreaticoduodenal artery (arrowhead) were also imaged. (Reproduced with permission from Liu et al.[22])*

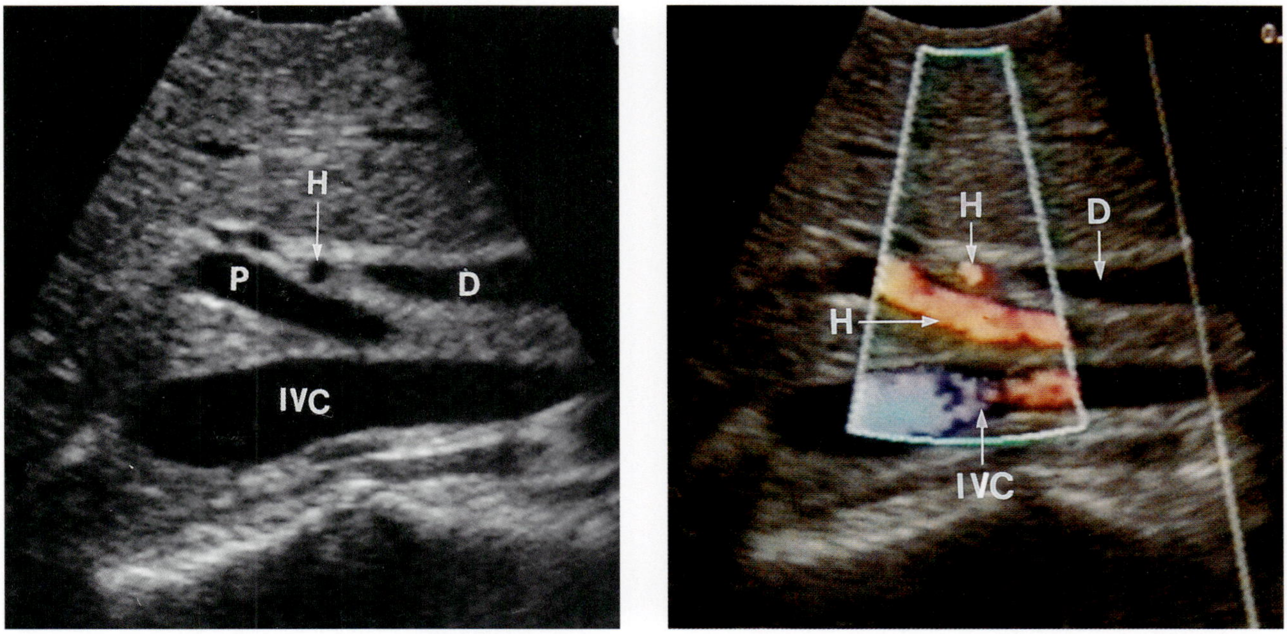

a *b*

Figure 11.33 *(a) Gray-scale ultrasound image showing the common bile duct (D), hepatic artery (H), main portal vein (P), and inferior vena cava (IVC). (b) Using color Doppler imaging, the bile duct is easily distinguished from the vascular structures.*

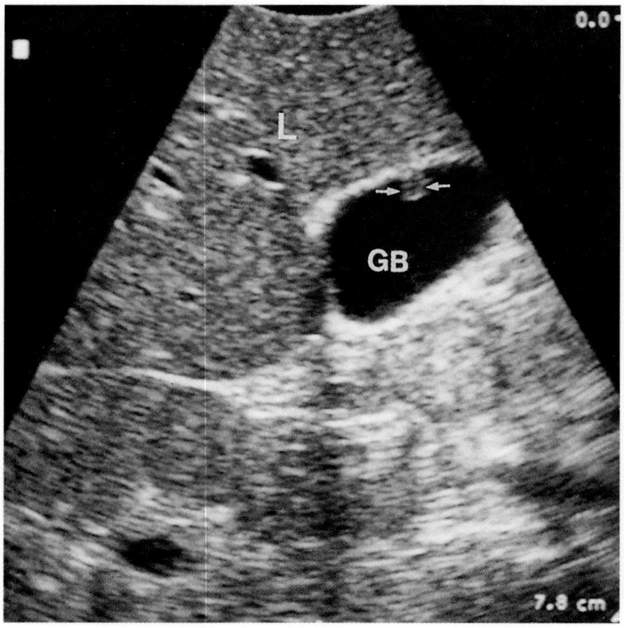

Figure 11.35 *Laparoscopic ultrasound image showing a small mass (arrows) arising from the anterior wall of the gallbladder corresponding with a polyp. L, liver; GB, gallbladder.*

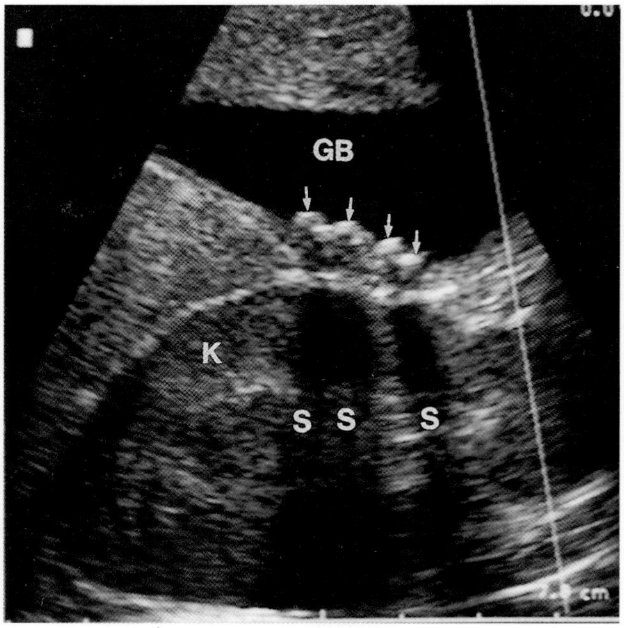

Figure 11.36 *Laparoscopic ultrasound image demonstrating multiple stones (arrows) within the gallbladder (GB). S, shadowing; K, kidney.*

With high-resolution laparoscopic ultrasound imaging, very small lesions within the gallbladder can be demonstrated (Fig. 11.35). Our preliminary results suggest that laparoscopic ultrasound is capable of delineating biliary anatomy and determining the presence or absence of gallstones (Figs 11.36 and 11.37) and duct calculi (Fig. 11.38). Laparoscopic ultrasound is a quick and reliable intraoperative diagnostic tool which could replace intraoperative cholangiography in laparoscopic cholecystectomy. In addition, laparoscopic ultrasound has been used to evaluate pancreatobiliary tumors in terms of tumor staging and stent patency in the biliary tract (Fig. 11.39).

PELVIC LAPAROSCOPY

Intraoperative ultrasound during pelvic laparoscopy has been used to demonstrate both normal and abnormal structures.[20,22,49] Normal ovaries with follicles and fallopian tubes can be imaged (Fig. 11.40). The pelvic vessels (such as the iliac, uterine and ovarian vessels) can be easily imaged using color and

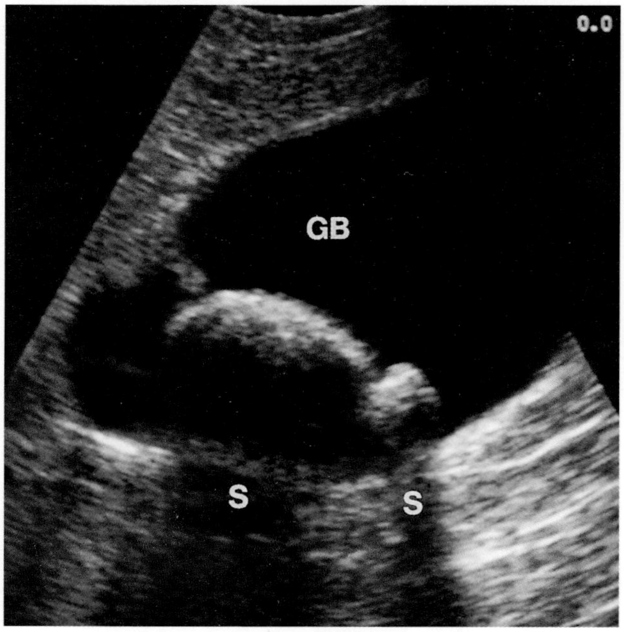

Figure 11.37 *Laparoscopic ultrasound image delineating two stones in the neck of the gallbladder (GB). S, shadowing.*

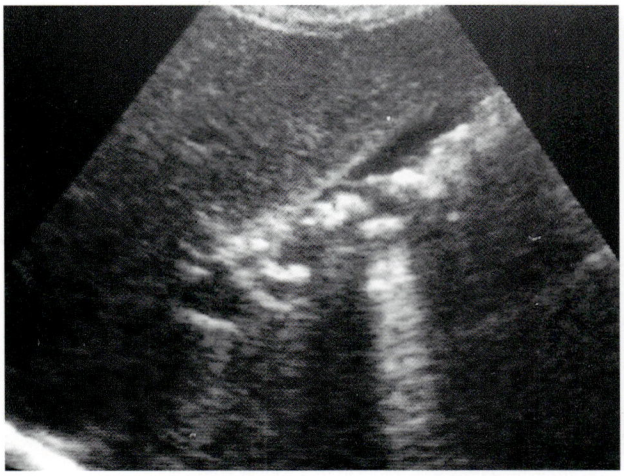

a

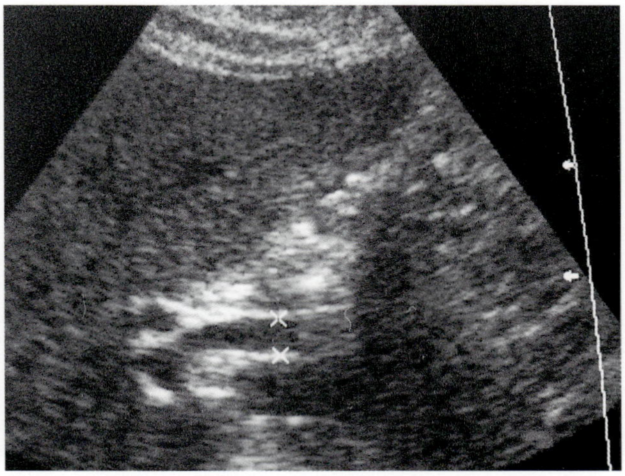

b

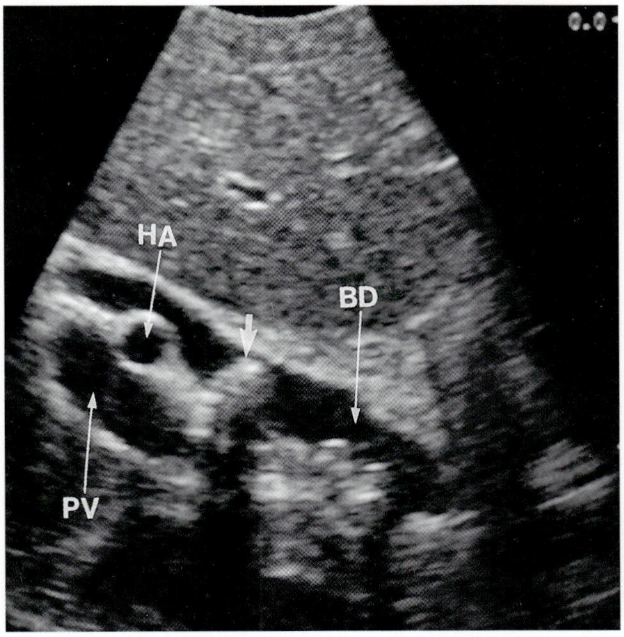

c

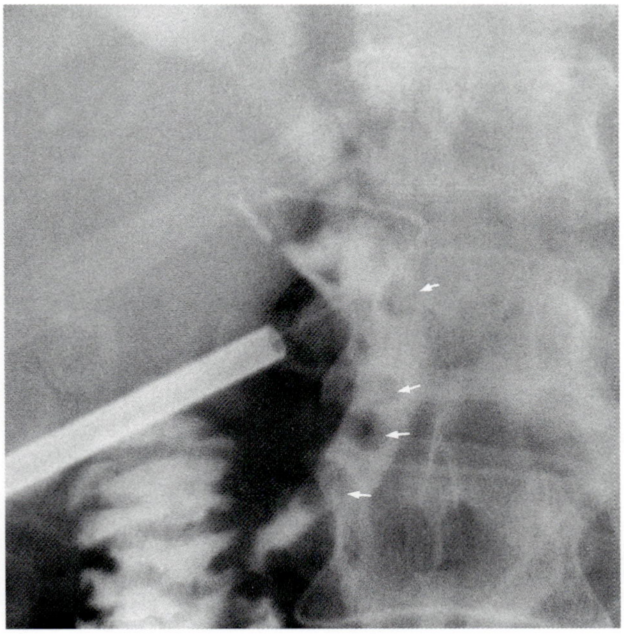

d

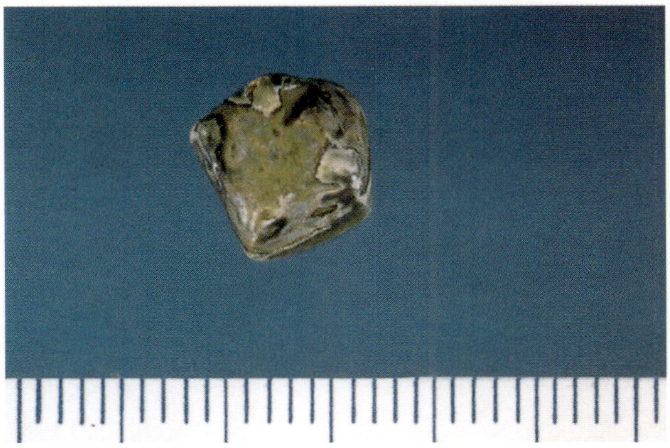

e

Figure 11.38 *In a patient with recurrent upper abdominal pain, preoperative transabdominal ultrasound scan depicts multiple gallstones (a) and slight dilation of common bile duct (x) with no evidence of stones (b). (c) Laparoscopic ultrasound identified multiple stones within the bile duct (BD); one stone is seen on this image (arrow). PV, portal vein; HA, hepatic artery. (d) The presence of the bile duct stones (arrows) was subsequently confirmed by intraoperative cholangiography. (e) Based on the ultrasound findings, open surgery was performed and stones were removed from the bile ducts. One stone specimen is shown in this picture. ((b), (c), and (d) reproduced with permission from Liu JB et al.[23])*

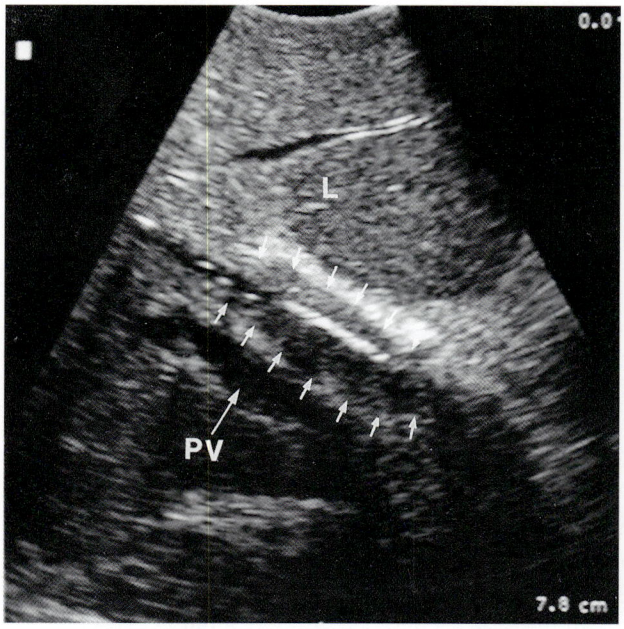

a

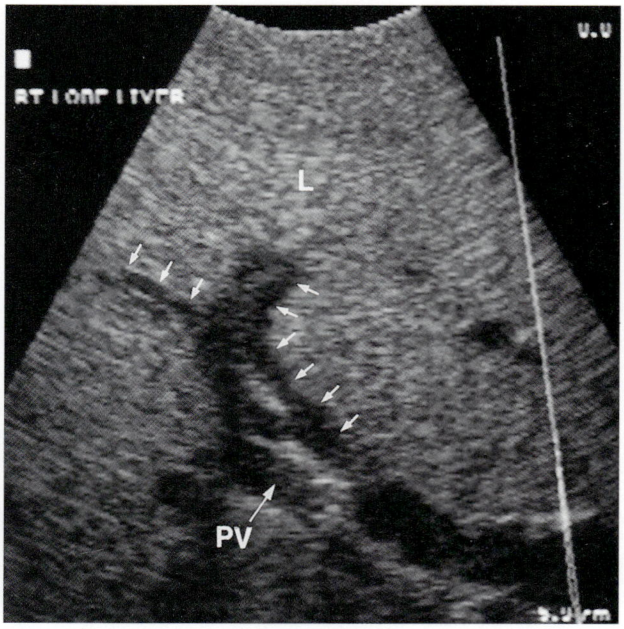

b

Figure 11.39 *In a patient with cholangiocarcinoma and post-statue biliary stent drainage, laparoscopic ultrasound was used to evaluate the patency of the biliary stent. (a) Laparoscopic sonogram showing that the stent was completely occluded by the tumor infiltration (arrows) and (b) the dilation of intrahepatic ducts (arrows) was associated with the obstruction of the distal bile duct. L, liver; PV, portal vein.*

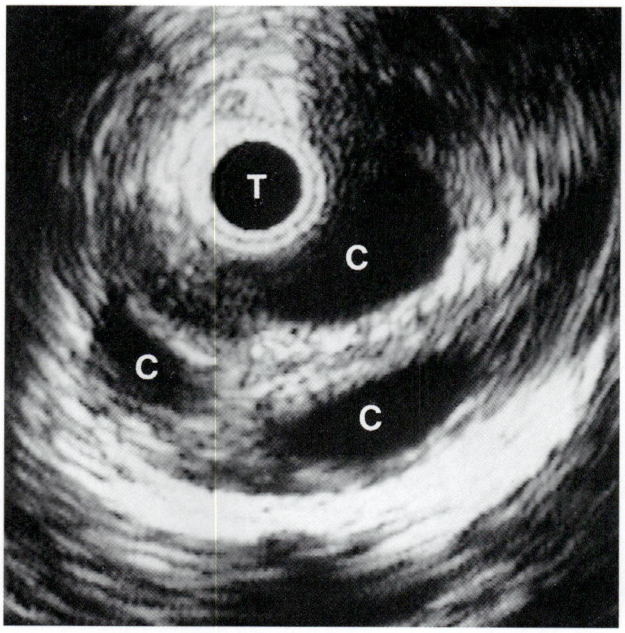

Fig. 11.40 *Laparoscopic ultrasound image obtained using a 20-MHz catheter-based transducer (T) showing the right ovary with several cystic areas (C) consistent with follicles. (Reproduced with permission from Goldberg et al.[20])*

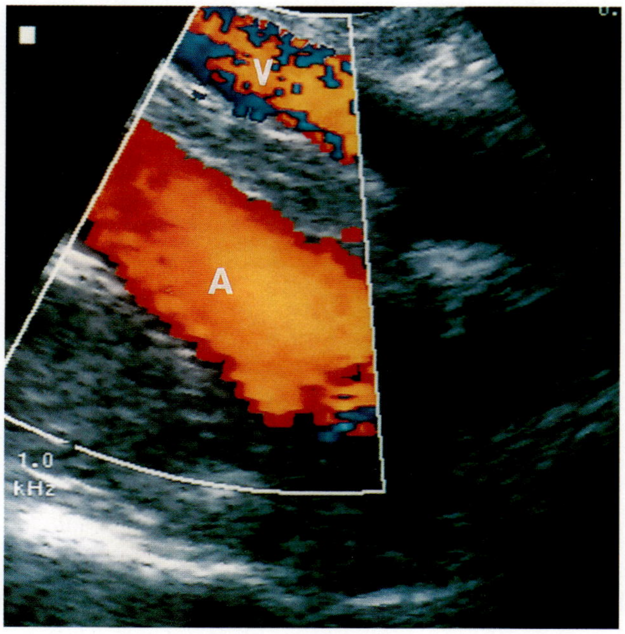

Figure 11.41 *Laparoscopic color Doppler image showing the iliac artery (A) and vein (V).*

spectral Doppler (Fig. 11.41). Vessels within ovarian tumors can also be identified.

By imaging beneath the exposed surface, it has been possible to identify lymph nodes and blood vessels, as well as establish their relationship to each other (Fig. 11.42). Clinically, pelvic laparoscopic lymph node biopsy has been used for staging of ovarian and prostatic tumors. The ability to image behind major blood vessels (such as the iliac artery and vein) enables dissection to be avoided when sonography fails to demonstrate any lymphadenopathy or masses.

With the use of this technique, we have been able to identify a small dermoid within a normal-sized ovary and to then guide removal of the tumor laparoscopically with a small incision on the ovary (Fig. 11.43).

LIMITATIONS AND FUTURE DEVELOPMENTS

The use of laparoscopic ultrasound has been technically successful in more than 97% of cases.[22,46,47] In some cases, however, abdominal adhesions prevented the positioning of the ultrasound probe over the target organ. Another technical limitation concerns the evaluation of the dome of the liver, where lesions may be beyond the reach of the probe, owing to the steep angulation necessary to make contact with that portion of the liver surface. Further experience in probe manipulation and improved probe design, along with better planning of trocar placement, should reduce this limitation. In some cases, the most distal common bile duct could not be adequately imaged, due to interference from bowel gas as well as scanning angle. Further modification of the probe, such as a combination of a side- and forward-viewing transducer along with more flexibility, should improve its capabilities in hepatobiliary imaging.

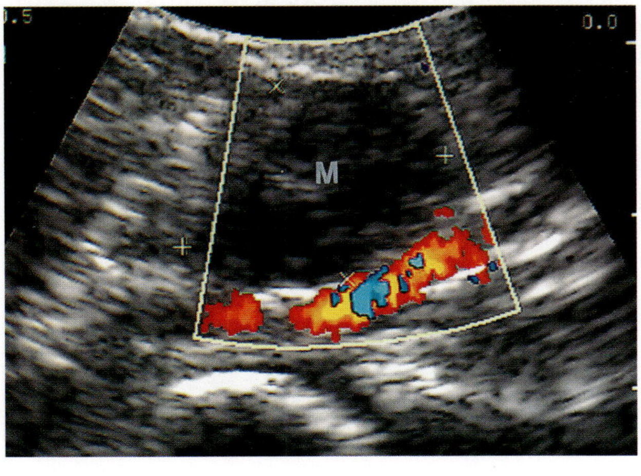

Figure 11.42 *A hypoechoic mass (M) measuring 1.6×1.2 cm was delineated adjacent to a branch of the iliac vessels corresponding with an enlarged lymph node.*

A biopsy working channel built into the laparoscopic ultrasound probe would make it easier to laparoscopically biopsy lesions, and should increase the accuracy of ultrasound-guided biopsy. This technique has been successfully used for biopsy of gastric lesions through flexible endoscopic ultrasound probes.[50,51]

Cryosurgery is a surgical procedure that employs an instrument containing liquid nitrogen to freeze the tumor in situ and leave the neoplasm for later internal absorption. Hepatic cryosurgery is important for patients with hepatic metastases abutting major vessels or involving multiple lobes, because only 25% of patients with hepatic metastases are eligible for surgical resection. Intraoperative ultrasound is crucial to locate deep metastases, to guide cryoprobe placement, to determine the size of frozen tissue, and to monitor the thawing process. Although the current cryosurgery requires an open surgical procedure, preliminary ultrasound-guided laparoscopic cryosurgery has been used in the treatment of hepatic tumors.[52] Further modification of laparoscopic ultrasound devices and refinement of cryosurgical probes may broaden the applications for laparoscopic cryodestruction.

CONCLUSION

Laparoscopic surgery has been accepted as the surgery of choice for many diagnostic and therapeutic abdominal procedures due to decreased morbidity, reduced cost and improvement in long-term outcomes compared with open procedures. This approach, however, has inherent limitations in the evaluation of diseases concealed within solid organs,

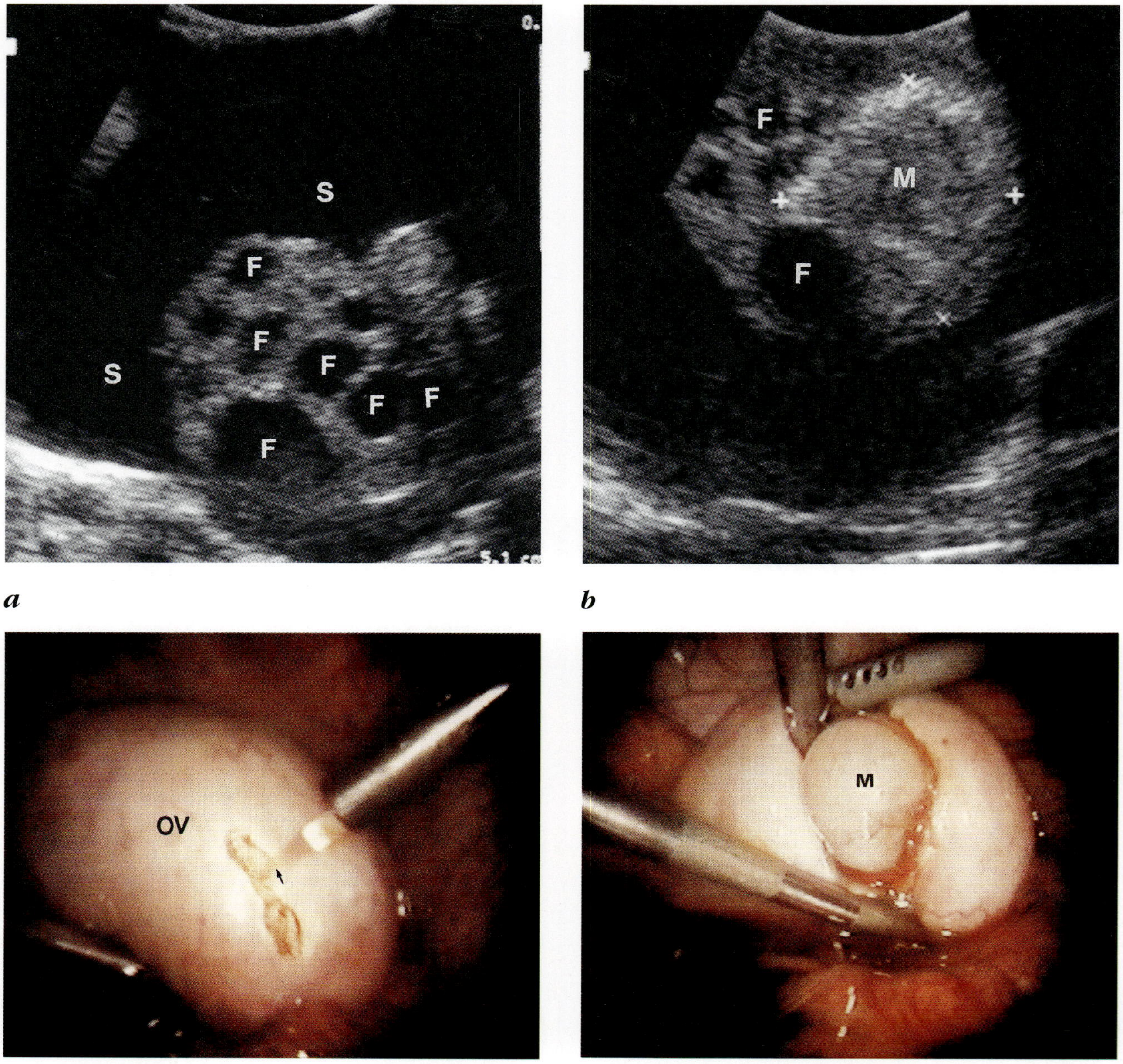

a *b* *c* *d*

Figure 11.43 *In a young patient with small right ovarian mass undergoing laparoscopic surgery to remove the mass, laparoscopic ultrasound was used to detect the lesion. (a) Laparoscopic sonogram of normal left ovary with follicles (F) surrounded with saline solution (S). (b) A hyperechoic mass (M) within a normal-sized ovary corresponding with an ovarian dermoid. F, follicles. (c) After ultrasound localization of the mass, a small incision was made using the laser knife (arrow). OV, ovary. (d) With minimal invasion of the normal portion of the ovary, the tumor (M) was removed laparoscopically.*

hollow viscera or the retroperitoneum. Laparoscopic ultrasound, which evolved from the concepts of intraoperative and endoscopic ultrasound, ceates a whole new range of possibilities for accurately diagnosing and treating conditions laparoscopically. Although a wide variety of uses for laparoscopic ultrasound have been demonstrated, continued development of laparoscopic ultrasound equipment and further investigation of this technique will be needed before its efficacy is fully established. We anticipate that this technique will prove to be a valuable new adjunct to a variety of laparoscopic procedures for the diagnosis and treatment of abdominal and pelvic abnormalities.

REFERENCES

1. The Southern Surgeons Club, A prospective analysis of 1,518 laparoscopic cholecystectomies performed by Southern US surgeons, *N Engl J Med* 1991; **324**:1073–8.
2. Soper NJ, Brunt ML, Kerbl K, Laparoscopic general surgery, *N Engl J Med* 1994; **330**:409–19.
3. Lightdale CJ, Laparoscopy and biopsy in malignant liver disease, *Cancer* 1982; **50**:2672–5.
4. Bass EB, Pitt HA, Lillemoe KD, Cost-effectiveness of laparoscopic cholecystectomy vs open cholecystectomy, *Am J Surg* 1993; **165**:466–7.
5. Bismuth H, Castaing D, Garden OJ, The use of operative ultrasound in surgery of primary liver tumor, *World J Surg* 1987; **11**:610–14.
6. Parker GA, Lawrence W, Horsely JS et al, Intraoperative ultrasound of the liver affects operative decision making, *Ann Surg* 1989; **209**:569–77.
7. Machi J, Takeda J, Kakegawa T et al, The detection of gastric and esophageal tumor extension by high-resolution ultrasound during surgery, *World J Surg* 1987; **11**:664–71.
8. Machi J, Sigel B, Overview of benefits of operative ultrasonography during a ten-year period, *J Ultrasound Med* 1989; **8**:647–52.
9. Sigel B, Coelho JCU, Machi J et al, The application of real-time ultrasound imaging during surgical procedures, *Surg Gynecol Obstet* 1983; **157**:33–7.
10. Yamakawa K, Naito S, Azuma K et al, Laparoscopic diagnosis of the intraabdominal organs, *Jpn J Gastroenterol* 1958; **55**:741–7.
11. Yamakawa K, Yoshioka A, Shimizu K et al, Laparoechography—an ultrasonic diagnosis under the laparoscopic observation, *Jpn Med Ultrasonics* 1964; **2**(2):26.
12. Kratochwil A, Vergleichende laparoskopie und ultraschalluntersuchungen bei hormonell stimulierten frauen, *Acta Endoscop Radiocinematograph* 1977; **7**(1):21–8.
13. Ohta Y, Yamazaki M, Torii M et al, A device of ultrasonic laparoscope, *Gastroenterol Endosc* 1981; **23**:1385–91.
14. Oda M, Development of ultrasonic laparoscope, *Gastroenterol Endosc* 1982; **24**:884–93.
15. Fukuda M, Mima S, Tanabe T et al, Endoscopic sonography of the liver—diagnostic application of the echolaparoscope to localize intrahepatic lesions, *Scand J Gastroenterol* 1984; **19**(S102):24–38.
16. Okita K, Kodama T, Oda M et al, Laparoscopic ultrasonography—diagnosis of liver and pancreatic cancer, *Scand J Gastroenterol* 1984; **19**(Suppl 94):91–100.
17. Frank K, Bliesze H, Honhof JA et al, Laparoscopic sonography: a new approach to intraabdominal disease, *J Clin Ultrasound* 1985; **13**:60–5.
18. Fornari F, Civardi G, Cavanna L et al, Laparoscopic ultrasonography in the study of the liver diseases, *Surg Endosc* 1989; **3**:33–7.
19. Miles WFA, Paterson-Brown S, Garden OJ, Laparoscopic contact hepatic ultrasonography, *Br J Surg* 1992; **79**:419–20.
20. Goldberg BB, Liu JB, Merton DA et al, Sonographically guided laparoscopy and mediastinoscopy using miniature catheter-based transducers, *J Ultrasound Med* 1993; **12**: 49–54.
21. Ascher SM, Evans SRT, Goldberg JA et al, Intraoperative bile duct sonography during laparoscopic cholecystectomy: experience with a 12.5 MHz catheter-based US probe, *Radiology* 1992; **185**:493–6.
22. Liu JB, Feld RI, Goldberg BB et al, Laparoscopic gray-scale and color Doppler US: preliminary animal and clinical studies, *Radiology* 1995; **194**:851–7.
23. Liu JB, Feld RI, Barbot DJ, Rosato FE, Goldberg BB, Laparoscopic ultrasound: its role in laparoscopic surgery, *Semin Laparosc Surg* 1996; **3**:50–8.
24. Spinelli P, Difelice G, Laparoscopy and abdominal malignancies, *Prob Gen Surg* 1991; **8**:329–47.
25. John TG, Greig JD, Crosbie JL, Miles WFA, Garden OJ, Superior staging of liver tumors with laparoscopy and laparoscopic ultrasound, *Ann Surg* 1994; **220**(6):711–19.
26. Barbot DJ, Marks J, Feld RI, Liu JB, Rosato FE, Improved staging of liver tumors using laparoscopic intraoperative ultrasound, *J Surg Oncol* 1997; **64**:63–7.
27. Feld RI, Liu JB, Nazarian L et al, Laparoscopic liver sonography: preliminary experience in liver metastases compared with CT portography, *J Ultrasound Med* 1996; **15**(4):289–95.
28. Makuuchi M, Hasegawa H, Yamazaki S, Clinical application of operative sonography for the liver, *Taisha* 1985; **22**(S):899.
29. Makuuchi M, Hasegawa H, Yamazaki S, Intraoperative ultrasonic examination for hepatectomy, *Jpn J Clin Oncol* 1981; **11**:367.
30. Nakashima T, Vascular changes and hemodynamics in hepatocellular carcinoma. In: Okude K, Petus RL, eds, *Hepatocellular Carcinoma* (John Wiley: New York, 1975) 196.
31. Fornari F, Civardi G, Cavanna L et al, Laparoscopic ultrasonography in the study of liver diseases, *Surg Endosc* 1989; **3**:33–7.
32. Boenhof JA, Frank K, Loch EG, Linhart P, Laparoscopic sonography, *Ann Radiol* 1985; **28**:16–18.
33. Frank K, Bliesze H, Hönhof JA et al, Laparoscopic sonography: a new approach to intraabdominal disease, *J Clin Ultrasound* 1985; **13**:60–5.

34. Murugiah M, Paterson-Brown S, Windson JA, Miles WFA, Garden OJ, Early experience of laparoscopic ultrasonography in the management of pancreatic carcinoma, *Surg Endosc* 1993; **7**:177–81.
35. Hann LE, Conlon KC, Bach AM, Dougherty EC, Brennan MF, Laparoscopic gray-scale spectral Doppler ultrasound: applications in management of pancreatic carcinoma, *J Ultrasound Med* 1996; **15**:S63.
36. Machi J, Sigel B, Schwartz JH, Zaren HA, Intraoperative laparoscopic ultrasound during exploratory laparoscopy, *J Ultrasound Med* 1996; **15**:S64.
37. Kane RA, Kruskal JB, Stone M et al, Laparoscopic ultrasound evaluation of hepatic biliary, and pancreatic tumors, *J Ultrasound Med* 1996; **15**:S64.
38. Pietrabissa A, Candio GD, Giulianotti PC, Mosca F, Laparoscopic exposure of the pancreas and staging of pancreatic cancer, *Semin Laparosc Surg* 1996; **3**(1):3–9.
39. Gadacz TR, Talamini MA, Traditional versus laparoscopic cholecystectomy, *Am J Surg* 1991; **161**:336–8.
40. Berci G, Sackier JM, Paz-Partlow M, Routine or selected intraoperative cholangiography during laparoscopic cholecystectomy? *Am J Surg* 1991; **161**:355–60.
41. Strasberg SM, Clavien P, Sanabria JR, Laparoscopic cholecystectomy, *Semin Roentgenol* 1991; **26**:232–8.
42. Machi J, Sigel B, Zaren HA et al, Technique of ultrasound examination during laparoscopic cholecystectomy, *Surg Endosc* 1993; **7**:544–9.
43. Yamamoto M, Stiegmann GV, Durham J et al, Laparoscopy-guided intracorporeal ultrasound accurately delineates hepatobiliary anatomy, *Surg Endosc* 1993; **7**:325–30.
44. Jakimowicz JJ, Ruers TJM, Ultrasound-assisted laparoscopic cholecystectomy: preliminary experience, *Dig Surg* 1991; **8**:114–17.
45. John TG, Banting SW, Pye S, Paterson-Brown S, Garden OJ, Preliminary experience with intracorporeal laparoscopic ultrasonography using a sector scanning probe: a prospective comparison with intraoperative cholangiography in the detection of choledocholithiasis, *Surg Endosc* 1994; **8**(10):1176–80.
46. Rothlin MA, Schlumpf R, Largiader F, Laparoscopic sonography: an alternative to routine intraoperative cholangiography? *Arch Surg* 1994; **129**:694–700.
47. Teefey SA, Soper NJ, Middleton WD et al, Imaging of the common bile duct during laparoscopic cholecystectomy: sonography versus videofluoroscopic cholangiography, *AJR* 1995; **165**:847–51.
48. Merlino R, Bezzi M, Orsi F et al, Laparoscopic ultrasound: results in 123 consecutive patients, *Gastroenterology* 1995; **108**(4):A427.
49. Kratochwil A, Vergleichende laparoskopie und ultraschalluntersuchungen bei hormonell stimulierten frauen, *Acta Endosc Radiocinematograph* 1977; **7**(1):21–8.
50. Chang KJ, Katz KD, Durbin et al, Endoscopic ultrasound-guided fine-needle aspiration, *Gastrointest Endosc* 1994; **40**:694–9.
51. Vilmann P, Hancke S, Henriksen FW, Jacobsen GK, Endoscopic ultrasonography-guided fine-needle aspiration biopsy of lesion in the upper gastrointestinal tract, *Gastrointest Endosc* 1995; **41**:230–5.
52. Stiegmann GV, Cohn AL, Nakano S, Cryodestruction of hepatic tumors. *Surgical Overview-Surgical Technology International III.* 61–6.

Chapter 12 Three-dimensional endoluminal ultrasound

Ji-Bin Liu, Larry S Miller, Demetrius H Bagley, Joseph Bonn, Flemming Forsberg and Barry B Goldberg

INTRODUCTION

Three-dimensional (3D) imaging by computerized tomography (CT) and magnetic resonance imaging (MRI) has been utilized in many aspects of diagnostic medicine and has been gradually integrated into routine clinical practice. Technical advances in image acquisition, processing and display have considerably facilitated the application of 3D imaging to the evaluation of many parts of the human anatomy.[1–3] Thus, it is not surprising that efforts have been made to develop computer-assisted systems for 3D display of ultrasound images.

Three-dimensional ultrasound was reported as early as 1961 by Baum and Greenwood for the evaluation of orbital lesions.[4] Since that time, researchers throughout the world have been working on developing computer systems that can produce 3D ultrasound images.[5–15] Three-dimensional reconstructed ultrasound images have been limited by the low dynamic range of the gray-scale ultrasound images and the large amount of computer power required. However, with the recent advances in computer technology, reports have appeared on 3D ultrasound reconstruction of the cardiovascular system, reproductive system, gastrointestinal tract and other structures.[5–15]

Endoluminal ultrasound in particular lends itself to 3D reconstruction. To date, most attempts at 3D imaging using catheter-based transducers have involved intravascular ultrasound. Reliable and consistent 3D reconstructions which correlate with angiography have been obtained.[7,8] Three-dimensional intravascular imaging allows evaluation of vascular pathology in multiple planes simultaneously. This advantage also applies to endoluminal nonvascular 3D ultrasound images.

In this chapter we will review and discuss current computer-assisted 3D methods and techniques for ultrasound imaging, in particular for 3D reconstruction of endoluminal images.

TECHNIQUE

DATA ACQUISITION

Three-dimensional images can be created using any digital tomographic medical imaging modality by stacking the two-dimensional (2D) slices, as in CT and MR imaging. Ultrasound imaging presents opportunities for 3D reconstruction, since the images are tomographic and frame rates are acquired at between 10 and 60 images per second. Data acquisition is the first, crucial step for all 3D ultrasound investigations. A number of techniques have been described for acquiring a sequence of ultrasound images, or data sets, so that they can later be combined into 3D volumes. Most 3D acquisition techniques share a common basis: during a scanning procedure, a data set of 2D ultrasound planes along with their relative spatial locations and orientations are saved into a computer memory. Knowledge of the spatial location and orientation of the scanned planes allows the visualization program to reconstruct the original geometry of the scanned object. The various 3D acquisition techniques differ in the ways in which the 2D planes are scanned and in how the spatial locations and orientations are determined. The acquisition methods can be optimized for various scanning situations such as organ location, acoustic window or pulsatile structures. Numerous instruments have been developed to meet the requirements of these

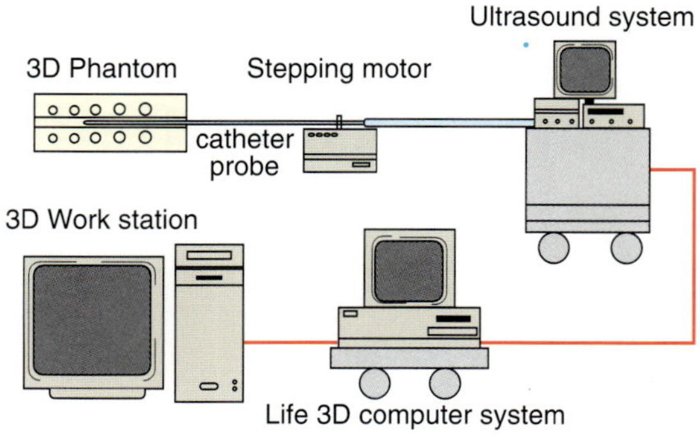

Figure 12.1 *Stepping motor, endoluminal ultrasound and the computer system set-up for 3D reconstruction.*

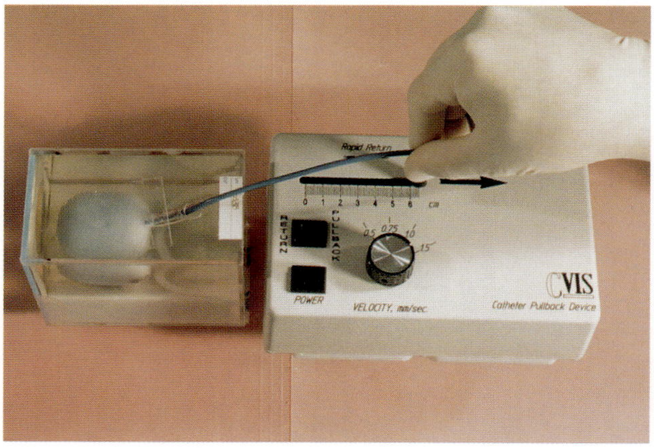

Figure 12.2 *The ultrasound catheter is positioned in the lumen of the 3D tumor phantom and is then attached to the stepping motor. The motor pulls the catheter at a set speed to acquire cross-sectional images on the IVUS system.*

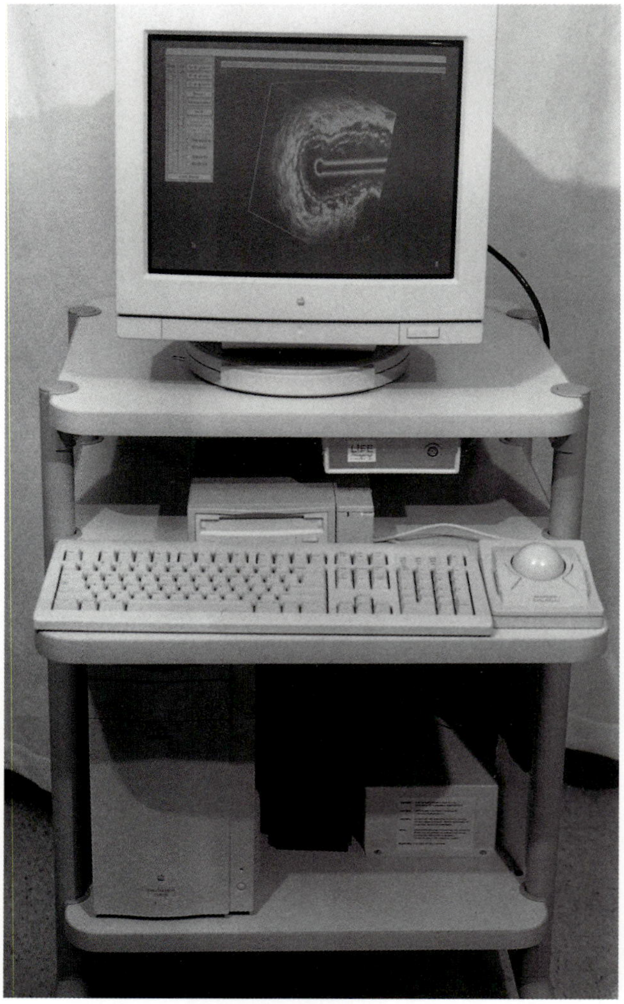

Figure 12.3 *The computer-based 3D reconstruction system (LIS 6000A, Life Imaging System Inc.).*

situations, including mechanical localizers, probe positioners, mechanical 3D probes, and remote localizers. More information about these techniques can be found in a review article by Rankin et al.[16]

Regardless of the acquisition methodology, it is essential to acquire the highest-quality data with the best available registration method, because the final reconstruction is completely dependent on the original data set. High-frequency endoluminal ultrasound provides excellent image quality which serves as a foundation for 3D reconstruction. In 3D endoluminal ultrasound, data sets are acquired by withdrawing (pulling back) an imaging catheter at a constant velocity while data are being acquired by the acquisition system. This pull-back can be performed either manually or mechanically by using a stepping motor device. At our laboratory we have assembled the acquisition system shown in Fig. 12.1 to obtain 3D endoluminal data.

During acquisition, the catheter-based transducer is first positioned in close proximity to the target (organ or phantom) being studied. It is then connected to an

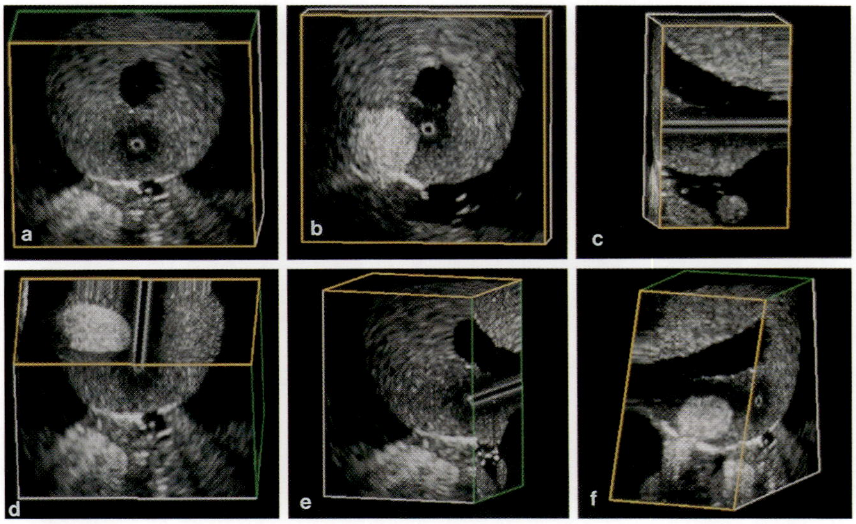

Figure 12.4 *When the 3D image is presented as a polyhedron, three perpendicular planes are displayed on the screen simultaneously (a). The multiplanar 3D image can be reviewed in any orientation, e.g. (b) transverse, (c) longitudinal, (d) coronal, (e) biplanar, (f) oblique. The polyhedron can be rotated to obtain the desired image orientation and then any of the planes can be selected parallel to the original and reformatted plane.*

endoluminal ultrasound system (IVUS, Diasonics, Santa Clara, CA) to produce 2D cross-sectional images. The stepping motor (also called pull-back device, CIVS, Boston Scientific Corporation, Sunnyvale, CA) is used to smoothly withdraw the catheter during the acquisition while images are continuously updated. The speed (ranging from 0.5 mm/s to 1.5 mm/s) and length (up to 6 cm) of the withdrawal can be preset (Fig. 12.2). The video output from the ultrasound system is connected to a dedicated 3D system (LIS 6000A, Life Imaging System Inc., London, ON, Canada) for acquisition, post-processing and visualization (Fig. 12.3).

To maximize acquired image quality, the internal frame grabber on the LIS 6000A is matched to the IVUS system's video output. This frame optimization permits each image slice to be collected at full resolution. For the IVUS data acquisition, a reasonable compromise in the acquisition parameters (data density, data set size and acquisition time) yields a slice-to-slice separation of 0.10 mm at a pull-back rate of 1.5 mm/s.

In practice, the acquisition process for an endoluminal data set is as follows: (1) place the ultrasound catheter slightly beyond the area desired to be imaged; (2) start the pull-back process; and (3) activate the frame-grabbing process at the same time as the withdrawal is started. A 3-cm scan length will contain 600 images and takes 20 s to acquire. Scan lengths up to 6 cm can easily be programmed and acquired. Immediately after acquisition, the data can be reviewed in 3D formats, and then stored in the LIS system so that another data set can be acquired.

VISUALIZATION AND IMAGING ANALYSIS

To review a particular data set, it is selected from the database and then transferred from the hard disk into the computer memory. It takes approximately 15 s to transfer a complete data set from the disk, after which 3D visualization can be initiated without any reconstruction delay. The 3D image is presented as a polyhedron representing the boundaries of the reconstructed volume. Each face of the polyhedron is rendered using a texture-mapping technique with the appropriate ultrasound image for that plane.[17] By using an intuitive interface with 3D clues, users can rotate the polyhedron and rapidly obtain the desired cut planes which display the anatomic and pathologic information in any orientation; e.g. transverse, longitudinal, coronal, oblique, etc. (Fig. 12.4).

The luminal profile can be projected, providing information similar to that obtained with an angiogram or a retrograde ureteropyelogram. In addition to the luminal profile, the 3D imaging system can also display the entire tubular structure with transmural morphology. This allows better identification and localization of lesions and, more importantly, better demonstration of the spatial relationship between the lesion and the surrounding structures.

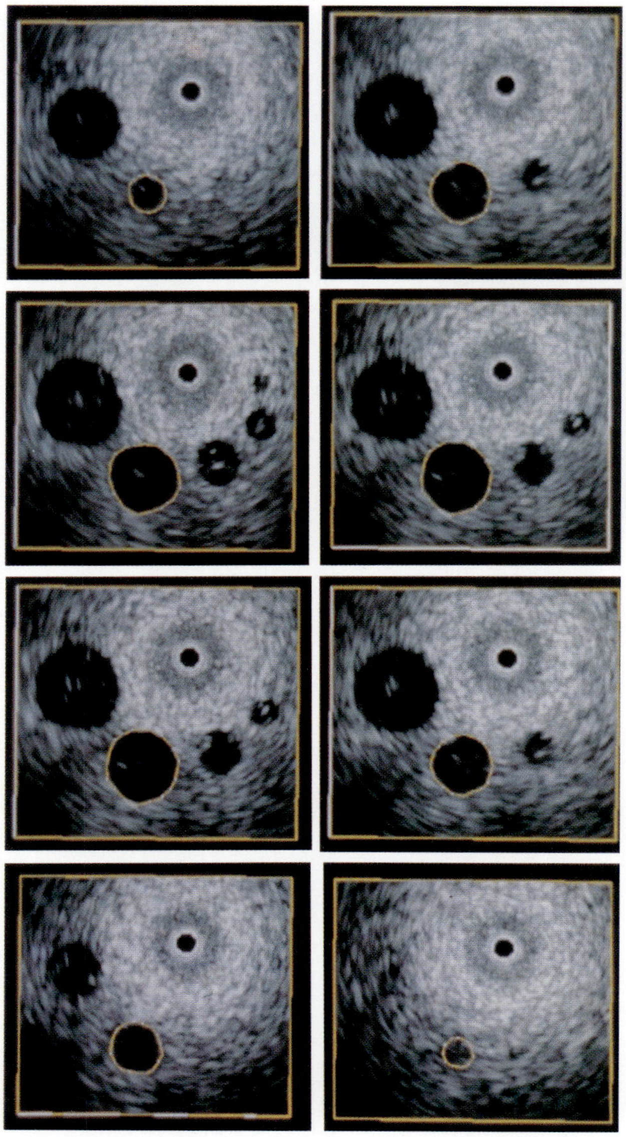

Figure 12.5 *The volume of an object is measured using a stack of equally thick slices. The surface area of the object on each slice is manually outlined using a cursor.*

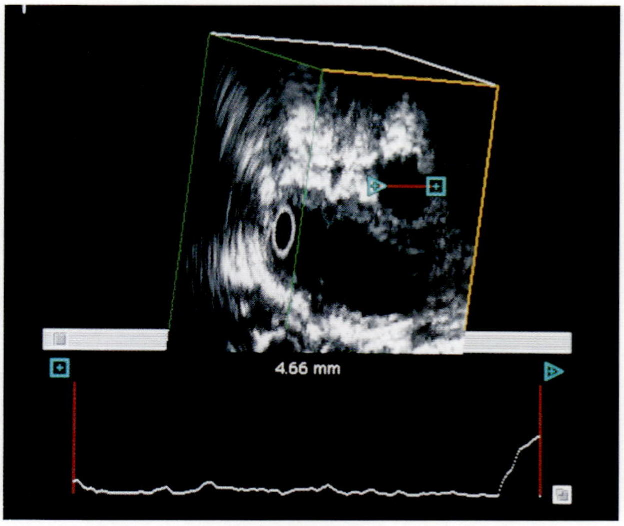

Figure 12.6 *With the A-mode technique for object selection, precise linear distance measurement can be obtained.*

Basic quantification tools are provided on the LIS 6000A computer system for the measurement of planar areas and path lengths as well as volumes. A stack of sequential 2D endoluminal ultrasound images is used for volume measurement. A computer mouse pointer is used to manually outline the circumference of the object to be measured on each slice. The computer software calculates the area of each outlined circumference by counting the pixels within the sector and multiplying that number by the area of each pixel. The volume is determined by summing the areas and multiplying by the interplane distance (Fig. 12.5). Additionally, a unique A-mode tool delivers very precise linear distance measurements (Fig. 12.6).

SEGMENTATION AND MODELING

Segmentation is the process whereby selected regions of interest are separated from the entire object.[18,19] Basically, there are three methods for segmentation: (1) extraction by visual inspection with manual tracking of the regions of interest, (2) semi-automatic separation based on input given by the operator and (3) and fully automatic computer-implemented segmentation. Automated segmentation is generally very difficult to perform on ultrasound images.

For reconstructing 3D endoluminal ultrasound, relevant objects such as vessel lumen, plaque lesions, dissection membranes or tumors have to be selected by the operator (i.e. segmentation). This step is very important, and errors in computer-assisted segmentation jeopardize the results of the 3D imaging process.

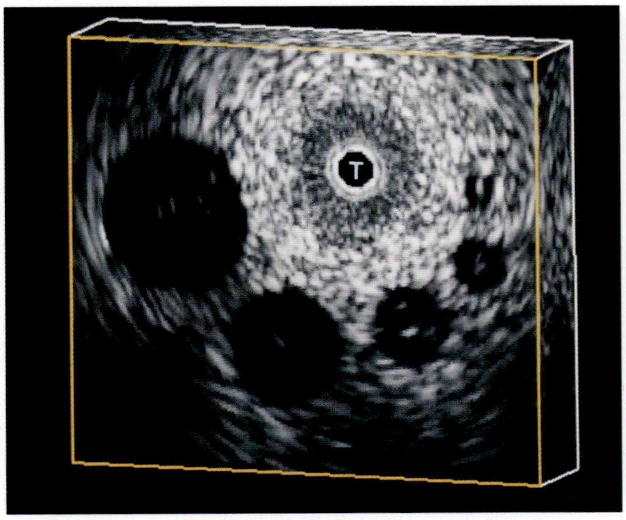

a

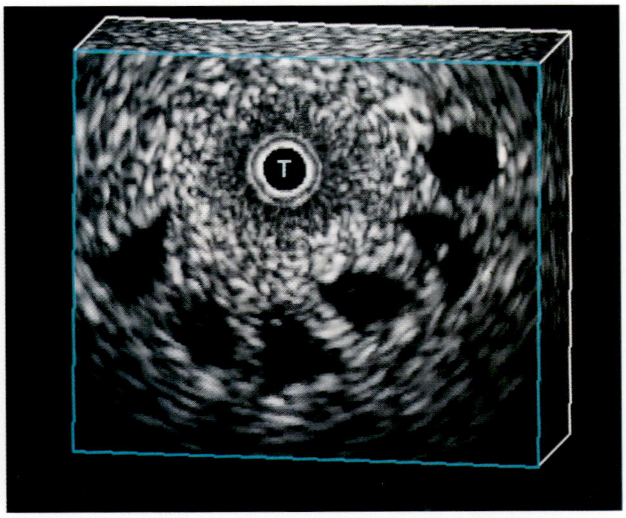

b

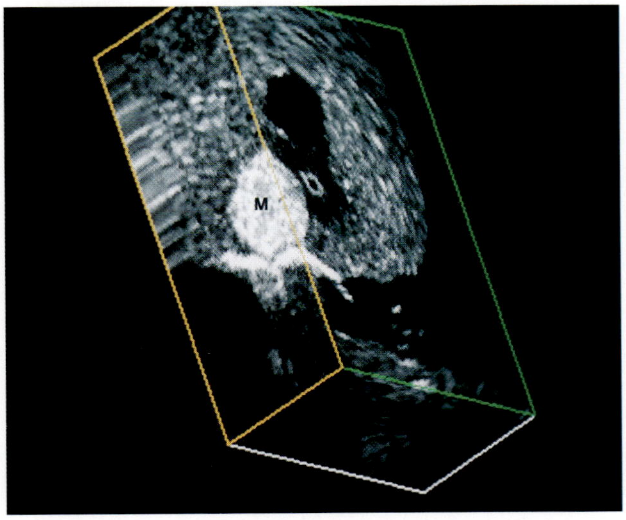

c

Figure 12.7 *A variety of 3D phantoms have been used for validating 3D reconstructed images and volume measurements. (a) Phantom with echo-free spheres ranging from 12 to 900 mm*^{3} *in size. (b) Phantom with echo-free objects of irregular shapes having approximately the same volume (mean 64.8 mm*^{3}*, range 58–72 mm*^{3}*). (c) Phantom with a hyperechoic mass (M) mimicking a tumor in the prostate. T, transducer.*

Three-dimensional reconstruction is a process by which a stack of consecutive 2D images are mapped and transferred into a volume display having dimensions in the x, y and z planes. Computer-based 3D renderings can be divided into two basic types: (1) surface rendering, and (2) volume rendering. In surface rendering, object surfaces are explicitly formed using techniques such as hidden-part removal, translucency, shading, dynamic rotation and stereo projection.[20,21] This is achieved by binary segmentation and/or thresholding of the digitized images. This format highlights the surfaces of the structure and the geometry. In volume rendering, object surfaces are not explicitly computed; instead, the entire data set is used throughout the reconstruction process. Volume rendering is based on the generation of interfaces and pseudosurfaces through a process of computed projections of the voxels.[22] Because all the information is retained in a voxel-based 3D image, one can assess the nature and extent of the disease process in addition to the geometry.

Among the various modeling techniques available, volume rendering is the most appropriate for modeling of anatomic structures (especially tubular structures). Voxel modeling can easily accommodate highly irregular structures and is able to demonstrate the internal characteristics of the lumen in great detail. In addition, voxel modeling is truly digital and, therefore, allows for rapid construction of multiplanar images from the 3D presentation in any orientation.

DOCUMENTATION

Endoluminal ultrasound images can be either stored on videotape for later digitization and reconstruction or directly digitized into a computer-based 3D system. Acquired stacks of 2D data sets can be archived onto a rewriteable magneto-optical disk for documentation. When needed, the data sets can be retrieved from the disk for 3D reconstruction and review. In addition, a video recorder can be connected to the 3D computer workstation to record real-time 3D manipulation for presentation.

VALIDATION

PHANTOM STUDIES

Quantitative assessment of a disease process is feasible only when computer-generated 3D images accurately represent original raw data. We have used custom-made 3D phantoms to validate voxel-based volume reconstruction on the LIS 6000A computer system. Three-dimensional computer images of objects or 'tumors' within the phantom were reconstructed in full voxel space using 9, 12.5 and 20-MHz catheter-based ultrasound transducers (Fig. 12.7).

A very high degree of correlation was found between the actual volume and the voxel-based volume reconstruction in the spherical phantom (Fig. 12.7a). Voxel-based volume reconstruction can be done at various slice thicknesses. When the objects are in the penetration range of the ultrasound transducer, an r value of 1.0 was generated at all thicknesses; e.g. 0.1, 0.5 and 1.0 mm. In addition, the interobserver variability was extremely low, with the correlation between two readers of $r = 1.0$. This demonstrates that the accuracy of volume measurements for 3D reconstruction is extremely high when the tumor is within the depth of penetration of the ultrasound transducer. However, these ultrasound transducers have a limited depth of penetration and as the objects are located farther away from the ultrasound transducer, the resolution decreases, thus decreasing the accuracy of the volume measurements.

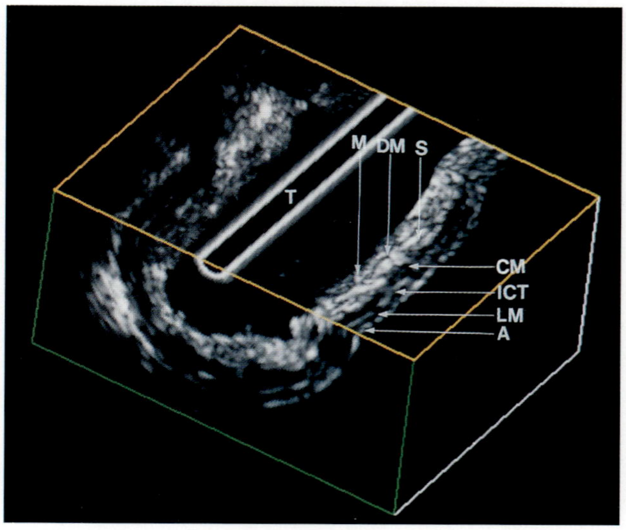

Figure 12.8 *Reconstructed 3D endoluminal image of the esophagus shows multiple layers of the esophageal wall, which are the mucosa (M), deep mucosa (DM), submucosa (S), circular smooth muscle (CM), intermuscular connective tissue (ICT), longitudinal smooth muscle (LM) and adventitia (A). T, transducer.*

ANIMAL STUDIES

As with previous studies using high-resolution endoluminal ultrasound, anatomic correlation between the high-resolution endoluminal ultrasound image and the actual histologic structure was sought.[23] Studies evaluating the canine esophagus and duodenum have revealed that 3D reconstruction can be accomplished using in vitro specimens filled with water to promote acoustic coupling. Steady pull-throughs were done using canine esophagus and duodenum. Specimens were hung in a water bath after the distal end was tied with a suture, and filled with water. A pulling device was used to pull either a 20-MHz or a 9-MHz catheter–transducer through the lumen of the specimen at a rate of 1.5 mm/s. The pull-through was done mechanically with the transducer attached to the pulling device in order to avoid any motion artifact due to pulling through by hand. As in 2D high-resolution endoluminal ultrasound, all of the wall layers were imaged (Fig. 12.8). The first hyperechoic layer represents the superficial mucosa; the second hypoechoic layer represents deep mucosa and muscularis mucosa. The third hypoechoic layer represents the submucosa. The fourth hyperechoic layer represents the circular smooth muscle. The fifth

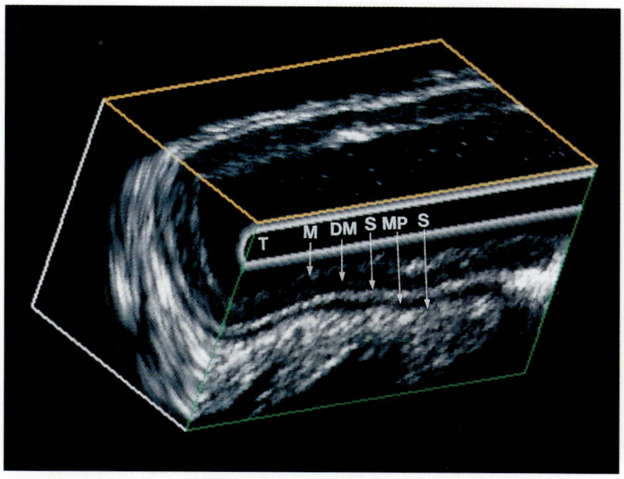

Figure 12.9 *A longitudinal view of a reconstructed 3D image of the duodenum demonstrates the layers of the duodenal wall, which are the villous mucosa (M), deep mucosa (DM), submucosa (S), muscularis propria (MP), and serosa (S). T, transducer.*

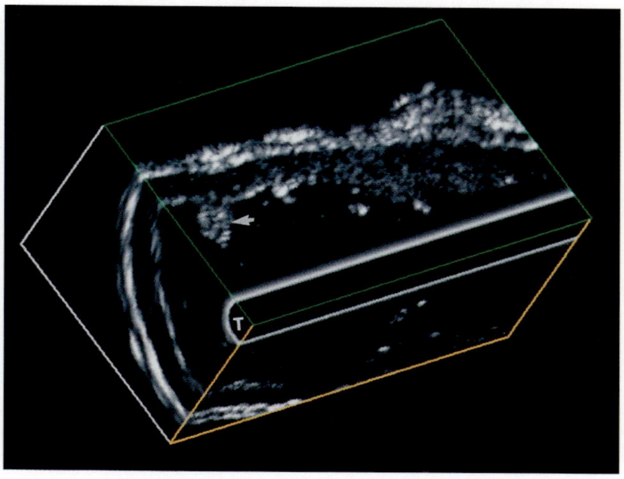

Figure 12.10 *A reconstructed endoluminal 3D image shows a small polyp-like mass (arrow), which was surgically created within the duodenum, and projects into the lumen of the bowel. T, transducer.*

hyperechoic layer represents the intermuscular connective tissue. The sixth hypoechoic layer represents the longitudinal smooth muscle and the seventh hyperechoic layer represents the adventitia in the canine esophagus.

Similar images were obtained in the duodenum; however, there is no intermuscular connective tissue layer, and only one layer of muscularis propria was imaged. In addition, in the duodenum the villous structure of the mucosa made the mucosa appear much thicker than in the esophagus (Fig. 12.9). Using the 3D reconstructed image, it was possible to observe relationships between the various sonographic layers that cannot be demonstrated longitudinally and coronally in two dimensions (i.e. the muscularis propria layers and the intermuscular connective tissue could be followed both in the sagittal and coronal planes and their relationships demonstrated).

Small and large pseudotumors can be created in vitro in animal specimens by inverting the tubular specimen, grabbing and raising the mucosa with a hemostat, and tying a silk suture around the base of the raised mucosa. The specimen is then everted. Imaging with a 9- or 20-MHz transducer is accomplished by pulling the transducer through the water-filled specimen at a rate of 1.5 mm/s. The images are then reconstructed in the 3D voxel format to evaluate the size of each pseudotumor and the relationship of the pseudotumor to underlying structures. There is a good correlation between measured 3D reconstructed images and the actual gross histologic specimens being imaged (Figs 12.10 and 12.11).

CLINICAL APPLICATIONS

INTRAVASCULAR USES

Angiography has been used for decades to provide the anatomic and pathologic information required for the application of vascular intervention. The introduction of intravascular ultrasound brought into use a new diagnostic tool. Two-dimensional intravascular ultrasound images have been shown to correlate with angiograms and histologic specimens and to be more accurate than angiography in determining cross-sectional areas in diseased arteries.[24,25] However, vascular structures and their related pathologies (plaque, aneurysm and dissection) are three-dimensional in nature. Accurate assessment of atheroma

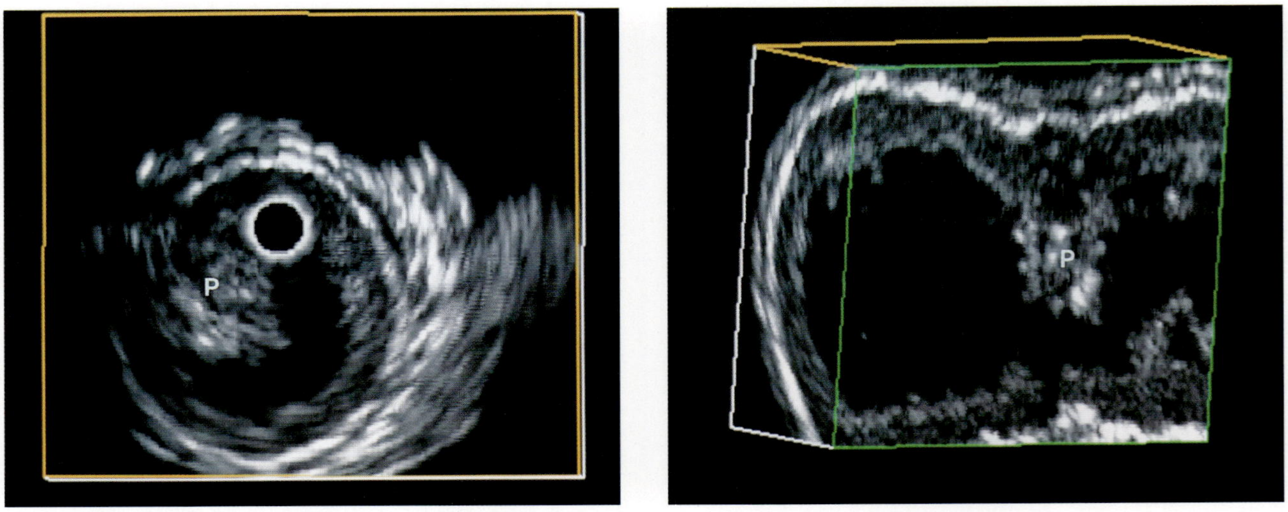

a *b*

Figure 12.11 *(a) A conventional 2D endoluminal image shows the pseudotumor (P) projecting into the lumen of the small bowel. (b) The same mass (P) is displayed in the longitudinal section of the reconstructed 3D mode. The relationship between the mass and wall structures is clearly demonstrated with 3D imaging.*

volume and comparison of adjacent segments requires repeated reviews of recorded images. The development of 3D intravascular ultrasound imaging offers a unique method for assessment of normal and diseased vascular structures.

Many investigators have developed 3D intravascular ultrasound techniques for efficient assessment of vascular geometry. These methods make use of a catheter-based probe that is inserted into the artery during the examination and advanced to the site of interest under fluoroscopic or ultrasound guidance. To obtain the data for reconstruction of a 3D image, catheter probes that provide 360° cross-sectional views of the vascular structures are then withdrawn either manually or mechanically.

Endoluminal 2D and 3D gray-scale images can reveal the three-layered appearance of medium-sized arteries; i.e. hyperechoic intima, hypoechoic muscular media and hyperechoic adventitia. The vascular branches and accessory vessels as well as their relationships to each other can be easily demonstrated with 3D imaging by selecting an angle, plane and section of the image (Fig. 12.12).

In the 3D reconstruction of atherosclerotic vessels, calcified plaque appears as a very bright reflection with acoustic shadowing behind the lesion, whereas

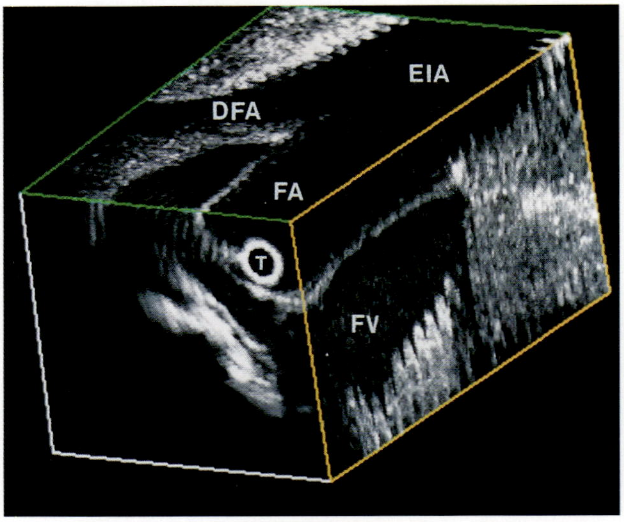

Figure 12.12 *A reconstructed 3D intravascular image of the iliofemoral artery demonstrates the vascular branches and accessory vessels as well as their relationships to each other. Note the sawtooth motion artifact along the wall of the vessel due to the arterial pulsation. T, transducer; EIA, external iliac artery; FA, femoral artery; DFA, deep femoral artery; FV, femoral vein.*

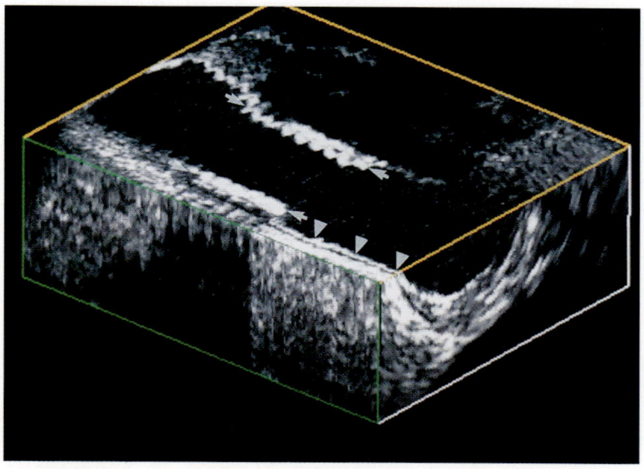

Figure 12.13 *A coronal view of the reconstructed 3D image of the common iliac artery demonstrates hyperechoic regions (arrows) with acoustic shadowing corresponding to calcified plaques. The normal appearance of the vascular layers (arrowheads) is seen in the noninvolved portion of the vessel.*

fibrous plaque appears as a bright or medium echogenic area without acoustic shadowing (Figs 12.13 and 12.14). The dimensions and shapes of the vascular lumen can be determined in the longitudinal view. By altering the viewing angle on the screen, the operator is able to examine the vessel segment in all possible orientations. This information is useful for determining the distribution and type of plaque in vessels (Fig. 12.14).

Three-dimensional intravascular ultrasound imaging is especially useful in the diagnosis of arterial dissections and aneurysms. Aortic dissection often results in a spiral or complex flap which is difficult to evaluate using angiography, CT and MRI or transabdominal ultrasound. Reconstructed 3D imaging allows global evaluation of the dissection entry site, extent of the flap, and the false lumen of the aneurysm (Fig. 12.15). Cavaye et al reported that 3D intravascular ultrasound plays an important role in the deployment of endovascular stents designed to treat aortic dissection in an animal model.[26,27]

The newest interventional radiologic tool for the treatment of certain pseudoaneurysms is the stent–graft, a merging of the sciences of vascular grafts and expandable vascular stents. By combining the relative impermeability of bypass graft material

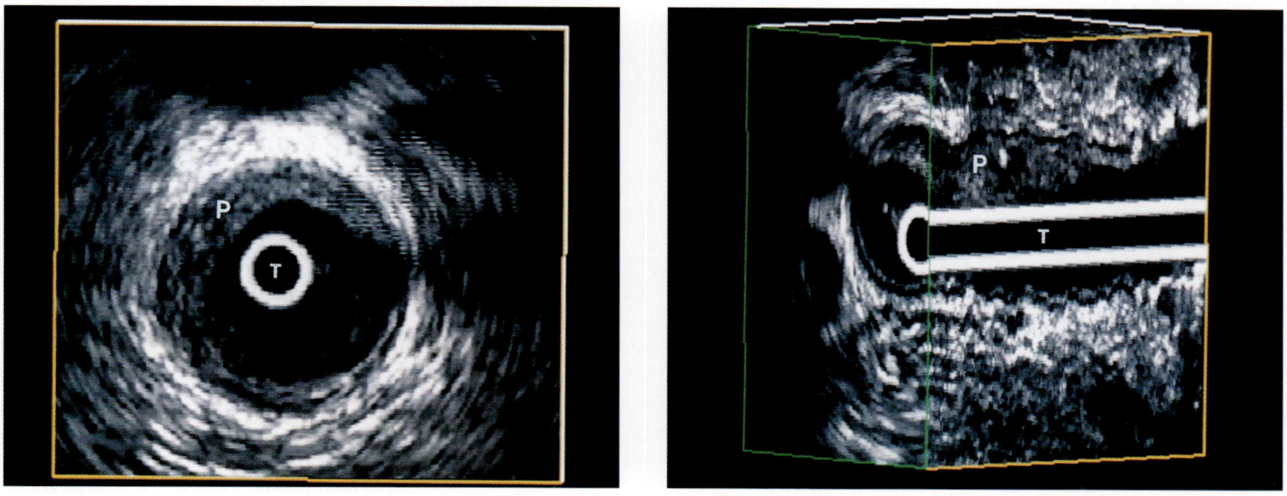

a ***b***

Figure 12.14 *(a) A conventional 2D endoluminal image of the iliac artery demonstrates a hypoechoic lesion (P) without acoustic shadowing corresponding to atherosclerotic plaque. (b) A longitudinal view of the 3D image of the same lesion provides more information for determining the distribution and type of plaque. Also, the dimensions and shapes of the vascular lumen can be demonstrated. T, transducer.*

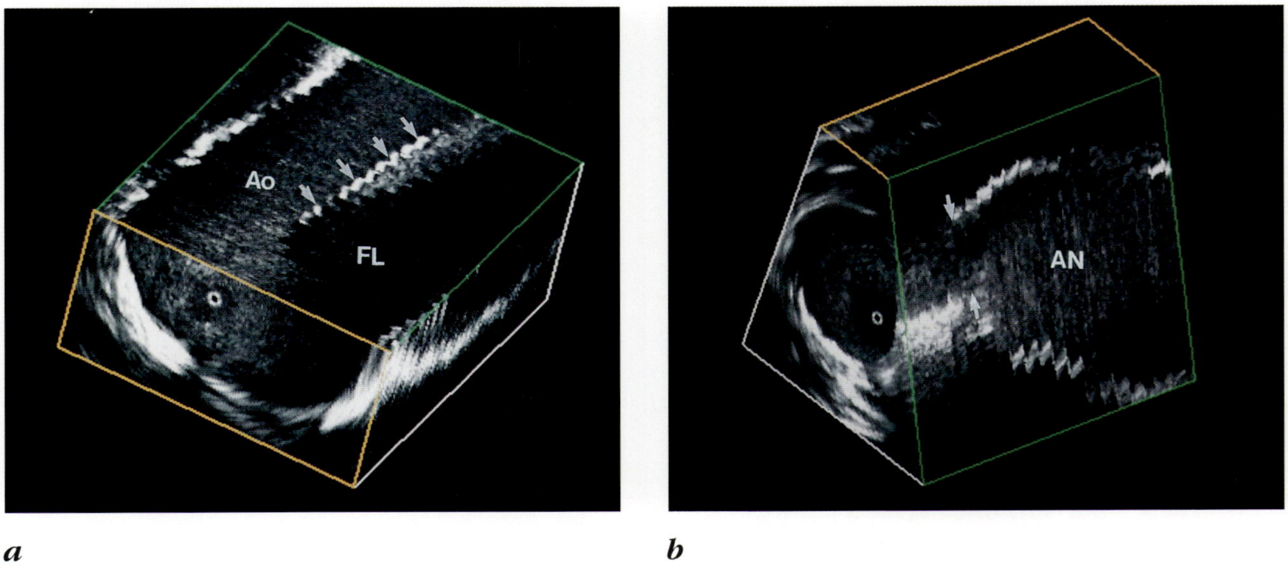

Figure 12.15 *In a patient with abdominal aortic aneurysm: (a) a 3D reconstructed image demonstrates the false lumen (FL) of the aorta (Ao) and dissection of the aneurysm (arrows); (b) an oblique view of the 3D image demonstrates the entry site (arrows) of the aneurysm (AN).*

with the percutaneous scaffolding properties of metallic stents, a device can be made which has the advantages of a small initial diameter to allow percutaneous insertion, and a significant expansion ratio to achieve large deployment diameters, with the force necessary to seal graft material against the endoluminal vessel wall, thereby excluding flow in the pseudoaneurysm while maintaining flow through the stent–graft, and distally in the vessel.

In a typical case, a pseudoaneurysm was discovered in a common iliac artery at the proximal aspect of a Palmaz balloon-expandable stent which had been put in place years earlier. It was speculated that the cause of the pseudoaneurysm was microperforation of the vessel wall during stent expansion, either by the metal struts of the stent or by the sharp edge of a calcified plaque. A stent–graft was made, comprising PTFE bypass graft material sutured to a medium Palmaz stent, which was crimped onto an angioplasty balloon. Prior to stent–graft deployment, the vessel lumen diameter had been measured. The location and extent of the pseudoaneurysm had also been mapped by contrast angiography, with the assistance of intravascular ultrasound; the latter provided more extensive and accurate information on the exact location and extent of the pseudoaneurysm than was possible with conventional angiography. In addition, the three-dimensional reconstructed intravascular ultrasound image demonstrated a parasagittal view of the pseudoaneurysm neck; this view was not possible with other imaging modalities (Fig. 12.16). Following successful stent–graft deployment, intravascular ultrasound was instrumental in analyzing the morphologic result, especially in determining the size of the new lumen, and whether the stent and its associated graft material had been adequately and fully apposed to the endoluminal surface to exclude flow in the pseudoaneurysm while maintaining flow distally in the artery. The exact apposition of the stent–graft to the inner vessel wall is one of the most important aspects of the device when used for this procedure. Three-dimensional reconstructed ultrasound images provide information not as readily or accurately obtained by other imaging modalities.

Another application has been in the diagnosis and treatment of the non-thrombotic venous cause of unilateral leg swelling known as May–Thurner syndrome, whereby the left common iliac vein is compressed between the posterior pelvic wall and the right common iliac artery as the latter crosses over from the aortoiliac bifurcation to the right inguinal region. Traditional therapy has been surgical correction of the vein compression, either by a vein

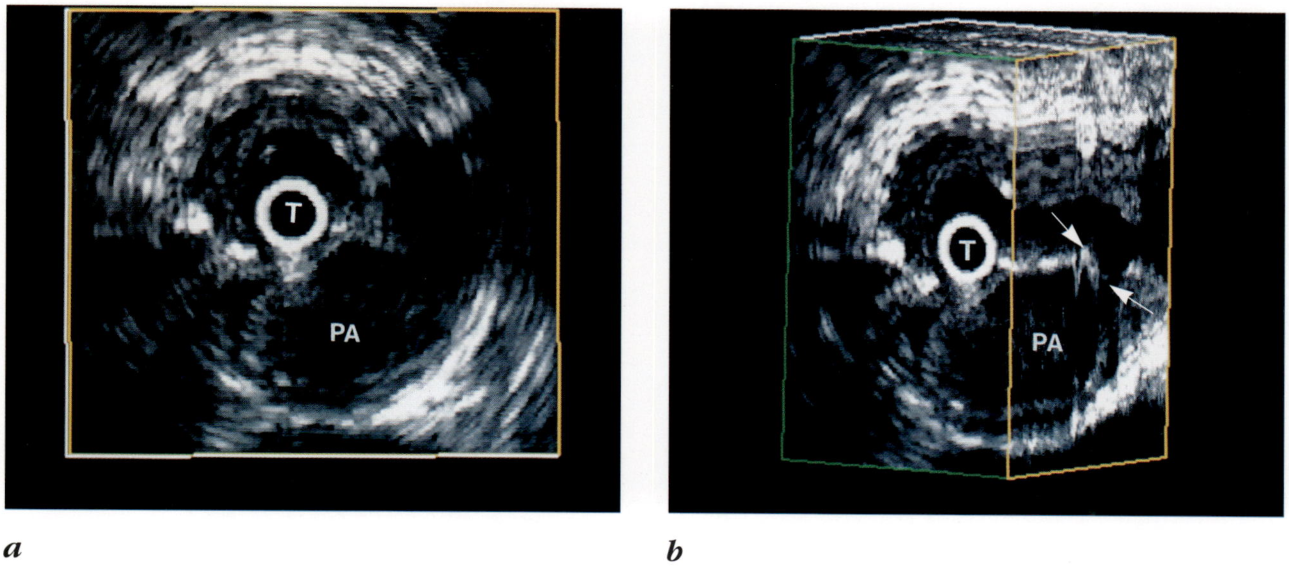

Figure 12.16 *The 2D (a) and 3D (b) intravascular ultrasound images demonstrate a pseudoaneurysm (PA) arising from the iliac artery. The information provided by the 3D image allows better evaluation of the lesion and helps guide the percutaneous stent–graft placement. Note that the neck of the pseudoaneurysm (arrows) can be seen on the 3D image. T, transducer.*

patch repair or a venous crossover bypass graft. More recently, interventional radiologic techniques, including percutaneous transluminal angioplasty (PTA) in combination with intraluminal stent placement, have provided a simple, durable, low-risk and low-cost solution. Although these techniques are typically performed under fluoroscopic guidance, intravascular ultrasound may be helpful in accurately depicting the length of the stenosis, the relationship to and quality of the adjacent artery, the diameter of the uninvolved vein proximal and distal to the stenosis, and the final outcome after stent deployment. In addition, 3D reconstruction of the standard intravascular ultrasound images may help in optimizing the location and size of the stent during treatment planning and after placement, as it provides the equivalent of a parasagittal view of the intimate relationship between the artery and vein, which is difficult to obtain with most other imaging modalities. In addition, intravascular ultrasound, including the 3D reconstruction, can be used after placement of the stent to evaluate the accuracy of the stent deployment, the size of the new lumen, the relationship of the stent to the vein wall, and the relationship of the newly expanded vein to the adjacent artery (Fig. 12.17).

We have also used intravascular ultrasound as an alternative method to guide deployment of inferior vena cava filter placement in patients who are not candidates for contrast venography.[28] These patients include pregnant women, patients with severe renal insufficiency, patients who are too heavy for the X-ray table, and patients with severe contrast allergy. Two-dimensional and three-dimensional endoluminal ultrasound has been used to calibrate the vena cava diameter, to detect the presence of vena cava thrombus, to identify the most appropriate site for filter placement, and, more importantly, to localize the origin of the main renal veins. Other potential applications of 3D intravascular ultrasound include assessment of interventional procedures such as PTA, atherectomy and thrombectomy.[29]

Despite mechanically assisted pull-back of the intravascular ultrasound catheter, there may still be artifacts within the reconstructed images due to cardiac motion and/or arterial pulsation as well as random motion of the catheter within the lumen of the vessel. These artifacts will be seen on the reconstructed longitudinal or coronal sections (Figs 12.12 and 12.13).

The major advantage of 3D intravascular ultrasound is that it provides high-resolution 3D images of both normal and abnormal vascular structures; the disadvantage is that geometric distortions may occur. For example, any vascular curvature, motion of the

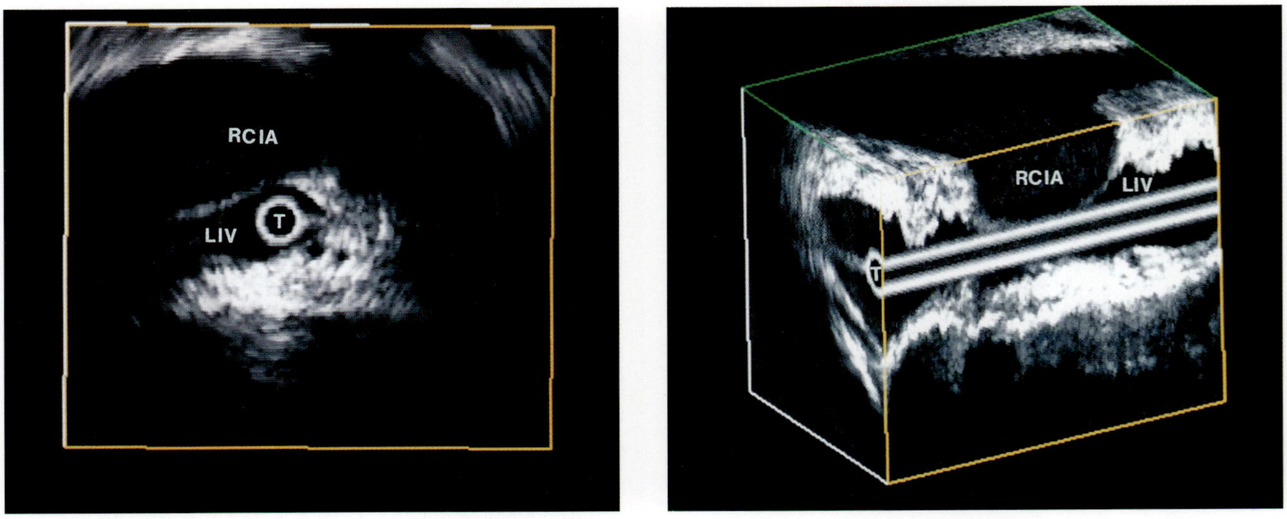

a *b*

Figure 12.17 *(a) Conventional 2D intravascular ultrasound demonstrates the left iliac vein (LIV) compressed by the right common iliac artery (RCIA), corresponding to the May–Thurner syndrome. (b) The 3D image provides comprehensive information regarding the location and length of the narrowing as well as the relationship of the vessels to each other. T, transducer.*

probe within the vessel or other geometric changes from a straight line are not represented accurately in the 3D image.

ENDOLUMINAL NONVASCULAR USES

The unique information provided by 2D endoluminal ultrasound imaging may be difficult to apply clinically because it is presented as a cross-sectional 'slice' of a 3D tubular structure. The radiologist may have difficulty in conveying critical anatomic information to the physician involved in the therapy. Computer-generated 3D ultrasound imaging has great potential for evaluation of hollow organs because it displays the luminal and transmural morphology with almost limitless available projections.

The multiplanar 3D image provides accurate transmural dimensions and a global view of tubular structures in an easily interpretable format. Lesions that arise from the lining of a lumen are imaged with far superior contrast resolution when using a transducer situated within the lumen. For tumors, this method presents the possibility of detection of smaller lesions, and the measurement of the depth, size and contour of the mass, an essential step in the staging of the tumor.

Esophagus

Three-dimensional imaging of the esophagus can be accomplished by placing the ultrasound transducer within the lumen of the esophagus and then by slowly withdrawing the transducer at a constant speed. A published study has demonstrated the use of this technique in the evaluation of the normal esophagus and esophageal abnormalities.[30] This study utilized a 7.5-MHz Olympus ultrasound endoscope which was withdrawn through the body of the esophagus for 3D imaging of mural and extramural structures surrounding the esophagus. Once the normal esophagus was defined, the technique was used to image and stage esophageal carcinoma.

With the advent of catheter-based transducers, it is obvious that the higher frequency will allow for much greater resolution with 3D reconstructive images, allowing for differentiation between the circular smooth muscle and longitudinal smooth muscle, and the intramuscular connective tissue within the wall of the esophagus. In addition, it can be hypothesized that the small size of these catheter-based transducers will not distort the normal anatomy of the esophagus, as do the larger endoscope-based transducers. Therefore, a much more natural and anatomically correct reconstruction of the mucosa and submucosa can be reconstructed. The catheter-

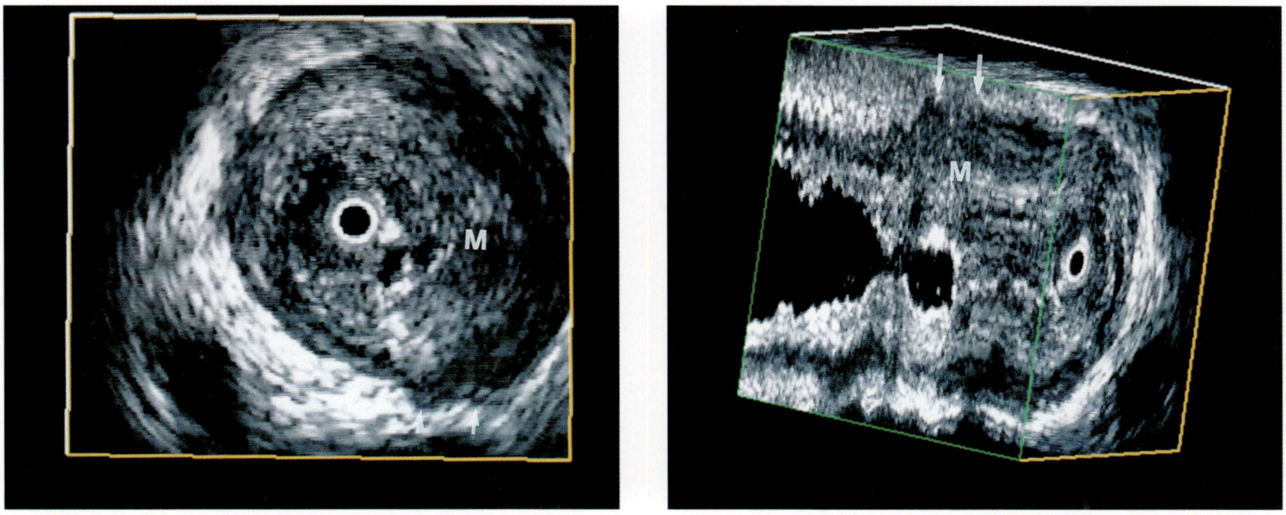

a *b*

Figure 12.18 *In a patient with advanced esophageal carcinoma, a conventional endoscopic ultrasound probe cannot be passed through the stricture of the esophagus. Conventional 2D (a) and reconstructed 3D images (b) using a catheter-based transducer demonstrated the mass (M) invading beyond the adventitia of the esophagus (arrows). The 3D image provides a longitudinal view of the lesion.*

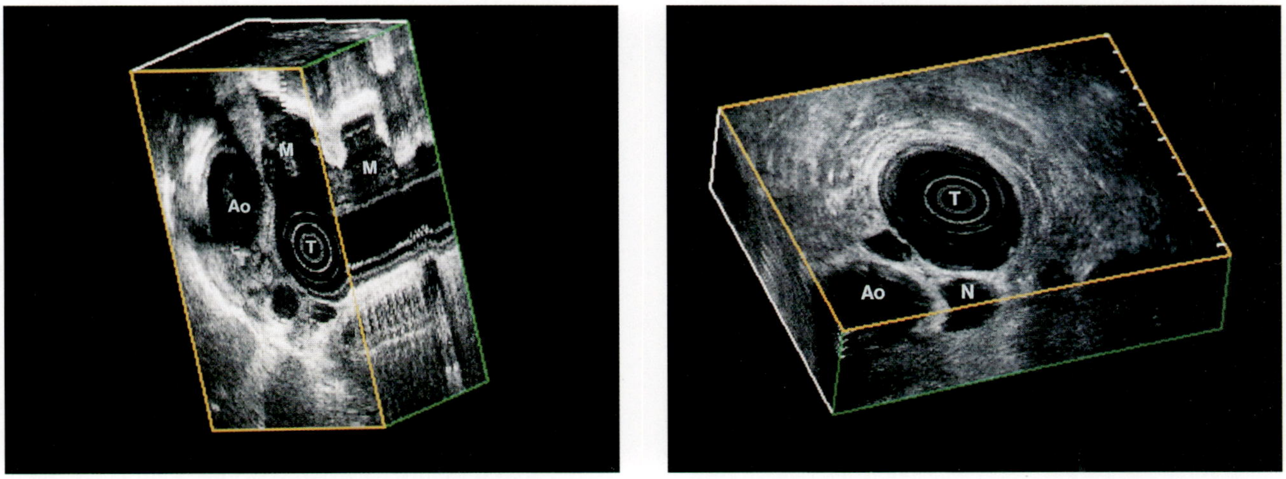

a *b*

Figure 12.19 *(a) A reconstructed 3D image using an endoscope-based transducer (7.5 MHz) demonstrates a hypoechoic mass (M) invading through the wall of the esophagus in both transverse and longitudinal views. (b) A lymph node (N) is confirmed by the 3D image through transverse and coronal views. T, transducer; Ao, aorta.*

based probe can be passed through narrow esophageal strictures to image mural abnormalities (Fig. 12.18). With the use of the 7.5-MHz endoscopic ultrasound probe, 3D reconstruction of the tumor and surrounding structures will allow evaluation of tumor, lymph node metastases and mediastinal abnormalities (Fig. 12.19). Because of the proximity of vascular structures that traverse the periesophageal area, it may be possible to noninvasively evaluate vascular structures such as the azygous vein and aorta without actually introducing a transducer into the lumen of the vascular structure.

Esophageal varices appear as hypoechoic fluid-filled structures in the submucosa of the esophagus on 2D endoluminal ultrasound images using a 20-MHz catheter-based transducer. Three-dimensional reconstruction of these images allows relationships of varices to each other and to other mural structures to be demonstrated as well as communications between varices to be evaluated. In addition, volume measurements for variceal segments can be followed after therapeutic procedures such as TIPS and/or sclerotherapy or after drug therapy with β-blockers or Octreotide.

One of the problems with this 3D imaging technology is that there is a great deal of movement artifact secondary to cardiac and respiratory motion. This motion artifact causes errors in 3D reconstruction. Since images can be acquired in a relatively short period of time (20–30 s), it may be possible to acquire esophageal images during breath-hold maneuvers. In addition, in the future it may also be possible to acquire images gated to the cardiac cycle, so that the movement artifacts from cardiac motion become negligible.

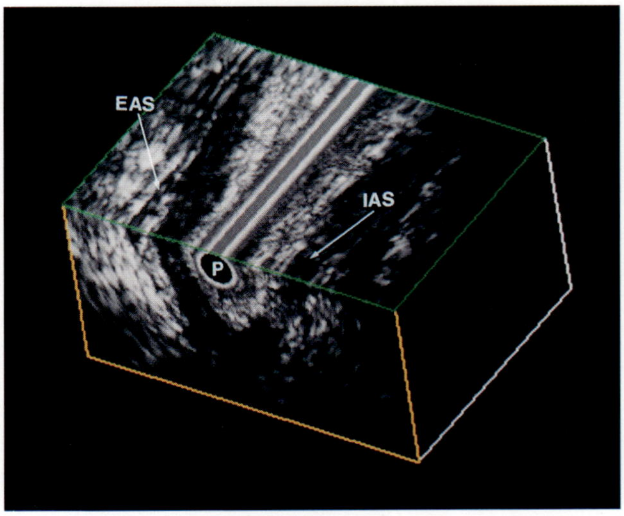

Figure 12.20 *With the use of a 9-Fr, 9-MHz catheter-based probe (P), a reconstructed 3D image of the normal anal canal demonstrates the internal (IAS) and external anal sphincters (EAS) in both transverse and longitudinal views.*

Anal canal

Three-dimensional imaging of the internal anal sphincter has already been accomplished using 12-MHz and 9-MHz catheter-based probes.[31] The internal anal sphincter appears as a tubular structure which is hypoechoic on high-resolution sonograms. This hypoechoic tubular-structure is surrounded by a hyperechoic mucosal–submucosal complex medially and a hyperechoic connective tissue plane laterally. The external anal sphincter is imaged as a mixture of hypo- and hyperechoic band outside of the internal anal sphincter. The entire anal sphincter complex is approximately 3–4 cm in length and can be imaged by pulling the transducer through the anal canal with a 9-MHz or 12.5-MHz transducer at a certain rate to reconstruct 3D images. The internal anal sphincter itself varies in thickness and in cross-sectional surface area, depending on the location within the anal canal. In the proximal portion of the internal anal sphincter, the cross-sectional surface area and thickness of the muscle are at their smallest. As the transducer is pulled more medially, the cross-sectional surface area and thickness of the internal anal sphincter increase to a maximum at approximately the center of the internal anal sphincter and then decrease again gradually as the transducer is pulled more distally.

Using a 9-MHz transducer, it is possible not only to image the internal sphincter but also to image the external anal sphincter, and to evaluate the orientation of the internal anal sphincter with respect to the external anal sphincter (Fig. 12.20). It can be clearly seen, using these relatively lower frequency transducers, that the internal anal sphincter ends in the distal aspect of the anal canal prior to the termination of the external anal sphincter. In addition to using 9 to 12.5-MHz transducers to evaluate the normal internal anal sphincter, abnormalities can also be evaluated.

Three-dimensional imaging is particularly well suited for the evaluation of fecal incontinence caused by obstetrical trauma or injury. Scar tissue and fibroconnective tissue within the internal anal sphincter appears as a hyperechoic defect within the normally hypoechoic internal anal sphincter. These abnormalities can be located very precisely using 3D imaging, and the length and severity of the defect can be accurately evaluated (Fig. 12.21). Three-dimensional imaging technology will provide surgeons with a precise map of the longitudinal and transverse location

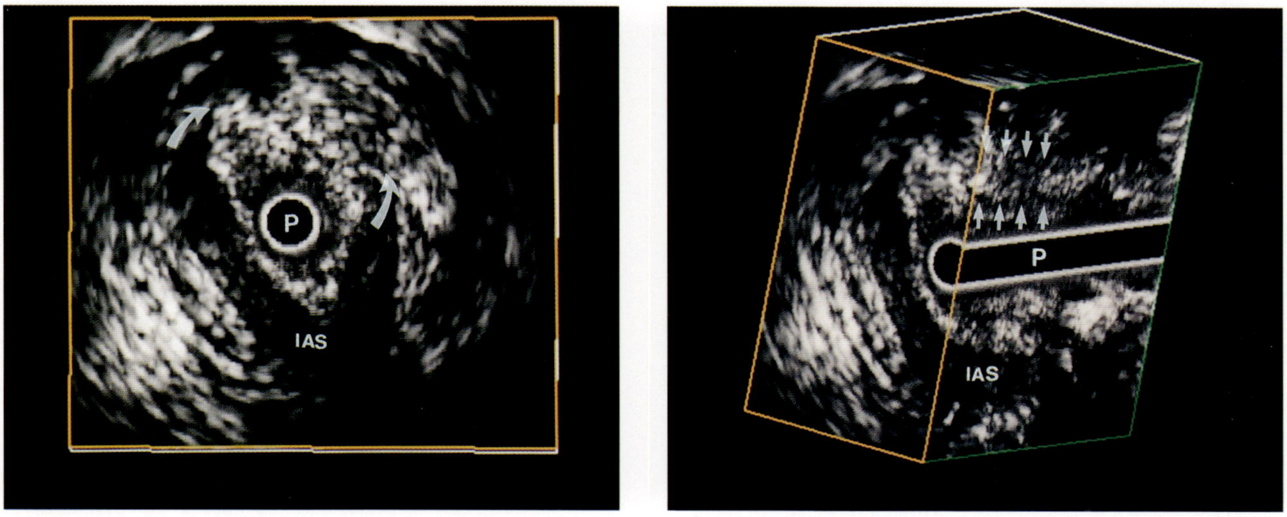

a *b*

Figure 12.21 *In a patient with fecal incontinence: (a) a conventional 2D endoluminal ultrasound image, using a 9-Fr, 9-MHz probe (P), shows a normally hypoechoic internal anal sphincter (IAS) replaced by a hyperechoic area (arrows), corresponding to scar tissue; (b) a reconstructed 3D image demonstrates the lesion (arrows) in a longitudinal view. P, probe.*

of the sphincter defect prior to surgically reconstructing the internal anal sphincter. In addition, these sphincter defects correlate very well with manometric abnormalities within the sphincter. It should be possible in the future to perform 3D simultaneous ultrasound and manometry to further delineate the abnormalities in the internal and external anal sphincters.

Urinary tract

The 3D acquisition techniques for imaging of the urinary tract are similar to those used for other endoluminal ultrasound studies. The catheter-based transducers are placed in the usual fashion and the specific site of interest is then identified and targeted, so that the transducer can be moved through the area of interest in a single, smooth motion. The most accurate pass of the catheter can be obtained by linking it to a mechanical, pulling device which can move the catheter at a predetermined, accurate rate. Alternatively, the catheter can be withdrawn by hand at a slow, steady rate, although this cannot give an accurate rate of withdrawal or allow dimensionally accurate 3D reconstruction.

One of the more difficult aspects of 3D imaging of the urinary tract is the selection of the exact segment for study. Since there is a limited memory capacity in the 3D program, it can be difficult to determine an appropriate starting point to include only the area of interest for reconstruction. Therefore, it is often more efficient to record the images on videotape first, and to then transfer the selected segment to the 3D computer system.

Another source of error with this method arises from patient movement during the imaging process. There can be considerable movement of the kidney and the proximal ureter with respiration. There is also some movement of the ureter at sites adjacent to arterial vessels. Any movement which changes the cross-sectional sonographic image during recording can give rise to artifacts within the 3D reconstruction.

The 3D image can be reconstructed in any plane. Therefore, a sagittal or coronal image can be reconstructed as easily as a cross-sectional representation. Since the ultrasound probes have been available only for cross-sectional imaging, this computer reconstruction may eliminate the need for development of a endoluminal linear transducer.

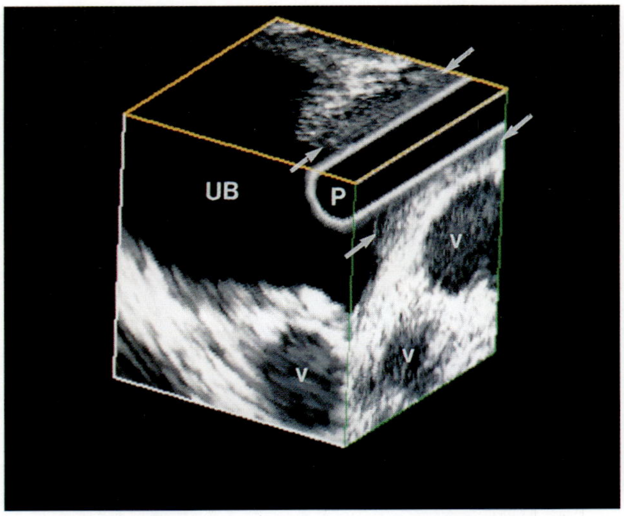

Figure 12.22 *The 3D reconstructed endoluminal ultrasound image of the normal ureterovesical junction, using a 6.2-Fr, 20-MHz probe (P), shows the transmural segment (arrows) of the ureter within the wall of the urinary bladder (UB). The vessels (V) adjacent to the junction are seen in different sections. T, transducer.*

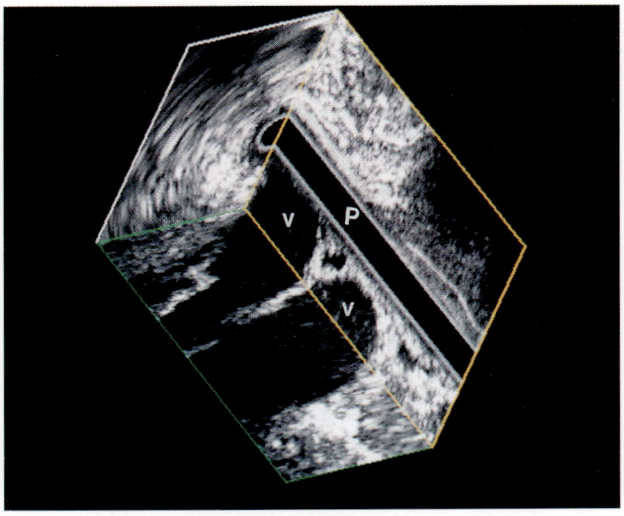

Figure 12.23 *A 3D reconstructed image obtained from the distal ureter, using a 6.2-Fr, 20-MHz probe (P), shows the longitudinal view of the ureter and adjacent iliac vessels (V) passing behind the ureter.*

Three-dimensional reconstruction of endoluminal images from several areas in the urinary tract has been employed. The different imaging perspectives available with this technique can give valuable information regarding anatomic and pathologic abnormalities. It appears to be of particular value for visualizing the upper urinary tract (Figs 12.22, 12.23, 12.24 and 12.25).

The ureteropelvic junction has been the segment most frequently studied with endoluminal ultrasound, both 2D cross-sectional and 3D imaging. The obstructed ureteropelvic junction can be treated by endoluminal incision; e.g. endopyelotomy. Therefore, it is a location at which endoluminal ultrasound has been useful to locate crossing vessels or define the anatomy of the high insertion of the ureter into the pelvis. When the cross-sectional images are converted to the 3D format, a different perspective is achieved (Figs 12.26 and 12.27). For example, two vessels crossing anterior to the obstructed ureteropelvic junction in a patient could be seen on the 2D cross-sectional views with the ultrasound transducer at two different positions. However, in the 3D presentation, it is apparent that both vessels are of a similar size and located anterior to the ureteropelvic junction. The course of vessels can also be determined by imaging

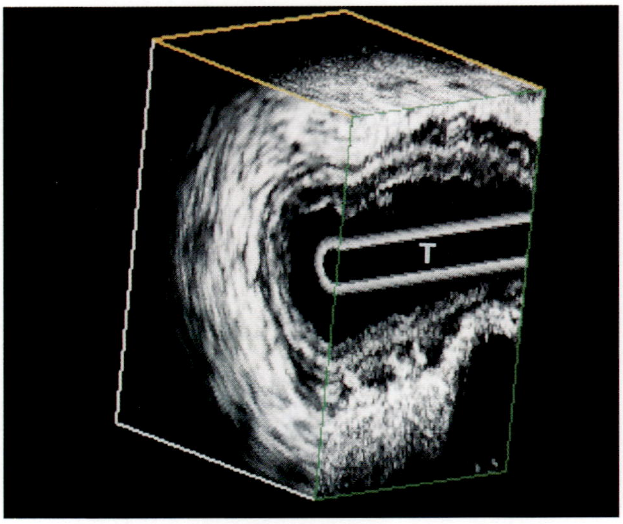

Figure 12.24 *A 3D image reconstructed from 2D endoluminal ultrasound images displays the longitudinal section of the normal ureter. T, transducer.*

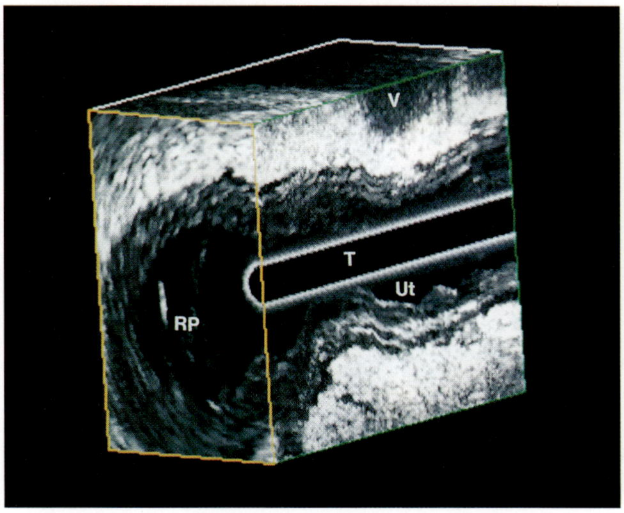

Figure 12.25 *A reconstructed 3D image acquired from the ureteropelvic junction (UPJ) shows the normal mural structure of the UPJ and an adjacent vascular structure (V). T, transducer; RP, renal pelvis; Ut, ureter.*

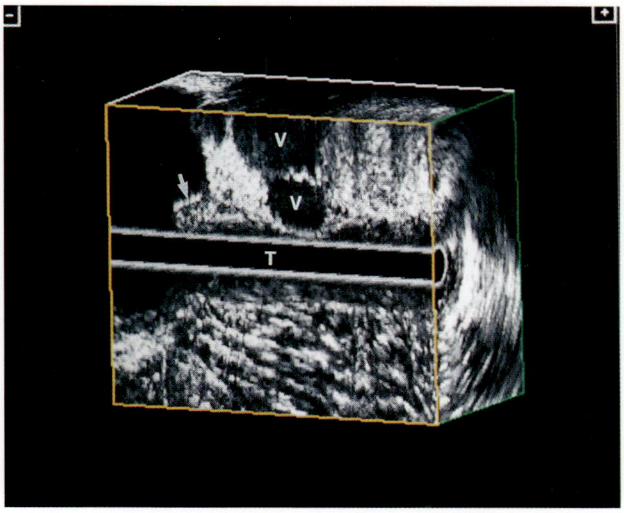

Figure 12.26 *A reconstructed 3D endoluminal image of the obstructed UPJ shows a septum (arrow) at the junction and crossing vessels (V) anteriorly. T, transducer.*

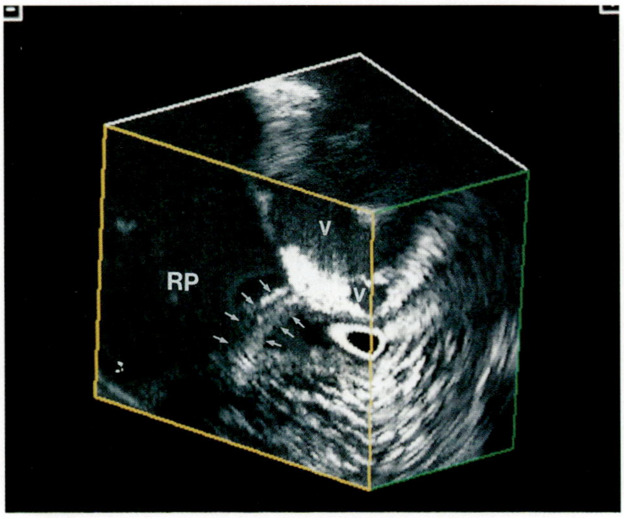

Figure 12.27 *An oblique section of a 3D image of the obstructed UPJ demonstrates the septum (arrows) and crossing vessels (V) anteriorly. The information provided by the 3D image is useful for endopyelotomy. The 3D format also offers an overview of the local anatomy by real-time rotation of the 3D model. RP, renal pelvis.*

the 3D reconstruction in different planes (Fig. 12.28). Similarly, reconstruction of an image of a ureteropelvic junction obstruction by a high insertion shows the septum separating the lumen of the ureter and the renal pelvis (Figs 12.26 and 12.27).

Variations in the ureteral lumen are also more apparent with a sagittal reconstruction. In this way, the length of a narrow segment can be more fully appreciated. Ureteral strictures seem to be represented more accurately by 3D reconstruction than by individual cross-sectional images alone. Although the variation in echogenicity which probably represents the density of the tissue can be appreciated in 2D cross-sectional images, subtle changes in the thickness of the ureteral wall or changes in the lumen are difficult to evaluate with 2D cross-sectional images alone. Three-dimensional reconstruction allows examination of longitudinal structures, and variations in wall thickness and lumen patency can be visualized along the strictured segment (Fig. 12.29).

Tumors within the ureteral lumen and renal pelvis can be shown well in a 2D cross-sectional mode with endoluminal ultrasound, but some features can be represented more accurately in other planes. For example, the distribution of tumor along the ureter can be shown more accurately with a 3D reconstruction

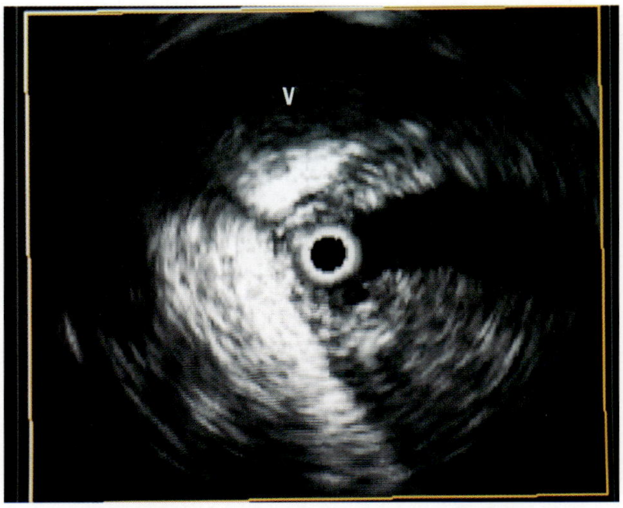

a

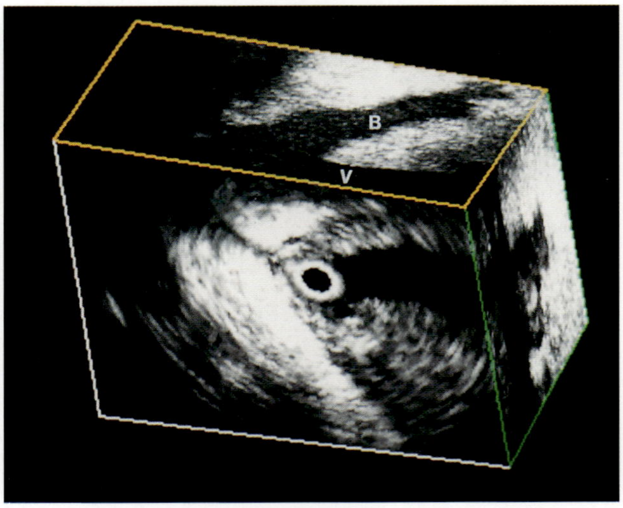

b

Figure 12.28 *(a) This 2D endoluminal ultrasound image obtained from a patient with UPJ obstruction shows a crossing vessel (V) at the level of the UPJ. However, the route of the vessel cannot be displayed by any single 2D image. (b) The 3D reconstructed image from the same area demonstrates the longitudinal view of this vessel (V) and its branches (B). The relationship between the UPJ and the crossing vessel can be more readily assessed.*

(Fig. 12.30). The presence of obstruction and the relationship of the tumor to crossing blood vessels can also be more accurately represented (Fig. 12.31). This information allows for more accurate staging and helps direct biopsy of the lesion to avoid damage to adjacent vessels.

There are numerous other potential applications for 3D reconstruction of endoluminal ultrasound images in urology. The ureterovesical junction can be demonstrated very accurately with endoluminal ultrasound. However, cross-sectional images alone do not represent the true anatomy at this site. The ureterovesical junction functions to prevent reflux from the bladder into the ureter. Thus, the 3D structure constitutes the functional entity. Appreciation of this function and any anatomic disturbance depends upon 3D reconstructed images (Fig. 12.22).

The use of computer-enhanced 3D reconstruction of ultrasound images in the urinary tract appears to have the potential for even greater accuracy in representing anatomic structures, particularly in the upper urinary tract. These images offer more accurate representation of the existing anatomy than do simple 2D cross-sectional images or radiologic representations. They may also reflect the pathophysiology of abnormal segments more accurately.

Prostate

Clinically, estimation of prostate volume is useful in a variety of clinical settings. An accurate estimation of prostate volume can provide important information in the evaluation of benign and malignant prostatic diseases and in determination of appropriate therapy. Also, the decrease in prostate mass after hormonal or radiation therapy can be used as an indication of therapeutic efficacy.

Although most prostate studies are performed using transrectal ultrasound with 5 to 7-MHz probes, the prostate can also be imaged transurethrally with a 9-MHz catheter-based ultrasound probe. The 9-MHz frequency allows a penetration depth of up to 4 cm. This allows full visualization of the entire prostate with higher resolution than can be obtained with transrectal probes. The cross-sectional images can be reconstructed in a 3D fashion. The 3D image can be viewed in multiple planes in different orientations, allowing visualization of coronal and oblique planes as well as biplanar and triplanar perspectives. The volume of the entire prostate or focal lesions within the prostate can be measured using special software on the 3D computer system. Studies on volumetric assessment of prostate demonstrated that 3D images

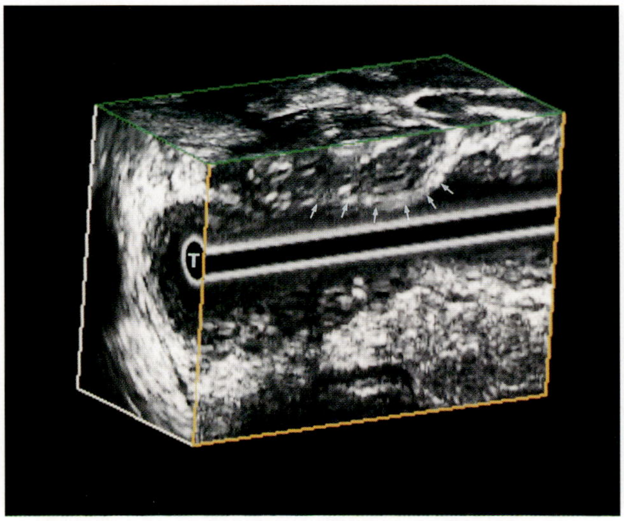

Figure 12.29 *A reconstructed 3D image of the ureter demonstrates a narrow segment of the ureter and mural structures in longitudinal section. The echogenic area (arrows) seen within the wall of the narrowed ureter represents fibro-connective tissue. T, transducer.*

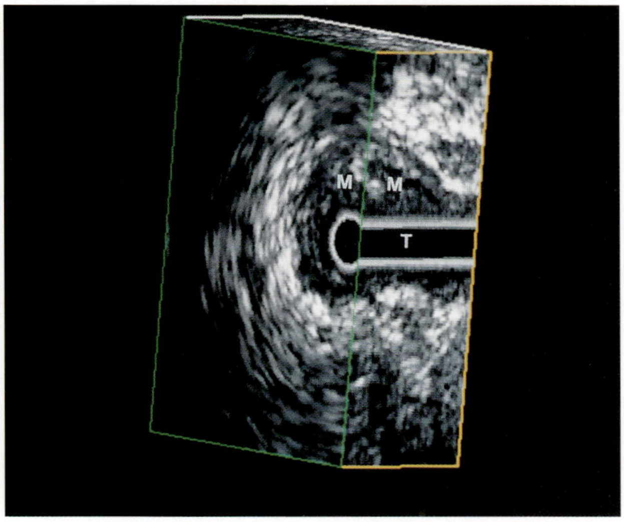

Figure 12.30 *A 3D endoluminal ultrasound image demonstrates a hypoechoic mass (M) arising from the wall of the ureter in both transverse and longitudinal views. There is no evidence of tumor invasion. T, transducer.*

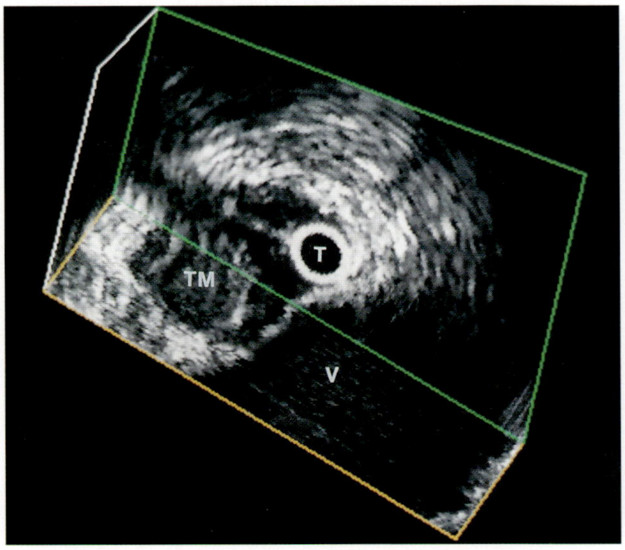

Figure 12.31 *A reconstructed 3D image demonstrates a ureteral tumor (TM) adjacent to the iliac vessel (V). These findings are useful for guiding biopsy of this lesion. T, transducer.*

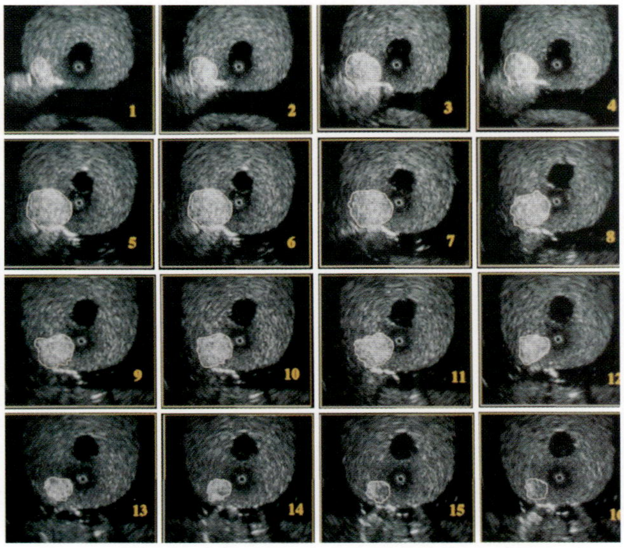

Figure 12.32 *Sequential 2D images obtained from the 3D prostate/tumor phantom were used to measure the volume of the tumor by the 3D computer system.*

allow more accurate assessment of volumes than standard 2D ultrasound images.[32,33] We have used tumor-bearing phantoms (mimicking a prostate tumor) to demonstrate the feasibility of 3D reconstructed images for tumor volume measurements (Fig. 12.32).

A relatively new ultrasound-guided procedure, radiation brachytherapy, has proven successful for treating prostatic cancer. The new procedure has been preferred by some patients and physicians because it has been reported to have fewer side-effects, such as impotence and incontinence, than surgical removal or external beam radiation. The procedure involves the insertion of tiny radioactive pellets into the prostate through the perineum. Reconstructed 3D transurethral ultrasound imaging has potential as an intraoperative tool in assessing the size of the prostate, localizing the tumor, and guiding the placement of radioactive seeds in the prostate. Our preliminary studies suggested that 3D endoluminal ultrasound may provide a unique imaging modality for evaluation of the prostate in a 3D fashion during brachytherapy.

CONCLUSIONS

Three-dimensional reconstruction of 2D ultrasound images is a unique method in the evolution of intraluminal imaging. It provides information about spatial relationships of anatomic structures that cannot be obtained using conventional methods. Although still in its infancy, 3D endoluminal ultrasound has the potential to become a dynamic tool in both the research and clinical areas. It has already been used clinically to diagnose and treat various luminal disease processes. With further improvements in computer technology, the rapid acquisition and reconstruction of 3D images may become routine in clinical practice.

ACKNOWLEDGMENTS

The authors acknowledge the financial support in part of the National Institutes of Health grant K08CA63494, which funded the research project leading to the results shown in this chapter. The authors also thank Richard M. Derman, Life Imaging Systems, Inc., and Michael Keegan, Microvasive, Boston Scientific Corporation, for their technical assistance and support.

REFERENCES

1. Fishman, EK, Magid D, Ney DR et al, Three-dimensional imaging, *Radiology* 1991; **181**:321–37.
2. Vannier MW, Marsh JL, Warren JO, Three-dimensional CT reconstruction for craniofacial surgical planning and evaluation, *Radiology* 1984; **150**:179–84.
3. Vannier MW, Gronemeyer S, Gutierrez FR, Canter CE, Laschinger JC, Knapp RH, Three-dimensional magnetic resonance imaging of congenital heart disease, *Radiographics* 1988; **8**:857–71.
4. Baum G, Greenwood I, Orbital lesion localization by three dimensional ultrasonography, *NY State J Med* 1961; **61**:4149–57.
5. Marx GR, Fulton DR, Pandian NG et al, Delineation of site, relative size and dynamic geometry of atrial septal defects by real-time three-dimensional echocardiography, *J Am Coll Cardiol* 1995; **25**:482–90.
6. Seward JB, Belohlavek M, O'Leary PW, Foley DA, Greenleaf JF, Congenital heart disease: wide-field, three-dimensional, and four-dimensional ultrasound imaging, *Am J Card Imag* 1995; **9**(1):38–43.
7. Roelandt JR, di Mario C, Pandian NG et al, Three-dimensional reconstruction of intracoronary ultrasound images. Rationale, approaches, problems, and directions, *Circulation* 1994; **90**:1044–55.
8. Chandrasekaran K, Sehgal CM, Hsu TL, Young NA, D'Adamo AJ, Robb RA, Three-dimensional volumetric ultrasound imaging of arterial pathology from two-dimensional intravascular ultrasound: an in vitro study, *Angiography* 1994, **45**:253–64.
9. Cavaye DM, White RA, Intravascular ultrasound imaging. *Int Angiol* 1993; **12**:245–55.
10. Hamper UM, Trapanotto V, Sheth S, DeJong MR, Caskey C, Three-dimensional US: preliminary clinical experience, *Radiology* 1994; **191**:397–401.
11. Kelly IM, Gardener JE, Brett AD, Riards R, Lees WR, Three-dimensional US of the fetus. Work in progress, *Radiology* 1994; **192**:253–9.
12. Gilja OH, Thune N, Matre K, Hausken T, Odegaard S, Berstad A, In vitro evaluation of three-dimensional ultrasonography in volume estimation of abdominal organs, *Ultrasound Med Biol* 1994; **20**:157–65.
13. Stiller MJ, Driller J, Shupack JL, Gropper CG, Rorke MC, Lizzi FI, Three-dimensional imaging for diagnostic ultrasound in dermatology, *J Am Acad Dermatol* 1993; **29**:171–5.
14. Hurter T, Hanrath P, Endobronchiale sonographie zur diagnostic pulmonaler und mediastinaler tumoren (Endoluminal sonography in the diagnosis of pulmonary and mediastinal tumors), *Dtsch Med Wochenschr* 1990; **115**(50):1899–905.

15. Cavaye DM, Tabbara MR, Kopchok GE, Laas TE, Cormier F, White RA, A new technique for intraluminal hollow organ imaging: three-dimensional ultrasound, *J Laparoendosc Surg* 1991; **1**(5):259–68.
16. Rankin RN, Fenster A, Downey DB, Munk PL, Levin MF, Vellet AD, Three-dimensional sonographic reconstruction: techniques and diagnostic applications, *AJR* 1993; **161**:695–702.
17. Robb RA, *Three-dimensional Biomedical Imaging: Principles and Practice* (VCH Publishers, Inc.: New York, 1995).
18. Wells PNT, The present status of ultrasonic imaging in medicine, *Ultrasonics* 1993; **31**(5):345–56.
19. Greenleaf JF, Belohlavek MB, Gerber TC, Foley DA, Seward JB, Multidimensional visualization in echocardiography: an introduction, *Mayo Clin Proc* 1993; **68**:213–20.
20. Cook LT, Dwyer SJ, Batnsitzky S, Lee KR, A three-dimensional display system for diagnostic imaging applications, *IEEE Comput Graph Applic* 1983; **3**:13–19.
21. Heffernan PB, Robb RA, A new method for shaded surface display of biological and medical images, *IEEE Trans Med Imag* 1985; **MI-4**:26–38.
22. Drebin RA, Carpenter L, Hanrahan P, Volume rendering, *Comput Graph* 1988; **22**:65–74.
23. Liu JB, Miller LS, Goldberg BB et al, Transnasal US of the esophagus: preliminary morphologic and function studies, *Radiology* 1992; **184**:721–7.
24. Tabbara MR, White RA, Cavaye DM, Kopchok GE, In vivo human comparison of intravascular ultrasound and angiography, *J Vasc Surg* 1991; **14**:495–504.
25. Davidson CJ, Sheikh KH, Kisslo K et al, Intracoronary ultrasound evaluation of interventional procedures, *Circulation* 1990; **82**(Suppl III):44.
26. Cavaye DM, White RA, Lerman RD et al, Usefulness of intravascular ultrasound imaging for detecting experimentally induced aortic dissection in dogs and for determining the effectiveness of endoluminal stenting, *Am J Cardiol* 1992; **69**:705–7.
27. Cavaye DM, White RA, Kopchok GE, Three-dimensional intravascular ultrasound imaging of normal and diseased human and canine arteries, *J Vasc Surg* (in press).
28. Bonn J, Liu JB, Winer LA, Sullivan KL, Shapiro MJ, Gardiner GA, Intravascular ultrasound as an alternative to contrast-enhanced vena cavography before filter placement, *J Vasc Intervent Radiol* 1994; **5**(1):6.
29. Rosenfield K, Losordo DW, Ramaswamy K et al, Three-dimensional reconstruction of human coronary and peripheral arteries from images recorded during two-dimensional intravascular ultrasound examination, *Circulation* 1991; **84**:1938–56.
30. Kalimanis G, Garra BS, Tio TL et al, The feasibility of three-dimensional ultrasonography: a preliminary report, *Gastrointest Endosc* 1995; **41**:235–9.
31. Alexander AA, Miller LS, Liu JB, Feld RI, Goldberg BB, High-resolution endoluminal sonography of the anal sphincter complex, *J Ultrasound Med* 1994; **13**:281–4.
32. Sehgal CM, Broderick GA, Whittington R, Gorniak RJ, Arger PH, Three-dimensional US and volumetric assessment of the prostate, *Radiology* 1994; **192**:274–8.
33. Basset O, Bimenez G, Mestas JL, Cathignol D, Devonec M, Volume measurement by ultrasonic transverse or sagittal cross-sectional scanning, *Ultrasound Med Biol* 1991; **17**:291–6.

Index

Page numbers in *italic* refer to the illustrations